AF782201

MINI DENTAL IMPLANTS

PRINCIPLES AND PRACTICE

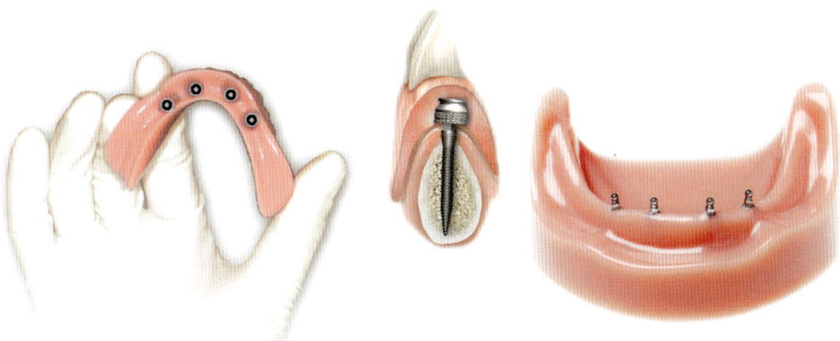

MINI DENTAL IMPLANTS

PRINCIPLES AND PRACTICE

Victor I. Sendax, BA, DDS, FACD, FICD

Diplomate, Past President
American Board of Oral Implantology/Implant Dentistry

Past President, Honored Fellow
American Academy of Implant Dentistry

Fellow
Royal Society of Medicine
Great Britain

Senior Attending Oral Implantologist
Roosevelt Hospital Dental Service
Department of Otolaryngology
New York, New York

First Director, Former Associate Professor
Implant Prosthodontics Research and Resident Training Program
School of Dental and Oral Surgery and Columbia-Presbyterian Hospital
Columbia University
New York, New York

Former Member Visiting Faculty
Dental Implant Department
Harvard University School of Dental Medicine
Boston, Massachusetts

Member
American and International Associations of Dental Research

ELSEVIER

ELSEVIER
MOSBY

3251 Riverport Lane
St. Louis, Missouri 63043

MINI DENTAL IMPLANTS: PRINCIPLES AND PRACTICE
ISBN: 978-1-4557-4386-5
Copyright © 2013 by Mosby, an imprint of Elsevier Inc.

No part of this publication may be reproduced or transmitted in any form or by any means, electronic or mechanical, including photocopying, recording, or any information storage and retrieval system, without permission in writing from the publisher. Details on how to seek permission, further information about the Publisher's permissions policies and our arrangements with organizations such as the Copyright Clearance Center and the Copyright Licensing Agency, can be found at our website: www.elsevier.com/permissions.

This book and the individual contributions contained in it are protected under copyright by the Publisher (other than as may be noted herein).

Notices

Knowledge and best practice in this field are constantly changing. As new research and experience broaden our understanding, changes in research methods, professional practices, or medical treatment may become necessary.

Practitioners and researchers must always rely on their own experience and knowledge in evaluating and using any information, methods, compounds, or experiments described herein. In using such information or methods they should be mindful of their own safety and the safety of others, including parties for whom they have a professional responsibility.

With respect to any drug or pharmaceutical products identified, readers are advised to check the most current information provided (i) on procedures featured or (ii) by the manufacturer of each product to be administered, to verify the recommended dose or formula, the method and duration of administration, and contraindications. It is the responsibility of practitioners, relying on their own experience and knowledge of their patients, to make diagnoses, to determine dosages and the best treatment for each individual patient, and to take all appropriate safety precautions.

To the fullest extent of the law, neither the Publisher nor the authors, contributors, or editors, assume any liability for any injury and/or damage to persons or property as a matter of products liability, negligence or otherwise, or from any use or operation of any methods, products, instructions, or ideas contained in the material herein.

The images on the front cover are courtesy of 3M™ ESPE™ MDI Mini Dental Implants. All rights reserved.

ISBN: 978-1-4557-4386-5

Vice President and Publisher: Linda Duncan
Executive Content Strategist: Kathy Falk
Senior Content Development Strategist: Brian Loehr
Publishing Services Manager: Julie Eddy
Senior Project Manager: Marquita Parker
Design Direction: Karen Pauls

Printed in China

Last digit is the print number: 9 8 7 6 5 4 3 2 1

Working together to grow
libraries in developing countries

www.elsevier.com | www.bookaid.org | www.sabre.org

ELSEVIER BOOK AID International Sabre Foundation

To the late Dr. Charles English, Board-Certified Prosthodontist, MDT, and Pioneer Advocate for the Sendax MDI System Protocol.

The mini dental implant (MDI) legacy of the late prosthodontist and master dental laboratory technician, Dr. Charles English, is the early adaptation of classic prosthodontic principles to mini implant applications that brought a sophisticated level of traditional discipline to MDI clinical technology and treatment planning at an early start-up period of development, when professional acceptance for the modality was still in its relative infancy. Inevitably, when a colleague of Dr. English's well-respected stature became a staunch MDI advocate, it gave an enormous boost to the MDI's inherent scientific credibility. His demise from cancer was tragic and premature; he still had much to offer the profession, with an increasingly bright future if he had survived. Those who labored by his side in a common cause will always treasure his memory and devoted friendship.

A representative sampling of Dr. Charles English's distinctive MDI philosophy and clinical mini implant enhancements can best be reviewed in the joint research paper he co-authored with our mutual colleague, Dr. George Bohle (also individually represented in this textbook), Memorial-Sloan-Kettering Hospital Maxillofacial Prosthodontist, as published in The long-term mini dental implant alternative: diagnostic, procedural, and clinical issues with the Sendax mini dental implant system. *Compendium* Nov. 2003, Vol. 24, No.11, pp 3-25.

CONTRIBUTORS

Burton E. Balkin, DMD
Clinical Professor (Adjunct)
Periodontology and Oral Implantology
Temple University
School of Dentistry
Philadelphia, Pennsylvania

Chapter 3: Background of Mini Dental Implants

Dr. Balkin demonstrates how the surface of the MDI osseointegrates comparably to traditional implants.

George C. Bohle III, DDS, FACP
Attending
Memorial Hospital/Sloan-Kettering Cancer Center
New York, New York

Chapter 8: The Maxillofacial Prosthodontist's Role in Postcancer Rehabilitation Using Mini Dental Implants

Dr. George Bohle, Maxillofacial Prosthodontist, attending at Memorial Hospital/Sloan-Kettering Cancer Center, New York City, provides an in-depth view of oral cancer surgery rehabilitation cases using MDIs for help in stabilization and support of obturators and a cross-section of maxillofacial applications. He provides a vivid demonstration of how minis can offer crucial linkage in this highly demanding area and how the aid of an in-house 3D cone beam CT scanner can offer added backup support for complex diagnostic and guidance considerations.

Gregory C. Bohle, MD, DDS
Fellow
Oral and Maxillofacial Surgery
L.I. Jewish Medical Center
New Hyde Park, New York

Chapter 8: The Maxillofacial Prosthodontist's Role in Postcancer Rehabilitation Using Mini Dental Implants

John B. Brunski, PhD
Senior Research Engineer
Stanford University School of Medicine
Stanford, California

Chapter 4: Biomedical-Engineering Analyses of Mini Dental Implants: Biomechanical Perspectives Relevant to the Use of Mini Implants

Prof. Brunski, in the course of a distinguished research and educational career at the Rensselaer Polytechnic Institute and currently at Stanford University, has devoted a substantial portion of his academic time to dental implant engineering principles, where he has earned the respect of his colleagues for a specialized focus on oral implant applications. In this chapter, he has provided both a primer on basic biomedical-engineering fundamentals and an overview of applied engineering for the oral implantology area, with a special technical perspective on the unique role that MDIs can fulfill in this rapidly evolving field.

Gordon J. Christensen, DDS, MSD, PhD
Consultant and Lecturer
CR Foundation and Clinicians Report
Provo, Utah

Essaying a pivotal role in educating and motivating the general practitioner (GP) to develop dental implant proficiency (via CRA and PCC) to insert and restore implants, Dr. Christensen has been a consistent advocate for MDIs as an optimal entry-level modality for GPs' introduction to clinical implant technology via his in-depth mini implant DVD presentations and internationally recognized MDI lecture-demonstrations. GPs' new-found ability to insert MDIs and more readily restore basic implant-prosthodontic cases should also encourage the referrals by GPs of more advanced complex cases to implant-experienced specialists, broadening the access of the public to the entire spectrum of oral implantology.

Dr. Christensen is arguably the most trusted contemporary voice for unbiased dental product, technique, and device evaluations; consequently, his gracious introductory forward to this first edition textbook is deeply appreciated.

Frans Currier, DDS, MSD
Presbyterian Health Foundation Professor
Program Director of Graduate Orthodontics
Member of Founding Faculty
College of Dentistry, Department of Orthodontics
University of Oklahoma
Oklahoma City, Oklahoma

Chapter 9: The Orthodontist's Role in MDI Therapeutics: ORTHO Transitional Anchorage Devices (TADs) and Related Applications

Dr. Frans Currier summarizes his extensive experiences with MDI Ortho applications. In association with Dr. Currier, Dr. Onur Kadidoglu, Assistant Professor of Orthodontics at OKU, has been instrumental in advancing the specialized research and development supporting the use of TADs.

Andrew Jaksen, CDT
Evolution/First Dental Laboratory
Buffalo, New York

Chapter 10: The Laboratory Technician's Key Role in MDI Prosthodontics

Andrew Jaksen, CDT and dentist-lecturer Dr. Benjamin Oppenheimer have been devoted to the process of consolidating advances in MDI laboratory coordination and work simplification via updated step-reduction techniques for fixed (and removable) applications and have pioneered advancing MDI education with specialized seminars specifically oriented to the dental laboratory community.

Onur Kadioglu, DDS
Clinical Assistant Professor
College of Dentistry
Department of Orthodontics
University of Oklahoma
Oklahoma City, Oklahoma

Chapter 9: The Orthodontist's Role in MDI Therapeutics: ORTHO Transitional Anchorage Devices (TADs) and Related Applications

Dr. Onur Kadidoglu, Assistant Professor of Orthodontics at OKU, in association with Dr. Frans Currier, has been instrumental in advancing specialized research and development supporting the use of TADs.

John Kirdahy, CDT
Innovation Dental Laboratory
Jersey City, New Jersey

Chapter 10: The Laboratory Technician's Key Role in MDI Prosthodontics

John Kirdahy's Innovation Dental Laboratory has consistently offered evolving lab techniques that have helped standardize the coordination of MDI chairside procedures with the implant-oriented dental laboratory and advanced the progressive design and processing of both fixed and removable MDI cases.

Jack E. Lemons, PhD
Professor, Department of Prosthodontics and Biomaterials
University of Alabama at Birmingham
Birmingham, Alabama

Chapter 4: Biomedical-Engineering Analyses of Mini Dental Implants: Biomaterial and Bioengineering Considerations in Conventional Implant and Mini Implant Design

Dr. Jack Lemons has been at the forefront of pioneer dental implant research and academic education from almost the onset of the oral implant discipline. He has been a key figure in promoting unbiased perspectives for this field, and we are indebted to him for his contributions to this textbook.

Bruce J. Lish, DDS
Chief, General Practice Residency
St. Luke's/Roosevelt Hospital Center
New York, New York

Chapter 5: The General Practitioner's Pivotal Role in Coordinating Therapeutics with Mini Dental Implants

Dr. Bruce Lish started the first comprehensive hospital-based MDI teaching and training program and "hands-on" surgical/restorative MDI seminars, emphasizing the pivotal role of the Sendax protocol in implant insertion and implant prosthodontics for the general practitioners' enlarged scope of practice.

Leonard R. Machi, DDS
Fellow
The American Academy of Implant Dentistry
Private Practice
Wauwatosa, Wisconsin

Chapter 5: Everyday Problem-Solving with Mini Dental Implants: A Private Practitioner's General Practice Retrospective

Dr. Leonard Machi is a well-rounded general practitioner with broad implant experience and is a Fellow of the American Academy of Implant Dentistry and a board-certified Diplomate of the American Board Of Oral Implantology. He presents a cross-section of MDI utilizations in diverse fixed and removable applications and emphasizes the types of useful salvage and repair techniques that Dr. Gordon Christensen has often emphasized in his MDI lectures and videos.

Leonard Marotta, CDT, MDT, PhD
Marotta Dental Studio, Inc.
Farmingdale, New York

Chapter 10: The Laboratory Technician's Key Role in MDI Implant Prosthodontics

Leonard Marotta, CDT, MDT, PhD, and associate Steven Pigliacelli, CDT, have been long associated with dental implant specialized requirements—from the inception of the Brånemark era to the present day high-tech manifestations—and recognized for working to encompass small-diameter implant restorative options that have been acknowledged by the profession to be at a premium quality level.

Ninian S. Peckitt, FRCS, FFD, RCS, FDS, RCS
Fellow
Australasian College of Cosmetic Surgery (FACCS)
Adjunct Associate Professor
Engineering Assisted Surgery

School of Engineering and Advanced Technology
Massey University
Wellington, New Zealand

Chapter 7: An Oral and Maxillofacial Surgeon's Role in Advanced MDI Therapeutics: Engineering Assisted Surgery™, MDIs in Functional Reconstructive Surgery within Great Britain and New Zealand Venues

Dr. Ninian Peckitt, Oral and Maxillofacial Surgeon of New Zealand and Australia, has furthered advanced biomedical tissue engineering by applying MDIs ingeniously as components of major trauma rehabilitation cases. Dr. Peckitt's most severely compromised patients have received a new lease on relative normality as a consequence of these uniquely sophisticated applied biotechnology procedures.

Murray Scheiner, CDT
Laboratory Technician
Office of Dr. Victor I. Sendax

Chapter 10: The Laboratory Technician's Key Role in MDI Implant Prosthodontics

Murray Scheiner, CDT, who has been Dr. Sendax's in-office personal lab technician for more than 40 years, dating from the earliest mini implant clinical trial cases, was initially exposed to the MDI restorative protocol at its inception in 1976 and since then has processed many fixed and removable MDI cases.

Victor I. Sendax, BA, DDS, FACD, FICD
Diplomate, Past President
American Board of Oral Implantology/Implant Dentistry
Past President, Honored Fellow
American Academy of Implant Dentistry
Fellow
Royal Society of Medicine
Great Britain
Senior Attending Oral Implantologist
Roosevelt Hospital Dental Service
Department of Otolaryngology
New York, New York
First Director, Former Associate Professor
Implant Prosthodontics Research and Training Program
School of Dental and Oral Surgery
Columbia University
New York, New York
Columbia-Presbyterian Hospital Resident Prosthodontic Program
Former member visiting faculty
Dental Implant Department
Harvard University School of Dental Medicine
Boston, Massachusetts
Member
American and International Associations of Dental Research

Chapter 1: Sendax Hybrid Mini Dental Implant Applications: Combining Natural Tooth Abutments with Conventional and Mini Dental Implants

Chapter 2: The Basic Insertion and Reconstructive Protocol Guidelines: Step by Step

Chapter 11: Concluding Postscript Analysis: The Role of MDIs in the Contemporary Imaging Evolution: A Current Assessment

Chapter 12: The Best of MDIs: Q and A

Dr. Victor Sendax is recognized as a leading pioneer in the field of Dental Implantology, and as the inventor and patent holder of the original Sendax Mini Dental Implant System (MDI), now a 3M Corporation acquisition.

Harold I. Sussman, DDS, MSD
Professor
Post-Graduate Periodontology
NYU College of Dentistry
Coler-Goldwater Specialty Hospital and Nursing
New York, New York

Chapter 6: MDI Solutions for the Medically Compromised Patient

Dr. Harold Sussman, Periodontist and NYU Professor of postgraduate periodontics, with his colleague Dr. Arthur Volker, presents the seminal MDI research project at Coler-Goldwater Memorial Hospital (Roosevelt Island, New York) using a simplified mandibular MDI insertion guidance technique, employing the aid of the Sussman Implant Guide (SIG) paralleling device, that demonstrated statistically significant MDI survival in the face of severe systemic morbidity in addition to ongoing negative byproducts of the aging process.

Stephen M. Taubenfeld, MD, PhD
Psychiatrist
Former Research Fellow
Mt. Sinai Hospital
New York, New York

Chapter 11: Concluding Postscript Analysis: Positive Patient Psychology In Relation to Mini Dental Implant (MDI) Therapy

Dr. Stephen Taubenfeld holds an MD/PhD degree in Neuroscience from Brown University School of Medicine. He completed an NIH-sponsored fellowship at Mount Sinai School of Medicine in New York where his research led to clinical trials for the treatment of post-traumatic stress disorder. Dr. Taubenfeld has authored numerous high profile research articles and reviews in the fields of psychiatry and neuroscience. He is currently a Partner at Iguana Healthcare Partners, LLC, a healthcare investment fund based in Greenwich, CT.

Arthur R. Volker, MSEd, DDS
Attending
Coler-Goldwater Specialty Hospital and Nursing
New York, New York

Chapter 6: MDI Solutions for the Medically Compromised Patient

Dr. Arthur Volker, in conjunction with Dr. Harold Sussman, developed a simplified mandibular MDI insertion guidance technique, employing the aid of the Sussman Implant Guide (SIG) paralleling device, that demonstrated statistically significant MDI survival in the face of severe systemic morbidity in addition to ongoing negative byproducts of the aging process.

Foreword

Nearly a quarter of a century ago, I attended my first course on root-form dental implants. It was delivered by Dr. Brånemark himself with a team of his colleagues. As a prosthodontist, I was limited at that time to learning only about the prosthodontic portion of his implant system. I was skeptical of the dental implant concept because I had been unsuccessful in making previously available oral implants serve well. After a few days of hearing about root-form pure titanium screw implants and seeing some cases that had served for a significant number of years, I was impressed that this type of implant was probably going to usefully serve patients.

On arriving home, I worked with several oral surgeons in an attempt to integrate this concept into my practice. We were able to place and restore implants in many patients with the original Swedish concept, inserting about 6 implants anterior to the mental foramen or anterior to the maxillary sinus and restoring the implants with a metal framework supporting denture base resin that held the denture teeth. Restorations for edentulous persons, who had the funds to pay for the implant-supported prosthodontic treatment, was indeed a revolution in patient care. Many of those patients continue to be seen by my practice, and their implants are still serving. Some of the prostheses have worn out and have had to be replaced, but using the same implants.

A few years after that course, I went to Sweden to learn more about the surgical aspect of oral implants, and I began to place at least some implants myself. Continuing improvements in implant alloys and surfaces and in implant placement and restoration procedures were being made. Currently, root-form implants approximately 3 mm in diameter and up to 6 mm in diameter are well proven and routinely used by the global dental profession. The serviceability of these implants and the prostheses they support is well known and accepted today.

However, several major problems related to dental implantology lingered in my mind since the introduction of root-form implants. Many of the patients I was trying to treat with implants did not have enough bone to allow placement of the standard 3.75-mm diameter implants without bone grafting. I found that the minimum amount of facial-lingual bone into which I could place a 3.75-mm implant was about 6 mm, and even that amount of bone required extreme care and a near-perfect technique. Additionally, those who did not have enough bone often could not afford the grafting procedures, or they were too debilitated physically to have bone grafting done. These challenges limited implant use to the wealthy or to those willing to go into debt to have the implant procedures accomplished for them.

The FDA cleared root-form dental implants, 3 mm in diameter or wider, for use in 1976. As a result, almost all root-form implants were made to be more than 3 mm in diameter, with most being close to 4 mm in diameter. A few companies provided 3.25-mm diameter implants, and I found that these smaller diameter implants were used frequently. Some dentists began researching screw-type implants less than 3 mm in diameter for "transitional" use to support prostheses while implants greater than 3 mm in diameter were "integrating" into place. Many of those practitioners using transitional implants occasionally found that when attempting to remove the transitional implants they could not be removed or were difficult to remove. Pioneers in the less than 3-mm implant concept, including Dr. Sendax, began to use these small diameter implants for "long-term" applications. In 1997, implants less than 3 mm in diameter were cleared by the FDA for long-term use. I began to use them for long-term applications around that time, and I have continued to do so with success.

At last I could place implants for patients who had minimal bone or who had adequate bone but were too physically debilitated to have typical flap procedures and greater than 3-mm diameter implants placed. Use of these small diameter implants required adequate radiographs, careful treatment planning, and more implants in number than the wider variety of implants.

I found that I could place 1.8-mm diameter implants in patients who had only 3 to 4 mm of bone in the facial-lingual dimension. Some of the patients with this limited amount of bone required a minimal "flap" procedure, but with 4 mm of bone or more present usually a flap was not necessary. I could also place the "mini" implants in patients with more bone than needed for these small implants, thus avoiding the surgical invasiveness of drilling an osteotomy that is required for the larger implants.

In the past several years, I have placed small diameter mini implants from 1.8 to 2.3 mm in diameter as support and retention for complete dentures, removable partial dentures, augmentation of tooth-supported long-span fixed partial dentures, as the sole support for selected fixed partial dentures, and for some single crowns with inadequate bone present between adjacent teeth. The success of these implants, properly placed and restored, has surprised me and has delighted patients.

A recent national survey we accomplished in CRA showed that the primary users of small diameter implants were general practitioners. This survey indicated a movement of general practitioners into implant placement and the extension of this service to more patients. The current generation of minimally invasive small diameter implants has allowed patients who previously could not have implants with the ability to be well served. The small diameter implant concept is growing, and success is observed on a routine basis. I congratulate Dr. Victor I. Sendax for his innovative thinking and being instrumental in the introduction of this clinical concept.

Gordon J. Christensen, DDS, MSD, PhD

Preface

MDI Introductory Perspectives

The creative process that results in something useful and substantial is typically the byproduct of a momentary deep insight, coupled with a huge input of serendipitous trial and error. This is certainly the case for the genesis of mini dental implants (MDIs). The particular epiphany that brought forth the MDI came in the frustration over a nagging oral implant stumbling block—our seeming inability to provide the well-accepted benefits of dental implants for an ever-expanding and aging population—without invasive surgical heroics and emphasizing rapid functionality at an affordable cost. What is indeed quixotic is that all of this innovation should have initially come about as a result of the Space Age popularization of a remarkable low-corrosive metal, *titanium,* which inevitably came to symbolize the great technologic advances and breakthroughs that were so vividly associated with that precedent-shattering era.

However, in its more humble manifestation as an endodontic titanium screw post in the mid-seventies of the last century, it certainly did not appear to be the forerunner of any major scientific breakthrough. In point of fact, ordinary root canal posts had, before that time, been (and continue to be) successfully fabricated out of diverse precious and base materials such as gold, brass, resins, and steel. Why had a few manufacturers turned to titanium in the mid-seventies, instead of sticking with those tried and true metals? The answer is probably based more on the glamour of orbiting satellite imagery than any inherent objective value that could be ascribed to endodontic posts machined out of commercially pure titanium. Unlike implants, standard endodontic posts never come into contact with bone or soft tissue and are confined to the essentially inert interior of sealed-off root canals where structural strength is the main requirement and biocompatibility has no critical significance.

What did, however, make titanium legitimately important for a dental implant application was its extremely low rate of corrosion. As a direct consequence, titanium, and particularly its less brittle alloy version (Ti-6Al-4Va), came to be recognized as an exceptionally strong, biocompatible implantable metal that was least likely to be rejected as a foreign body. Only chrome-cobalt steel alloy dating from the World War II era had a comparably favorable track record of low corrosion and successful implant-ability in a host of body replacement part applications, from skull plates, hips and knees, to limbs and jaws. One problem, however, in using steel alloy for relatively small dental implants was that chrome-cobalt steel was exceptionally hard and typically had to be waxed up and cast rather than machined, like titanium.

When the Swedish vascular/orthopedic researcher P.I. Brånemark discovered by happenstance that bone bonded to titanium in an arcane process he dubbed "osseointegration," he fostered a seemingly new and ultimately well-accepted use for titanium, which, in fairness, had been applied previously in the United States and elsewhere but without the benefit of the formally-controlled, Swedish government-sponsored studies and funded applications that helped put titanium oral implants scientifically on the map internationally. These seminal studies and the data they supplied helped set the stage for a specialized new technology, waiting only to be developed and applied for the greater good of humankind.

Sadly, prohibitive costs have often placed dental implants out of reach for a most needy and rapidly aging patient population: the worldwide millions of fully or partially edentulous patients with unstable, loose, and often painful dentures that typically required gobs of adhesive to hold them in place and make them minimally tolerable.

An analysis of the earlier attempts at dental implantation reveals several key limitations to patient success. A particularly unsettling factor that diluted professional and public acceptance of previous oral implants was the unpredictability of the result, owing largely to a relatively imprecise insertion technique, typically associated with pre-osseointegration-era implants, such as the blade design favored by several of the original implant pioneers, such as Linkow, Lew, and Pasqualini. This blade type required flap surgery followed by a longitudinal channel cut deeply into the bone, slightly wider and deeper than the blade implant itself. Tapping the blade-shaped implant into this long, uneven groove was a relatively imprecise operation, leaving the blade in contact with variable amounts of supportive bone. When performed by a skillful operator, the implant became sufficiently stable so that it could provide a reasonable degree of immediate function via its typically preattached post abutment(s). Although this blade system could be successful and many of these blade devices persevered over long time spans without significant morbidity, they could also be associated with a nagging unpredictability and variable outcomes over different time spans.

A drastic change in protocol occurred with the advent of precise cylindrical-shaped osteotomy drills revolving at carefully controlled moderate speeds with copious water irrigation to avoid overheating the bone. This technique advancement, with P.I. Brånemark's then strict advocacy of burying the implant bodies in bone anywhere from 4 to 12 months before permitting a second uncovering surgery to connect abutment posts, helped provide patients with a screw-in fixed-detachable prosthesis, but which was initially limited to the anterior mandible This unique perspective bequeathed the profession a high degree of predictable oral implant outcomes (confirmed by well-respected Swedish state-supported research studies) that were welcomed by clinicians internationally and, to an oddly quixotic degree, also promoted a virtually religious fervor on behalf of the Brånemark regimen that was deemed by its proponents as essentially inviolate. This also included at the time a strict prohibition of any immediate postoperative x-ray implant evaluation, based on the wholly untested theory that the radiation could inhibit or compromise the supposedly vulnerable osseointegration process, which seems fortunately to have been relegated nowadays to the dustbin of untenable restrictions.

Needless to say, looking forward to today's clinical setting shows that the original Brånemark precepts have been considerably modified, most notably the lengthy waiting span before implant activation and the near absolute requirement to fully bury the implant during a nonfunctional latent bone gestation period. Why this current break with a once rock-like tradition? That can be answered succinctly: the public's newly emergent outcry and hunger for more *immediate* function! Of course, this was aided and abetted by that portion of the dental profession that desired simpler, quicker results for an increasingly demanding patient population.

Coincidentally, this patient push for speedier prosthodontic results provided a timely opening opportunity for acceptance of the MDI concept. This relates in turn to the prime difference between osseointegration and the Sendax MDI insertion protocol: namely the divergent manner in which bony connection is achieved in these two approaches to implant stability. For the MDI approach, it is not achieved by a variable waiting period for bone to fully grow into supportive biomechanical contact with the newly inserted implant. Rather, for an ultra-narrow streamlined 1.8-mm titanium implant, it was only necessary to open directly through the overlying keratinized soft tissue with a small starter entry hole, employing a minimal 1.1-mm drill penetration through the denser crestal cortical bone, followed by just a moderate extension into the underlying medullary bone. The MDI could then be inserted and auto-advanced into this minimal starter entry hole (without a bone-eliminating osteotomy) until it self-taps its way into solid apical bone. This process can be properly classified as *osseoapposition* because the MDI comes into immediate direct contact with *mature supportive bone* over its threaded length from day 1 of insertion and does not require the complex biochemical process of osseointegration for bone to grow gradually into contact with the implant over a substantial surface area before it can achieve stable functionality. This is the essential and distinctive element in the Sendax MDI insertion protocol that permits predictable immediate function followed by long-term favorable outcomes (see related histologic illustrations elsewhere in this textbook by Balkin, Steflik, Lemons, and Sendax for confirmative study details).

The other major factor that accounts for the immediate stability and functionality of MDIs lies in the key concept of *bicortical stabilization*. For conventional implants, this stability factor is achieved by buttressing the wider-bodied implants variably between the buccal or labial and lingual bony cortical plates during the insertion process. For 1.8-mm MDIs, the width dimension is usually too narrow to gain any support from widely separated cortices, whereas the MDIs can gain bicortical stabilization in the maxilla by starting initially from crestal cortex and thens after traversing variable medullary bone densities, biting into solid basal bone apically (without perforating) into the floor or walls of the maxillary sinus, or nasal cavity, or pyriform rim, as well as the tuberosity and even the dense midline cortex (in the incisive foramen region). Without this crest to apex cortical buttressing, the MDI must be realistically regarded as a limited-term transitional implant rather than the long-term abutment that can perform on a par with a traditional osseointegrated "fixture" (as per the original Brånemark coinage; see Glossary for details of fixture versus implant).

Of course, to maintain this desirable osseoapposition and ultimate functional supportiveness, MDIs also required balanced and controlled prosthodontic occlusal management to avoid lateral shear overload. Excessive iatrogenic and parafunctional/habitual forces are often prime culprits that may readily destroy otherwise healthy periimplant bone contact—the key breakdown elements found in the presence of traumatic occlusion or coincident infectious bone damage, often associated with a consequent loss of support for any implant system—and MDIs are no exception to this fundamental hazard. A saving grace for MDIs, however, when lost under these negative occlusal overload/inflammatory conditions, is the minimal morbidity and rapid healing closure routinely encountered upon removal compared with the more invasive (and costly) standard-sized implant bodies and their equivalently expansive abutments.

The First Complete-Arch MDI Case (1976)

The jolting transition from dentate to edentulous state has always put a psychologically demanding burden on patients at whatever stage in life it occurs and is accompanied by a sense of lost youth and of physical decline, with a reduced ability to masticate and enjoy food, and with phonetic handicap and speech discomfiture.

And so it was when late in the office day (as so often is the case) an elderly woman presented with terminally failing dentition, with a plea to secure a removable prosthesis so she could cope with a highly important occasion scheduled for the very next morning. Her desperation was palpable, and the potential embarrassment engendered by the near hopeless oral condition was driving her into a severe emotional crisis.

In searching my mind rather feverishly for a rational solution to this patient's dilemma, I fortunately recalled a concept that I had been recently testing, which brought into play an unusual approach to implant design. All of our intrabony oral implants to date had required an incision down to the periosteum and reflection of a full epithelial soft tissue flap to expose the crestal cortical bone to permit drilling a sufficient opening into the underlying medullary bone, which would allow the insertion of a mechanical replacement for the lost tooth root in that site. My thought had been to try to find a minimally invasive technique for inserting an ultrathin implantable device directly through the overlying soft tissue into the bone without a flap or typical osteotomy, so that a transitional prosthesis could be immediately secured and rendered functional. My difficulty was to find or construct a device that could be deployed in this manner. The only existing shape that seemed to be a modest candidate for such employment was that of endodontic screw posts that were then available as sold in dental supply depots. The limiting problem with such posts, however, concerned the metallic materials from which they were typically fabricated—gold, brass, stainless steel, etc.—none of which could be considered acceptably biocompatible for human implant application.

Fortunately, as was acknowledged in the opening remarks, the advent of titanium as a spin-off of

Space Age engineering brought forth screw posts made of this remarkable metal, undoubtedly with the manufacturers' hope that they would be viewed by the profession as an advance over previous mundane endodontic posts.

To my mind, however, these machined titanium posts also came to represent, in relatively crude form, the ideal implantable entity for a nonsurgical approach to a streamlined insertion protocol. Therefore, in 1976, I came to offer the fruits of my brainstorming to Mrs. Beverley Johnson (now sadly deceased) when she appeared at my office at day's end with her desperate cry for help.

Mrs. Johnson was a senior voice teacher at the eminent Juilliard School of Music in New York city, who later became the voice teacher/vocal coach for the celebrated American operatic soprano Renee Fleming (who subsequently also become a patient of mine, referred by Mrs. Johnson), and was set to teach a master class in operatic vocal technique the next day when her residual dental prosthesis failed and painfully exfoliated. When I tried to explain to her, as she arrived with this critical emergency, that I knew of no plausible way to quickly secure her prosthesis then and there, except possibly by way of my relatively untried and minimally tested "mini" implant technique, she immediately opted without reservation to have me put the system into practice and signed off to that effect on an improvised consent form.

The sole surviving support elements in her mandible consisted of two small blade-type implants, situated perilously close to the neurovascular bundle and mental foramen, with scant bone in what was left of an extremely atrophic arch. In contemplating the challenging strategy for inserting some of the titanium screw posts, I chose the narrowest posts that I reckoned would fit between the narrow labiolingual and buccolingual bony plates without perforations and with still enough occlusal loading resistance to avoid fracture. My tentative previous trials with the titanium screw posts in the existing post kits led me to have some confidence in the 1.8-mm width as the best overall sizing compromise, although I acknowledged that the height would be limited posteriorly by the available bone above a perilously close inferior alveolar canal or the sparse anterior symphyseal bone from crest to inferior mandibular border, if that could be accessed.

As to the number of inserted titanium screw posts, I elected to place as many around the arch as could be reasonably accommodated, postulating that one mini implant might replace one lost tooth root (a concept which, I might add, has since produced viable MDI outcomes). Radiographs of this historic early case and clinical views of its associated prosthodontics may be seen in Figures1 and 2 of this textbook's Section on Hybrid MDI Applications.

The real test of the insertion concept came when it was time to decide how much drilling would be needed to permit directly screwing these devices into the bone. I had previously come to the realization that it might be possible to avoid incising and laying back a flap for these ultrathin devices and to drill a minimal opening entry directly through the soft tissue into the crestal cortex and then into medullary bone just enough to allow the mini implant to then self-tap its way to its final depth, just like a wood screw into a plank. (This was precisely the analogy that Dr. Gordon Christensen chose to apply many years later to describe the direct simplicity of the basic MDI insertion process!)

I was particularly encouraged in thinking about how to avoid a conventional surgical flap approach by the realization that my patient had always demonstrated an extreme aversion to local anesthetic injections and "shots" in general and a consistently low pain threshold that was only partially ameliorated by the use of ample nitrous oxide-oxygen relaxation gas. It occurred to me that I might be able to avoid the hated mandibular block injection completely by employing minimal deep crestal infiltrations to the periosteum; this proved to be precisely the case not only for Mrs. Johnson's procedures but happily for most subsequent patients having MDIs placed in the maxilla as well as the mandible, proving to be a distinct advantage of this often key antianxiety feature of an evolving MDI insertion protocol.

Additionally, avoiding the patient-averse inferior alveolar block injection provided an unforeseen advantage in that it helped avoid impingements on the nerve and potential paresthesias. Gradually deepened rotational advancement of the MDI during insertion rarely caused any patient pain awareness if local infiltration anesthesia was used unless the MDI was coming progressively close to the mandibular nerve or mental bundle. A periapical progress x-ray could then assess the proximity factor and further insertion could either be aborted with the implant permitted to remain at the attained depth, reinserted in a less vulnerable proximate location, or backed out and replaced with a shorter implant. In any case, the likelihood of excessive drilling depth was mitigated by the fact that only a "starter" depth in medullary bone was usually needed to initiate the insertion process, and the subsequent finger and thumb-driver phase could be readily calibrated to avoid overt compressive neurologic impairment.

It could also be observed that the ultra-narrow 1.8-mm dimension was an added safety factor during insertions because it could easily slip between the cortical plates of thin ridges, avoiding potential perforations. It applied equally as well for perilously close adjacent tooth roots in single tooth replacement applications, for which the MDIs turned out to be the ideal, and often the only, realistic implant choice for treacherously narrow interradicular spaces that would otherwise require significant orthodontic intervention.

As to the insertion technique implementation, the standard screw post kits in use at the time fortunately came with simple knurled drivers that allowed moderate clockwise finger rotation with concurrent intraosseous pressure to adequately accomplish the insertion maneuver. Subsequent instrumentation design modifications and refinements made the placement process considerably more efficient, with finger driver, thumb wrench, and ratchet/torque wrench tools specifically fabricated for dedicated MDI insertion procedures.

Dr. Victor I. Sendax

ACKNOWLEDGMENTS

To my estimable colleague Dr. Ronald Bulard, who, at an incipient stage of mini implant evolution, grasped the unique potential of the Sendax MDI Insertion and Reconstructive Protocol and provided the personal and corporate energy to put it decisively on the professional map, with the invaluable assistance of Stephen Hadwin, who engineered and machined the original MDI devices and related instrumentation.

Suzanne W. Vivino: for her skilled secretarial and computer assistance in organizing and preparing the extensive material that was essential to developing this MDI textbook.

Gary J. Ruth, DDS: oral and maxillofacial surgeon, for his generous and collegial contribution of professional time on the front line of clinical MDI research projects.

Raymond Choi, DDS: for his Global Mini Implant Institute consistently embracing MDI teaching and training as an ongoing in-depth project.

ABOUT THE AUTHOR

Dr. Victor Sendax is recognized as a leading pioneer in the field of Dental Implantology, and as the inventor and patent holder of the original Sendax Mini Dental Implant System (MDI), now a 3M Corporation acquisition.

He has served as President of the American Academy of Implant Dentistry, and as Diplomate-President of the American Board of Oral Implantology/Implant Dentistry. He is the recipient of both the AAID's Gershkoff Special Recognition Award, and the AAID's Lew Research Foundation Award for Oral Implant Research. He is also the 2012 recipient of the American Academy of Small Diameter Implants Lifetime Achievement Award.

Academically, he trained and also served as a faculty member, at both NYU College of Dentistry and the Harvard University School of Dental Medicine, and more recently as Associate Professor and First Director, Implant Prosthodontics Research and Resident Training Program at Columbia University School of Dental and Oral Surgery and Columbia-Presbyterian Hospital, and currently as Emeritus Senior Attending oral implantologist in the Department of Otolaryngology and General Dentistry at St. Lukes/Roosevelt Hospital Center, NYC.

As an officer in the US Air Force Dental Corps he graduated from the School of Aviation Medicine at Gunter Air Force Base in Alabama and served as Captain and Base Dental Surgeon on active duty in Japan from 1955 to 1957.

His professional fellowships include the American College of Dentists, the International College of Dentists and the Royal Society of Medicine (Great Britain).

He is internationally recognized in the Marquis Who's Who In America, Who's Who In The World, Who's Who In Medicine & Healthcare, and Who's Who In Frontiers of Science & Technology.

Musically, he is an alumnus of the Tanglewood Study Group at the Berkshire Music Center, and has served as a Board Member of the NY City Center for Music and Drama (a constituent of Lincoln Center for the Performing Arts and the parent organization of the NYC Ballet and NYC Opera). He has also been a member of the board of directors for the Schola Cantorum under Maestro Hugh Ross, and the Society for Asian Music with sitarist Ravi Shankar and violinist-conductor Yehudi Menuhin.

Magically, he is a life member of both the Society of American Magicians and the International Brotherhood of Magicians (Order of Merlin), and the S.A.M.'s 2012 choice as "Magician of the Year!" As a member of The London Magic Circle he has been recognized as the sleight-of-hand magician who puzzled His Royal Highness Prince Charles with the Interlocked Hands Rising Card Production, which Dr. Sendax first invented and perfected as a young teen-age magician.

He is a member of the Century Association in New York City and has produced the Century Club's Magic Night in conjunction with his Co-Centurion, Dick Cavett, who prior to his Talk Show Host career also got his start as a magician, as did fellow-luminaries Johnny Carson, Woody Allen and Orson Welles.

CONTENTS

Chapter 1

Sendax Hybrid Mini Dental Implant Applications

Combining Natural Tooth Abutments with Conventional and Mini Dental Implants

VICTOR I. SENDAX

Outline

> The primary operational basis for hybridizing three diverse abutment support systems is the underlying critical need to maximally offset potentially traumatic force overload.
>
> *Victor I. Sendax*

Benefits of Mini Dental Implants (MDIs) and Hybrid Combinations

1. Ultra-small diameter MDIs will slip into minimal-width islands and columns of bone, allowing MDI insertions to proceed even in sites where standard-width conventional implants might be considered too bulky and consequently contraindicated as too risky without major grafting.
2. Minimally invasive starter drill openings through bony cortices and into medullary bone, for only one third to one half of the implant length, means that direct drill encroachment should never occur on any vulnerable adjacent tissues, including mandibular neurovascular canal, mental foramen, inferior border of mandible, adjacent tooth roots, lingual, labial, and buccal cortical bone plates, floor of maxillary sinus, floor of nasal cavity, and posterior wall of maxillary tuberosity.
3. Auto-advancement of the MDI, driven slowly into medullary bone with finger and thumb wrench rotations and compressive pressure until biting into denser bone apically, helps stabilize the MDI but does not require overt penetration of any cortical wall. Additional gradual force can be marshaled by using a ratchet wrench or an adjustable torque wrench (in Newton-centimeters) to improve the mechanical advantage but not to apply excessive force that might snap the implant or fracture very dense Type 1 basal cortical bone typically found in the mandibular symphysis region.
4. MDI crestal emergence profiles through small islands of keratinized gingival soft tissues attached to crestal bone significantly improve the prognosis for the periimplant environment of the MDIs and, by extension, enhance the predictability of the entire hybridized prosthesis.

5. Ponabut design MDIs encourage optimal esthetic outcomes because they can be contoured to provide normal ridge laps in the esthetic zone as well as open embrasures for hygiene maintenance.
6. Occlusal management for MDIs is straightforward and can be harmonized with typical morphology common to conventional implants as well as anatomic variables of natural teeth.
7. MDI affordability can play a significant role in patient acceptance of a restorative treatment plan wherein the need for additional implant abutments to render an improved case predictability may tip the balance into a rejection of an entire important rehabilitative program. The MDI can supplement conventional implants in select cases that can be made more readily cost-effective in such a hybrid combination.

The following images (Figures 1-1 to 1-23 and Box 1-1), starting with the first hybrid MDI case, are sequentially designed to impart an orderly instructional basis for implementing hybrid MDI applications and gradually reinforce the learning curve on a pathway to more advanced MDI combinations.

BOX I-I **Rationale for MDI and Natural Tooth Abutment and Hybridization**

- Rationale for hybridizing MDIs with natural tooth abutments is the subject of a proposed research study by Dr. John Brunski et al of Rensselaer Polytechnic Institute and Stanford University in conjunction with Dr. Victor I. Sendax.
- Ongoing clinical case reports have demonstrated minimal morbid complications from splinting MDIs with supportive dentition compared with anecdotal reports of incompatibility between conventional implant abutments and natural tooth abutments.
- A working hypothesis to explain these different outcomes hinges on the varied bending stiffness of a 1.8-mm wide titanium alloy MDI compared with the 3.0-mm width—plus increasingly greater widths—of conventional implants. It is assumed that the narrower 1.8-mm width of the MDI permits a degree of flexibility that becomes increasingly unrealizable as the width of a metallic implant enlarges. The greater flexibility of the ultra-small-diameter MDIs may mimic to some degree the cushioning effect of the periodontal ligament and possibly account for the apparent compatibility of the minis with natural dental supports.

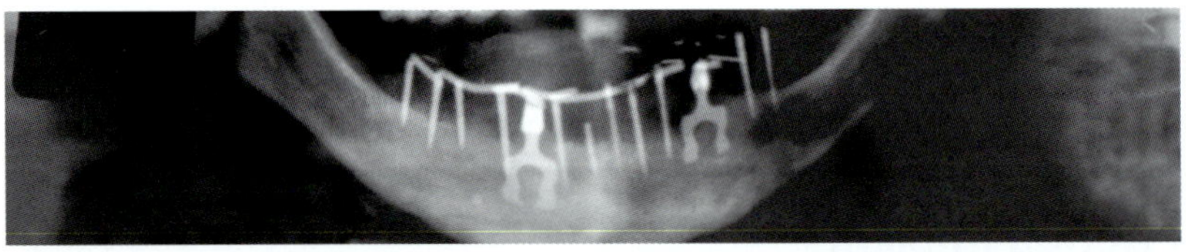

FIGURE 1-1. **Historic First "Mini Implant" Hybrid Case.** Titanium endodontic screw posts used as prototype mini implants, hybridized with two mandibular preexisting (blade-type) implants circa 1976.

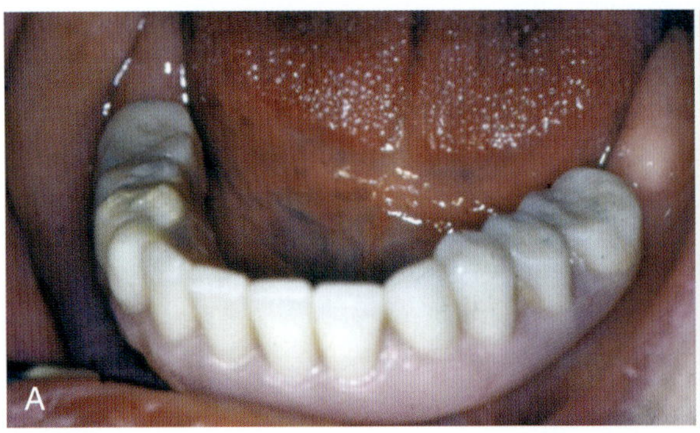

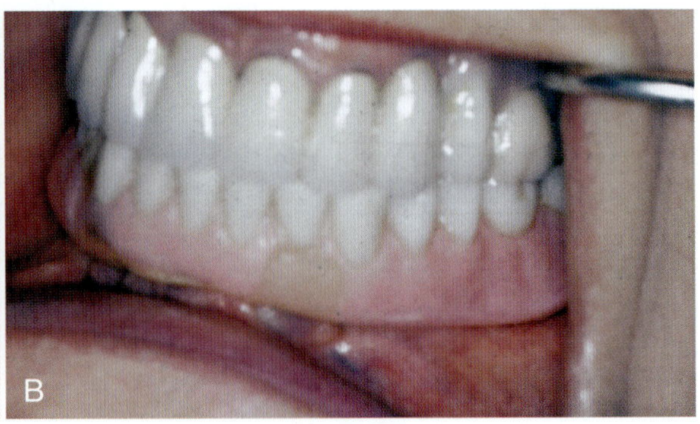

FIGURE 1-2. **First Mini Implant Case with Prosthesis.** Mandibular prosthesis and underlying mini implants (titanium screw posts) survived intact for 25 years until patient's demise.

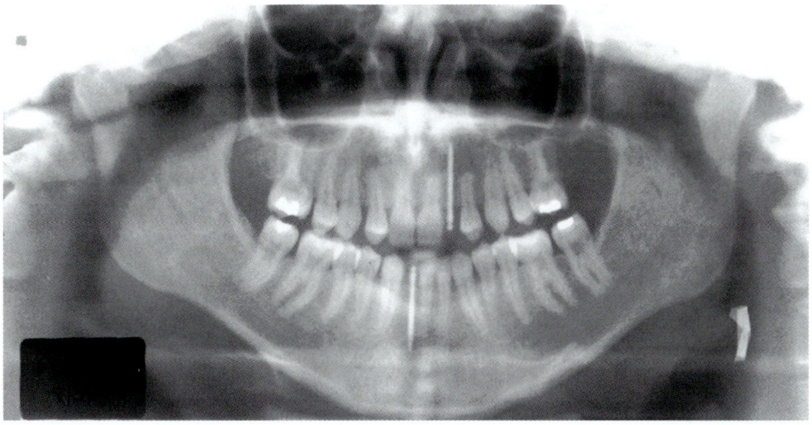

FIGURE 1-3. MDIs (1.8 mm) for ideal ultra-small diameter, maxillary and mandibular, single tooth replacements.

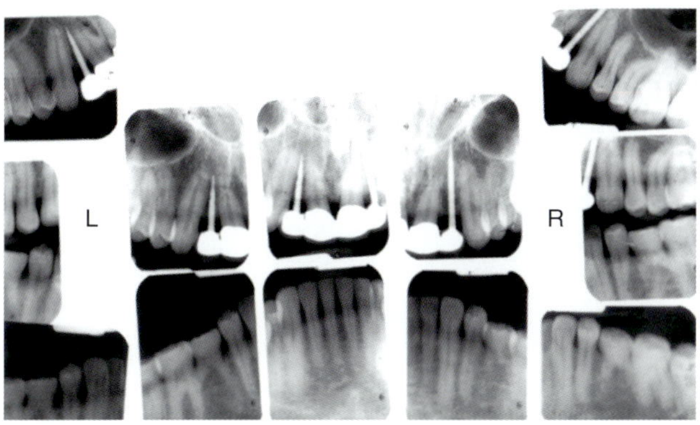

FIGURE 1-4. MDIs for congenitally missing lateral incisors.

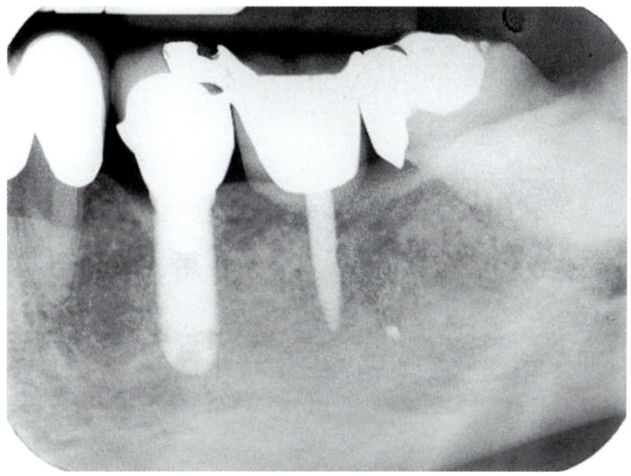

FIGURE 1-5. Maryland-type MDI bridge hybridized with conventional implant.

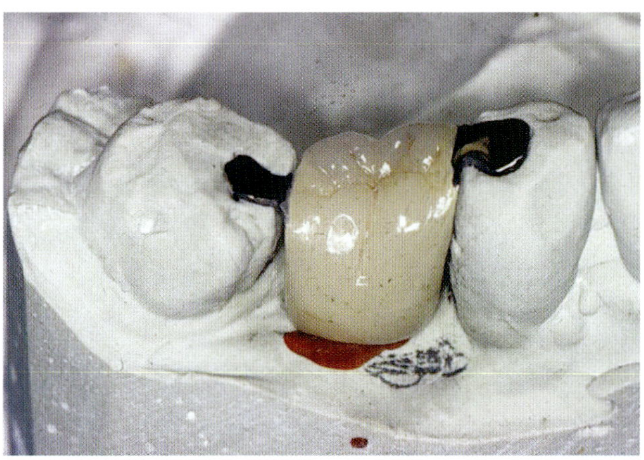

FIGURE 1-6. Maryland-type hybrid MDI bridge single tooth replacement.

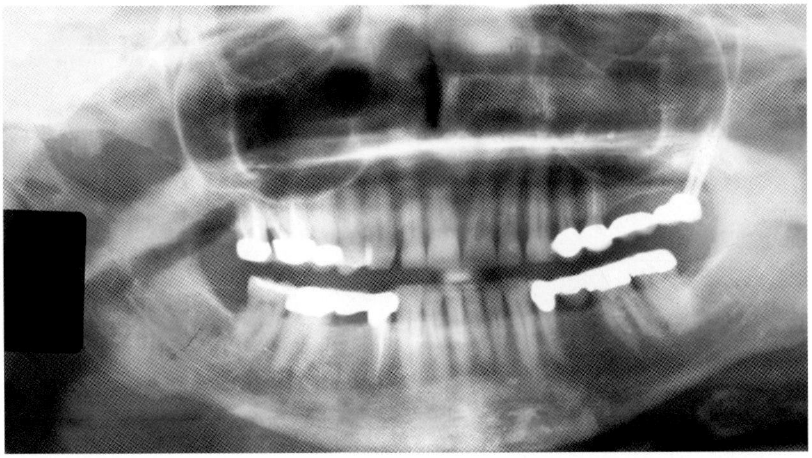

FIGURE 1-7. Dual tuberosity MDIs hybridized with natural tooth abutments.

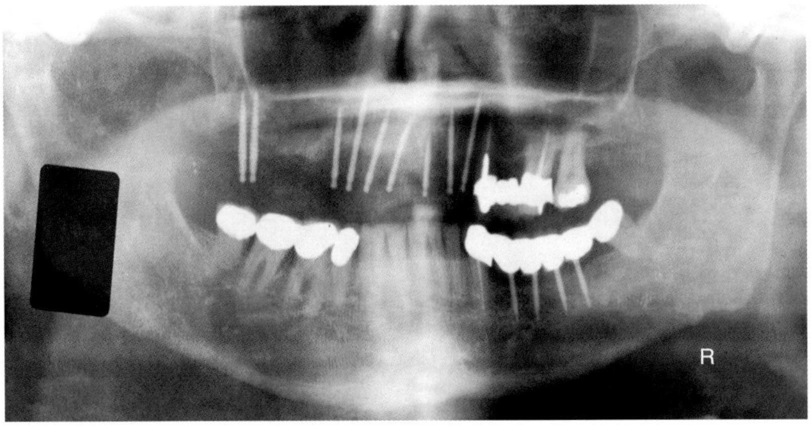

FIGURE 1-8. Dual maxillary MDIs anchored in tuberosity cortical wall, hybridized with supportive mandibular interdental MDIs.

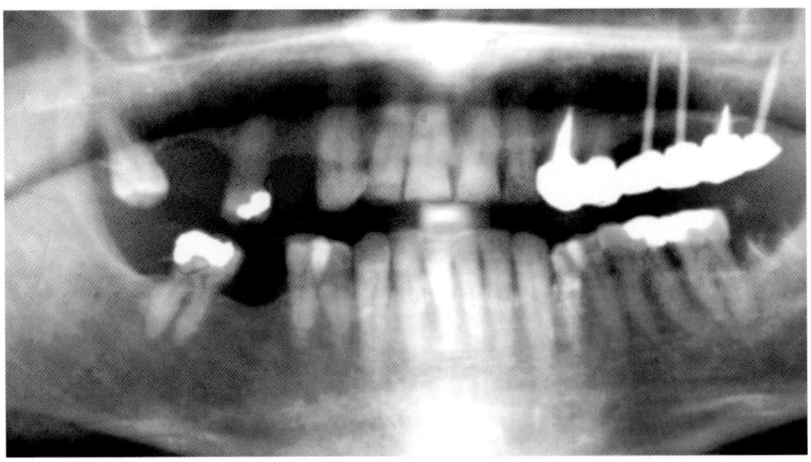

FIGURE 1-9. MDIs anchored in tuberosity cortical wall and cortical floor of sinus hybridized with natural tooth abutments.

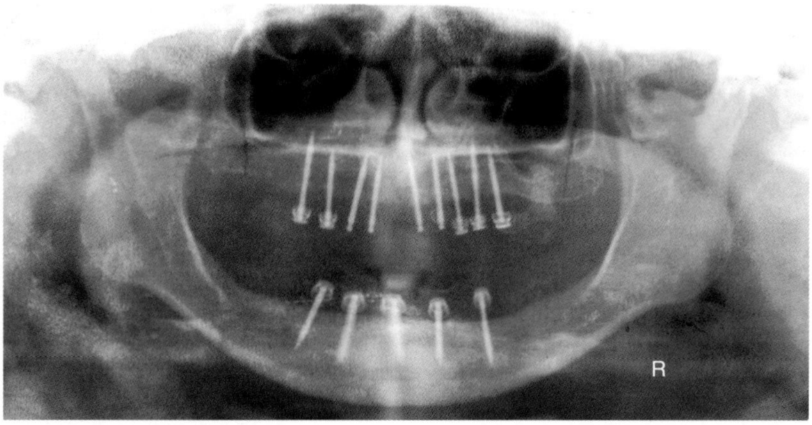

FIGURE 1-10. Bicortical stabilization is key to maxillary and mandibular long-term MDI functionality.

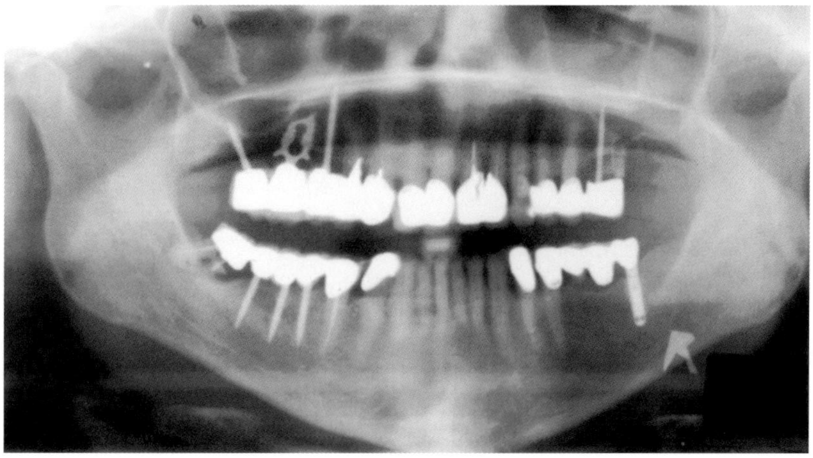

FIGURE 1-11. MDI hybridized with classic (25 years in situ) blade implant, conventional implant, and natural tooth abutments.

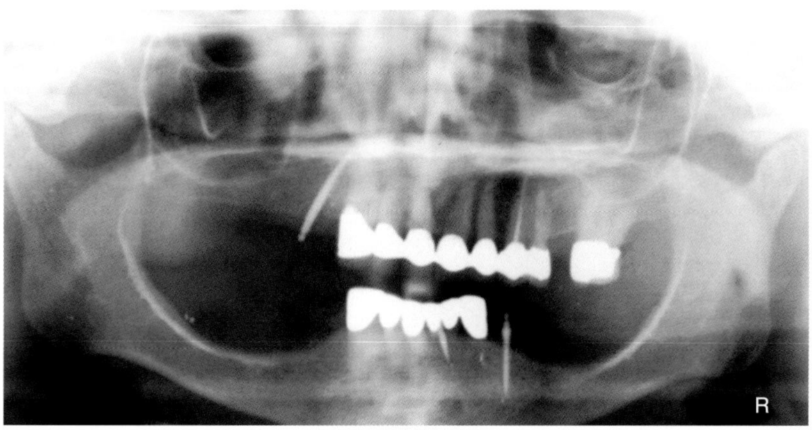

FIGURE 1-12. Hybrid removable and fixed MDI applications.

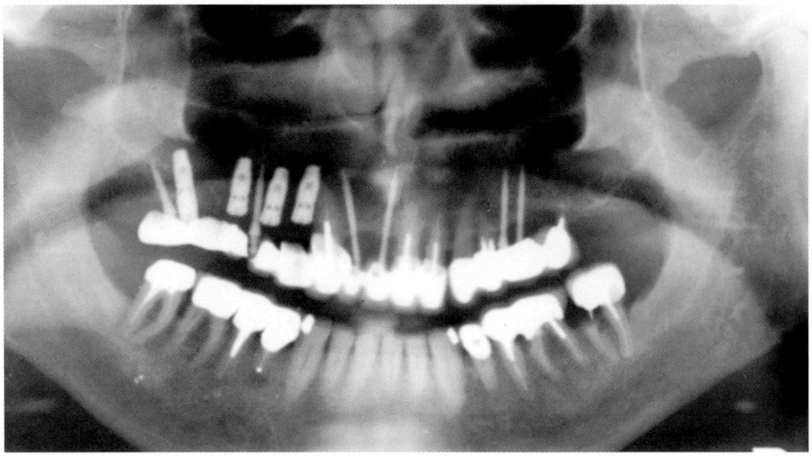

FIGURE 1-13. MDIs hybridized with natural tooth abutments and conventional implants for both transitional and long-term definitive applications.

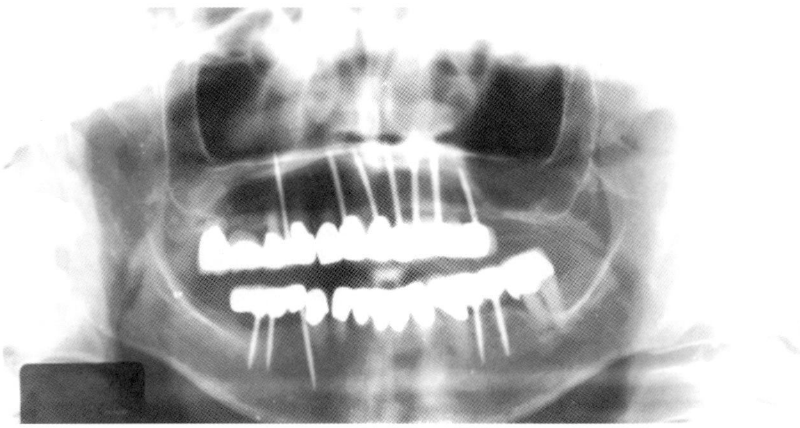

FIGURE 1-14. Maxillary MDIs "biting" into floor of nasal cavity and sinus for immediate bicortical stabilization, and mandibular MDIs hybridized with natural tooth abutments.

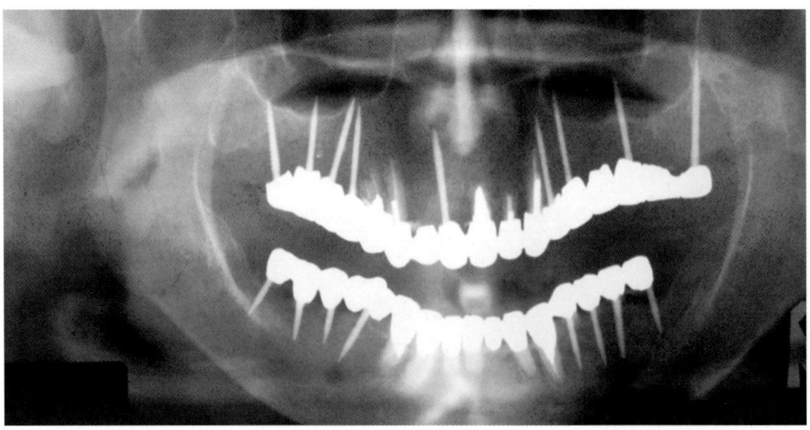

FIGURE 1-15. MDIs anchored in maxillary cortices and mandibular dense lingual mylohyoid ridge bone, hybridized with natural tooth abutments.

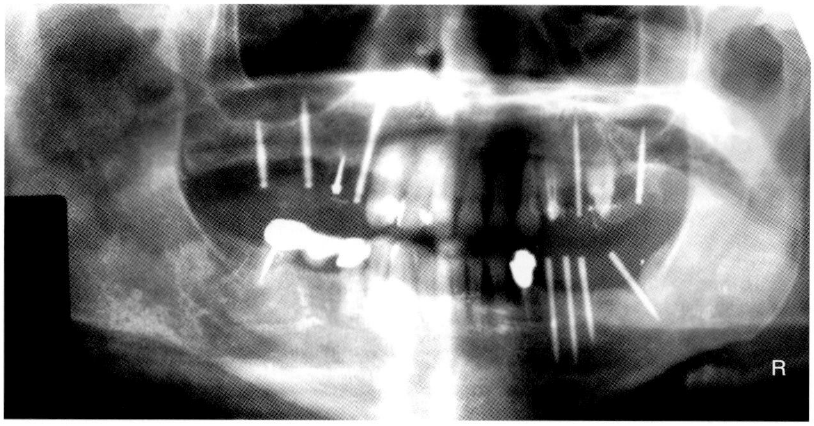

FIGURE 1-16. Tall, cortically anchored maxillary MDIs hybridized with shorter natural tooth abutments.

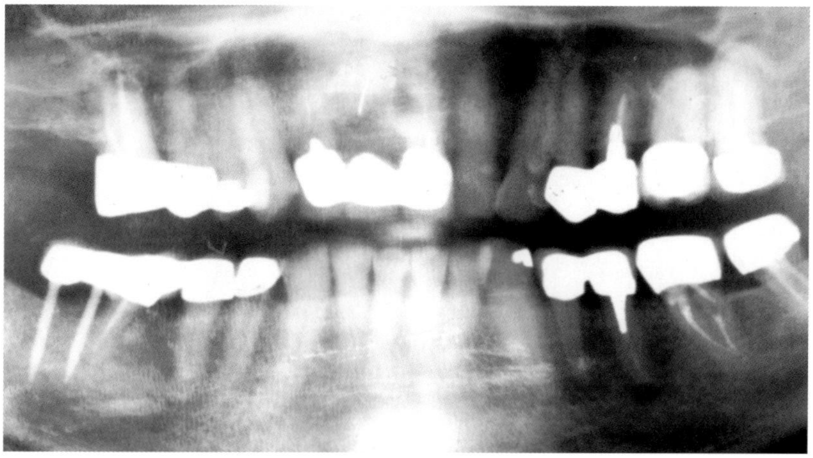

FIGURE 1-17. Dual mandibular terminal-abutment MDIs hybridized with natural tooth abutments.

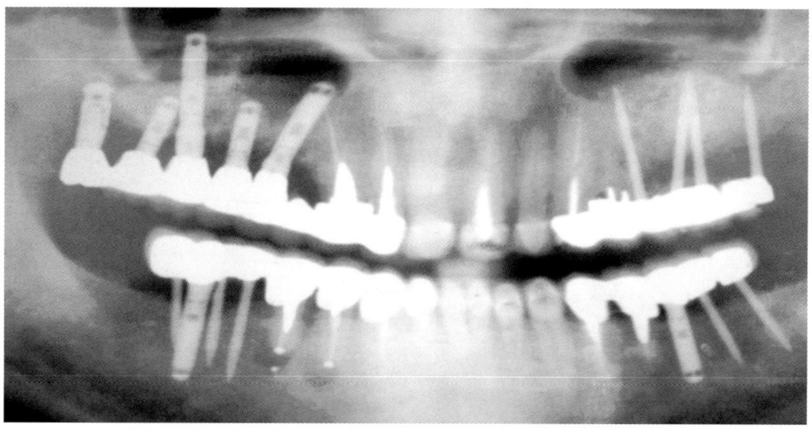

FIGURE 1-18. MDIs and conventional implants inserted in bilateral sinus grafts, hybridized with natural tooth abutments, and mandibular conventional implant abutments corestored with MDIs and natural dentition.

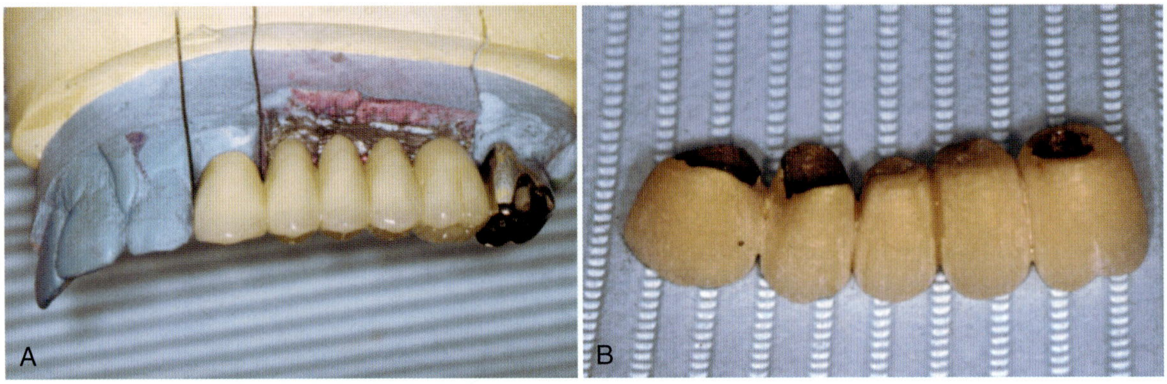

FIGURE 1-19. MDI maxillary Ponabut-design ceramic-metal units hybridized with conventional crown units.

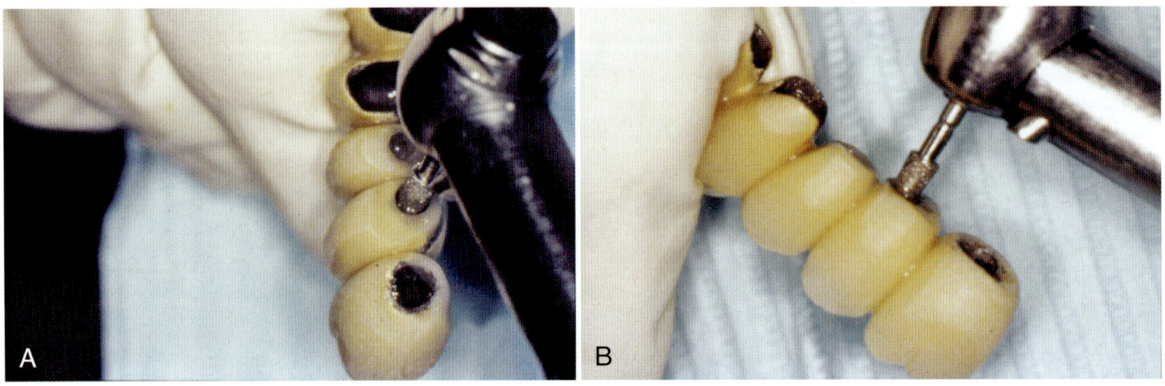

FIGURE 1-20. Ponabut internal modifications with medium speed diamond drill and water spray.

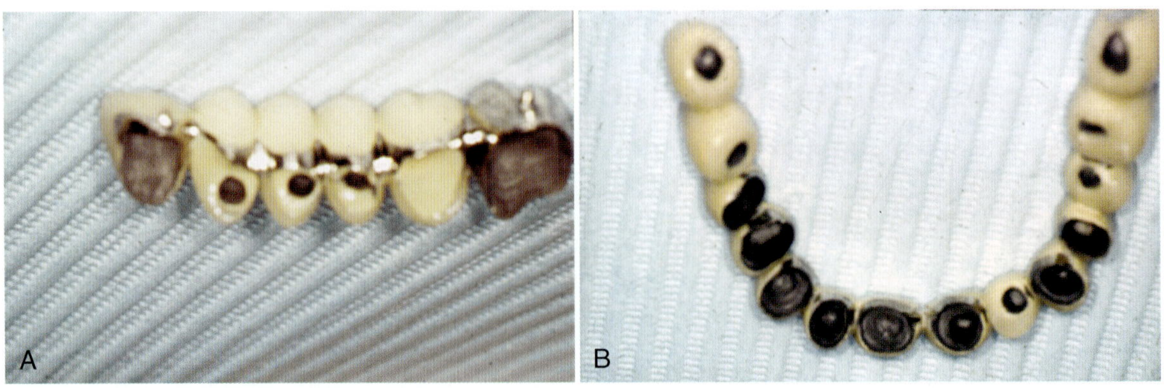

FIGURE 1-21. Ponabut units hybridized with natural tooth abutments.

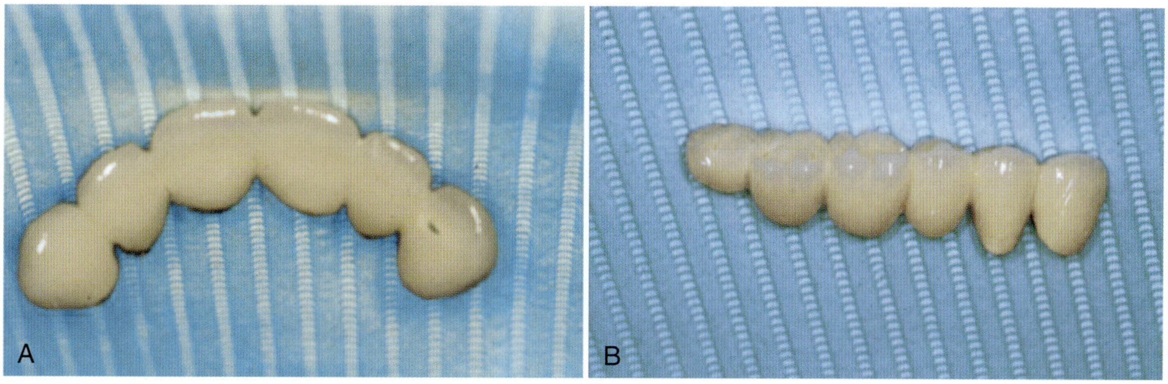

FIGURE 1-22. Glazed MDI hybrid Ponabut bridge/splint.

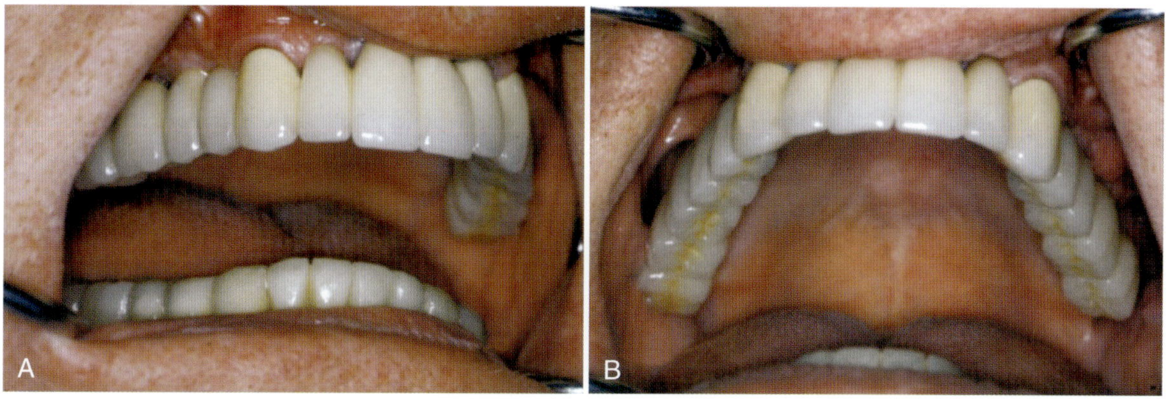

FIGURE 1-23. Complete hybrid maxillary and mandibular MDI case.

Chapter 2

The Basic Insertion and Reconstructive Protocol Guidelines

Step by Step

VICTOR I. SENDAX

Outline

Key Elements of a Minimally Invasive, Immediately Functional Mini Implant System

After making a minimal starter drill opening directly through attached crestal gingiva, then use a 1.1-mm bone drill through dense crestal cortical bone and drill farther into the more porous medullary bone, and terminate drilling in denser basal bone found typically in mandibular symphysis or posterior dense basal bone layers close to buccal-lingual cortices, buccal external oblique ridges, and lingual mylohyoid ridges. In the maxilla, apical terminus locations should end in the floor of the nasal cavity, floor and bony septa of the antra, cortical walls of the tuberosities, sinuses, pyriform rim, and nasal cavity. Dense midline suture bone may also be a useful destination for apical termination, providing a solid bite-in surface for the apical tip of the mini dental implants (MDIs). Bicortical stabilization is the essential principle.

A standard width 1.8-mm MDI with O-Ball Head or rectangular head (sometimes referred to as square head) abutment should be the most useful size for exploration of bone density, quality, and supportiveness during function and/or parafunction. Wider-threaded MDIs can be employed if a greater "bite-in" is needed than can be provided by the ultra-narrow standard 1.8-mm MDI. One can always change from the 1.8-mm standard MDI to a wider type, using the same starter opening without stripping bone, but not vice versa because the 1.8-mm implant will no longer be in sufficient oppositional contact with mature unprepared bone and consequently will be less likely to be useful as a long-term supportive implant.

Orthodontic Note

Mini implants that are narrower than 1.8 mm typically used in orthodontic TAD applications will not be in immediate contact with enough bone to qualify as anything more than the transitional anchorage for which they were originally designed and dedicated (see Chapter 9).

Summary Guidelines Governing Widths of Mini Dental Implants

The wider the mini implant the greater the challenge for that implant to be immediately and sufficiently bone-appositioned for predictable functionality without observing the gradual healing delay once considered essential for classic Branemark-defined osseointegration to occur. As a direct consequence of this working rule of thumb, it is suggested that the surgeon routinely start by inserting a standard 1.8-mm width MDI, the slowly-evolved optimal diameter derived during the early clinical trials period by Sendax, Balkin, and Ricciardi, and an exploratory technique to determine the bone quality and quantity in the placement site before actually inserting the MDI into its final desired location.

Clinical Tip

Only after this initial step using the 1.8 mm width mini implant should one proceed to try wider diameter 2.1 to 2.5 mm examples in hopes of gaining increased osseous surface area stability and functional supportiveness in Type IV bone sites of poor density and trabeculation.

Another advantage of starting the procedure with the standard width 1.8-mm MDI is the conservation of bone achieved by only gradually "upping the ante" with increasing width implants. The simple but essential choice of osteotomy avoidance with the narrower diameter mini will go a significant way towards avoiding undue loss of valuable bone resource during the critical osseoapposition insertion process.

The following basic step-by-step training presentation is offered to demonstrate basic contemporary sequential training for the Sendax MDI System technology in visually accessible terms.

Editor's Comment

Nothing presented herein is considered technically "set in stone" because operational variations in MDI pedagogy and training continually evolve with experiential outcomes being gleaned from broad-based clinical settings and from ongoing feedback from laboratory, industry, and research domains. Representative examples are to be found throughout this textbook, some with considerable modifications from this core presentation.

Benefit Highlights

Long-Term

- MDI Long-Term Solution: The original mini implant to first earn FDA Acceptance for Long-Term Use to Stabilize Upper and Lower Dentures, Crowns and Bridges

Simple Technique

- 5-step placement protocol
- Basic finger and thumb driven instrumentation

Minimally Invasive

- No flap for most cases
- No osteotomy (1.1-mm starter pilot hole)

Immediate Load

- Denture is stabilized the day MDIs are placed
- Existing dentures are retrofitted chairside
- Soft tissue is supported and/or implant is retained

Cost Effective

- Affordable materials for dentists
- Affordable procedure for patients

Indications

- Patients who are medically compromised
- Patients who are financially compromised

- Patients who are anatomically compromised
- Patients with diabetes that is controlled

Lower Denture Stabilization (Figure 2-1)

The Primary MDI Application

- Patient's chewing function is immediately and dramatically improved.
- Bone height is retained due to presence of implants.
- Tissue is supported, and implant is retained!
- A predictable treatment option (approximately 97% implant success rate).
- 4 MDIs can be placed in the anterior mandible (between the foramina) for immediate stabilization.
- Bone is typically dense but often lacking in height and width.
- For MDI, only 10-mm bone height and 4-mm buccolingual width is needed.
- From implant placement to denture retrofitting, the procedure lasts an average 90 minutes.

Lower Denture Stabilization: From Case Planning to Postoperative Care

Preoperative Planning

Applicable Radiographs

- *Panoramic*: best jaws overview
- *Lateral-Cephalic* or equivalent view
- *CT scan*: 3D collimated
- *Periapical*: good detail but may have a limited field of view (FOV)

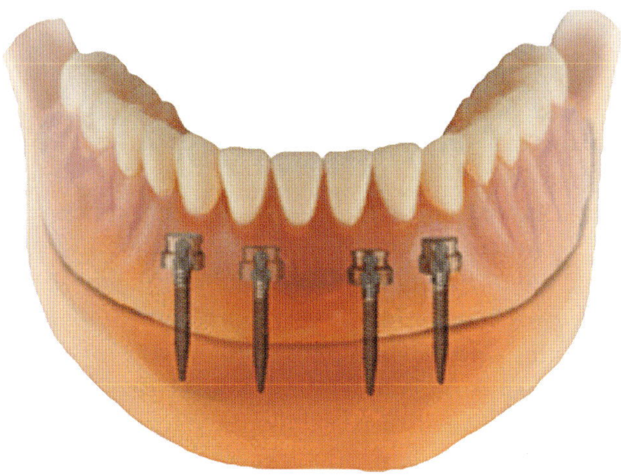

FIGURE 2-1

Treatment Planning Guidelines

- Choose length with radiographs and MDI template.
- Choose thread design: Standard 1.8 mm or maximum width? (Typically, standard in mandible and maximum in maxilla).
- How many implants?
  Mandible: Four is *advisable*
  Maxilla: Six is *advisable*
- Locate mental foramen on panoramic x-ray.

Day of Surgery

- Mark left and right mental foramen with intraoral skin marker.
- Measure 7 mm anterior of the mental foramen and mark the ridge to map the most distal implant site.
- Mark remaining sites, leaving approx. 4.5 to 5 mm between each.
- Inject minimal local anesthetic at each implant crestal site down to periosteum covering cortical bone.

Placement Protocol

Step 1. Drill Pilot Hole (Figure 2-2)

- Objective: To penetrate crestal cortical bone.
- Use up and down pumping motion while drilling and irrigate to cool bur.
- Avoid drilling a full-length osteotomy.

During the drilling process, monitor depth and angulation for two reasons:

1. To ensure that the length of implant chosen during treatment planning will approximate the length of implant placed in bone; and
2. To be sure the divergence of neighboring implants is within a reasonable degree of abutment parallelism for ease of O-Ring insertion and removal.

Step 2. Insert Implant Using Finger Driver

- Turn clockwise until resistance calls for increased torque (Figure 2-3).

Step 3. Advance Implant with Winged Thumb Wrench

- In many cases, the implant can be fully seated by using a winged thumb wrench (driver) to reach and bite into dense supportive bone (Figure 2-4).

Step 4. Final Seating of Implant using Ratchet Wrench or Torque Wrench

Slow Down To avoid fractures!

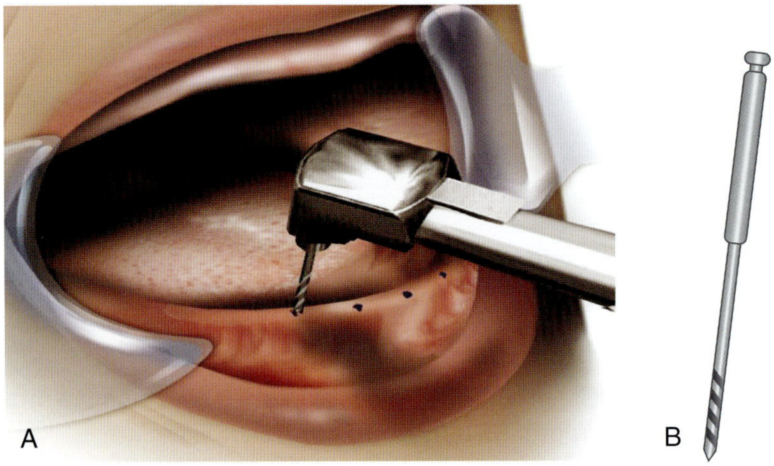

FIGURE 2-2. Drill pilot hole.

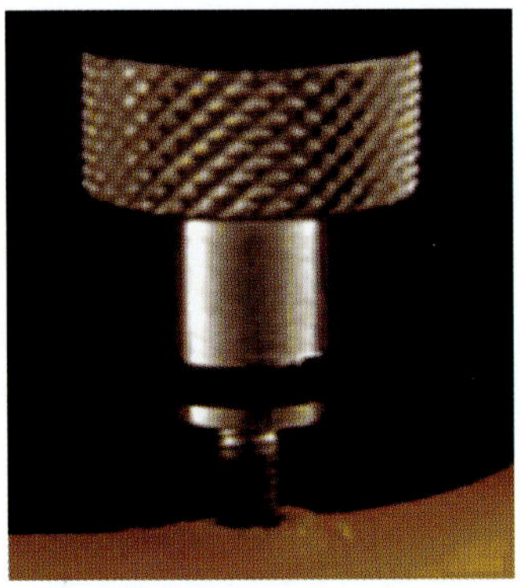

FIGURE 2-3. Finger driver.

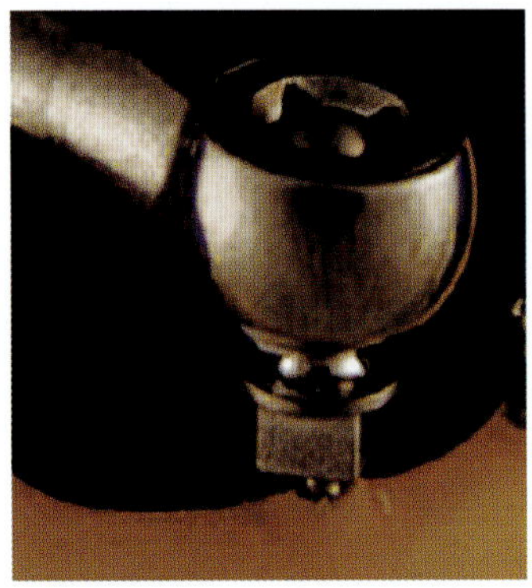

FIGURE 2-5. Ratchet wrench.

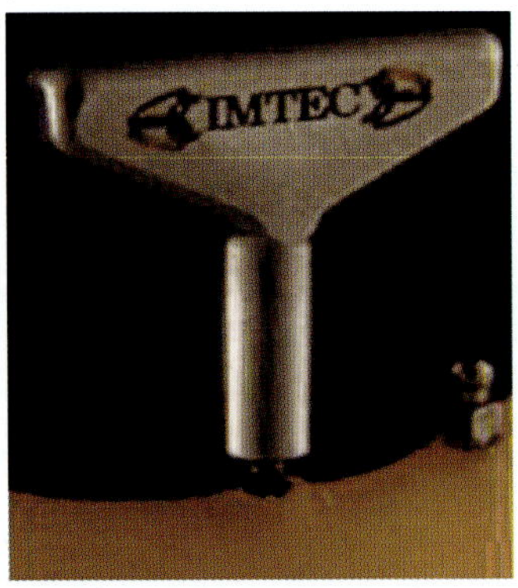

FIGURE 2-4. Winged thumb wrench.

- Use MDI ratchet adapters with ratchet wrench (or torque wrench with adjustable Newton-centimeter [Ncm] settings) (Figure 2-5).

Guideline: Insert Slowly

The ratchet (or adjustable torque) wrench is most necessary when the bone is *very* dense. Thermal trauma created by excessive friction can damage bone, and torque could fracture mini implant if MDI is too aggressively and rapidly inserted.

- MDI is best advanced in slow, measured stages! Dense bone resists self-tapping insertion.
- Carefully avoid lateral forces, which can cause fracture even with torque levels in a safe range.

Potential implant fractures can be minimized by:

1. Using an adjustable torque wrench set at the recommended 30 Ncm to maximum 45 Ncm depending on bone density and resistance, which is especially useful for very dense Type I bone.
2. Taking approximately 7 seconds for each quarter turn and waiting 5 to 10 seconds or more between turns (allowing viscoelastic bone to accommodate and expand for immediate osseoopposito n).

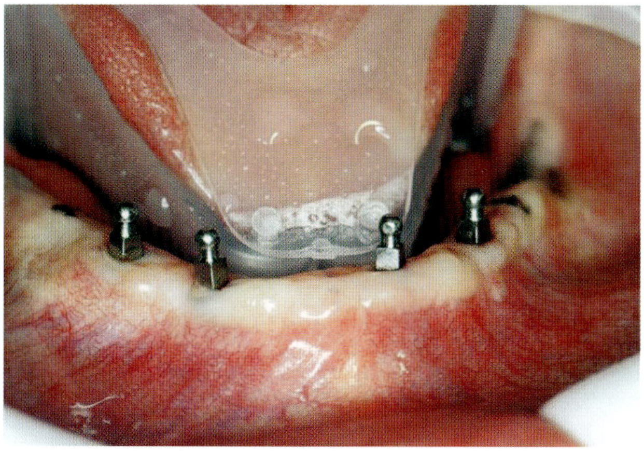

FIGURE 2-6. Fully seated implants.

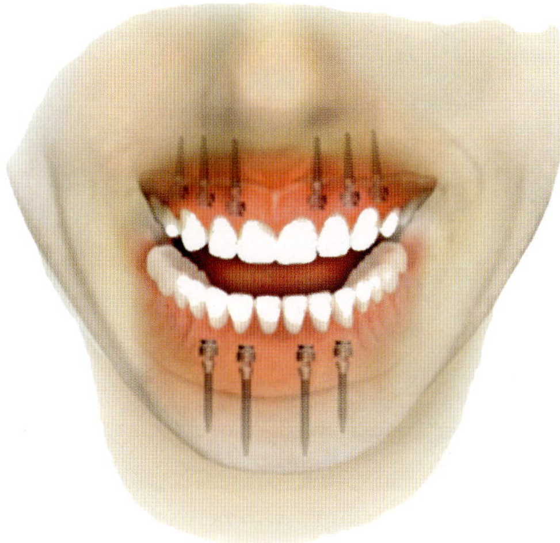

FIGURE 2-7. Prosthetic protocol.

IMPORTANT

Use the thumb or forefinger of opposite hand supporting jaw to apply downward pressure to the head of the ratchet or torque wrench during use. This will limit excessive lateral forces that can also contribute to implant fractures and be more comfortable for patient and doctor.

Ready for the Denture

Implants are fully seated only when:

1. All *or most* threads are engaged in bone.
2. The apical tip of each mini implant is stabilized by biting into dense mandibular symphyseal bone (Figure 2-6).

Prosthetic Protocol (Figure 2-7)

Step 1. Place Block-Out Shims

Trim soft elastomeric shims into approximately 2-mm pieces and push each piece over O-Ball Head to cover square neck base completely.

Step 2. Place Metal O-Ring Housings

Use downward and rotational pressure to ensure housings fit passively over slightly compressed soft elastomeric shims.

Step 3. Trough Denture and Check for Critical Internal Clearance

- Use an acrylic bur to make a trough in the anterior portion of the denture (Figure 2-8).
- Dot each housing with white disclosing paste or correction fluid or indelible marker and replace denture over housings.

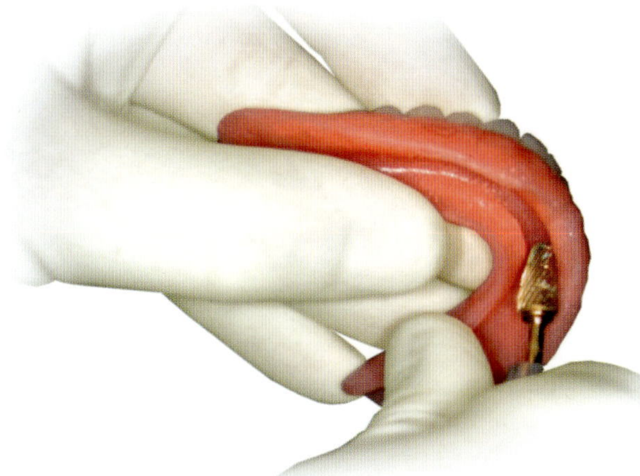

FIGURE 2-8. Create trough in denture with acrylic bar.

- Remove and check denture interior for transfer markings.
- Relieve all areas of housing interferences as indicated to obtain unobstructed internal fit!

To Save Time Later

After roughening the interior of the denture with an acrylic bur, coat the exterior of the denture with standard petroleum jelly. This will prevent acrylic bonding to that denture surface and teeth and save valuable time during the cleanup phase.

Step 5. Fill Trough with Fast-Set Acrylic Mix

After setting, Cold-Cure Acrylic Resin can also function as a hard reline material, so a full denture reline can be done simultaneously with O-ring housings pick-up for improved functional stability (Figure 2-9).

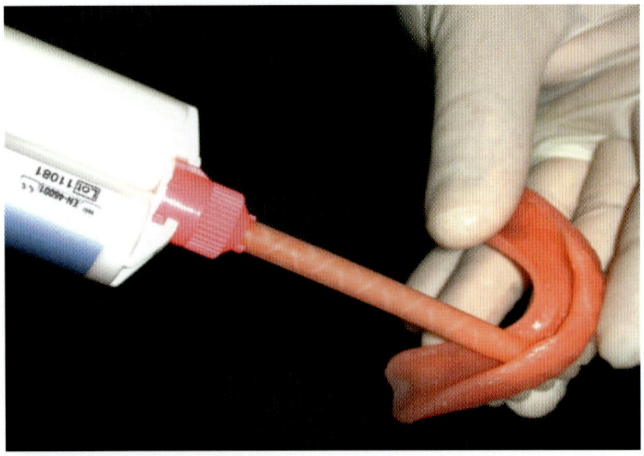

FIGURE 2-9. Fill trough with fast-setting acrylic mix.

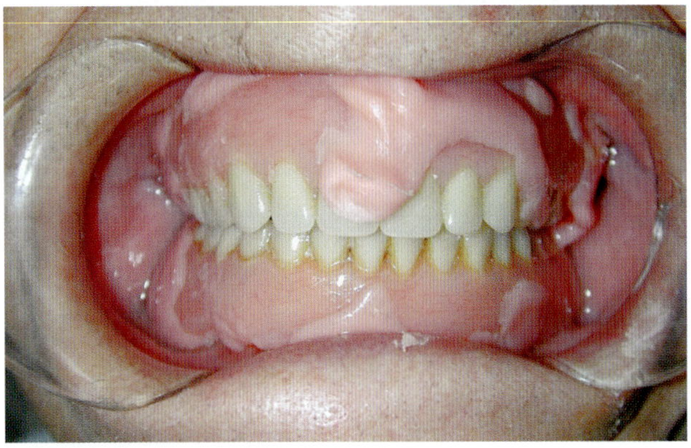

FIGURE 2-10. Patient provides 6 to 8 minutes of normal occlusion while secure hard acrylic sets.

Step 6. Insert Relined Over-Denture Orally

- Patient provides normal occlusion for 6 to 8 minutes while **secure** hard acrylic sets (Figure 2-10).
- Support patient's chin and monitor bite.
- Bite register can be made before surgery to be used at this time *(blue mousse).*
- Trim excess reline resin and polish denture (Figure 2-11).
- Re-insert for patient try-in and any border and internal O-ring relief.

Choosing the Right Length

Bi-Cortical Stability: The apical tip of the implant should engage and bite into dense cortical bone.

MDI Threads: All threaded implant surfaces should preferably be engaged in bone rather than soft tissue.

Soft Reline

Soft relines are used for progressive loading without metal housings/O-rings to test for questionable bicortical stabilization

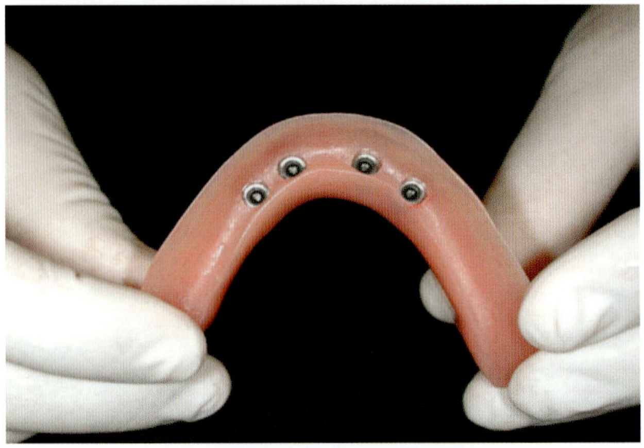

FIGURE 2-11. Denture after trimming excess reline resin and polishing.

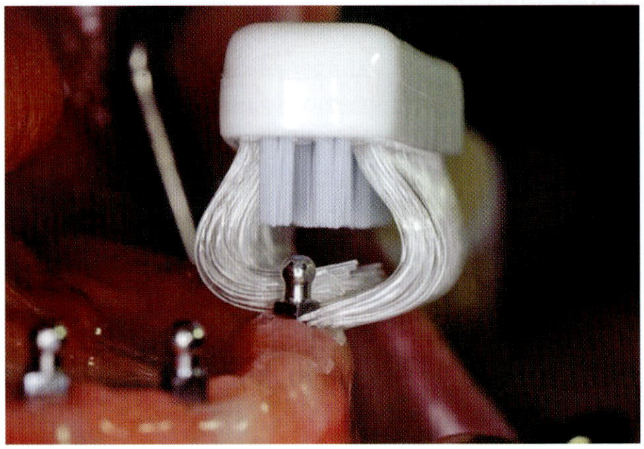

FIGURE 2-12. Access dedicated implant toothbrush.

Access Home Care Brush for Patients with MDIs, Conventional Implants, and Natural Teeth

Access Dedicated Implant Toothbrush

An access dedicated implant toothbrush cleans implant and soft tissue interface and prosthetic abutment portion of the MDI with its unique curved-bristle memory (Figure 2-12).

Basic Mandibular Step-by-Step Overdenture Stabilization Review

(Case Provided By Dr. Charles English*)

1. Marked Ridge (Figure 2-13)
2. Drilling the Starter Pilot Hole (Figure 2-14)
3. Insertion of MDI Using the Finger Driver (Figure 2-15)

---

*deceased

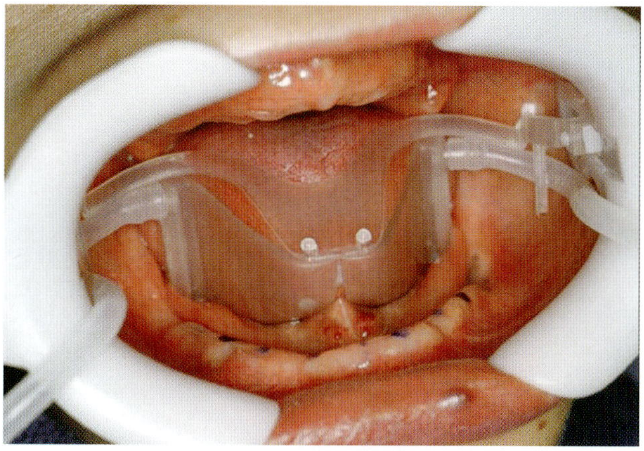

FIGURE 2-13

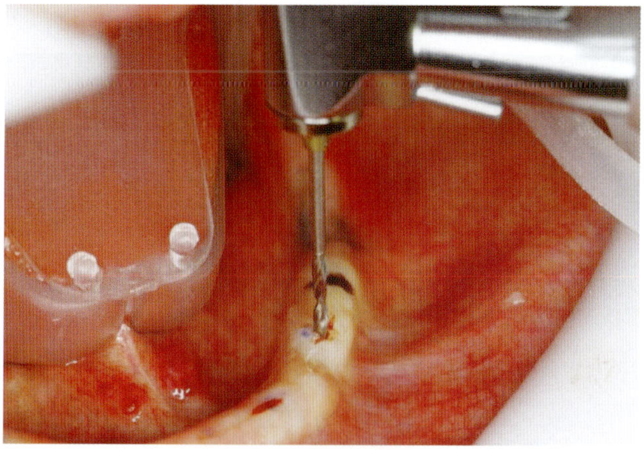

FIGURE 2-14

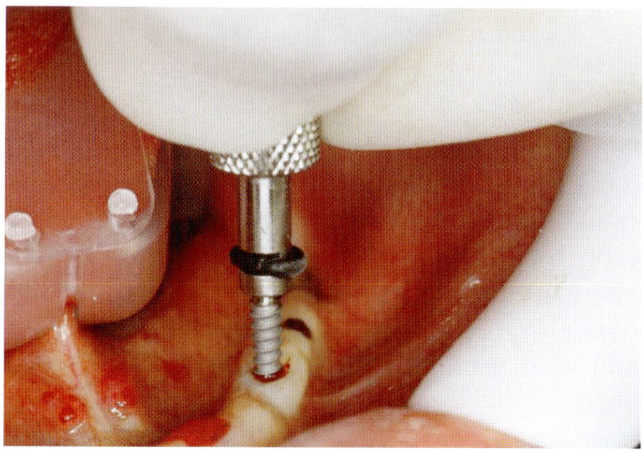

FIGURE 2-15

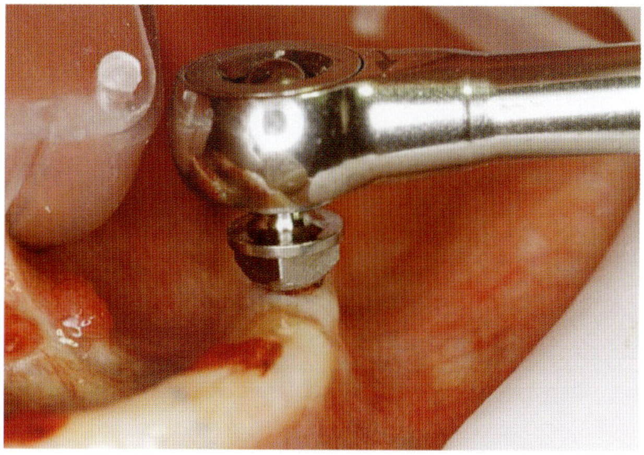

FIGURE 2-16

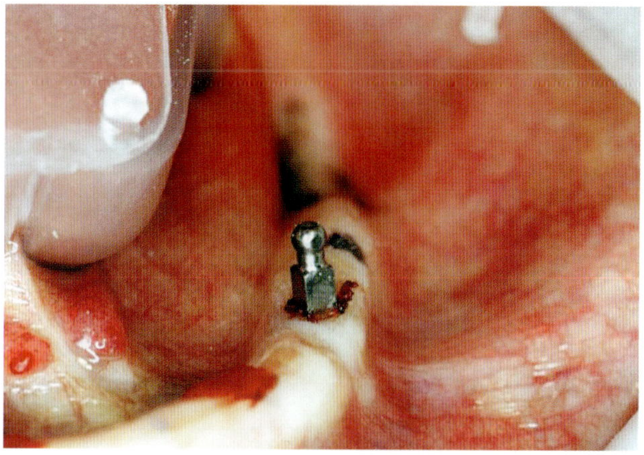

FIGURE 2-17

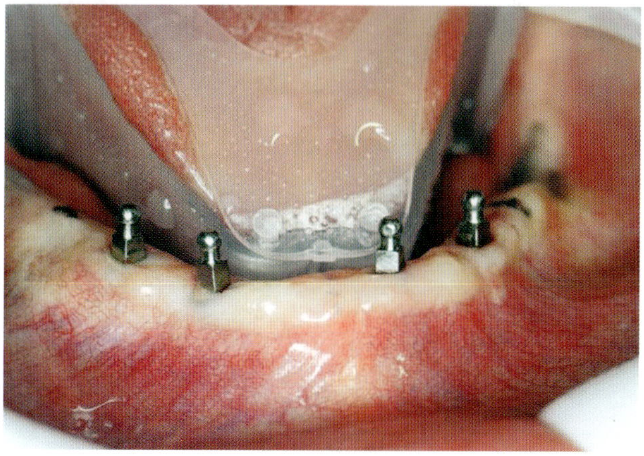

FIGURE 2-18

Winged thumb wrench continues insertion until significant bony resistance is felt.

4. Final Minimal MDI Seating with the Ratchet Wrench (approximately 30 Ncm) (Figure 2-16)
5. First Implant Fully Seated (Figure 2-17)
6. Repeat Steps 1 to 4 for all four MDIs (Figure 2-18)
7. Silicone Elastomeric Block-Out Shims (Figure 2-19)
8. Seating the Metal Housings Over Block-Out Shims (spacers) (Figure 2-20)
9. Relieve Anterior of Denture, Roughen Tissue Born Surface, and Apply Adhesive (Figure 2-21)

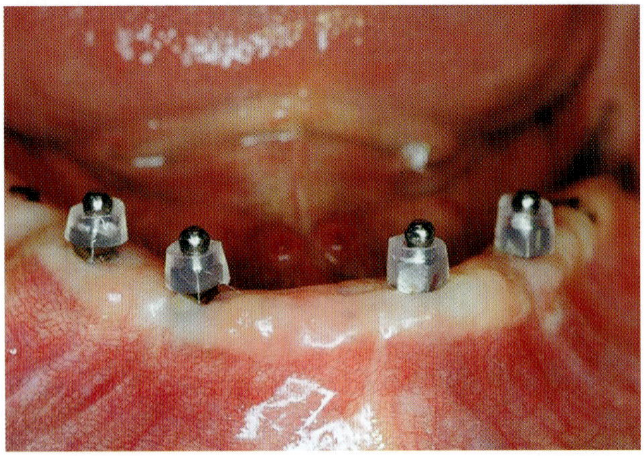

FIGURE 2-19

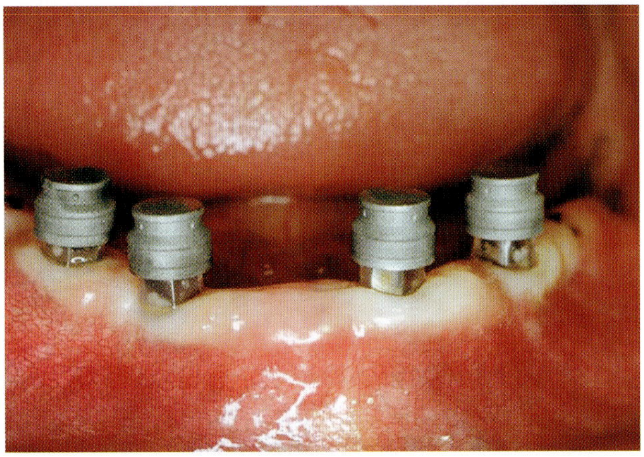

FIGURE 2-20

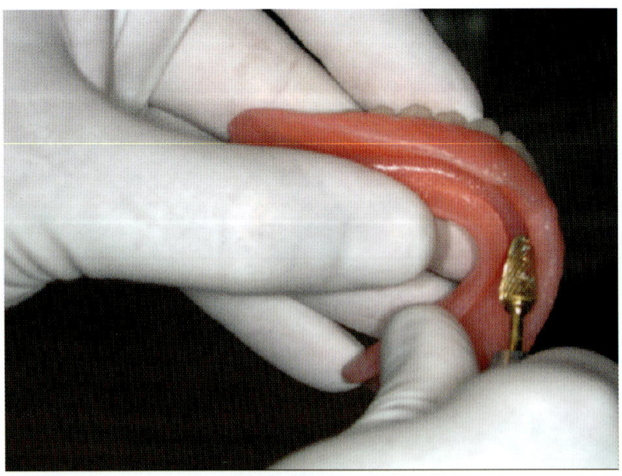

FIGURE 2-21

10. Fill with Hard Pick-Up Resin Mix (Figure 2-22)
Seat denture and allow to set for 6 to 8 minutes over O-ring housings. *Note:* Block-out shims prevent pick-up acrylic from getting trapped and set under housings and dangerously locking on to MDIs.

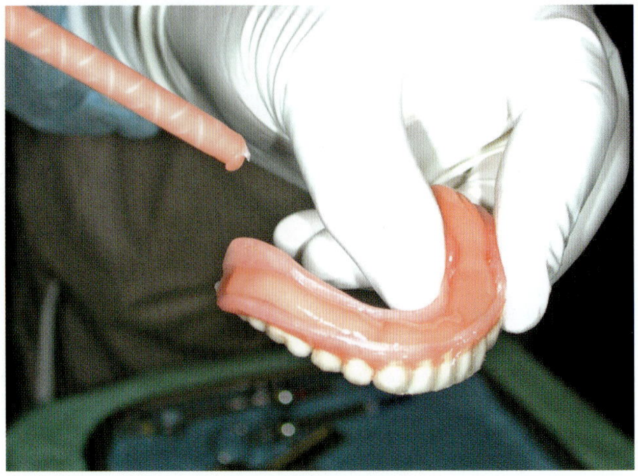

FIGURE 2-22

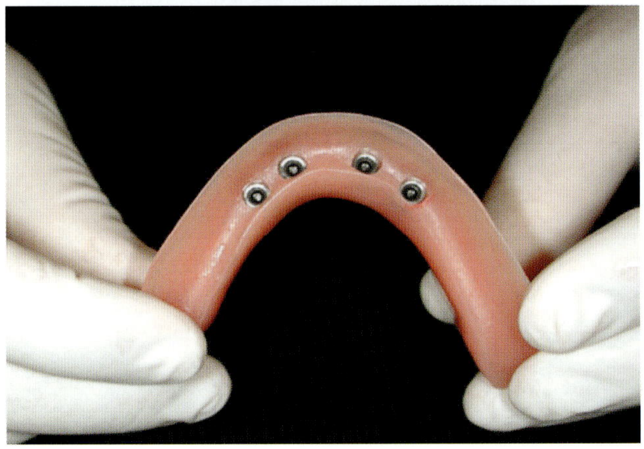

FIGURE 2-23

11. Retro-Fit Denture (Figure 2-23)
12. Soft Reline:
Perform a soft reline for trial progressive load period to test mini implants viability, before use of efficient, definitive O-rings, which is especially applicable for questionable maxillary porous bone implant sites, or for ultra-short mandibular implants tenuously secured in dense, resistant bone strata, and with marginal prognoses, especially if secure bicortical stabilization is not achievable.

Chapter 3

Background of Mini Dental Implants

BURTON E. BALKIN

Outline

The Early Historical Perspective: Sendax, Balkin, and Ricciardi

History

Dental implants date back to the ancient Egyptian and South American civilizations. Recorded progress commenced in the 1880s and progressed into the 1900s, and the Harvard and National Institute of Health's consensus development conference on dental implants indicated acceptance as a mode of treatment in 1988.[1]

In 1970-80 Brånemark and associates advocated an extended, soft-tissue covered healing period after implant insertion to allow for what came to be termed *osseointegration* and maintained in an unloaded environment for optimum predictability.[2,3] In the 1980s implantologists gradually saw a need to try to accommodate the desire of patients for more immediate implant support. Thus narrow-diameter mini dental implants came into use initially as a provisional treatment during healing/integration periods of traditional endosteal root-form implants. However, during this period, while utilizing mini dental implants for provisionalization, it was noted that these immediately loaded mini implants were often difficult to remove and appeared to have become clinically integrated. This led to an ongoing development of applications and to the current use for long-term restorative cases. The initial concept was developed and tested by Dr. Victor Sendax with further development of use, trials, and applications by co-investigators Dr. Burton Balkin (Professor of Periodontology and Oral Implantology, Temple University School of Dentistry) and Dr. Anthony Ricciardi (New Jersey College of Medicine and Dentistry). Dr. Balkin demonstrated bone stability with mini implants inserted via the auto-advance technique and immediately loaded. Supportive information was obtained from a human histologic study and a human subtraction radiography study.

The Sendax insertion protocol included preparing a minimal receptor site for a 1.8-mm implant by drilling directly through the attached gingiva into the bone for the part of the length of the implant portion that would be inserted but without the classic osteotomy that removed substantial bone to provide premeasured space for stabilizing traditional implants. The mini implant would then be turned

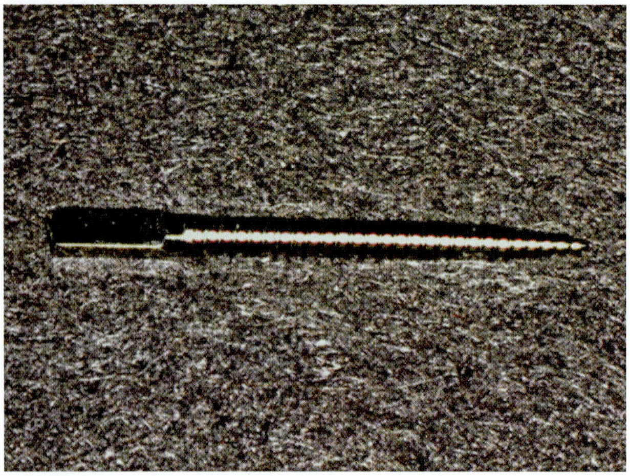

FIGURE 3-1. Example of 1.8-mm titanium alloy implant.

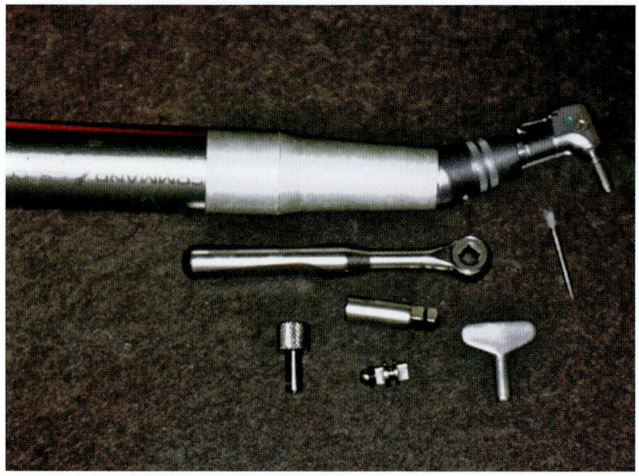

FIGURE 3-2. Instrumentation for auto-advance technique insertion of mini dental implant.

and threaded into the bone with pressure from finger and thumb drivers until the threads were fully inserted.

The auto-advance technique was a modification initiated by Balkin and colleagues[4] to enhance immediate implant stability for both ongoing and long-term applications and to refresh the well-used self-tapping concept with a newly dynamic image of the narrow-width mini implant feeling drawn into the bone automatically during guided insertion. The technique used only a minimal starting point opening in bone, and then the 1.8-mm implant was inserted by turning into the bone without a deeply drilled receptor site. This insertion was performed by using either an ultra-slow high-torque machine driver and/or hand drivers (Figures 3-1, 3-2). Cases were immediately loaded and anecdotal evidence indicated a more predictably stable result with the auto-advance insertion technique in accommodating bone of varied trabeculation and density (Box 3-1). Very dense Type 1 bone and extremely osteoporotic Type 4 bone required limited compensatory deviation from this basic underlying process.

To further test the validity of the clinical protocol, the mini implant system was subjected to histologic and radiographic scrutiny in two studies:

1. Histological specimens of minis were obtained by Dr. Balkin at 4 to 6 months after insertion and placement into immediate function while other traditional root-form implants integrated. Mini implants that supported the transitional prostheses were removed by trephination. The specimens were prepared and read by histologist David Steflik, M.S., EdD. Results indicated osteointegration to the surface of the implants based upon close adaptation of bone to the surface of the implants without interposition of soft tissue. This information was published in *The Journal of Oral Implantology* in 2001 and was the first human histologic report on the auto-advance insertion technique with immediate loading of mini dental implants, demonstrating feasibility for ongoing applications.[4]

BOX 3-1 Mini Dental Implant Insertion with Auto-advance Technique

- Starting point in bone
- Auto-advancing into position without preparation of a receptor site
- Ultra low-speed machine driver
- Hand driver

Description of Histologic Preparation

Two mini dental implants were fixed in 10% neutral buffered formalin for at least 72 hours. The samples were dehydrated in ascending concentrations of ethenol (50%, 75%, 90%, and 100% twice). Samples were transferred through acetone and infiltrated with methacrylate. Initially samples were immersed into a 50/50 mixture of methyl methacrylate, and samples were immersed into a 50/50 mixture of methyl methacrylate monomer and acetone for 24 hours, followed by 100% methacrylate monomer for 24 hours. The samples were

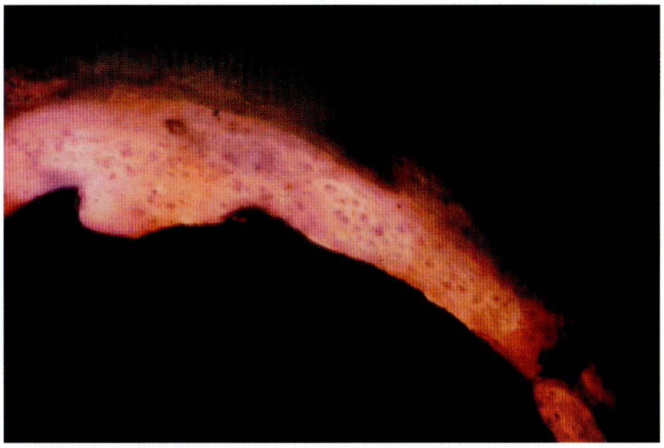

FIGURE 3-3. Core of bone interposed between the implant and the drill bit. (From Balkin BE, Stefik DE, Navel F: Mini dental implant insertion with the Auto-Advance Technique for ongoing applications. *J Oral Implantol* 27:32, 2001)

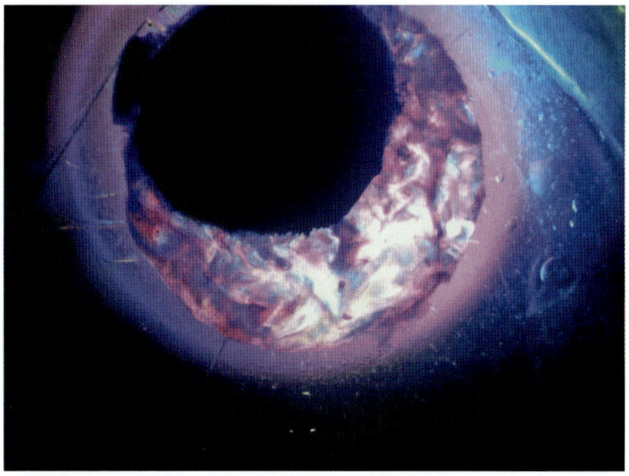

FIGURE 3-4. Low magnification photo micrograph shows close bone congruency to the implant surface. (From Balkin BE, Stefik DE, Navel F: Mini dental implant insertion with the Auto-Advance Technique for ongoing applications. *J Oral Implantol* 27:32, 2001)

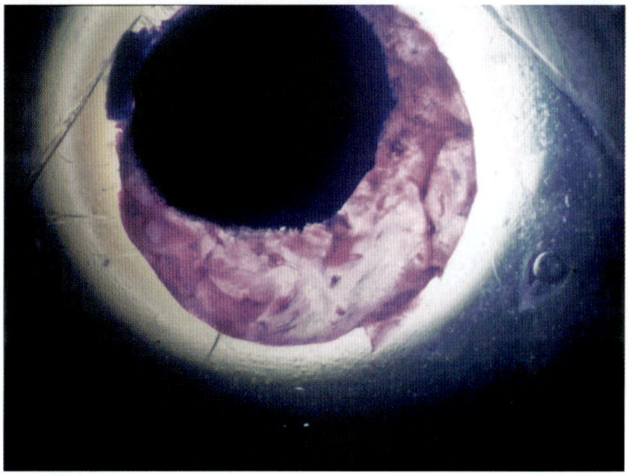

FIGURE 3-5. Bone apparent with routine light microscopy. (From Balkin BE, Stefik DE, Navel F: Mini dental implant insertion with the Auto-Advance Technique for ongoing applications. *J Oral Implantol* 27:32, 2001)

then vacuumed and infiltrated with methacrylate at room temperature for 14 days. Thereafter, they were placed in a vacuum oven, as per our previous report. As embedded blocks, they were then sectioned on an Isomet low-speed saw (Buehler Ltd., Lake Bluff, Ill.). The low-speed saw was affixed with a diamond wafering blade. Sections were cut in serial cross sections at thicknesses of 150 UM if necessary. They were ground to 80 UM if there were irregularities in the surface texture. The sections were stained with warmed toluidine blue and basic fuchsin, cover slipped, and viewed with a Zeiss Axiophat photomicroscope (Carl Zeiss Microscopy, LLC, Thornwood, N.Y.). Images were taken at various magnifications using Nomarski deferential interference imagery or polarized microscopy and routine light microscopy.

Results

Two implant samples were prepared. The samples were cut in situ with a trephine over the implant and bone. In one sample the trephine remained fixed over the implant and bone, and the bone and implant were unable to be retrieved from the trephine. Figure 3-3 shows a core of bone interposed between the implant and the trephine drill bit, which prohibits the trephine drill from being removed. The osseous core consisted of cortical bone with osteonal bone apparent. In the second sample, the trephine was able to be removed from the bone and implant. The low magnification photomicrograph (Figure 3-4) depicts close bone congruency to the implant surface. Bone is clearly apparent with both routine light microscopy (Figure 3-5) as well as corresponding Nomarski differential interference, microscopy (see Figure 3-4), which showed the morphology of the osteone bone. Higher magnification of the similar area (Figure 3-6) demonstrated the osseointegration of the implant with osteonal bone directly interfacing the implant. The interstitial lamella, as well as the corresponding circumferential lamellae of the remodeled bone, is apparent.

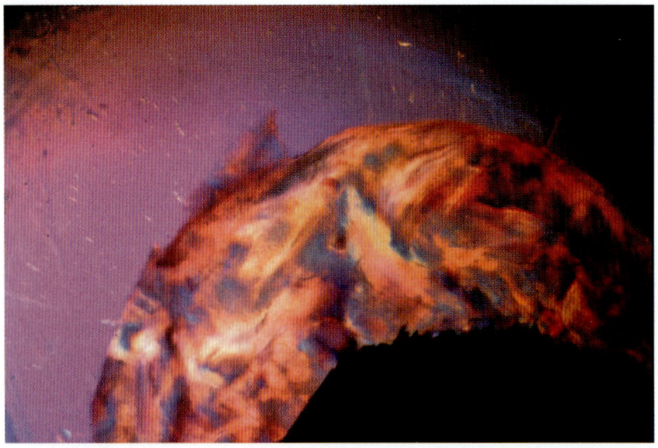

FIGURE 3-6. Integration of the implant with osteonal bone. (From Balkin BE, Stefik DE, Navel F: Mini dental implant insertion with the Auto-Advance Technique for ongoing applications. *J Oral Implantol* 27:32, 2001)

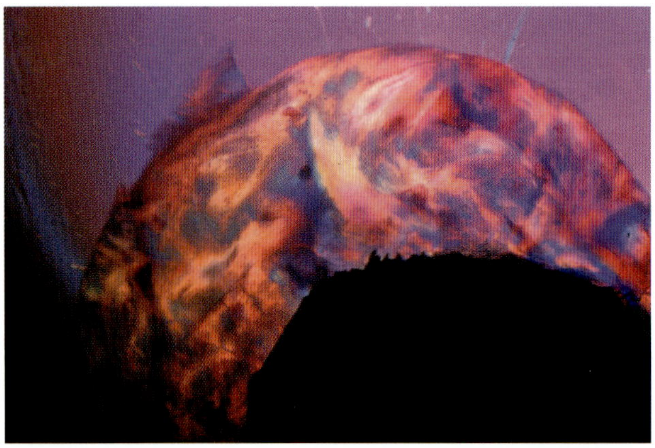

FIGURE 3-7. Demonstration of the concentric lamellae of the formed osteon and interstitial lamellae. (From Balkin BE, Stefik DE, Navel F: Mini dental implant insertion with the Auto-Advance Technique for ongoing applications. *J Oral Implantol* 27:32, 2001)

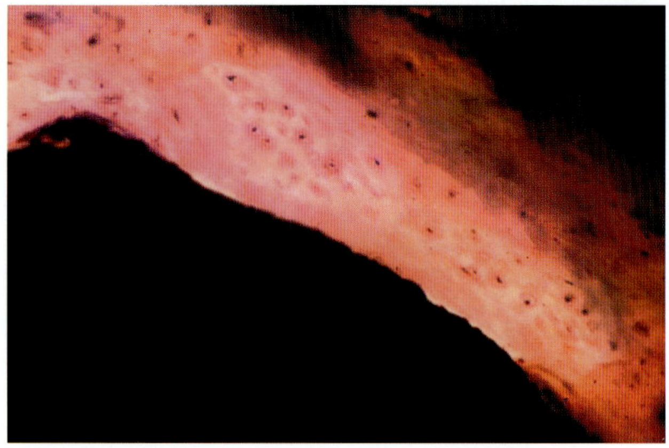

FIGURE 3-8. Osteocytes revealed within their lacunae. (From Balkin BE, Stefik DE, Navel F: Mini dental implant insertion with the Auto-Advance Technique for ongoing applications. *J Oral Implantol* 27:32, 2001)

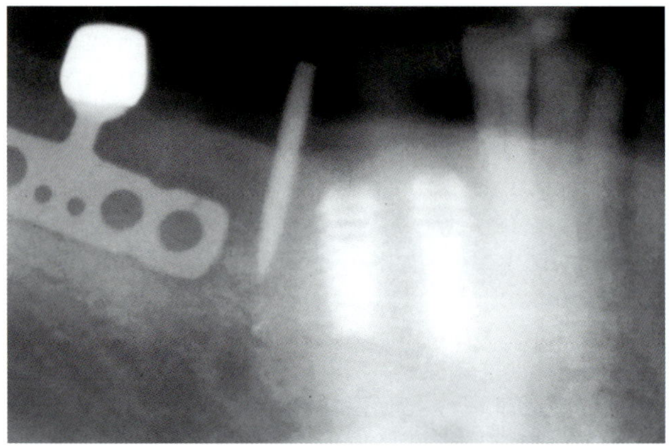

FIGURE 3-9. Mini implant inserted as transitional support during integration of cylindrical implants #27, #28.

Higher magnification (Figure 3-7) of the same area clearly shows the concentrical lamellae of the formed osteon and the interstitial lamellae. Such an image suggests the intimate association of the remodeled bone to the implant and the osseointegration of the implant. Higher magnification (Figure 3-8) shows osteocytes within their lacunae.

This remodeled bone is closely placed to the implant surface. Vascular elements within this remodeled bone are apparent (Figure 3-9), providing the nutritional requirements for the healthy-appearing remodeled bone interfacing this dental implant.[4]

2. Based upon the observations that mini dental implants may function better and longer than originally anticipated, in 2004 a pilot study examined the outcomes with digital subtraction radiography of human mini dental implants subjected to long-term fixed prosthetic function at least 3 years after their immediate loading after surgical placement.[6]

Methods and Materials (Subtraction Radiography)

Subjects and Dental Implants

In three systemically-healthy adults requiring multiple tooth replacement, a total of 14 mini titanium screw dental implants were surgically inserted with an auto-advance technique,[4] and then immediately loaded with fixed prosthetic bridges and followed for at least 3 years after treatment.

Digital Subtraction Radiographic Analysis

Conventional periapical radiographs were taken of each of the 14 mini dental implants at the time of surgical placement, and at least three years after treatment, providing 14 serial radiographic pairs for digital subtraction analysis. Changes in crestal alveolar bone mass between the serial radiographic pairs were assessed using a United States Federal Drug Administration (FDA) approved, computer-assisted, digital subtraction radiography program (DSRTM, Electro Medical Systems, Richardson, Tex.), which compensated for geometric projection and film contrast differences between the pairs of radiographic images before the subtraction. A board-certified oral and maxillofacial radiologist independently scored the computer-generated digital subtraction images at 27 proximal surfaces on the 14 mini dental implants as either exhibiting a gain (indicated by the appearance of a white color in the area of interest), no change (seen as a gray coloration), or a loss (black color) in crestal alveolar bone mass over the 3-year period subsequent to immediate fixed prosthetic loading and function on the mini dental implants.

Results (Subtraction Radiography)

None of the 14 mini implants were lost over the 3-year observation period. Of the 27 proximal implant surfaces examined with digital subtraction radiography, 8 (29.6%) mini implant surfaces exhibited a gain in crestal alveolar bone mass, 18 (66.7%) showed no change, and 1 (3.7%) surface revealed a loss in crestal alveolar bone mass. Representative digital subtraction images are presented in Figures 3-10 to 3-16.

Conclusions (subtraction radiography)

This pilot study demonstrates that human mini dental implants subjected to immediate fixed prosthetic loading and function for at least 3 years survived and exhibited a remarkably high degree of stability in crestal bone mass, as indicated by the occurrence of only one of 27 viewed proximal surfaces exhibiting a loss in crestal alveolar bone mass as seen with digital subtraction radiographic analysis.

Further research with larger patient sample sizes is indicated to additionally assess the capability of mini dental implants to successfully anchor fixed bridge restorations over extended periods after their surgical placement and immediate prosthetic loading.

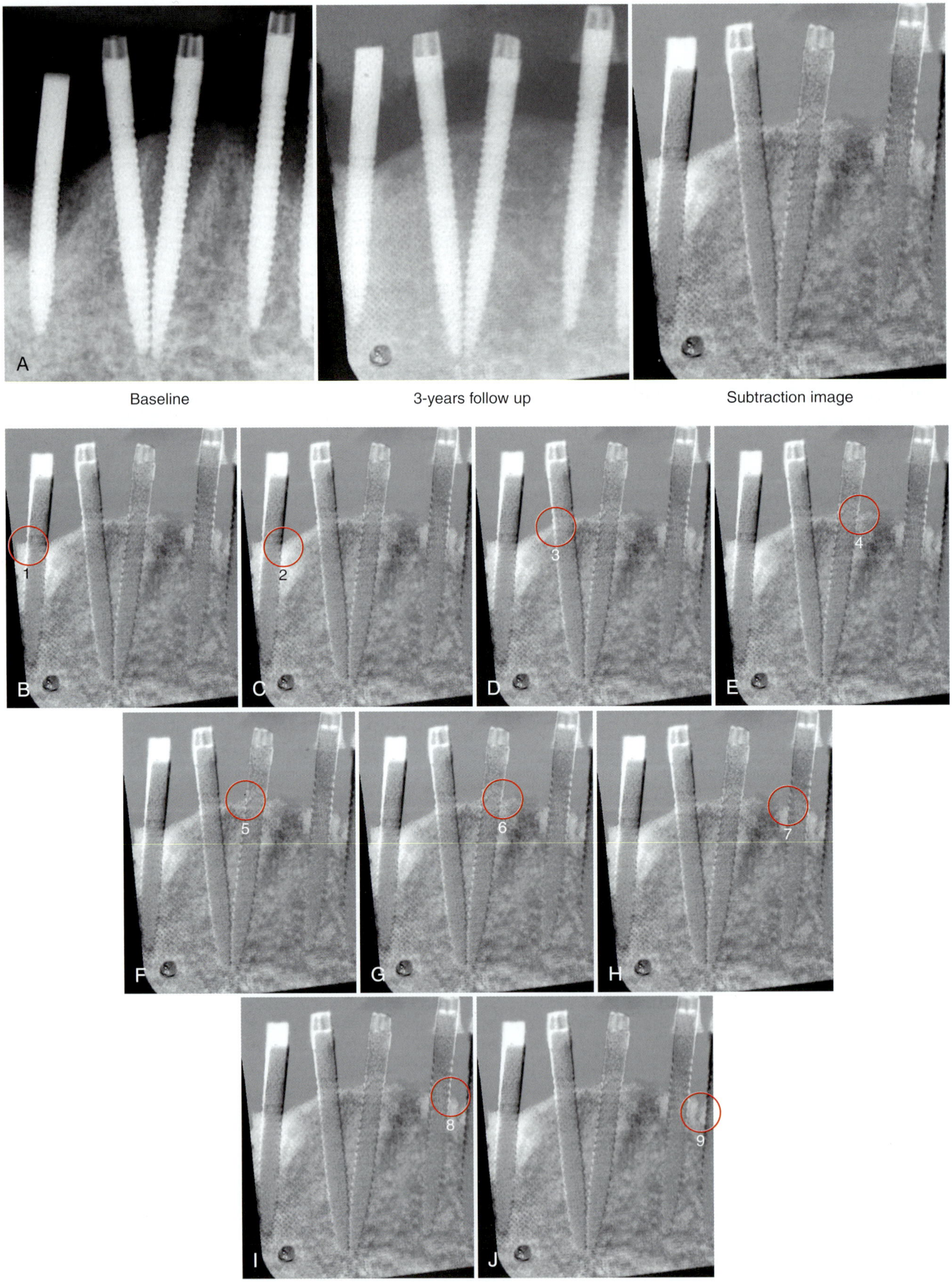

FIGURE 3-10. Subject D01, sites 24-26

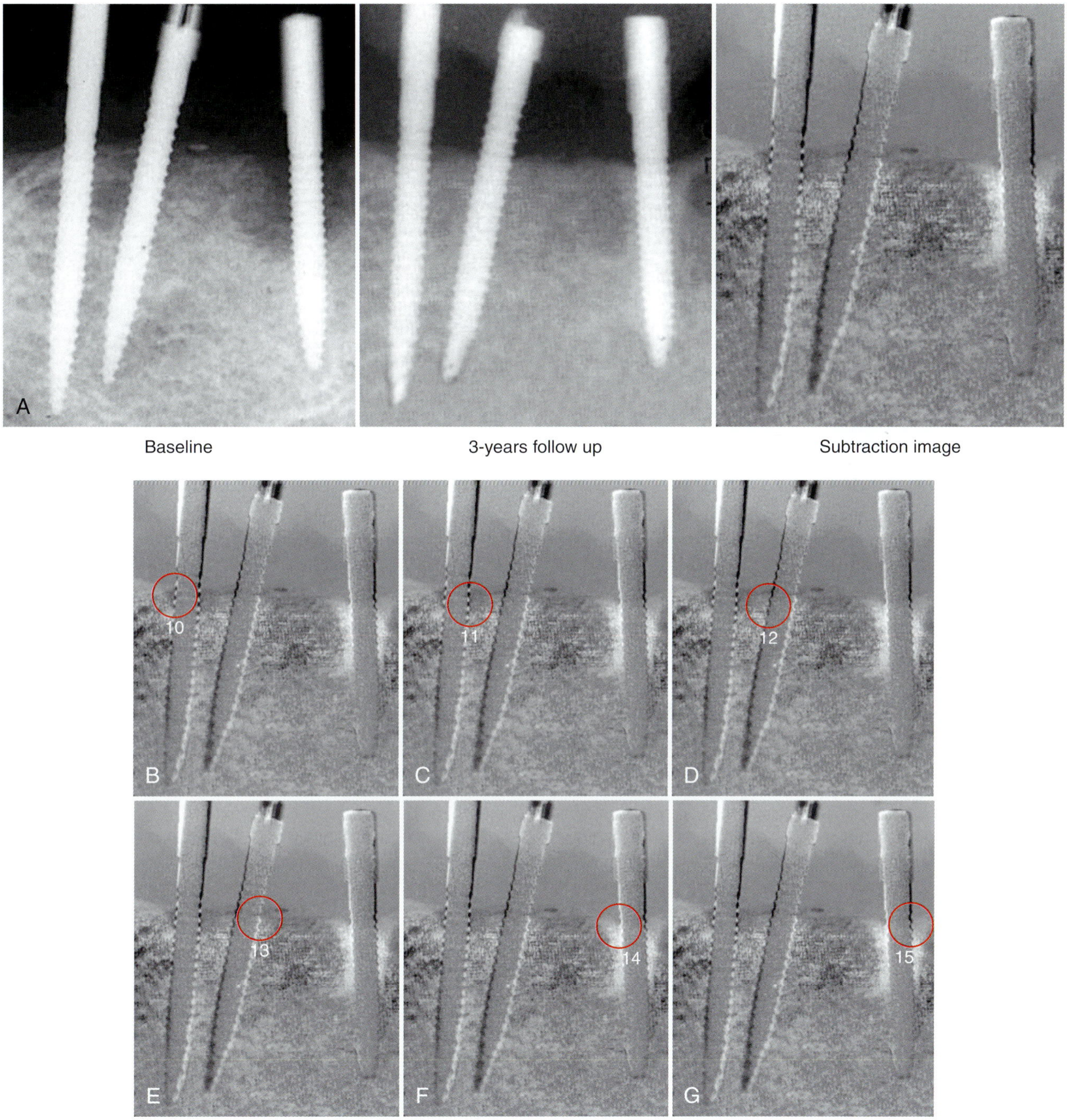

FIGURE 3-11. Subject D01, sites 27-30

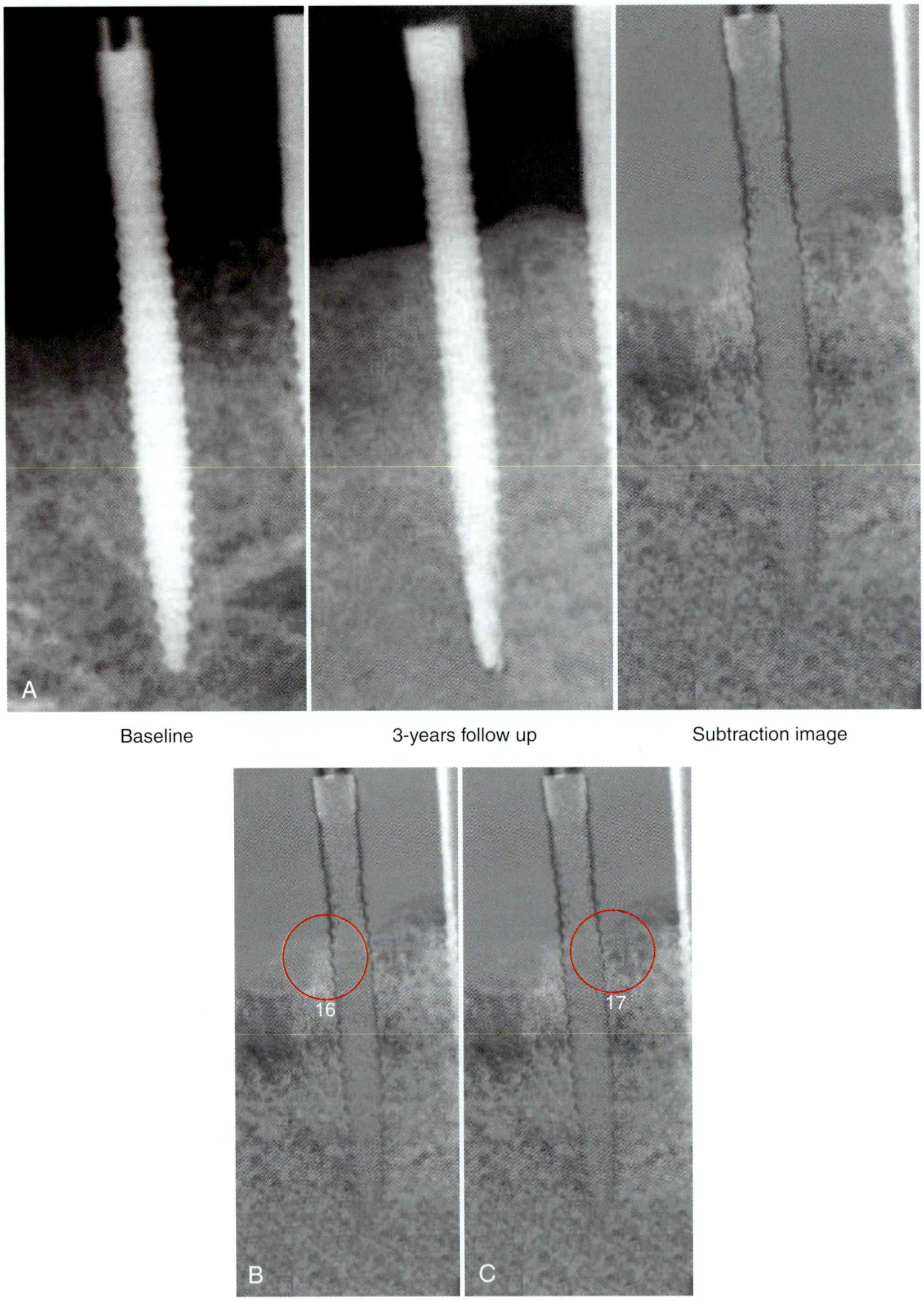

FIGURE 3-12. Subject D01, site 19

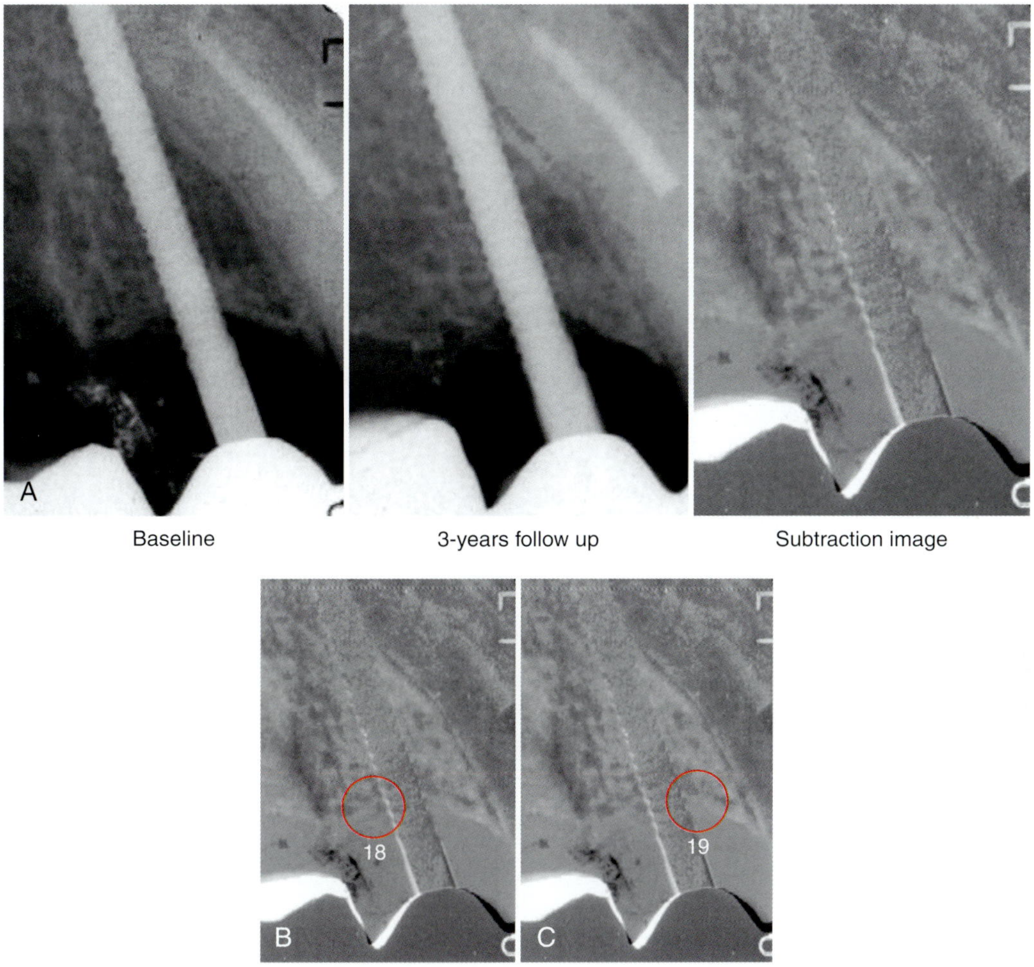

FIGURE 3-13. Subject D02, site 5

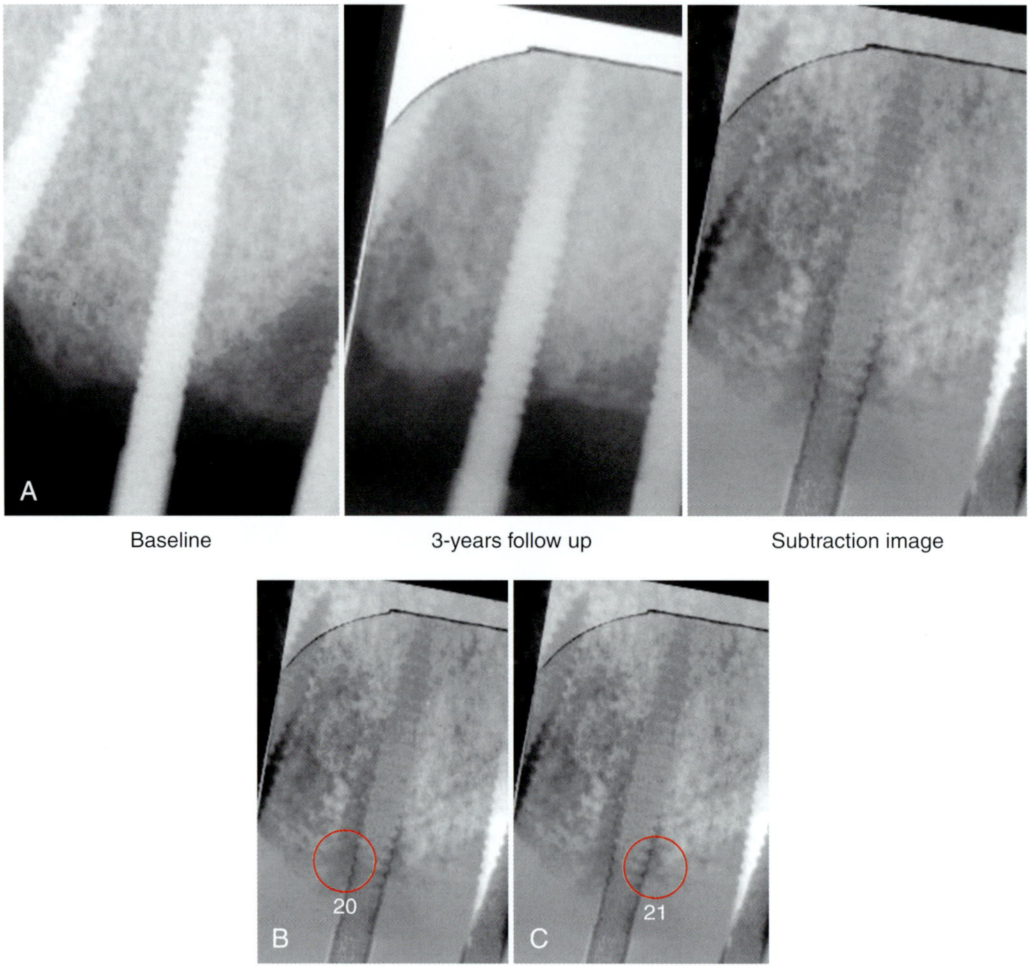

FIGURE 3-14. Subject D03, site 12

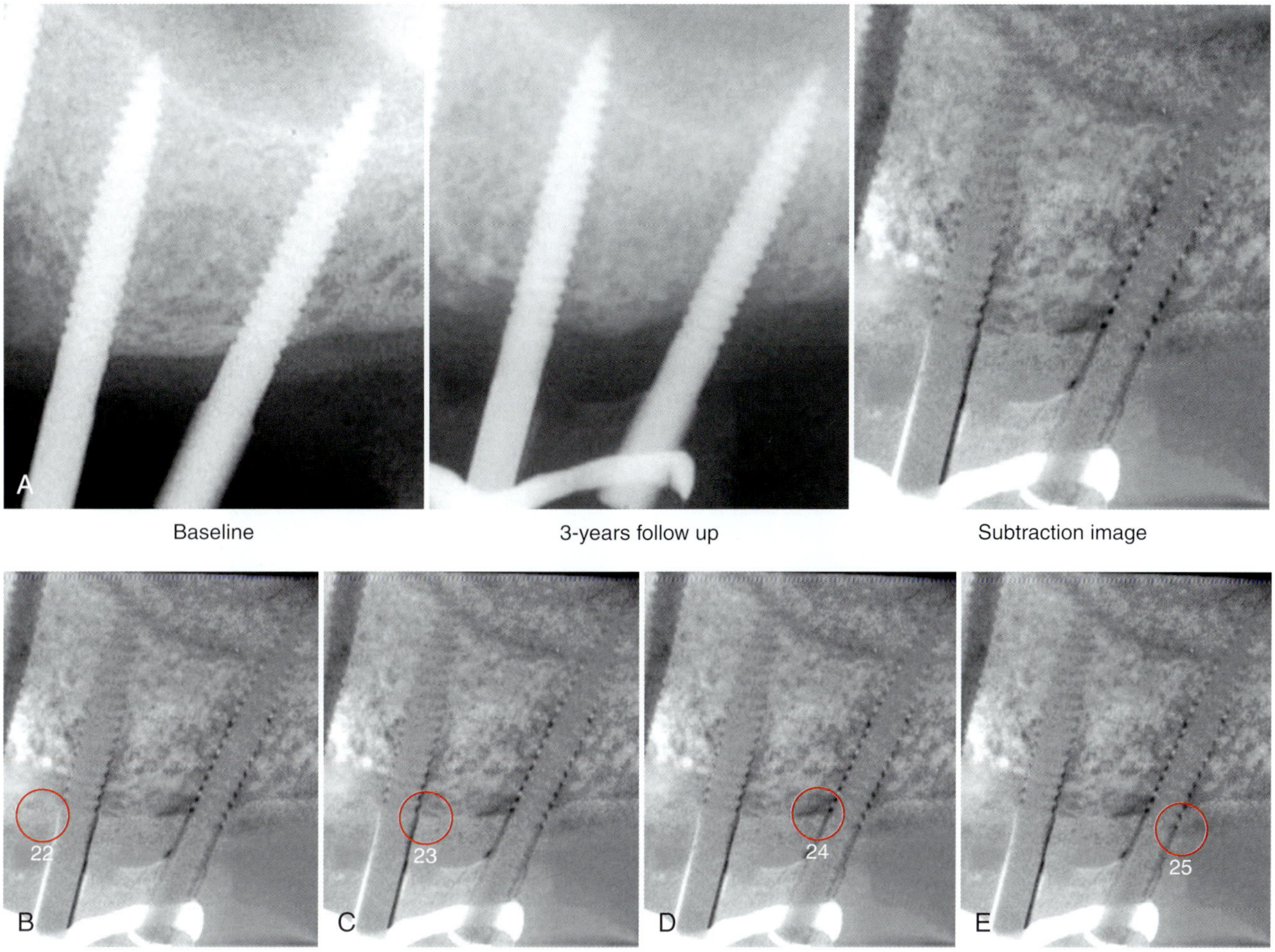

FIGURE 3-15. Subject D03, sites 14-15

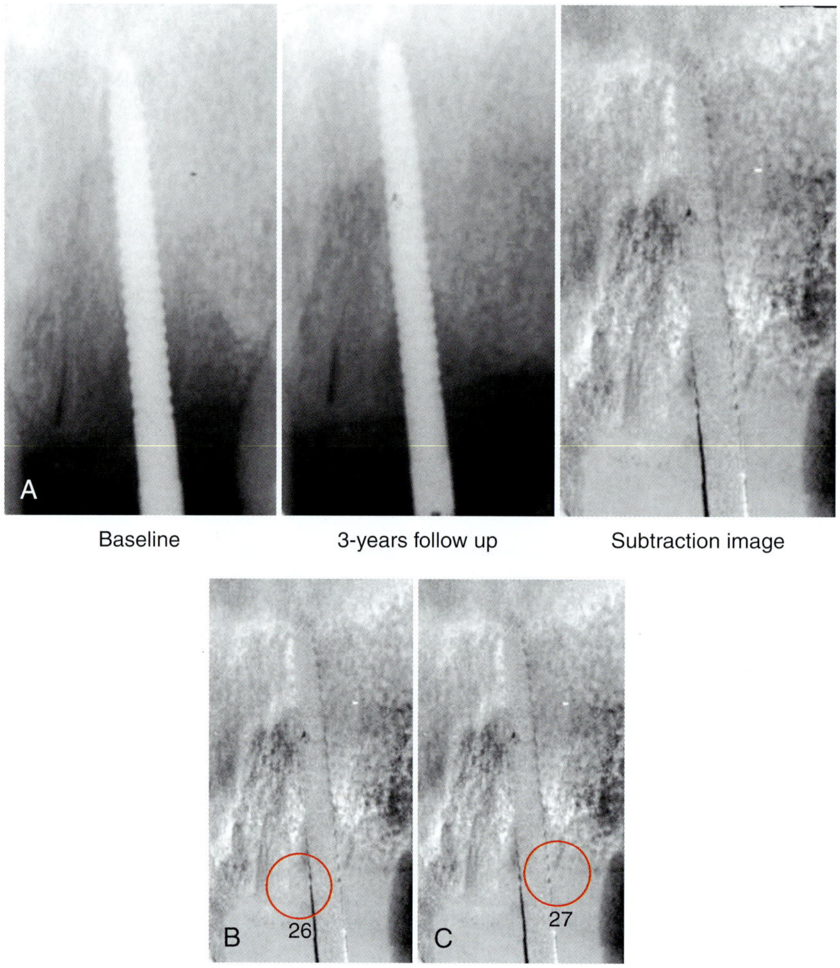

FIGURE 3-16. Subject D03, site 10

Early Clinical Applications

Initial use was for support/stabilization of fixed temporization (see Figure 3-9 and Figure 3-17). This was followed by support/stabilization of removable prosthesis (Figure 3-18). Uses in ongoing and long-term applications (Figures 3-19 to 3-21) followed as experience and information accrued.

Subsequent development by Bulard, Sendax, and Hadwin of the O-ball abutment allowed for O-ring attachment of a removable prosthesis to the mini implants, while also being partially tissue-supported (Figures 3-22 to 3-26).

Use of mini implants rather than traditional implants could be considered in cases of:

- Compromised health with minimal surgery and trauma,
- Minimal bone where grafting or bone regeneration is considered contraindicated,
- Desired immediate loading and function,
- Minimal financial resources.

Highlights include reduced chair time, simplified conventional restorations, and reduced cost to both patient and doctor.

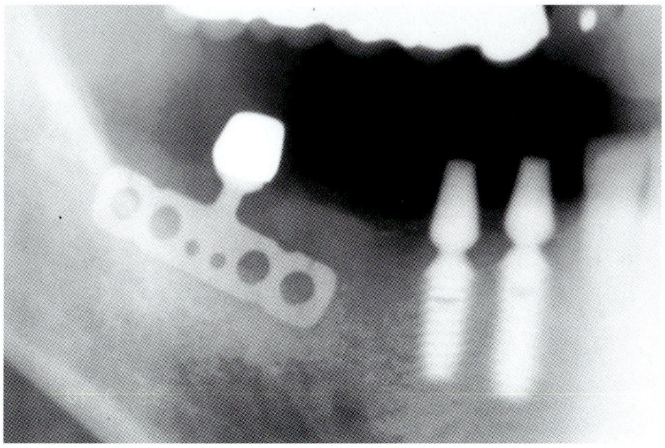

FIGURE 3-17. Transitional implant removed and abutments inserted.

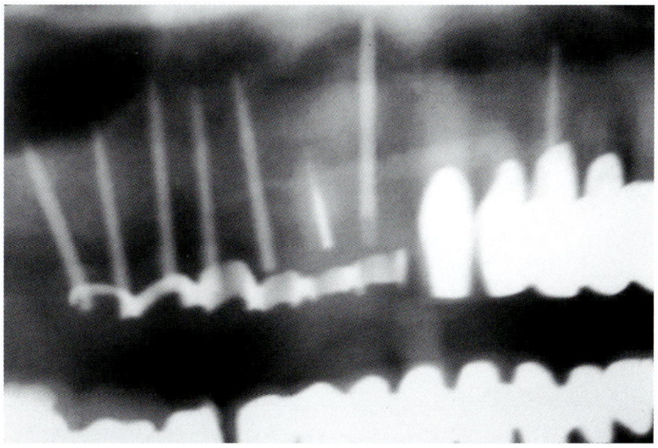

FIGURE 3-18. Implant supported ongoing fixed prosthesis of reinforced processed acrylic for an elderly patient with compromised health.

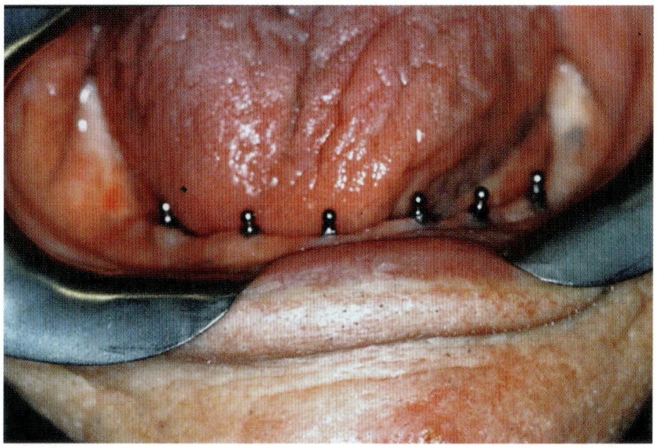

FIGURE 3-19. O-ball mini implants for mandibular overdenture.

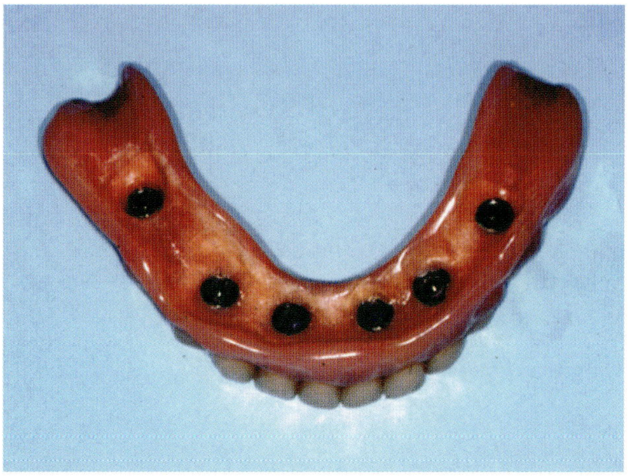

FIGURE 3-20. O-ring retention for mandibular overdenture.

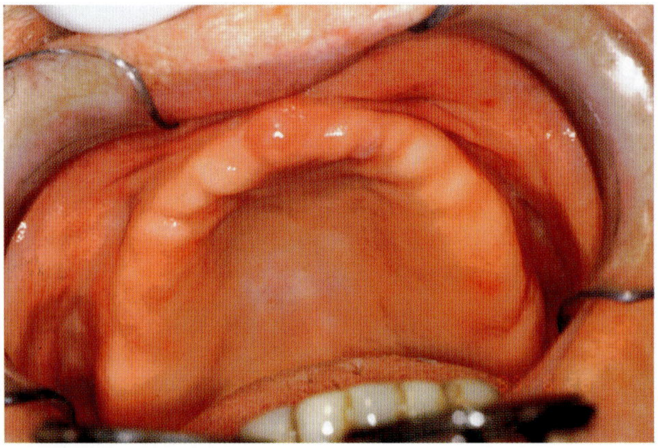

FIGURE 3-21. Edentulous maxilla, before operation.

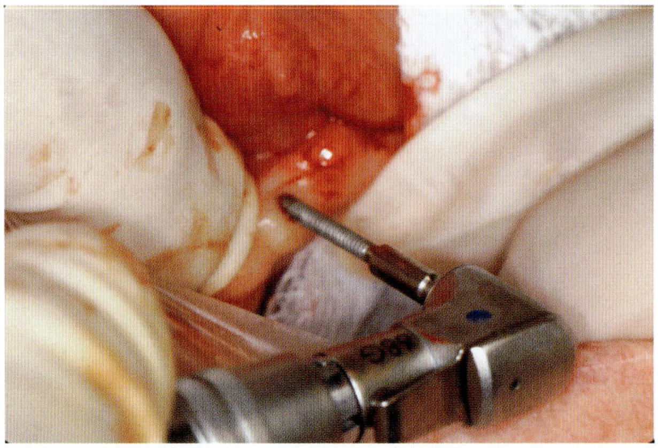

FIGURE 3-22. Insertion of mini implant with machine driver.

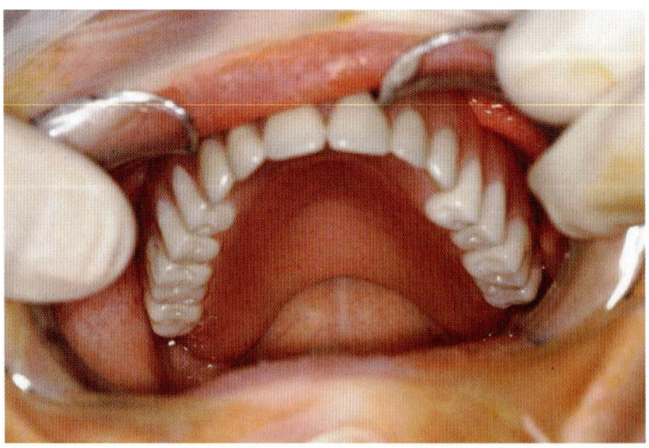

FIGURE 3-23. Maxillary implant overdenture.

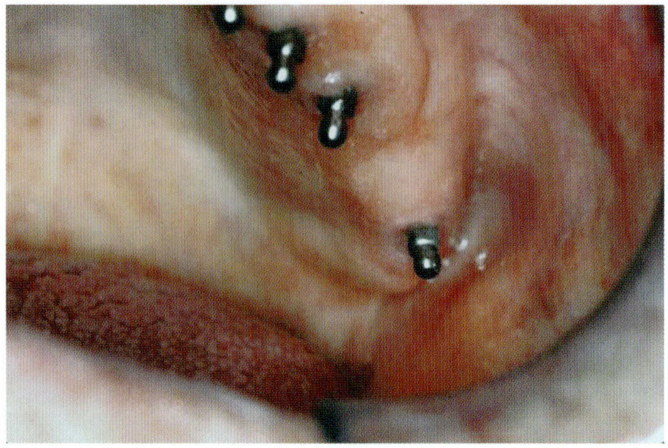

FIGURE 3-24. Maxillary implants for overdenture without palate and with O-ball abutment heads for O-ring retainers.

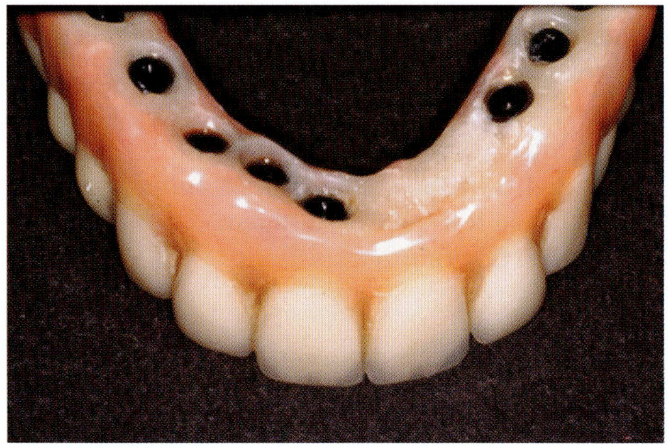

FIGURE 3-25. Maxillary overdenture without palate with multiple O-ring retainers.

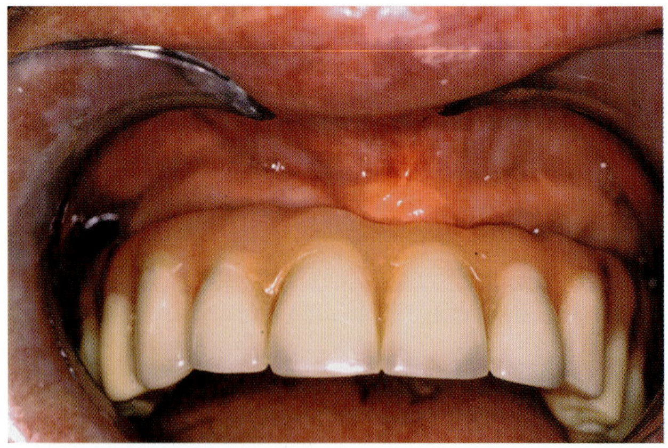

FIGURE 3-26. Postoperative with prosthesis insertion.

Conclusion

Early findings of case reports, including histology and subtraction radiography, suggest the successful utilization of an auto-advancing threaded implant of titanium 6Al 4V alloy[5] with adequate strength to penetrate the bone without a fully prepared receptor site while at the same time using a minimum diameter to avoid fracture of surrounding bone.

Such a construct with auto advance insertion may also diminish implant fractures and provide a stable mini dental implant which when placed in adequate numbers for stress distribution and with immediate loading in mature bone may indeed provide interim transitional support, ongoing applications, and ultimately long-term use.

Histology demonstrates healthy integrated bone in the areas of concern immediately surrounding the mini dental implants 4 to 5 months postoperatively. Subtraction radiography of cases with mini dental implants in immediate function demonstrates bone integration around the implants, including regeneration of previous intraosseous and soft tissue defects after a 3 year elapsed time period.

This information, plus markedly expanded use of mini dental implants in the years since the early review was completed, indicates that the potential use of mini dental implants, using the auto-advance technique protocol, can provide immediate loading with integration for transitional use, ongoing applications, and long-term use. Further comparison studies with other implant designs and techniques in similar circumstances are indicated and to be encouraged.

Thus mini dental implants have demonstrated an additional venue in dental implant treatment within the context of adequate knowledge, skill, and experience.

References

1. Balkin BE: Implant dentistry: historical overview with current perspective, *J Dent Educ* 52:683, 1988. (NIH Consensus Development Conference on Oral Implants).
2. Adell R, Lekholm U, Rockler B, Brånemark PI: A 15-year study of osseointegrated implants in the treatment of the edentulous jaw, *Int J Oral Surg* 10:387, 1981.
3. Brånemark PI: Osseointegration and its experimental background, *J Prosthet Dent* 50:399, 1983.
4. Balkin BE, Steflik DE, Navel F: Mini-dental implant insertion with the auto-advance technique for ongoing applications, *J Oral Implantol* 27:32, 2001.
5. McCracken M: Dental implant materials: commercially pure titanium and titanium alloys, *J Prosthodont* 8:40, 1999.
6. Balkin BE, Diaz JH, Yang J, Rams TE: Mini dental implants in human long-term fixed prosthetic function, *J Dent Res* 84(Special Issue A):2081, 2005. [Abstract].

Chapter 4

Biomedical-Engineering Analyses of Mini Dental Implants

JOHN B. BRUNSKI JACK E. LEMONS

Outline

Biomechanical Perspectives Relevant to the Use of Mini Implants: John B. Brunski

The last two decades have seen increasing interest in biomechanical principles for treatment planning with dental implants. Although these principles can assist in a satisfactory treatment outcome, they are obviously only one part of any comprehensive treatment. Eventually a key aim is to have a well-tested, proven architectural and structural "building code" for treatment with oral implants.

As will be clear to anyone reading recent journals on dental implants, the implant field is highly dynamic, with many new implant systems being developed and used along with many different loading protocols for implants (e.g., single-tooth versus full-arch restorations; delayed versus immediate loading). Although we do have the beginnings of a biomechanical basis for predicting how loads are supported by dental implants and how these loads create stresses and strains to the surrounding bone, none of these load-prediction methods has been thoroughly tested and verified against actual in vivo data from patients, nor do we yet have a deep understanding of exactly what stress and strain states should be avoided—or perhaps even promoted—in bone around an implant. Hence, considerably more needs to be done to better understand implant biomechanics and the full implications of implant loading in relation to bone biology at the bone-implant interface. That said, progress has been made.

The use of mini implants has been evolving in this biomechanical context. This chapter outlines some biomechanical ideas pertaining to all oral and maxillofacial implants, including mini implants. Unfortunately, in-depth discussion of important topics such as load-sharing among multiple implants supporting bridgework, stress and strain, material failure, stress transfer at the bone-implant interface, and interrelationships between bone biology and mechanical loading, etc., are beyond the scope of this introductory chapter; recent publications can be consulted if a reader wants more detailed information about these and other topics.[1-3] Useful topics to help understand the performance and potential of mini implants include the following:

- A review of osseointegration;
- A primer on implant loading by forces and moments;
- Predicting implant loading during case planning;
- An introduction to safe versus dangerous loading, which depends upon:
  - An implant's initial stability in bone;
  - Size, shape, material, and surface texture of the implant;
  - Nature of the bony site (e.g., dense cortex or porous cancellous bone);
  - How the implant is splinted to other teeth or other implants.

Review of Osseointegration

There is an implicit biomechanical meaning of the term *osseointegration*. Brånemark and Skalak[4] originally noted that an oral implant may be called osseointegrated if "it provides a stable and apparently immobile support of a prosthesis under functional loads without pain, inflammation, or loosening." Going farther, a second definition suggested that an implant may be termed osseointegrated if "there is no progressive relative motion between the implant and surrounding living bone and marrow under functional levels and types of loading for the entire life of the patient." Third, from a microscopic, biophysical point of view:

> … osseointegration implies that, at the light microscopic and electronmicroscopic levels, the identifiable components of tissue within a thin zone of an [implant] surface are identified as normal bone and marrow constituents that continuously grade into normal bone structure surrounding the fixture [implant]. This implies that mineralized tissue is found to be in contact with the [implant] over most of the surface within nanometers [1 nm = 10^{-9} m] so that no functionally significant intervening material exists at the interface.[4]

A point that is often missed in these definitions—especially when considering the third one alone—is that the histological finding of bone-implant apposition at an interface does not necessarily mean that there is "osseointegration"; recall that the full meaning of osseointegration includes the idea of having "stable and apparently immobile support of a prosthesis under functional loads without pain, inflammation, or loosening" as well as "no progressive relative motion between the implant and surrounding living bone and marrow under functional levels and types of loading for the entire life of the patient." In other words, there is an important functional connotation to the term osseointegration.

Beyond these attempts at definitions, the literature has established that the osseointegration approach has allowed highly predictable, long-term functional clinical performance of implant-supported prostheses in both fully and partially edentulous patients. However, it cannot be over-emphasized that this statement applies mainly to the use of commercial purity titanium screw-shaped implants of a typical size of roughly 3.75 mm diameter × 7-18 mm in length and mainly refers to clinical studies with implants used in the so-called *delayed loading protocol*, where the implants are not built into full function until about 4 to 6 months after surgical implantation. On the other hand, there is accumulating—but not always conclusive—evidence of comparable performance in immediate (as opposed to delayed) loading.[5]

Another key point is that the literature also provides some general rules about biomechanical problems in osseointegration, which will also extend to the use of any new sort of implant, including mini implants.

First, it is well known that bone healing can be disturbed if the clinical conditions of implant use permit excessive *relative motion* (also called *micromotion*) at the bone-implant interface during the early healing period. A more detailed discussion of relative motion appears elsewhere.[1,6-9] But the basic idea is that micromotion occurs when an implant has excessive instability, if it is not fixed firmly enough within the surgical site, therefore allowing relative motion of the implant with respect to the bony site when the implant is either directly or indirectly loaded. Observations show that a consequence of such early, postoperative implant instability in the wounded surgical site is that the interface does not heal via bone regeneration but instead attempts to repair itself with nonmineralized fibrous tissue encapsulation—the latter being an undesirable result because such fibrous tissue is not as predictable as osseointegration for implant function in the long term. Interestingly, evidence exists that formation of fibrous tissue in cases of micromotion is largely independent of the biomaterial used for the implant,[10] but otherwise a full understanding is still lacking about the exact type and amount of micromotion that leads to such nonosseous tissue formation and the cell and molecular mechanisms underlying such tissue formation. Currently the focus of much research, micromotion is especially pertinent to the increased interest in immediate loading of implants, which carries the risk for implant micromotion.

The second biomechanical problem that can occur with any implant is that a successfully healed-in and functioning implant can still be lost if the implant is subsequently "overloaded." That is, it has been observed[11-14] that if there are excessively large forces and/or moments on the implant, there can be a progressive loss of interfacial bone-implant contact, which can worsen in a period of weeks to months if the excessive loading conditions continue unabated; eventually the implant and/or interfacial bone fails, and the implant can no longer function as a fixed support for a prosthesis. As with relative motion, the cellular and molecular details underlying failure by overload have yet to be fully determined, although strain levels in the bone and the bone remodeling cycle are likely candidates.[3]

In any case, both of these biomechanical failure modes are pertinent in any clinician's understanding of how to treat patients appropriately with implants of any type. The obvious questions from this analysis are how to predict loadings on implants and how to tell which loadings are safe versus dangerous.

A Primer on Forces and Moments

A common clinical question about, say, a full-arch restoration is determining how many implants to install and how they should be spaced and oriented around the jaw to produce the best results. Although current knowledge makes it difficult to solve this problem conclusively for all the various implants on the market, the problem can be boiled down to the three basic questions:

- First, what are the forces and moments on the prosthesis and supporting implants?
- Second, during early case planning (or after the prosthesis is inserted on existing implants), how can we predict the load distribution across the one or more implants that support the prosthesis? What factors influence the load distribution among the implants?
- Third, what are safe versus dangerous loads on implants and surrounding bone?

Answers to these questions can help prevent failure of any part of the implant case, including the prosthesis, supporting implants, and supporting biologic tissues. In the next several sections we consider the nature of implant loading and how to predict it when several implants are involved. Then in the last section we make observations about safe versus dangerous loading.

Forces and Moments on Implants

The purpose of any oral or craniofacial implant is to act as a *fixed support*—much like a common household nail or screw driven into a piece of wood acts as a fixed support for hanging a picture on the wall. A fixed support *is anchored* in such a way that it can resist forces and twisting actions (moments) applied to it in all directions. Moreover, the implant should be anchored strongly enough in bone so that neither the implant nor the surrounding interfacial bone fails under the expected loadings. So, what are the expected loadings?

Forces

The masticatory muscles act to move the jaws during mastication, which allows the teeth to produce forces to crush food into particles. Defined loosely as a push or a pull, a force is measured in the units of pounds (lb, in the U.S. Customary System of Units) or Newtons (N, in the *Système International d'Unités* or SI system), with 1 lb converting to 4.448 N. Force is a *vector* quantity, meaning that its definition includes both magnitude and direction. For example, a 10-lb force acting downward on a tooth or implant does not have the same effect as a 10-lb force acting sideways. The intuitive idea that chewing forces always act parallel to the long axes of teeth and implants is an oversimplification; although it is often true that the largest component of a force is the vertical component, the vertical component is not necessarily the only component; it depends also on the facets and inclines on the surface of the crown or prosthesis.

Moments (Torques)

Another essential concept is the idea of a moment or torque. A moment or torque is a loading action that tends to rotate a body. Most commonly, moments on a body such as an implant or a tooth are produced by the actions of forces. So why is the concept of moments needed in the first place? The explanation is that moments are inherent in the definition of equilibrium of a rigid body; that is, for static equilibrium of a rigid body, the sum of forces must be zero *along with the sum of the moments about any point.* So moments are inherent in defining equilibrium. The dimensions of a moment are force multiplied by distance; hence, typical units are N·m or N·cm in the SI system, and lb·ft or oz·in in the U.S. Customary System. Examples of moments arise in the use of an ordinary screw driver, where a hand supplies a pair of equal and opposite forces (called a *couple* or *couple-moment*) to the screwdriver handle, which tends to turn the screwdriver; there is also usually a small axial "pushing" force that is usually directed along the axis of the screwdriver. Just focusing on the torquing action on the screwdriver's handle, that couple or couple-moment is a good example of a *moment*, or *torque*, around the axis of the screwdriver. A similar situation arises when one uses a torque wrench with a handle, where the torque around the axis of the screw or nut that is being turned is created by a force on the handle multiplied by the perpendicular distance from the line of action of the force to the axis of the screw. In a more clinically relevant example of a moment, a lateral force of, 10 N acting 7 mm above the level of a conventional Brånemark-style screw joint abutment would produce a moment of 70 N·mm, or 70 N·cm, at the base of the abutment. To illustrate the significance of this magnitude of a moment, a traditional Brånemark system abutment plus gold cylinder and gold screw tends to undergo opening at about 50 N·cm, so the 70 N·cm is actually large enough to cause a problem.[15] Although in mechanics a moment is a vector quantity, it serves our purposes to simply speak of the moment around a point as being a scalar magnitude equal to the force times the perpendicular distance between the point and the force's line of action.

Biting Forces In Vivo

Normal human patients without dental implants or dentures, and with opposing natural teeth in health, can typically exert axial components of biting force in the range of 100 to 2400 N, which is 27 to 550 lbs in English units (Table 4-1). However, exact bite force values depend on location in the mouth, nature of the food, chewing versus swallowing, degree of exertion by the patient, presence or absence of parafunctional habits of the patient, etc. The term *axial* refers to the force component acting parallel to the long axis of a natural tooth or implant. Axial force components on natural teeth tend to be larger at more distal locations in the mouth, which is explained by idealizing the mandible as a class 3 lever, in which all forces (i.e., those due to biting, joint reaction force at the temporomandibular joint [TMJ], and jaw muscle forces) are assumed to act in the sagittal plane.

Typical magnitudes of axial forces on natural teeth during mastication (see Table 4-1) should be regarded only as rough estimates for the typical magnitudes of axial forces on natural teeth in humans. One limitation of these data is that the experimental methods by which they were obtained can sometimes change the details of chewing so that the resulting data do not necessarily pertain to natural chewing events. Accordingly, the data in Table 4-1 represent what might best be termed as *closure forces* (i.e., forces exerted on an object when the patient closes the teeth on the object); these data at least provide some "ball-park" estimates of the magnitudes of expected axially-directed biting forces in vivo.

Data on the lateral force components in the natural or restored human dentition are scarce (see Table 4-1). One study reported that typical lateral components were approximately 20 N for the special case of a prosthesis in the first mandibular molar region. This value is relatively small compared with typical axial force components as detailed in Table 4-1. Because axial forces during biting can also end up

TABLE 4-1

Bite Forces and Related Data

Description of Data	Typical Values	Reference
Vertical component of biting force in adults, averaged over several teeth	200-2440 N	Craig[39]
Vertical component of biting force in adults, molar region	390-880 N	Craig[39]
Vertical component of biting force in adults, premolar region	453 N	Craig[39]
Vertical component of biting force in adults, incisor region	222 N	Craig[39]
Vertical component of biting force in adults wearing complete dentures	77-196 N	Meng and Rugh[40], Ralph[41], Colaizzi et al.[42], Haraldsson et al.[43]
Vertical component of biting force in adults with a maxillary denture opposed by natural teeth in mandible	147-284 N	Meng and Rugh[40]
Vertical component of biting force in adults with dentures supported by implants (patients asked to exert max force)	42-412 N (median 143 N)	Carlsson and Haraldsson[44]
Vertical component of biting force in adults with dentures supported by overdenture attachments	337-342 N	Meng and Rugh[40]
Lateral components of bite forces in adults	~ 20 N	Graf[45]
Frequency of chewing strokes	60-80 strokes/min	Harrison and Lewis[46]
Rate of chewing	1-2 strokes/sec	Ahlgren[47], Graf[45]
Duration of tooth contact in one chewing cycle	0.23-0.3 sec	Graf[45]
Total time of tooth contact in a 24-hr period	9-17.5 min	Graf[45]
Maximum closure speed of jaws during chewing	140 mm/sec	Harrison and Lewis[46]
Maximum contact stresses on teeth	20 MPa	Carlsson[48]

acting on the curved occlusal surfaces of teeth or crowns over implants, it is possible that the lateral component of such a force could end up being on the order of 100s of N; therefore for design purposes with implants, it could be prudent to assume that lateral forces on teeth and implants could sometimes be as large as this.

Common experience shows that biting is a dynamic (time-varying) process rather than a static event. Table 4-1 shows that the maximum closure speed of the mandible relative to the maxilla is estimated at about 140 mm/sec. While this speed appears to be moderately fast, nevertheless, a working assumption of most mechanical analyses of implants is that dynamics and related inertial effects are not significant at such closing speeds and do not appreciably affect biting loads. This means that analyses based on statics alone appear to be sufficient for most design purposes.

The net "chewing time per meal" has been found to be about 450 sec (see Table 4-1), so if the chewing frequency is about 1 Hz with a 0.3-sec duration of tooth contact during each chewing stroke, chewing forces will act on teeth approximately 9 min per day. If other activities such as swallowing are considered, the time might increase to about 17.5 min per day. Obviously, these are estimates only. Parafunctional habits such as bruxism could significantly increase this time.

Values of Moments In Vivo

Moments develop on implants largely from the action of forces, as noted earlier. As with forces, there are components of the moment vector, for instance, components about the occlusoapical, buccolingual, and mesiodistal axes in the mouth. Unfortunately, few studies have determined typical values of moments applied in vivo to implants in various sorts of clinical situations. From direct measurements by several groups working with human subjects having implants[16-20] and from simulations with finite element models,[21,22] it is known that typical values of the buccolingual and mesiodistal bending moments can be in the range of 0 to 40 N·cm, with maximal values estimated in computer models as large as 70 N·cm. Values for the moment component about the long axis of an implant are of the order of 10 N·cm. So far, these data at least serve as a guide to the expected moments on implants in various situations in the mouth.

Predicting Forces and Moments on Dental Implants

A First Example

Given information on the biting forces, the problem then becomes to estimate the loadings on multiple supporting abutments (natural teeth or implants). The methods here are not very dependent on the exact type of implant being used. In general, for a multiple implant case, the force on an abutment will not be the same as the bite force exerted on the prosthesis. A quick way to see that this is true comes from the following example. Suppose a downward force *P* acts at the end of an implant prosthesis with a cantilever section (Figure 4-1). The distance between the line of action of *P* and the nearest implant (#2 in the diagram) is *a*, the length of the cantilever portion of the prosthesis. The bridge is assumed to be a rigid (undeformable) body supported by two implants (#1 and #2) that are spaced *b* apart. The problem is to predict the forces on implants #1 and #2.

The simplest solution to this problem is to use a model involving rigid-body static equilibrium in two dimensions (2D). The analysis starts with a *free body diagram* of the prosthesis, which is drawn in Figure 4-1 as a simple beam at the top right of the figure. This beam is isolated (removed from the implants), and all forces acting on the beam are shown. (The beam is assumed to have no appreciable weight.) Forces F_1 and F_2 represent the forces that the implants exert on the beam. The true directions of the forces do not have to be known at this stage of the analysis; the correct directions will emerge from the solution. (However, in this example the forces are drawn in the actual directions in which they act.) The assumption that only forces—and no moments—exist at the prosthesis-implant connection(s) comes from the idealization that the implants are connected to the prosthesis by pin-joints in this 2D model; pin-joints transmit only force components and not moments. (In the 3D analog of this example, a ball and socket joint would be the comparable connection.) Force *P* is the biting force. The next step is to recognize that the beam is in static equilibrium, which means, according to Newton's Laws, that the sum of the forces and the sum of the moments on the beam are each equal to zero. The application of equilibrium allows us to solve for the two unknown forces F_1 and F_2, which is done by solving the two equations of static equilibrium (note sign conventions according to the coordinate system in Figure 4-1):

$$\begin{aligned} \sum F_y &= 0: -F_1 + F_2 - P = 0 \\ \sum M_Q &= 0: +F_1 b - aP = 0 \end{aligned} \qquad (1)$$

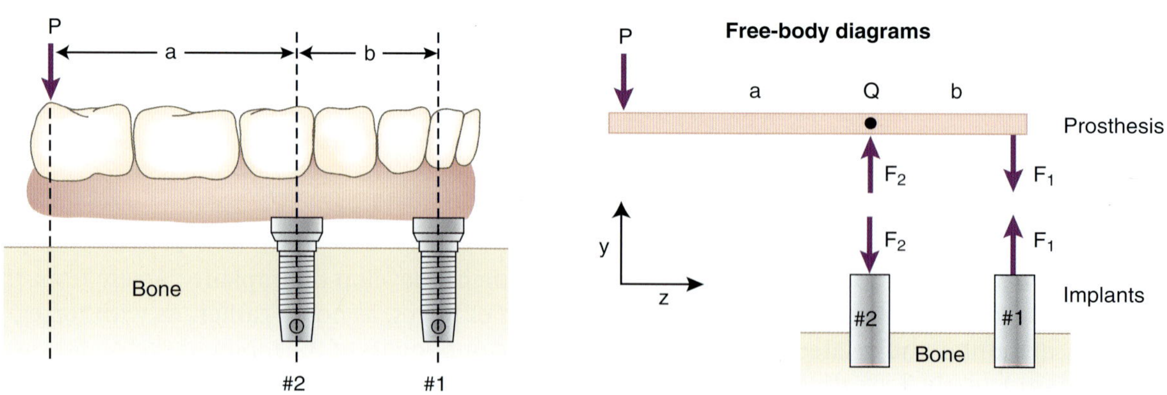

FIGURE 4-1. A method for predicting the forces on two fixtures supporting a cantilever portion of a prosthesis. At left is a diagrammatic view of the situation in 2D; at the right are free body diagrams of the prosthesis *(top)* and the implants *(bottom)*.

The notation ΣF_y means "summation of forces in the y-direction", while ΣM_Q means "summation of moments around point Q." (Point Q is not unique; any point could have been chosen with the same final result.) The solution of these two equations in two unknowns is

$$F_2 = (1 + a/b)P \text{ and } F_1 = (a/b)P \qquad (2)$$

The above analysis has several important messages. First, it shows that although the bridge is loaded by a biting force of magnitude *P*, *the implants are loaded by forces for which the magnitudes can be larger than* P, *depending on the ratio a/b*. For example, if a/b = 2—which is not an uncommon value in clinical practice—the forces on the implants will be 3P and 2P. Second, the analysis shows that the forces F_1 and F_2 do not act in the same direction; implant #2, nearest to the point at which *P* acts, experiences a compressive load (tending to push it into the bone), while implant #1 experiences a tensile load (tending to pull it out of the bone). So the key result from this introductory analysis is that the forces on the implants can sometimes exceed the value of the biting force on the prosthesis.

A numerical example helps drive home the point: If we have a moderately low biting force *P* of 250 N, and an a/b ratio of 2, then the tensile force on implant #1 will be 2P = 2 × 250 N = 500 N, whereas the compressive force on implant #2 is 3P = 3 × 250 N = 750 N. As a quick indication of the clinical significance of such force levels on dental implants, it is known that implant loadings of 250 to 500 N can exceed the absolute failure strength of many implants that have been tested in various animal models. Two examples of this are Block and Kent[23] measured maximal pull-out strengths of about 150 N for hydroxyapatite (HA)-coated cylindrical implants that had healed in dog mandibles for 32 weeks, and Burgess et al.[24] measured mean pullout forces of about 200 N to 350 N at 3 weeks and 15 weeks, respectively, after implanting cylindrical HA-coated implants in dog bone. Although many factors influence the strength of the bone-implant interface, including healing time, cancellous versus cortical bone site, and size and shape of the implant,[1] unfortunately, for human cases the implant field does not yet have an extensive database of strengths of bone-implant interfaces for various implants in different types of bone quality and quantity, etc. However, exactly this sort of database is part of what is needed to establish safe versus dangerous applied force levels on implants.

More Complicated Examples

As noted above, the two-implant case is obviously only one of many ways that implants can be used. In general, there is a need to be able to compute the expected forces and moments on more than two implants supporting a loaded prosthesis of arbitrary shape, size, and material (e.g., regular size implants or mini implants). A number of factors can arise in trying to solve this more general problem, including:

- A full or partial prosthesis; number and location of implant (and/or natural tooth) abutments; angulations of the implants; nature of the bridge-abutment connection; use of overdentures supported by a mixture of soft tissue and implants, etc.
- The mechanical properties of the material(s) and structure of the bridge or prosthesis, implants, and bone (e.g., elastic moduli, structural stiffnesses); deformability of the mandible or maxilla; misfit of the prosthesis relative to the supporting implants.

There is now a large literature on these factors, and only a limited discussion is supplied here with a few examples to illustrate how the models work. Generally, models for predicting implant loading fall into two categories. The first category includes analytical models—those that provide explicit equations allowing calculation of implant loading via pencil and paper, pocket calculator, or personal computer. A good example of this sort of model is the Skalak model from the early 1980s.[25] The second category of model consists of more complicated computer models such as finite element (FE) models, some of which now can run on ordinary personal computers. Ideally, such FE models should only be used by operators with a reasonably advanced understanding of solid mechanics and stress analysis.

Whatever the model, the most important point is that both analytical and computer models are indeed *models*, or *idealizations*, of reality and must be used with a full understanding that some models may come closer to reality than others. Whether one analysis method is "better" than another does not depend on the inherent complexity of the model as much as it depends on the goals of the analysis and the assumptions that go into the model. In general, the best advice is that a clinician must understand the underlying assumptions and methods of a particular model in relation to reality. Also, to gain confidence in a model, it is essential to check how the model's predictions stack up against reality.

The 1983 Skalak Model for Cases Involving Three or More Implants

In the language of mechanics, the problem of predicting loads on *all* implant abutments in a multiple implant distribution is a statically indeterminate problem; the abutment loadings can be obtained using the theory of rigid body statics together with some assumptions about mechanical properties of the system. Skalak's 1983 model[25] was based on an established method in mechanical engineering for predicting the load distribution among bolts or rivets joining rigid plates. When applied to the oral implant situation, this approach idealizes the prosthesis and the jaw as two rigid "plates" joined by spring-like bolts; the model predicts the vertical and horizontal force components on spring-like implants supporting the prosthesis (plate) subjected to vertical and horizontal loadings. Essentially, the model assumes that the implants in the bone act as elastic springs with known spring constants. The detailed equations for the model are available in Skalak[25] (see also Brunski and Skalak, 1998[1]), but a main result is that a purely vertical force on the prosthesis (i.e., acting perpendicular to the plane of the prosthesis) is counterbalanced by a distribution of purely vertical forces among the *N* supporting abutments. Similarly, for a horizontal load on the prosthesis (i.e., acting in the plane of the prosthesis), the model predicts that there will be a counterbalancing distribution of horizontal forces among the *N* abutments. In the general case of an arbitrary force vector on the prosthesis, with *both* vertical and horizontal components, the resultant loading on each implant can be found by resolving the force into vertical and horizontal components and then using the Skalak model to compute the results for each component. Likewise, if there are several points at which forces are applied to the prosthesis, the Skalak model can be run for each of these situations independently, with the final loading on any one implant found by superposition of results from the various loading calculations. Some example results with the Skalak model have been presented in other sources[26] and will not be further discussed here.

Implant "Stiffness"

The stiffness of an implant (or natural tooth, for that matter) is related to the clinical term *mobility* and becomes important when predicting the load-sharing among implants and/or teeth supporting a bridge. Here, "mobility" does not mean orthodontically-induced movement resulting from biological activities around a tooth or implant, but rather it means relatively small (e.g., 10s or 100s microns), reversible displacements of teeth or implants caused by temporarily applied forces. At the clinical level, mobility describes tooth or implant movement in axial or lateral directions with respect to a fixed reference such as the fixed bone of the jaw. When testing tooth mobility, a dentist often applies a lateral force to a tooth with a dental instrument (such as a mirror handle) and then estimates the lateral movement of the tooth by the naked eye. While movements greater than 1 mm are easily detected by eye and would suggest an advanced degree of breakdown in periodontal support, movements of, 0.020 mm (20 microns) would be imperceptible by the naked eye yet could also be important when it comes to implant behavior, especially when it comes to predicting how implants (and teeth) behave when splinted together in supporting a bridge.

For example, in the case of a prosthesis supported by both teeth and implants, complications arise because natural teeth and implants do not have the same mobility characteristics (Table 4-2). Moreover, some workers[27,28] suggest that combining implants with natural teeth seems to carry with it a greater rate of complications. Such studies point to differing mobility of teeth and implants as a causative factor in predisposing these cases to complications. Although so far we have not discussed models for predicting abutment loading that account for differing mobility among abutments, a modification to the Skalak model[29] actually does do this. Before discussing it, it is useful to explore a more complete definition of stiffness.

Teeth and implants can displace intrusively, extrusively, buccolingually, and mesiodistally, and tooth displacements can occur in more than one direction even when the applied force only acts in one direction. (We shall ignore this last complication.) Second, when a constant force is applied to a tooth or implant, the displacement

TABLE 4-2

Data on Stiffnesses* of Dental Implants and Teeth

Implant or Tooth	Stiffness (N/micron)	Reference
Implants alone		
IMZ implant with IME	2.57	Hoshaw & Brunski[49]
"Flexiroot" implant with polymer insert and attachment (per A. Haris)	4.11	Hoshaw & Brunski[49]
Brånemark fixture (7 mm) plus abutment screw, abutment, and gold cylinder	4.55	Hoshaw & Brunski[49]
Driskell Bioengineering (Stryker) implant, with abutment (precursor to Bicon implant)	5.50	Hoshaw & Brunski[49]
Implants in bone or in plastic, in vitro		
Brånemark in polycarbonate plastic	3.66	Hoshaw & Brunski[49]
Ti bladevent implant in fibrous tissue, retrieved sample from dog mandible	0.22-0.88	Brunski and Schock[30]
Bioglass cylindrical implants in fibrous tissue, retrieved dog mandible	1.9	Weinstein et al.[31]
Bioglass cylindrical implants with a direct bone-implant interface, retrieved dog mandible	8.5	Weinstein et al.[31]
Nobel Biocare, 14 mm-long "immediate provisional implant" in cancellous bone	0.42 (axial) 0.0798 (lateral)	Brunski, unpublished data
Nobel Biocare prototype of the Mark IV in trabecular bone (10 mm length of implant)	0.180 (axial) 0.122 (lateral)	Liu and Brunski[50]
Nobel Biocare regular implant in trabecular bone (10 mm length of implant)	0.157 (axial) 0.098 (lateral)	Liu and Brunski[50]
Implants or teeth, in vivo [data estimated from slopes of graphs in publications]		
Tubingen Al_20_3 implant, human mandible	10	Shulte[51]
Human molar	0.1-1.0	Richter et al.[52]
Human incisor	0.1-3.0	Picton[53]
Tooth 24	0.1-1.0	Schulte[51]

IME, Intramobile element
*Axial stiffness except where noted.

of the tooth or implant may increase slowly with time in a process called *creep*. With implants, creep is probably not significant unless there is a fibrous tissue around the implant (see references to Brunski and Schock[30] and by Weinstein et al.[31] in Table 4-2). Third, intrusive tooth displacement is not always linear with intrusive force; data for maxillary incisors show an approximately bilinear relationship between intrusive displacement and intrusive force on a tooth, with the tooth displacing less per unit load when loaded beyond about 49 N.

In defining stiffness, then, it is necessary to define tooth or implant *displacement*. Displacement is a vector quantity, having both magnitude and direction. For example, if one pushes laterally with a 1 N force on the tip of a tooth, the tip of the tooth might move (displace) 0.2 mm in a direction parallel to the applied force. Alternatively, a 1 N force in a different direction— say, downward, parallel to the tooth's long axis (i.e., an intrusive force)—might cause an intrusive displacement of 0.1 mm. In either case, a coordinate system is needed to describe both the force and displacement, and often one picks an x-y-z coordinate system fixed with respect to some reference point such as nearby bone of the jaw. Although data on tooth and implant mobility in the literature show that they do not behave exactly like simple, linear springs, for present purposes this ideation is sufficient. So here we can assume that when a force F is applied on a tooth or implant, the displacement from its equilibrium position, Δx, is related to the force by the following simple equation for a spring:

$$F = k\Delta x \qquad (3)$$

Here *k* is a spring constant, or *stiffness*, having the units of force/displacement (for example, N/mm or N/μm). The stiffness *k* depends on the material and structural properties of the tooth or implant as well as the mechanical properties of the tissues supporting the tooth or implant. Assuming that the tooth or implant stiffness is one spring (with spring constant k_{tooth} or $k_{implant}$) attached with a second spring representing the tissue interface (with spring constant $k_{interface}$), then these two springs can act in series or in parallel (depending on various factors) and have the net spring constant, k_{net}. The meaning of the *k* value is that as the spring constant *k* increases, there will typically be less displacement for the same applied force.

Based on this idealization, Table 4-2 shows typical axial (and also some lateral) stiffness data for teeth and implants as estimated from test data reported in a variety of sources. Values of about 3 to 5 N/μm have been determined for the old-style IMZ (press-fit) implant system (nonthreaded and titanium-plasma-sprayed, or hydroxyapatite-coated), which involved a titanium implant having a deformable inner element called an intramobile element (IME) made of a polymer. Most implants in bone are characterized by a stiffness in the axial direction that is larger than that for natural teeth. However, if there is a soft tissue interface (fibrous nonosseointegrated interface) around an implant, the stiffness value is less than those for implants with an osseointegrated interface. Likewise, based on preliminary testing of only one example mini implant in bone, the axial stiffness value was comparable to that for larger-diameter implants in cancellous bone, but the lateral stiffness was smaller—as might be expected from the smaller diameter (1.6 mm) of the mini implant versus the normal implants (4 mm).

The Role of "Stiffness" of an Implant in Load Distribution

Based on the concept of stiffness, the problem of predicting the distribution of forces and moments among natural teeth and implants supporting a prosthesis can be revisited. Experimentally, it can be demonstrated (see Figure 4-1) that implant stiffness is important. Figure 4-2 shows that if low-stiffness implants are located bilaterally at the two most distal locations in, for example, a six-implant distribution, they support less force than they do if they have the same stiffness as the other implants. In effect, when the two most distal implants are less stiff than the other four implants, a *six*-implant distribution becomes more like a *four*-implant distribution. To incorporate stiffness into a Skalak-type model, one assumes or measures the axial and lateral stiffness of each implant, and then uses that data in a modified version of the original Skalak model.[29] Results from this approach show good agreement with data from laboratory testing (see Figure 4-2; see also Brunski and Skalak[1]).

Another good example of the role of implant stiffness arises in the area of connecting natural teeth to implants. For some time, questions about whether it is wise to connect implants (which are generally "stiffer" in bone than natural teeth) to natural teeth have been asked; the original biomechanical concern was that a stiff osseointegrated dental implant might take too much load relative to the tooth (surrounded by its periodontal ligament) when the two structures were splinted together.[32] On the other hand, it has been suggested that the issue is moot due to some flexibility inherent in some of the screw joint connections in some implant systems (e.g., see Rangert et al.[15,33]). In any event, some of the pertinent issues in this discussion were first outlined biomechanically by Skalak[32] and illustrated in Figure 4-3, which shows how load-sharing between a natural tooth and an implant can be influenced by the implant's axial and lateral stiffness. (See Brunski and Skalak[34] for more details on the assumptions and computer modeling involved in the results shown in Figure 4-3.) Here an FE model explored whether load–sharing between an implant and natural tooth supporting a prosthesis depended upon whether the implant did, or did not, have a so-called intramobile element (IME) made of polymer inside the implant—which had the effect of decreasing both the axial and lateral stiffness of the implant (i.e., it "softened" the implant, making it more like the tooth). The results of the modeling showed that as the stiffness of the implant decreased and approached that of the natural tooth, the load-sharing between the two bridge supports

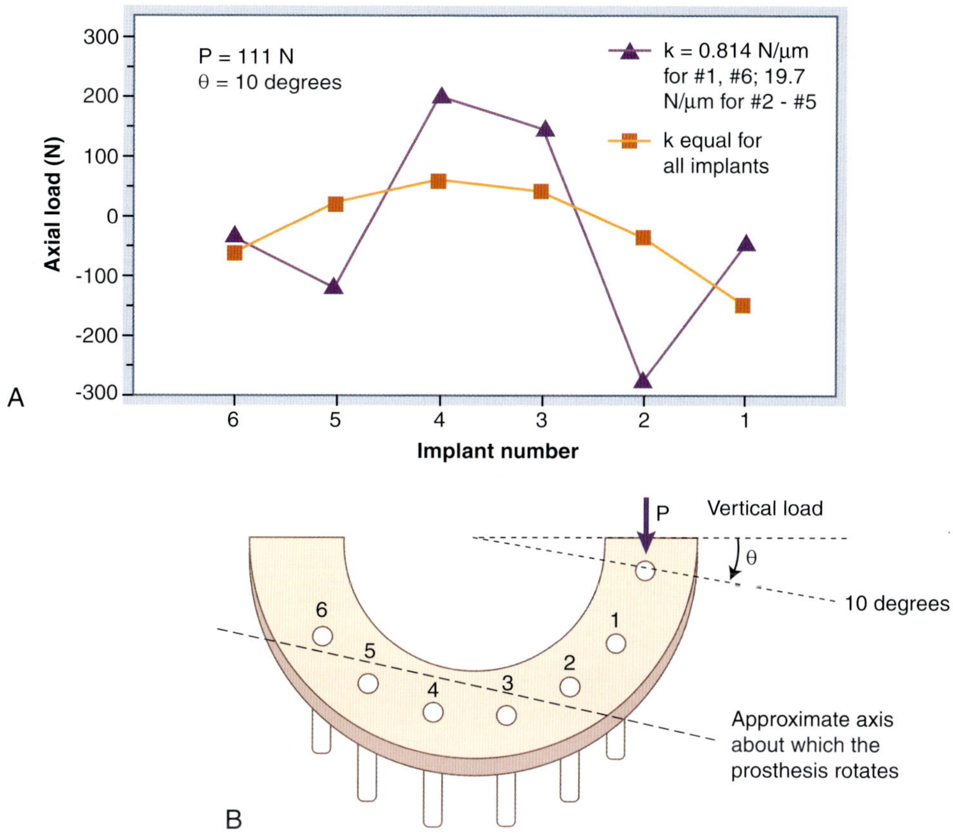

FIGURE 4-2. **A,** Illustration of changes in force distribution among the implants when all six implants have the same stiffness *(square marks,* ■) versus when implants #1 and #6 are assigned an approximately 10-fold lower stiffness (i.e., are more compliant) than implants #2, #3, #4, and #5 *(triangular marks,* ▲*)*. The results were generated with the Skalak et al.[29] model, which can account for differing stiffness values among the implants. The effect of lower stiffness at #1 and #6 is to increase the forces on implants #2, #3, #4, and #5—in a sense converting a six-implant case into a four-implant case. **B,** Perspective view of the loading situation analyzed in A: The prosthesis is shown as a large U-shaped bridge supported by six implants and loaded at a distal location on the left side.

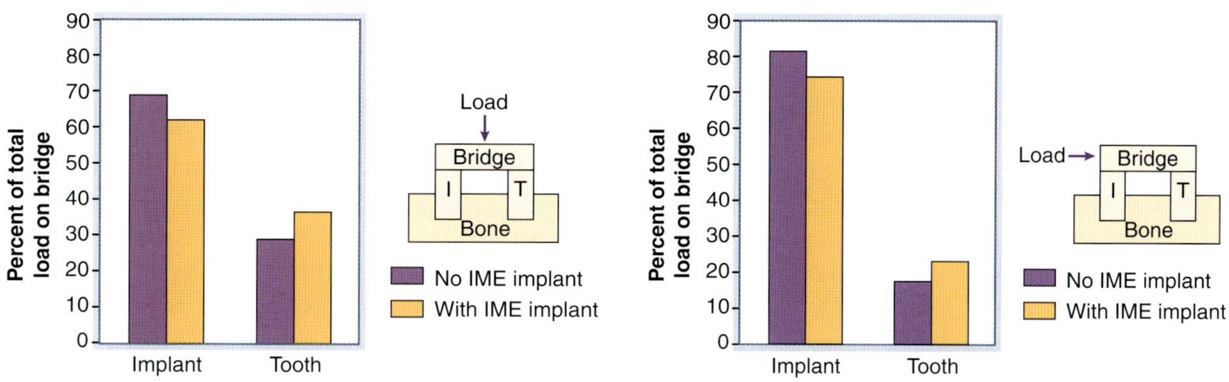

FIGURE 4-3. Results of 2D finite element models of a bridge supported by a natural tooth and an implant, in which the implant does, or does not, have a decreased axial and lateral stiffness due to its internal construction (i.e., in this example, the implant did, or did not, have a built-in "intramobile element" made of Delrin polymer, the presence of which decreased the stiffness). It can be seen that decreasing the implant's stiffness relative to the tooth tends to even out the load-sharing between the two supports. Because a mini implant's lateral stiffness tends to be less than for a regular implant, the same trend as seen in this figure could be hypothesized to exist when splinting mini implants to natural teeth.

become more even than it was when the implant lacked the IME. What this suggests for the use of mini implants is as follows: Because a mini implant's lateral stiffness seems to be less than that of a regular implant (see Table 4-2), we can hypothesize that the same trend as seen in Figure 4-3 will apply; for example, there could be a more even load-sharing between the tooth and the mini implant compared with the situation of splinting the tooth to a regular-sized implant. Of course more work needs to be done to prove that this is a clinical reality, but the mechanical analysis suggests that the idea is plausible.

Deformability of the Prosthesis

Analyses of forces and moments on implants supporting bridgework have also been accomplished by the computer method called FE modeling. FE methods allow the investigation of factors that cannot yet be easily addressed with analytical models, such as the mechanical properties of the prostheses, implants, and the bone. For example, an FE model by Elias and Brunski[35] (see also Brunski[26])—together with laboratory testing and analytical modeling—leads to the conclusion that the structural rigidity of the prosthesis is another factor that can affect the way loading is shared among the abutments. As an example, the load distribution among six implants did not exactly follow the predictions of the 1983 Skalak model[25] if the prosthesis was made out of either 100% acrylic or 100% casting alloy; for both the acrylic and the alloy, FE models and direct measurements showed that forces were more concentrated on those implants nearest to the loading point—which would not be predicted if the prosthesis were truly infinitely rigid (undeformable). Evidently, neither the all-acrylic nor the metal frameworks were infinitely rigid. Other FE models of actual prostheses show the same trend as discussed above.[20,22,36] Along the same lines, direct testing of examples of clinical prostheses was conducted in the author's laboratory using three-point bending tests. The results showed that acrylic-veneered, cast-metal frameworks were slightly stiffer than all-acrylic prostheses in terms of the engineering property known as bending rigidity, which is the product of Young's elastic modulus (E) and the moment of inertia (I) of the prosthesis' cross section, EI. Results showed EI values for two clinically used acrylic-veneered, cast-metal framework prostheses were 0.91 (± 0.53) and 0.57 (± 0.2) Nm^2, and values for two similar-sized all-acrylic prostheses bridges were 0.74 (± 0.47) and 0.39 (± 0.06) Nm^2. So, interestingly, the two types of frameworks were not markedly different. This point, together with the previous discussion of FE models and laboratory testing of load distributions among abutments supporting all-acrylic versus cast-metal frameworks, supports the idea that neither all-acrylic nor all-metal frameworks are infinitely rigid in the sense of the assumption in the Skalak theory.

Frameworks, Screw Joints, and Misfit

Another factor that can influence how implants are loaded is the quality of fit between the prosthesis and the implant abutments. In common implant systems, a metal framework of a full-arch or partial prosthesis is held onto the abutments by screw joints. For example, in the original Brånemark system, two screw joints exist, one at the gold cylinder (which is cast into the framework) and a second at the abutment cylinder. The biomechanics of both screw joints are important in determining the loading of the component parts of the implant system, which in turn influence the likelihood of problems and failure. Also, the screw joints play a role in misfit and in the implant loading that can occur as a result. Because this topic is not as relevant with the use of mini implants, the reader can examine other sources for more details if needed.[26]

The Issue of Safe Versus Dangerous Loading

The most difficult problem in the implant field is defining exactly what constitutes safe versus dangerous loading of an implant and surrounding bone. An answer to this question is, in principle, straightforward because—as in any engineering problems involving mechanical loading—*it all comes down to the levels of stress and strain in the materials involved, and how they compare with known danger limits for those materials*. So for implant cases, the answer involves the levels of stress and strain in the bone, the implants, and the prostheses. In conventional engineering, one does a stress or strain analysis of the materials of interest and then compares the computed stresses or strains to known danger levels for the material involved, for example, danger levels such as the yield strength, ultimate tensile strength, ultimate compressive strength, shear strength, or fatigue strength (to cite just a few of the possible material properties that need to be considered, depending on the problem. The big difficulty with implant cases is that for bone especially, we do not yet have a full database of what constitutes safe versus dangerous stresses and strains. Certainly the literature is reasonably large and expanding about the properties of different types of bone, but when it comes to bone that has healed to varying extents next to an implant after surgery, little data are actually available. This makes it virtually impossible, or at least speculative, to make firm conclusions about the meaning of certain computed stress/strain states around an implant. Certainly analyses are possible, but there are always shortcomings and qualifications. This subject is beyond the scope of this short chapter, but a chapter by Brunski et al.[3] and a textbook by Renouard and Rangert[38] provide a useful review. In the meantime, some precautionary rules to keep in mind when using any implant in bone—including mini implants—are as follows:

1. As the diameter of the implant *decreases* (as it does with mini implants compared with regular-size implants), the stress and strain levels in the bone around that implant will *increase* for the same applied loading. This is true because a smaller diameter implant has a smaller surface area in the bone (stress is force divided by area).
2. The bone around a healed-in implant will have better mechanical properties than the bone around an immediately loaded implant, because the surgery inevitably produces mechanical and biological damage to the bone, which takes time to be repaired. Although immediate loading on this damaged interface is not necessarily an obstacle to success, the challenge for the bone is to heal and remodel properly—and keep the implant properly stabilized—while the implant is being loaded. Note that the loading of the implant will produce stresses and strains in the bone that could, in some cases, create more damage beyond the initial damage.
3. In a typical full-arch situation involving six regular-size implants versus six mini implants supporting the same loaded bridge, the force distribution among the implants is probably not very different. However, what will likely be different is the stress and strain in bone around the smaller implants for the reason outlined in rule 1 above.
4. As noted in rule 2, immediate loading is not necessarily a problem if the implant remains properly stabilized in the bone and excessive micromotion of the implant is avoided. Unfortunately, a definition of how much micromotion is "excessive" is an ongoing research question that in all likelihood also centers on stresses and strains in the healing tissues.[8]

Summary

Biting forces on fixed prostheses are of the same order of magnitude as the forces in the natural dentition, and, when implants are used to support multiple-unit prostheses, biomechanical analyses show that forces on individual implants can be larger than the biting forces on the prosthesis due to geometry effects from the prosthesis. Estimates of implant loading can be made using approximate analytical and computer models. In general, there will be forces and moments on implants. Naturally, adjustments in the number of implants, cantilever length, and/or interimplant spacing can improve or worsen the situation. Factors such as (a) implant stiffness in the bone, (b) framework rigidity, and (c) misfit between bridge and abutment, can influence the manner in which loads are distributed among the abutments. As a general rule, if the goal is to involve as many implants as possible in sharing load support, all implants should have the same stiffness in the bone, and the prostheses ought to be as rigid as possible. When it comes to exactly what levels of force and moment are safe versus dangerous to the implant and the bone-implant interface, a firm answer continues to be a major research question.

Postscript Comment by Dr. Sendax

One issue under scrutiny in clinical oral implantology that has seemingly eluded definitive resolution is the question of whether it is possible to splint natural teeth to dental implants without incurring troublesome complications. Investigation of bending stiffness variables are under current consideration as perhaps a key to unlocking the apparent ability of ultrathin MDIs to be mated to natural tooth abutments while displaying few of the perplexing mobility and instability issues often encountered when conventional-width implants are comparably splinted to periodontally viable teeth intraorally. Research inquiries conceived by me and my coinvestigator Dr. John Brunski are designed to test the hypothesis that ultrasmall-diameter 1.8-mm IMTEC/Sendax MDIs have a degree of latitude in their bending stiffness at least analogous to that of a natural tooth's periodontal ligament, thereby serving as a protective mechanism helping to safeguard the restorative system from the unequal loading and bite instability that may characterize the force impact of natural tooth abutments connected to unyielding conventional-width implants. The hope is that this evolving direction of investigation will provide reasonable guidance for clinicians as they are called upon to treat increasingly complex oral profile cases and require sophisticated treatment options, including the use of MDIs in hybrid permutations and combinations. A working corollary to this issue is the proposition that, as the width of a small diameter implant increases, its inherent ability to flex sufficiently decreases proportionate to its increased thickness and may thereby end up lessening its protective potential, making this a likely subject for further investigation.

Biomaterial and Bioengineering Considerations in Conventional Implant and Mini Implant Design: Jack E. Lemons

The evolution of synthetic origin substances (metals, ceramics, and polymers) as replacements for human organs, such as teeth, has included a compilation of extensive experience often based on need and invention. Most advances have included in vitro and in vivo laboratory and human clinical studies. Within the modern era of synthetic substances to replace hard and soft tissues, selections have been made from detailed analysis of the historical, scientific, technical, and clinical aspects of interpreting tissue interface conditions in terms of biomaterial and biomechanical properties. Since the 1950s implant dentistry's early supporting studies in biomaterials and biomechanics have now matured into accepted disciplines and brought about significant advances in the process.

Key to these advances has been the multiple contributions of dental practitioners, who have always been striving to maintain and improve health conditions through the restoration of normal oral function. In part because of access to the oral cavity, number of teeth per person, and educational background of dentists, many advances in musculoskeletal implant treatments at large have originated within the dental community.

Loss of teeth and the supporting bone and soft tissues has been and continues to be a significant health care issue. In this regard, surgical implants have been developed and applied to address many of these needs with current uses exceeding millions per year. In the times before the 1950s, most efforts were attempts to develop analogs of teeth in terms of shapes, sizes, and materials. Although some success existed, in general, function of the devices used for earlier approaches were limited with respect to quantity and quality.[55-57]

Biomaterials

From a historical perspective, many different biomaterials were investigated for dental implants during the period 1950 to 1980 with several of the metallic alloys and high purity ceramics continuing as the biomaterials of choice for specific systems. However, in general, most dental implant devices are now fabricated from titanium and alloys of titanium. Some of the body portions (endosteal) of these implants have been coated with biometallic or bioceramic substances, but most are intended for function where the metallic surface oxide interfaces directly with the host tissues. This has been called osteoosseo or fibroosseo integration.[58]

Using published and unpublished studies, this portion of the chapter will focus on the shape and size (design geometry) of the endosteal portions of dental implants of one alloy composition utilized to provide initial osteoapposition and long-term osteointegration. Considerations of biomaterial and biomechanical principles related to dental implant designs from a bioengineering perspective will be supported by a brief presentation of terminology and the basis for function utilizing integrated (direct implant-to-bone force transfer) conditions.

Biomechanics

When an intraoral load (force) is applied to an implant through a dental crown (a single crown and implant construct), the applied forces are transferred through the body section of the implant into the supporting bone. This applied force results in a mechanical response in terms of substrate deformation. As the force increases so does the deformation as long as the force and deformation are within the biomechanical elastic limits of the system. Under these conditions and at lower magnitudes, the force can be applied repetitively millions of times, without causing mechanical breakdown of the construct. Also, if the dental implant is titanium or alloy, the overall properties of the crown are different than the implant, and the implant is different than bone and very different than soft tissues. In terms of longer-term functional stability, these relative differences in properties have presented a significant challenge to the disciplines associated with dental implant research, development, and clinical applications.

To interpret what happens during applications of force and deformation, the force is considered in terms of the area over which the force is applied (*mechanical stress*). The deformation is considered in terms of the dimension (along the force direction) that the deformation takes place (*mechanical strain*). From an engineering/bioengineering perspective a very significant science exists in terms of the mechanical stress and strain aspects of synthetic material and human tissue properties.

Titanium, alloys of titanium and bone have been shown to be capable of function in an elastic manner (in terms of stress and strain for implant systems) under normal intra oral functional conditions. Thus when considering the response of bone to functional stress, the interactions at the contiguous implant biomaterial and bone interface are a central consideration.

Osseous Integration

Considering the interface, titanium and alloys used for surgical implants are finished normally to produce a thin and amorphous titanium dioxide surface. This oxide is always present on titanium under normal physiological conditions. Thus the implant-to-bone interface is titanium oxide that is directly in contact with the normal structural components of bone. It is well established that titanium and alloy oxide surfaces fabricated to a wide range of surface roughness, can remain stable (nonfractured) at relatively high strain magnitudes (more than hundreds of microstrain units). Thus the biomedical consideration is what happens to the directly associated bone, especially because bone has a lower elastic modulus and strength compared with titanium and alloys. One critical aspect is that the bone transfers applied stresses and strains that are within the functional stability limits of the elastic and physiologic properties of the local host tissues and regional anatomy.[59]

Decades of laboratory and clinical experience show that specific designs of titanium and alloy biomaterials fabricated into dental implant devices, can function at the macroscopic and microscopic assessment levels in a bone integrated condition. Returning to the issue of elastic strain induced into bone, studies have determined estimates of the limits (lower and upper) of bone strain magnitudes for normal clinical function. Therefore before proceeding to a discussion of dental implant shape and size (design geometry), a brief summary of important results established from previous investigations[60] is given:

1. Dental implant biomaterials, including titanium and alloys of titanium, have been used successfully for bone integrated dental implants.
2. Dental implant-supported crowns and bridges can exist in a condition of stable function for decades.
3. The literature on the science of biomaterials and biomechanics of implant-to-tissue interfaces provides key information related to force transfer along integrated hard and soft tissue dental implant interfaces.

Dental Implant Designs and Osseous Integration

Interface Biomechanics

Related to the design aspects of smaller dental implants, there are key questions: What is the interfacial bone contact area of one implant, and is it necessary to have more than one implant supporting the intraoral crown/bridge construct when smaller (mini) implants are utilized?

In general, endosteal bone integrated dental implants are designed as rods, cylinders, and threaded screws. Surface area, therefore, depends upon implant length and diameter plus the number of thread surfaces interacting with the tissues. The critical factor related to forces transferred through a threaded screw type of implant, once again, is that the stress and strain aspects are within the elastic response limits of the local (interface) and regional bone. In this regard, because mechanical stress is force per area, the larger the implant-to-bone contacting diameter, length and threads, the greater the surface area. The greater the surface area the lower the stress and strain magnitudes for any given applied force.

When considering more than one implant design, a critical biomechanical question is how much dental implant body section surface area is necessary for stable functional conditions. The immediate and obvious simple answer from a biomechanical standpoint is that the surface area must be enough to keep the stress and strain magnitudes within the elastic limits of the bone. Therefore, the initial factors are the capacity of the patient to apply intraoral force including magnitude, cycles, and directions; the intraoral crown and bridge construct that influence force transfer; and the local anatomy (bone dimensions and density) of the host location into which the force is transferred.

The experience and literature provided in this book supports the ability of small size (mini) dental implants to provide stable and long-term function. This, of course, from a biomechanical viewpoint, depends on the patient selection, the intraoral prostheses and the diameter, and length and number of threads of the specific implant within the bone. Therefore, this next section on biomechanics will emphasize the mini implant design and conditions of local force transfer from a bioengineering perspective using examples of histologic sections developed by our laboratory some years ago.

Example: Osteoapposition and Mini Implant Design

Midline nondecalcified histological sections taken from an explanted mini implant that had been used as a part of human dental treatment[61] are shown in Figures 4-4 to 4-8. These figures show similar unstained and stained sections (section numbers 1 and 2) from the same mini implant specimen. Conditions at the time of treatment resulted in exfoliation of the local bone segment containing the mini implant and thus this specimen. Overall these images show the complex characteristics of the dental implant surface-to-bone regions. Relatively dense bone exists at the implant site with some trabecular (lower bone density, modulus, and strength) bone within the structures shown in these particular sections.

In more detail, the lower magnification images shown in Figures 4-4 and 4-8 demonstrate the mini implant shape with bone engaging the implant threads and central shaft implant tip, some direct bone to implant contact along most surfaces and the implant-to-bone interface along the length of the implant. It must be recognized that these midline sections do not represent a bone condition after healing and functional loading or apposition versus integration. Therefore, the following discussion is also based on many other dental implant and bone sections that have been analyzed in our laboratories plus general information from textbooks and published journal literature.

Considering force transfer, the implant-to-bone contact (BIC) is the amount of mineralized bone in direct contact with the titanium alloy surface. Any

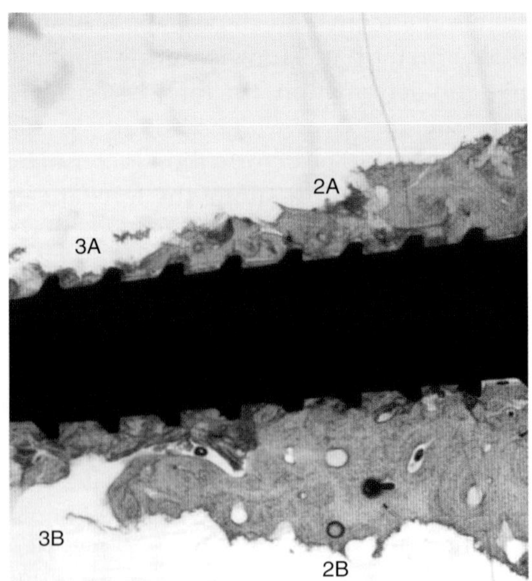

FIGURE 4-4. Longitudinal nondecalcified section 1; Sanderson red bone stain.

nonbone soft tissues at the implant interface would not transfer a significant amount of force on a relative basis due to known differences in modulus of elasticity magnitudes. Also, if the implant were loaded (applied force) from the oral cavity (top) and along the longitudinal axis of the implant, the undersides of the threads and the implant tip would be in a position to transfer the most force as stress and strain due to conditions of local "compressive loading." If intraoral loading was extractive or at an angle, different BIC regions would become more active and exhibit different stress magnitudes.

Another aspect shown in these sections is the "initial" BIC condition of the implant at the time of placement. The close (interface) fit of the implant into the bone (osseoapposition) is important

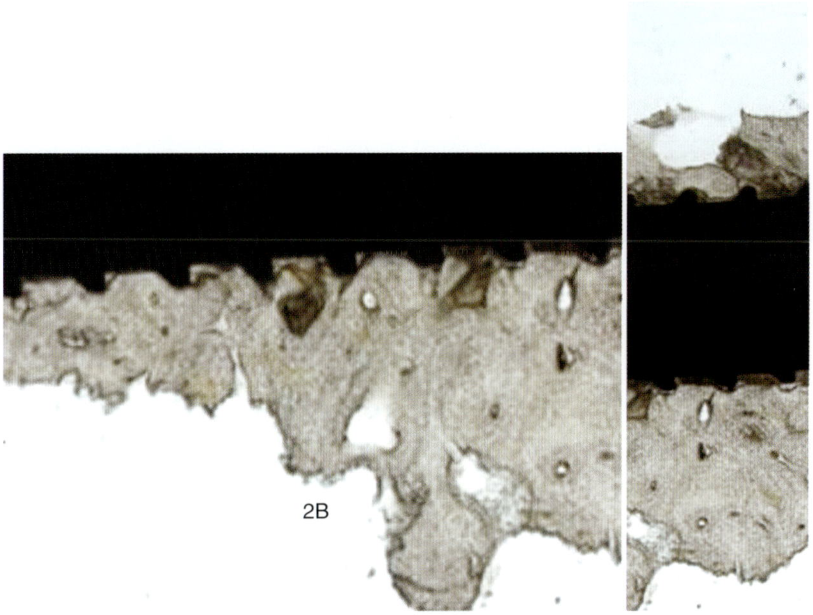

FIGURE 4-5. Longitudinal nondecalcified section 2; unstained.

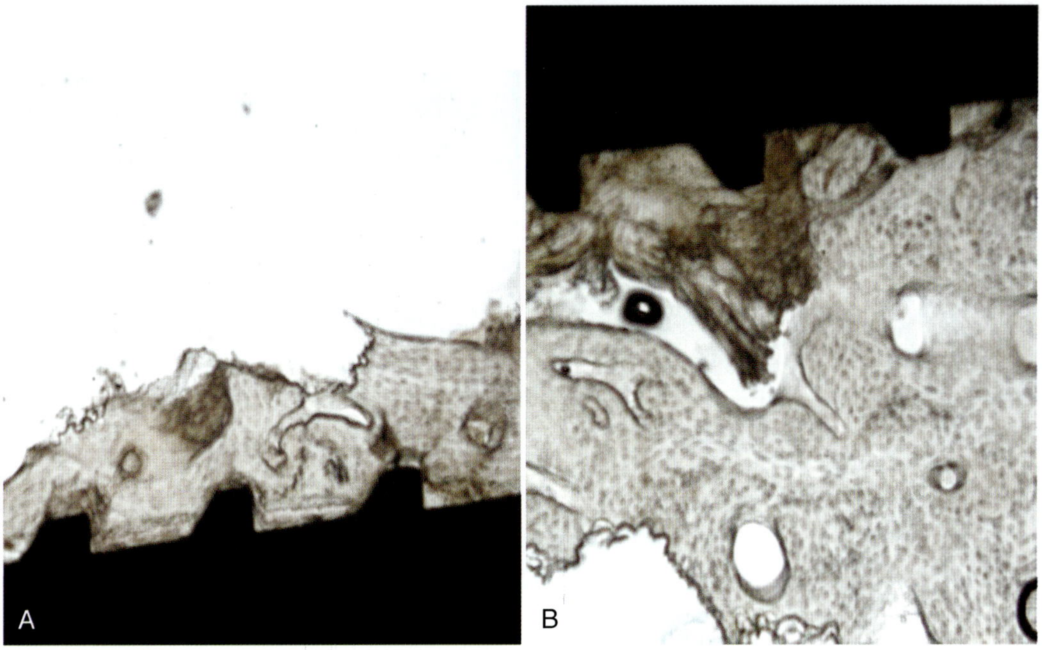

FIGURE 4-6. Details of section 1; unstained.

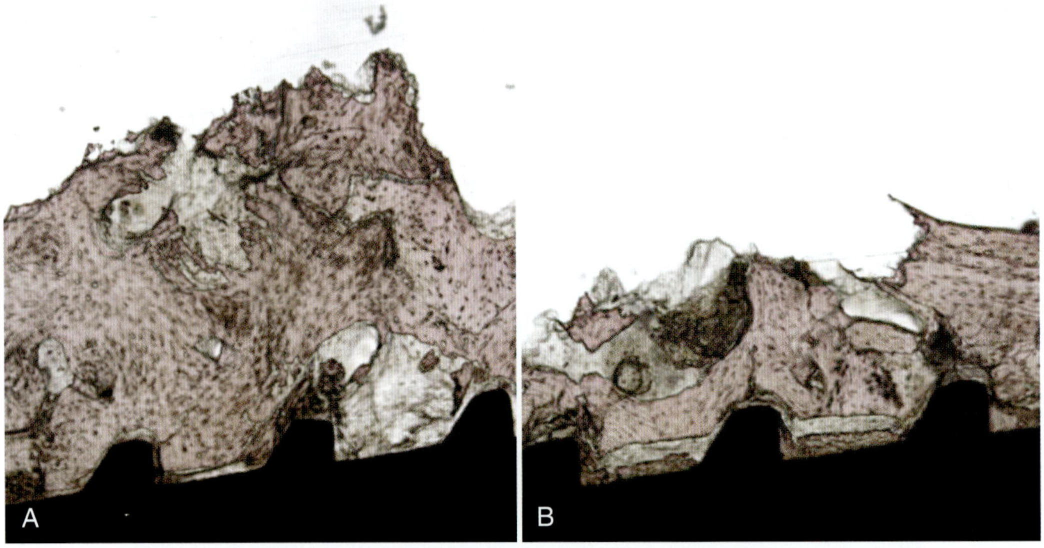

FIGURE 4-7. Details of section 1; stained.

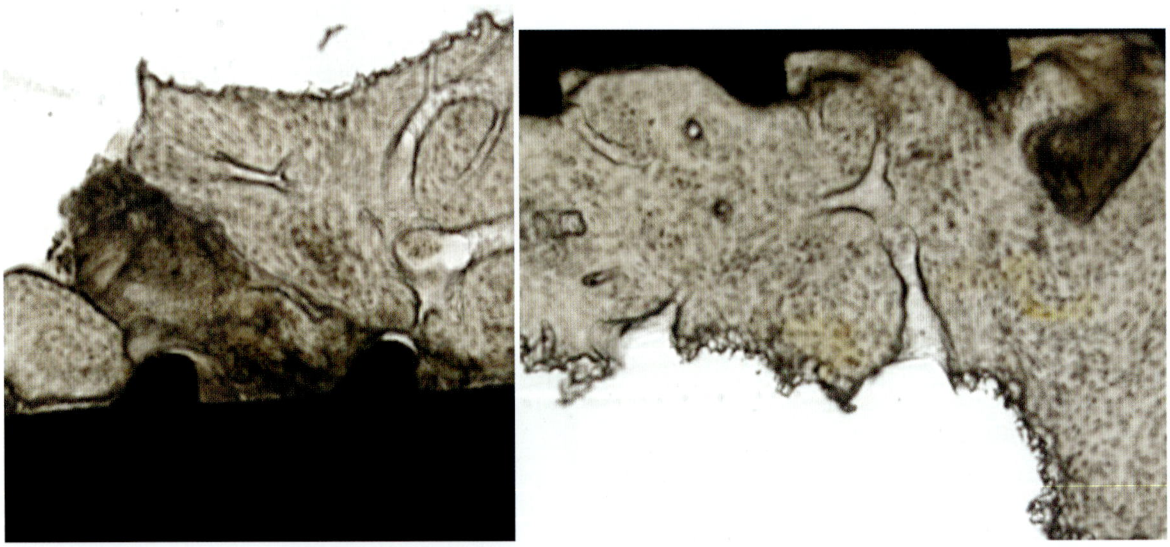

FIGURE 4-8. Details of section 2; unstained.

to mechanical stability at times before and during bone modeling/remodeling to reestablish the longer-term bone integrated BIC support. When the implant fits directly into the bone, the bone will be supportive in proportion to the area of immediate contact. In this regard, studies have shown that, after surgical placement, the initial bone response (crestal die-back zone) occurs for weeks. This response is proportional to the amount of thermal (heating), chemical (nonphysiologic solutions), and mechanical (microfracture) damage at the implant site, and most importantly, at the implant interface from surgical preparation and implant placement. In general, smaller implants and associated insertion procedures may result in less damage to bone and soft tissue (as covered in other sections).

Example: Force Transfer of Dental Implants

In terms of the mini implant design concept, simple examples of intraoral loading, implant design, implant surface area, bone density, BIC, and microstrain at the BIC are presented for discussion purposes. Previous measurements have shown that average loading along the longitudinal direction of implants in regions of the oral bones ranges from approximately 10 to 400 Newtons(N) in force.[62,63] If we assume that forces of this magnitude are applied to the upper surface (top) of a mini implant, that the force is along the long axis of the implant, and that all threads and the tip equally transfer the applied force, simple estimates of the contact stress and strain (microstrain) can be calculated from the implant-to-bone-surface area.

Previous studies have shown that direct correlations exist between microstrain magnitudes and bone stability/instability conditions. This has been summarized by Frost.[64] Interpretation of the results show that if microstrain magnitudes are less than 500, bone undergoes disuse atrophy (loss of bone). A transition range of 500 to 1500 microstrain leads to the range of normal stability (functional status) at microstrains of approximately 1500 to 4000. Again, with increased microstrain, a transition region leads to bone damage at magnitudes above 4000 (often called *biomechanical trauma-induced change*).

Written contact was made with a mini implant manufacturer (IMTEC) with a request to provide some design engineering details on surface areas. Calculations of endosteal body section areas were made by the company using CAD software and solid models created in Solidworks 2008 (personal communication, S. Hadwin, 2008). The request was for areas from the smallest and largest mini implant designs. The company selections were the ORTHOC-6 implant (1.8-mm diameter) to the longest OB-18 (1.8-mm diameter). Also included were the MOB-18 (2.4-mm diameter) and the IDB-10 (2.9-mm diameter).

Theoretical Interpretations

The application of this information to "theoretical" interpretations of the mini implant system will include an initial example of one free standing implant and associated crown. The approach will be to make simplifying assumptions leading to calculations of bone interface microstrain using patient applied forces, implant surface areas, and known (published) moduli of lower and higher density regions of oral bone.

Endosteal surface areas (totals) for the mini implants listed in this study ranged from 30.2 to 158.2 millimeters squared or approximately 30 to 158 mm^2. These areas were utilized in calculations of force per unit area in stress. The interfacial conditions were considered to be fully integrated and within the mechanical elastic properties of the bone (modulus equals stress divided by strain, or strain equals stress divided by modulus). At one extreme, a "worst case condition" would include higher forces and lower elastic modulus (lower density) bone. The average modulus of the trabecular bone was estimated at 100 MPa and the applied forces were estimated at 10 and 400 Newtons (N) axial loading.[62,63] Calculations for interfacial microstrain (stress divided by modulus) gave magnitudes of 300 to 30,000 microstrains for the 158 to 30 mm^2 surface areas and these applied forces.

Clearly, these microstrain magnitudes demonstrate, as anticipated, a condition of bone trauma at the higher forces and lower surface areas and therefore, interfacial instability of the bone.

A general review and presentation in a recent book edited by Misch[57] lists selected implant surface areas from 73 to 213 mm^2 for implants of 3 to 4 mm in diameter and 7 to 16 mm in length. Estimates of tooth surface areas are also given as 154 to 433 mm^2. Thus the surface area magnitudes for mini implants is somewhat smaller than most other larger implants and teeth, however, the numbers are within the same order of magnitude.

It is recognized that under intraoral functional conditions, strain magnitudes will not be equally distributed along implant length and diameter and that the BIC, local bone density, and orientation(s) of surfaces would result in somewhat different microstrain magnitudes. However, this assumption of isotropy and a single crown/implant unit does provide an estimate of extreme limits for microstrain magnitudes with calculated magnitudes into the thousands.

Because these estimated magnitudes in the previous example represent an extreme condition and it is also recognized that mini implants are often utilized as multiple units, are often stabilized during force transfers through bridgework, and are often placed in higher density bone, a simple division by numbers of implants and/or a higher density bone could decrease the microstrain calculations by 10 times multiplied by the number of implants used. This would therefore lead to calculations of microstrain magnitudes within the normal functional range of bone, which is the experience presented in the literature of mini implants and detailed in this book. In more detail, as another example, if we assume that the intraoral force is equally distributed to four mini implants, that the bone modulus is 1000MPa due to higher density bone, and one half of each implant area transfers force (orientation and BIC), the microstrain magnitudes presented previously would be changed from 300 and 30,000 to 15 and 1500 respectively for these surface areas used in the calculations. Within these examples, the microstrain magnitudes, compared with the numbers from Frost[64], show possibilities of trauma and disuse atrophy at the extremes and opportunities for normal bone maintenance (integration) under controlled conditions of treatment.

These examples, including extremes, are correlated with the clinical aspects of mini implant applications as presented in this textbook; that is, free standing single mini implant constructs are to be avoided if occlusal forces (especially lateral vectors) cannot be adequately controlled and balanced to offset traumatic overload.

This history and examples are a significant simplification of overall clinical circumstances; however, the importance of the decisions made by the dentist providing the implant treatment is clearly demonstrated. These examples have been presented to introduce some basic principles and are intended to provide insights into what is needed to provide biomechanical conditions of dental implant function and stability from a theoretical viewpoint. Dentists have achieved an understanding of critical and important circumstances specific to the biomechanics of function from experience with multiple patient intraoral prostheses, and bone anatomy conditions. The future of enhanced dental implant treatment opportunities and selection of the best implant system for each patient should be continuously improved as we continue to better understand the detailed relationships between dental implant function as related to basic biomaterial and biomechanical properties of implants and tissues.

References

1. Brunski JB, Skalak R: "Biomechanical Considerations for Craniofacial Implants, " in Osseointegration. In Brånemark P-I, Tolman DE, editors: Craniofacial Reconstruction, Carol Stream, IL, 1998, Quintessence Publishing Co., Inc, pp 15–36. Chapter 2.
2. Brunski JB, Puleo DA, et al: Biomaterials and biomechanics of oral and maxillofacial implants: current status and future developments, *Int J Oral Maxillofac Implants* 15(1):15–46, 2000.
3. Brunski JB, Glantz P-O, Helms JA, et al: "Transfer of mechanical load across the interface", Chapter 10 in The Osseointegration Book. editorial board, In Brånemark P-I, Chien S, Gröndahl H-G, Robinson K, editors: pp 209–249, 2005, Quintessenz Verlags-GmbH.
4. Brånemark P-I, Skalak R: Definition of osseointegration. In Brånemark P-I, Rydevik BL, Skalak R, editors: Osseointegration in Skeletal Reconstruction and Joint Replacement, Chicago, 1997, Quintessence Pub., Inc. (Second International Workshop on Osseointegration in Skeletal Reconstruction and Joint Replacement, Rancho Santa Fe, CA, Oct. 1994) p. xi.
5. Jokstad A, Carr AB: What is the effect on outcomes of time-to-loading of a fixed or removable prosthesis placed on implant(s)? *Int J Oral Maxillofac Implants* 22(Supp l):19–48, 2007.
6. Brunski JB: Influence of biomechanical factors at the bone-biomaterial interface. In Davies JE, editor: The Bone-Biomaterial Interface, Toronto, 1991, University of Toronto Press, pp 391–405. 1991.
7. Brunski JB, Nanci A, Helms JA: Implant stability and the bone-implant interface, (invited editorial), *Applied Osseointegration Research* 2:3–5, 2001.
8. Leucht P, Kim J-B, Wazen R, Nanci A, Brunski JB, Helms JA: Effect of mechanical stimuli on skeletal regeneration around implants, *Bone Apr* 40(4):919–930, 2007.
9. Szmukler-Moncler S, Salama H, et al: Timing of loading and effect of micromotion on bone-dental implant interface: review of experimental literature, *J Biomed Mater Res* 43(2):192–203, 1998.
10. Soballe K, Brockstedt-Rasmussen H, et al: Hydroxyapatite coating modifies implant membrane formation. Controlled micromotion studied in dogs, *Acta Orthop Scand* 63(2):128–140, 1992.
11. Hoshaw SJ, Brunski JB, et al: Mechanical loading of Brånemark implants affects interfacial bone modeling and remodeling, *Int J Oral Maxillofac Implants* 9:345–360, 1994.
12. Isidor F: Histological evaluation of peri-implant bone at implants subjected to occlusal overload or plaque accumulation, *Clin Oral Implants Res* 8(1):1–9, 1997.
13. Duyck J, Ronold HJ, et al: The influence of static and dynamic loading on marginal bone reactions around osseointegrated implants: an animal experimental study, *Clin Oral Implants Res* 12(3):207–218, 2001.
14. Kozlovsky A, Tal H, et al: Impact of implant overloading on the peri-implant bone in inflamed and non-inflamed peri-implant mucosa, *Clin Oral Implants Res* 18(5):601–610, 2007.
15. Rangert B, Gunne J, Sullivan DY: Mechanical aspects of a Brånemark implant connected to a natural tooth: an in vitro study, *Int J Oral Maxillofac.* 6:177–186, 1991. Implants.
16. Duyck J, Van Oosterwyck H, et al: Magnitude and distribution of occlusal forces on oral implants supporting fixed prostheses: an in vivo study, *Clin Oral Implants Res* 11(5):465–475, 2000a.
17. Duyck J, Van Oosterwyck H, et al: Three-dimensional force measurements on oral implants: a methodological study, *J Oral Rehabil* 27(9):744–753, 2000b.

18. Glantz PO, Rangert B, et al: On clinical loading of osseointegrated implants. A methodological and clinical study, *Clin Oral Implants Res* 4(2):99–105, 1993.
19. Gunne J, Rangert B, et al: Functional loads on freestanding and connected implants in three-unit mandibular prostheses opposing complete dentures: an in vivo study, *Int J Oral Maxillofac Implants* 12(3):335–341, 1997.
20. Richter EJ: In vivo horizontal bending moments on implants, *Int J Oral Maxillofac Implants* 13(2):232–244, 1998.
21. Mailath G, Schmid M, Lill W, Miller J: 3D-Finite-Elemente-Analyse der Biomechanik von rein implanatatgetragenen Extensionbrucken, *Z Zahnnarztl Implantol* 7:205–211, 1991.
22. Mailath-Pokorny G, Solar P: Biomechanics of dental implants. In Watzek G, editor: Endosseous Implants: Scientific and Clinical Aspects, Chicago, IL, 1996, Quintessence, pp 291–318.
23. Block MS, Kent JN: The integral implant system and the science of hydroxylapatite coated implants. In Block MS, Kent JN, editors: Endosseous Implants for Maxillofacial Reconstruction, Philadelphia, 1995, WB Saunders Co, p 223.
24. Burgess AV, Story BJ, et al: Highly crystalline MP-1 hydroxylapatite coating. Part II: In vivo performance on endosseous root implants in dogs, *Clin Oral Implants Res* 10(4):257–266, 1999.
25. Skalak R: Biomechanical considerations in osseointegrated prostheses, *J Prosth Dent* 49:843–848, 1983.
26. Brunski JB: "Biomechanics", Chapter 6 in Osseointegration in Dentistry – an Overview. In Worthington P, Lang B, Rubenstein J, editors: ed 2, pp 49–83, 2003.
27. Pesun IJ: Intrusion of teeth in the combination implant-to-natural-tooth fixed partial denture: a review of the theories, *J of Prosth* 6:268–277, 1997.
28. Naert IE, Duyck JAJ, Hosny MMF, van Steenberghe: Freestanding and tooth-implant connected prostheses in the treatment of partially edentulous patients, *Clin Oral Impl Res* 12:237–244, 2001.
29. Skalak R, Brunski JB, Mendelson M: "A Method for Calculating the Distribution of Vertical Forces Among Variable-Stiffness Abutments Supporting a Dental Prosthesis." 1993 Bioengineering Conference, BED-Vol 24. In Langrana NA, Friedman MH, Grood ES, editors: NY, 1993, ASME, pp 347–350.
30. Brunski JB, Schock RB: Mechanical behavior of a fibrous tissue interface of an endosseous dental implant, *Trans 5th Ann Meeting Soc*, p 41, 1979. for Biomaterials.
31. Weinstein AM, Klawitter JJ, Cook SD: Implant-bone characteristics of bioglass dental implants, *J Biomed Mater Res* 14:23–29, 1980.
32. Skalak R: "Aspects of biomechanical considerations." Chapter 5, pp. 117–128, in Tissue-Integrated Prostheses. In Brånemark P-I, Zarb G, Abrektsson T, editors: Chicago, IL, 1985, Quintessence.
33. Rangert B, Jemt T, Jorneus L: Forces and moments on Brånemark implants, *Int J Oral and Maxillofac*. Implants, 4:241–247, 1989. .
34. Brunski JB, Skalak R: "Biomechanical Considerations for Osseointegrated Fixtures, " in Advanced Osseointegration Surgery: Applications in the Maxillofacial Region. In Worthington P, Brånemark P-I, editors: 1992, Quintessence Publishing Co., Inc, pp 15–39, (1992).
35. Elias JJ, Brunski JB: Finite element analysis of load distribution among dental implants. In Vanderby R Jr, editor: 1991 Advances in Bioengineering, 1991, American Society of Mechanical Engineers, pp 155–158. BED-Vol. 20.
36. Brooke-Smith M: The study of fatigue life of small gold locating screw used in osseointegrated implant technique, 1988. B. Eng. Thesis, University of Sheffield [also see pp. 63–64 in White, GE (1993) Osseointegrated Dental Technology. Quintessence, Chicago IL.].
37. Ashby MF: Materials Selection in Mechanical design, ed 3, Burlington, VT, 2005, Elsevier, Butterworth-Heinemann.
38. Renouard F, Rangert B: Risk factors in Implant Dentistry, ed 2, Paris, 2008, Quintessence International.
39. Craig RG, editor: Restorative Dental Materials, ed 6, St. Louis, MO, 1980, C.V. Mosby, pp 60–61.
40. Meng TR, Rugh JD: Biting force on overdenture and conventional denture patients, *J Dent Res* 62:249, 1983. (Abstract No. 716).
41. Ralph WJ: The effects of dental treatment on biting force, *J Prosth Dent* 41:143, 1979.
42. Colaizzi FA, Javid NS, Michael CG, Gibbs CJ: Biting force, EMG, and jaw movements in denture wearers, *J Dent Res* 63(1984):329, 1984. (Abstract No. 1424).
43. Haraldsson T, Karlsson U, Carlsson GE: Bite force and oral function in complete denture wearers, *J Oral Rehabil* 6:41–48, 1979.
44. Carlsson GE, Haraldsson T: Functional response. In Brånemark P-I, Zarb G, Albrektsson T, editors: Tissue Integrated Prostheses, Chicago, 1985, Quintessence, pp 155–163.
45. Graf H: Occlusal forces during function. In Rowe NH, editor: Occlusion: Research on Form and Function, Ann Arbor, 1975, University of Michigan, pp 90–111.
46. Harrison A, Lewis TT: The development of an abrasion testing machine, *J Biomed Mater Res* 9:341–353, 1975.
47. Ahlgren J: Mechanism of mastication, *Acta Odontol Scand* 24(Suppl 44):100–104, 1966. 1966.
48. Carlsson GE: "Bite force and chewing efficiency." Front, *Oral Physiol* 1:265–292, 1974.
49. Hoshaw SJ, Brunski JB: Mechanical testing of dental implants with and without "intramobile elements", *J Dent Res* 67:314, 1988. (Abstract No. 1612).
50. Liu C, Brunski JB: Axial and lateral mobility of standard vs. experimental Brånemark fixtures, *J Dent Res* 1999(78):246, 1999. (Abstract #1123), 1999.
51. Schulte W: The intraosseous Al2O3 (Frialit) Tuebingen implant. Developmental status after eight years (I), *Quintessence International* 15(1984):1–39, 1984.
52. Richter E-J, Orschall B, Javanovich SA: Dental implant abutment resembling the two-phase tooth mobility, *J Biomech* 23(4):297–306, 1990.
53. Picton DCA: Vertical movement of teeth during biting, *Arch Oral Biol* 8(1963):109–118, 1963.
54. Natiella J, Armitage J, Meenaghan M, et al: Current evaluations of dental implants, *J Am Dent Assoc* 84:1358, 1972.
55. Cranin N, editor: Oral Implantology, Springfield, IL, 1970, Thomas, C.
56. McKinney R. Jr, editor: Endosteal Dental Implants, St. Louis, MO, 1991, Mosby.
57. Misch C, editor: Contemporary Implant Dentistry, ed 3, St. Louis, MO, 2008, Elsevier.

58. Van Steenberghe D, editor: Tissue Integration in Oral and Maxillofacial Reconstruction, Amsterdam, 1986, Excerpta, Medica.
59. Cowin S, Biomechanics Bone, CRC Press, Boca Raton Fl, 1989.
60. Fritz ME: Overview of clinical trials on endosseous implants, *Ann Periodontol* 2(1):270–283, 1997.
61. Sendax V: submission of mini dental implant /human bone specimen for analysis by Dr. J. Lemons and laboratories, 1990s.
62. Lemons J, Misch-Dietsh F, and Bidez M: Chapters 24. In Brånemark P-I (ed): The Brånemark Novum Protocol for Same-Day Teeth. Chicago, IL, Quintessence.
63. Chapter 25 In P-I Brånemark (ed) The Brånemark Novum Protocol for Same-Day Teeth. Chicago, IL, Quintessence: 9–30.
64. Frost H: Bone "mass" and the "mechanostat": a proposal, *Anat Rec* 219:1–9, 1987.

Chapter 5

The General Practitioner's Pivotal Role in Coordinating MDI Therapeutics

BRUCE LISH LEONARD R. MACHI

Outline

The General Practitioner's Pivotal Role in Coordinating Therapeutics with Mini Dental Implants – Bruce Lish

Mini Dental Implants in a General Practice Hospital Residency Setting

Although the restoration of dental implants is becoming more commonly taught in hospital based general practice residency programs, the instruction for insertion of implants has lagged behind. The surgical placement of endosseous implants is usually limited to residents in oral maxillofacial departments or fellows in oral implantology. The scope of implant surgery will be determined by the patient pool and curriculum of that program. The guidelines for accreditation of general practice residency programs include a standard to teach general practice residents to *manage* implants. Manage is defined as coordinating the delivery of care using a patient-focused approach within the scope of their training. Patient-focused care should include concepts related to the patient's social, cultural, behavioral, economic, medical, and physical status." There is no requirement to teach the placement of or restoration of implants. Many programs now teach both placement and restoration. It is currently a luxury often seen as an attractive privilege by general practice residency applicants.

Dental implants are not just the domain of specialists but are becoming routine practice for many general practitioners. Classically, to place implants one needed a large initial investment, both financial and in terms of dedicated office space. This is no longer the case.

The continuing success of small-diameter dental implants as a treatment modality has become increasingly clear.[10,13,8,15,14,5] The mini dental implant (MDI) system has provided a cost-effective, time-efficient, patient-satisfying option that can be easily integrated into a general practice. This supports the philosophy that implantology is a science driven primarily by the restorative phase and not the surgical phase. The surgical aspects of implants are a means to an end: the restoration of form and function for the patient. Any implant therapy needs to have the patient's specific needs addressed in the treatment plan.[9] What better group to be trained in the placement of implants than the general practitioner who will be doing the final restorations? The number of general practitioners placing implants has increased over the last decade.[4] Mini dental implants are a minimally invasive treatment option that serve as a rational place for general practitioners to begin their implant experience. The philosophy of a general practice residency is to expose the residents to all areas of dentistry. This provides a springboard from which they can begin to mold their own treatment philosophy. They can acquire proficiency in many areas and still retain the insight into what to refer to specialists. The positive result for our profession of general practice residency training is that more general dentists are trained to treat patients with more complex problems.[3] As we see in all areas of dentistry, the general practitioner is seeking further training to achieve a higher level of skill in any given field, and implant dentistry is an increasingly significant part of that learning equation.

The general practice residency at St. Luke's-Roosevelt Hospital Center in New York city, to illustrate one specific example of this educational trend, is a 1-year postgraduate program with three general practice residents. The hospital also has an Oral and Maxillofacial Surgery residency program. The general practice residents are based in the outpatient clinic of the Roosevelt Hospital Division. They do participate in various rotations throughout the institution, but their main dental clinical experience is at the Roosevelt Division's outpatient dental clinic. The clinic is a five-chair office with standard equipment in each operatory. The curriculum of the program includes training in the placement and restoration of mini dental implants; specifically the 3M/IMTEC-Sendax Mini Dental Implant System. As a host hospital for training courses, our residents are able to be trained before treating patients with these implants. Early in the academic year the MDIs are introduced. Lecture time is dedicated to information about the placement and restoration of all implants. During the training, the case selection criteria are reviewed for MDIs and conventional implants.

The patients that the residents are encouraged to treat are based on their clinical experience and comfort level with the protocol for these implants. They are highly supervised during the early months of the program and then are encouraged to work independently as the academic year progresses and they have shown competency and gradual proficiency.

The residents are asked to locate a lower lateral or central incisor, single tooth replacement case as their first patient experience. Often these cases are simple with few problems and give the residents the basics they need to treat larger more complex cases. Before treating patients with the MDI, the residents must complete training in the surgical protocol for their placement. This consists of either participating in a one day training course or having the same lecture material presented as part of the regular curriculum during the residency. The goals are for each resident to plan treatments and treat one or more single tooth replacements and one or more implant overdenture cases. There is no limitation on the clinical experience available to the residents in this area.

Curriculum

The curriculum for the placement and restoration of MDIs in the general practice residency program is broken up into three categories: single tooth restoration, complete overdentures, and combination tooth/implant cases. Combination hybrid cases also include crown and bridge salvage cases, which can be rather complicated but nonetheless ideal for the MDI application.

The didactic curriculum includes basic lectures on case selection, surgical protocol, and prosthodontic restoration procedures for MDIs.

After a case is identified by the resident, it is reviewed by the clinical faculty. The proper diagnostics are performed and the implant(s) ordered. The day of the scheduled procedure, consent is obtained, treatment plan is verified, and the resident performs the implant placement with the clinical faculty acting as assistant. The prosthetics are then performed the same way.

MDIs are useful solutions in cases for which conventional implants are not possible, either due to prosthetic restrictions, surgical restrictions, or medical restrictions. The dental clinic in a hospital setting treats a large medically compromised population. Often hospital clinics treat a financially compromised population as well. These two parameters combine to make the ideal patient population for the use of the MDI in both fixed and removable restorations. The initial training in oral implantology needs to begin with complete diagnosis. It is the foundation for the success of any procedure. The criteria for MDIs as well as for conventional diameter implants are taught and clearly understood by the residents. This allows them to properly identify patients who may benefit from MDIs or whose restorative needs would be better met with larger diameter, conventional implants. Patients who might also be candidates for a conventional implant approach are typically referred to the Oral and Maxillofacial Surgery residents for treatment, and then they return for restoration. Recently the placement of MDIs has also been introduced into the oral surgery teaching curriculum, but currently only general practice residents are placing and restoring them.

Medically compromised patients who have all of their care, including dental care, in hospital outpatient clinics tend to have a number of complex medical issues and comorbidities. These are the same conditions that would preclude them from being able to safely tolerate invasive dental surgical procedures without increased medical risks. Conventional dental implant surgery is often in this category. With the use of the MDIs for these patients, we can provide them the life quality improvements that come with implant enhancement of existing prosthetics. The minimally invasive surgical protocol for the MDIs assure decreased stress during placement, during restoration, and minimal to no discomfort during recovery.

Resident Case Selection

When selecting a first MDI case for restoration, the residents are encouraged to limit as many variables as possible. As their experience and training progress, more complicated patient profiles and procedures are selected. Hospital dental clinics fabricate a large number of complete dentures. This is usually due to the patient populations' financial limitations and dental history. For the same reasons, these patients are usually not offered or, if offered, able to accept conventional dental implants. Others have avoided anything but dentures due to fear of surgery, fear of pain, or, again, for lack of finances. Moreover many of the patients are kept from surgical implant therapy by their medical status. Often consultations from cardiology, hematology, and many other medical specialties advise against invasive procedures on certain patients. These cases are where MDIs shine as an option. As a first case, the residents are asked to select patients with few complicating medical conditions (ASA 1 to ASA 2) (Box 5-1).[2]

Our patient population is vast and diverse. Any hospital service will draw patients from within the

BOX 5-1 American Society of Anesthesiology (ASA) Physical Status Classification System

ASA 1: a normal healthy patient
ASA 2: a patient with mild systemic disease
ASA 3: a patient with severe systemic disease
ASA 4: a patient with severe systemic disease that is a constant threat to life
ASA 5: a moribund patient who is not expected to survive without the procedure
ASA 6: a brain dead patient whose organs are being harvested for donation purposes

institution as well as from the community. The patients are varied both medically and socioeconomically. Over time we have become a center for small diameter implants, with regard to both their placement and their restoration. For the purposes of this chapter, we will focus on the medical and dental parameters of our patients. We are faced daily with many different situations that require a complete understanding of the patient's past medical history and how it will affect the proposed treatment plan.

Patients With Medical Complexities

A multitude of our patients are referred from neighboring medical clinics. The use of hospital outpatient clinics for primary care medicine will benefit a patient because all of their primary care and specialty care is under one roof. This allows and encourages better coordination of therapy and communication between the various medical and dental practitioners. Many of our regular patients will fall into the ASA 2 category. These people have one or more medical conditions that are well controlled by lifestyle, diet, and/or medications. These patients are to be treated with a clear understanding that as long as their medical conditions are managed well, and they are in "control," they have low risk for complications from either small diameter minimally invasive procedures or conventional larger diameter implant placement surgeries. As we look at more complex medical histories in our patients, extensive surgical procedures such as might be needed in some cases for multiple conventional implant placement may put them at risk for greater postsurgical complications.

Patients With Cardiac Conditions

The hospital dental clinic setting is a common place for referrals of patients seen for other services in the hospital. Many patients have some form of cardiovascular disease. Arteriosclerosis and hypertension make up 40% of all organic heart diseases.[9] Recent protocols for patients in cardiac rehabilitation who have medication releasing stents dictate that they must stay on oral anticoagulants for the rest of their lives. In some cases, these patients are treated with a combination of anticoagulant and antiplatelet therapies.[12] These patients are at risk during surgical procedures for excessive bleeding. They are at times poor candidates for large incisions and flap reflections. Due to the vascularity, cutting osteotomies into medullary bone causes bleeding. Increasing the diameter of the osteotomy opens more vasculature to increase bleeding. Wide full thickness mucoperiosteal flaps causes bleeding as well. Both procedures can cause changes in crestal bone that can adversely affect implant healing.[9,11] A far better option for this group of patients is the simplified nonsurgical protocol of the MDI. Because no flap is created, bleeding is minimal. The hole through the soft tissue made by the pilot drill is only 1.1-mm wide. The pilot hole is taken one-third the length of the implant (in moderately dense bone) and removed. The implant is then placed into the hole and engages bone. As the implant is progressed to full length, it is not removing bone as an osteotomy would, but rather compressing the bone around it. This tamponade stops medullary vessels from bleeding. This also contributes to its initial stabilization. This generally stops any bleeding from bone, and the procedure is completed with little or no postoperative bleeding.

Patients After Radiation Therapy

Another common referral to our dental clinic is from the departments of Medical and Radiation Oncology. These patients often present after surviving various forms of cancer and having had radiation and chemotherapy. The bone and soft tissue will be affected directly. The associated medical issues and compromised immune system place them in a fragile category in which conventional implant therapy to replace missing teeth or to stabilize a removable prosthesis is not an option. Radiation therapy has much longer lasting consequences that chemotherapy. Patients who have had radiation therapy directly to the mandible or maxilla due to oral and head and neck cancers or metastasis to the head and neck region are particularly fragile. These patients are often faced with few options for improvement of quality of life in the area of their oral health, both in form and function.[6] Often radiation to the head and neck results in destruction of the salivary glands, both major and minor. Complete denture retention relies heavily on oral moisture to develop "suction."

Without this moisture denture retention suffers and denture function is severely impaired. With the concurrent loss of stability, denture sores are common and heal poorly due to decreased tissue vascularity. The minimally invasive protocols for MDIs are again of great benefit in these cases. Using the MDI to stabilize complete upper and lower dentures gives these patients the ability to function with their dentures normally.

For patients who have received radiation therapy to the mandible or maxilla, conventional implants would not be an option. The process of healing relies on the formation of a stable clot from healthy bleeding bone. Higher doses of radiation therapy decreases the ability of bone to heal properly. Radiation therapy also results in compromised vascularity of the overlying, soft tissue. Large, full thickness flaps show poor healing and are at risk for breakdown, exposing underlying bone. The margins of a surgical flap and the cut bone walls of a conventional osteotomy will have poor healing. The MDIs are placed into the pilot hole, and they are self threading and compress the bone as they engage it. After the pilot hole there is no cutting of bone when using the MDIs, and the compromised vascularity will not adversely affect the healing.[1]

Patients After Chemotherapy

Many types of cancer are treated with a combination of radiation and chemotherapy. Although radiation therapy may not affect the prospective implant surgical sites, if chemotherapy is used in conjunction to treat the cancer, the systemic effect is a concern. The severe neutropenia that accompanies chemotherapy places a patient at much greater risk for postoperative complications. The best option of course is to wait a prescribed amount of time before beginning any elective dental surgery. The healing of the soft tissue, response of bone to surgical trauma, and the risk for infection will benefit from waiting.[7]

Patients With Developmental Disabilities

In a large segment of the developmentally disabled population, the only treatment for advanced caries is extraction. As one would expect, this would leave a large portion of that population either partially or completely edentulous. To further complicate dental rehabilitation, there are often advanced medical conditions and multiple medications for both systemic disease and emotional or psychological support. The range of developmental disabilities is vast. Any combination of symptoms can lead to any number of issues regarding a patient's ability to function.

In many cases these patients are treated in a routine dental setting for restorative procedures, but for any more invasive procedures such as oral surgery, soft tissue surgery, or even implants, general anesthesia is indicated.

Patients who cannot tolerate dental care in a routine setting will benefit from general anesthesia. In some cases, the outcomes will be better than if only conscious sedation is used. After these patients have any unrestorable teeth removed, they are left partially or completely edentulous. That leads to the next great challenge of restoring the patient to function with prosthetics. Often fixed prosthetics involving castings and porcelain are not practical due to the rather technique-sensitive nature of tooth preparation and impression making and a patient's inability to sit and tolerate such procedures. Often a sufficient impression for an acrylic removable prosthesis is all that is possible. Fabrications of all-acrylic removable prostheses are therefore often easier for both the patient and practitioner. The next challenge lies in the patient's ability to retain and then function with these prosthetics. MDIs greatly increase the success of these prostheses by increasing retention and stability. Once again, the simple and minimally invasive nonsurgical protocol for MDIs makes them the solution of choice. After the prosthesis is fabricated, a return to general anesthesia or sedation will allow the placement and attachment of the implants to the prosthesis. This allows a patient immediate ability to function with the prosthesis, without waiting for surgical healing and a third visit under anesthesia.

In this same vein, because there are fewer postoperative complications with these implants, the postoperative problems that are much harder to manage in these cases can be avoided.

If a patient presents with a small edentulous area a greater number of implants can be placed and used to retain a fixed prosthesis. The nonsurgical protocol lends itself to the treatment of patients for whom a larger more invasive and longer implant surgery is not ideal. In these cases, a laboratory processed long-term provisional bridge is the restoration of choice. A processed temporary is serviceable for repair or modification, can be removed if needed for evaluation, and replaced at reasonable cost.

Clinical Applications

It is best to examine the clinical applications of small diameter implants by looking at their various applications separately. The remainder of the chapter will be looking first at removable applications in various types of patients, then the uses for fixed prosthetics, and finally salvage operations of fixed prosthetics.

The place to begin in the review of the versatile uses of the small diameter MDI is with the most exciting solution for a patient with a complete lower denture: overdenture support. As any lower denture wearer will willingly share with anyone who asks, a lower denture does not stay still during function. Even the best fitting, properly extended, and well maintained lower denture will move during function. Upper dentures are to some degree better in terms of retention due to the support of the full palatal coverage. During function, however, both dentures will dislodge and move. The classic prosthetic adage "enter bolus, exit balance" clearly defines the reality that dentures at rest and in occlusion do not move, but during function they move readily.

With the advance of implant dentistry, overdentures retained in place with various types of fixtures have become standard. Their benefit however has not become universally accepted due to obstacles to many patients. Some of these obstacles are cost, fear, lack of understanding (by both patients and dentists), and the inability for the patient to have the implants placed due to medical, surgical, or anatomic limitations. MDIs have been able to overcome many of these obstacles for many patients, taking dentistry one step closer to making implant-supported overdentures the standard of care.

It is important to remember that regardless of the simplicity of placement and use of small diameter implants, they require the same preparation, both diagnostically and in patient preparation. The preoperative workup of a potential patient needs to adhere to the current standards.

Patient Interview

Any patient who is being interviewed and who is seeking implant dentistry needs to completely understand their options. A review of expectations and final treatment goals need to be done to assure that they can be met. Some of the most successful cases could be considered failures if patients' expectations are not met. A complete informed consent covering all implant options and restorative options must be done. It is during this process that the benefits of small diameter implants will be clear. In some cases, a patient's needs and restorative goals may not be suited for MDIs, and either conventional implants or even a combination of MDIs and conventional diameter implants may be appropriate. It is recommended that a written consent form is provided to the patient that reviews the details of the discussion. The patient should be allowed to review the document and initial each specific paragraph and sign at the end. The treating dentist and a witness, usually a dental assistant, should also sign the consent.

Radiographic Studies

Radiographic studies of the proposed implant sites will provide the basic information needed to plan the placement and help in the selection of the proper implant type and length. A combination of panoramic and periapical radiographs will provide a clear indication of a patient's oral maxillofacial anatomy and dental anatomy.

In most cases, CT scans are not needed. In cases where the anatomy is unclear, or space for implants is very limited, these higher level studies can be useful. With the advent of cone beam tomography, a comprehensive 3D image can be constructed to allow clear diagnostics in the selection of the implant and placement.

With the panoramic and periapical radiographs mounted properly, a clear overlay template can be used to visualize what various implants will look like after placement. Issues of angulations, depth, even implant diameter can be decided.

Other critical diagnostic information can be determined by close inspection of the radiographs. Mainly, anatomical landmarks and possible limitations to implant placement can be visualized. In some cases

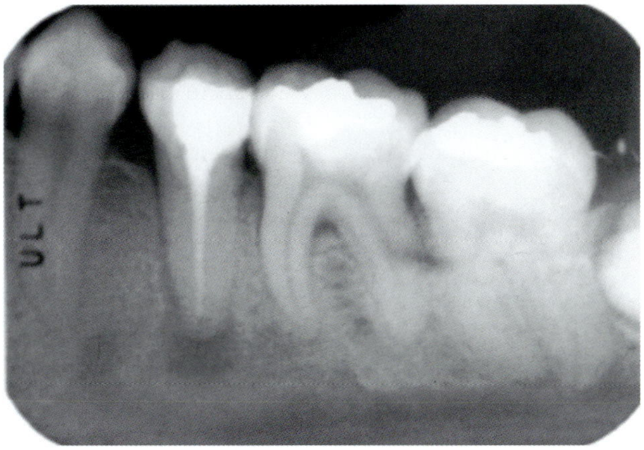

FIGURE 5-1. Periapical view showing anterior mental loop of inferior alveolar nerve (IAN).

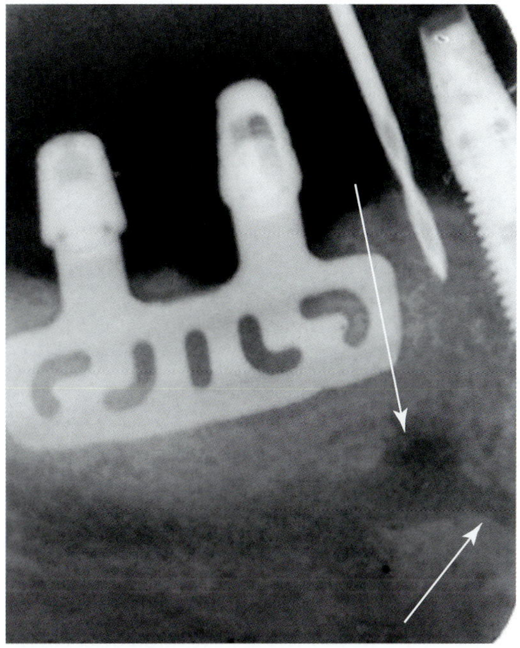

FIGURE 5-2. Another example of anterior loop of the IAN.

the quality of the bone at the implant site can be assessed before placement from the appearance of the bony architecture on radiographs. Of course the overall health of the bone is evaluated to assure there are no lesions, malignancies, or other pathologies present.

In most cases, the main anatomical structures that must be identified on radiographs and subsequently avoided during placement are the anterior loop (Figures 5-1 and 5-2), the inferior alveolar canal (Figure 5-3), the mental foramen and the floor of the nose (Figure 5-4), and the floor of the maxillary sinus (see Figure 5-3). There are occasions when engaging the floor of the maxillary sinus is beneficial, resulting in bicortical stabilization and enhanced initial stability of the implant. Radiographic examples of this bicortical stabilization can be seen in Figures 5-5 and 5-6.

The implants should always remain within the periosteum; a perforation of the buccal or lingual plate can lead to implant failure.

The use of radiographs and the clear overlay template are keys to the successful planning of even the most routine cases. No matter how routine a case may seem, these diagnostic steps need to be taken to help insure predictability.

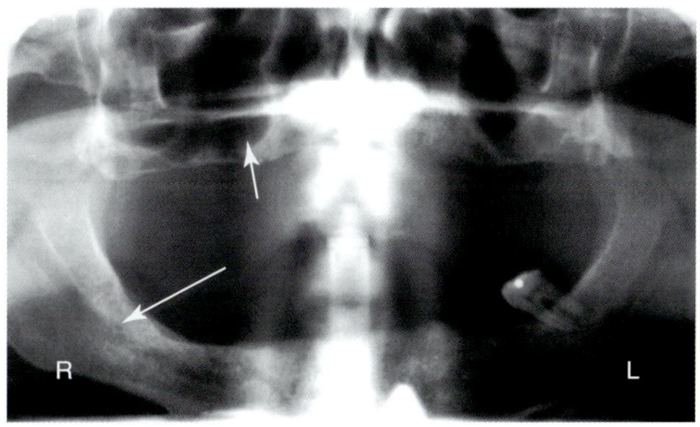

FIGURE 5-3. Anatomy that was of concern in treatment planning: maxillary sinus and IAN.

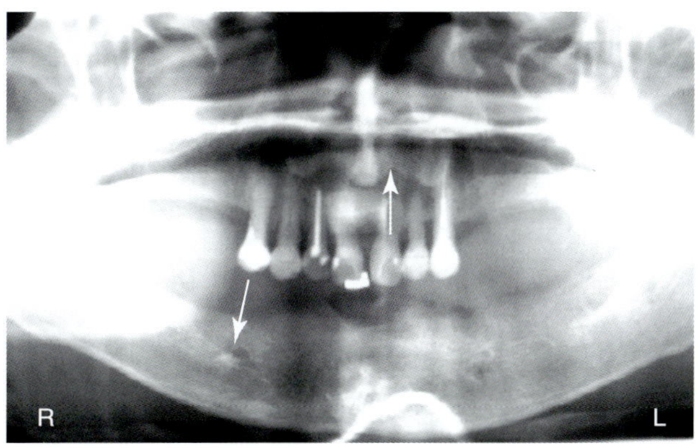

FIGURE 5-4. Anterior loop of IAN and floor of nasal cavity.

Clinical Exam

After radiographs have been reviewed, a clinical evaluation of the proposed implant sites needs to be done. The needs for evaluation for a removable retention case or a fixed prosthesis is not very different.

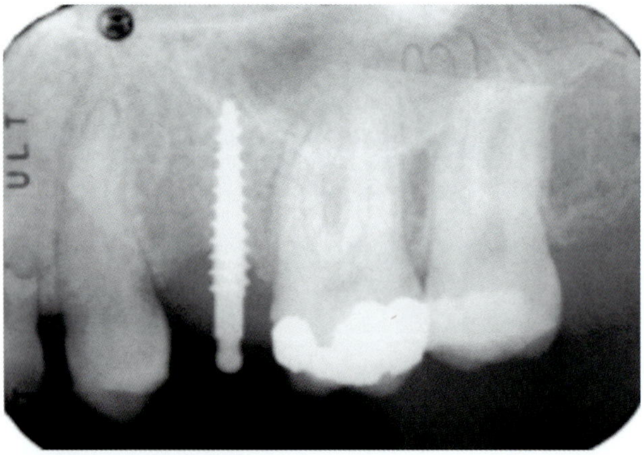

FIGURE 5-5. Bicortical stabilization using floor of maxillary sinus.

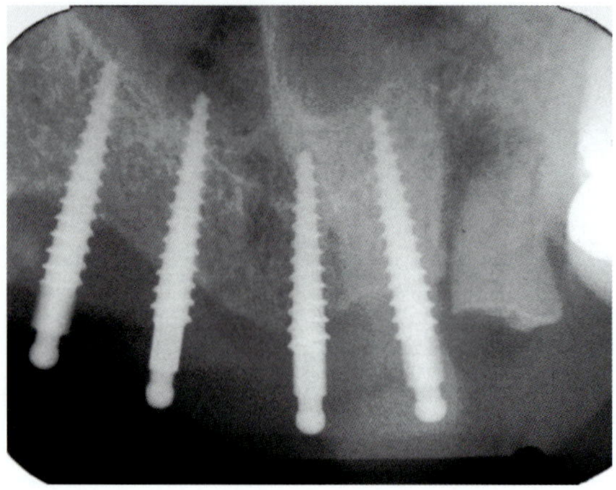

FIGURE 5-6. Bicortical stabilization using floor of maxillary sinus.

The size, height, width, and location of the bone at the implant site needs to be evaluated and correlated with the radiographic surveys. Combining these two diagnostic tests is the best way to get a clear picture of what will be encountered when placing any implants. Aside from manual palpation of the bony ridge, the use of bone calipers or other thickness measuring devises that can be used to gauge bone width are very useful. The practitioner can create a very accurate bone width map, which can assure proper implant placement for success.

These techniques also give valuable information about the thickness of the tissue on the alveolar ridge through which the implants are being placed. The use of a periodontal probe through the tissue down to the crest of bone will give a better indication of tissue height than any other diagnostic test.

After all the diagnostic data are collected, the case can be planned effectively and accurately.

Treatment Planning

After all diagnostic information is gathered and the patient interview is complete, the final treatment plan can be constructed to meet the patient's needs and treatment goals. Use of any implant as a treatment modality must be considered within the overall condition of the patient's dentition. If the patient is edentulous and wears a prosthesis, the process is certainly easier, and the treatment goals are clear; to retain the patient's dentures and provide better function and quality of life. If a dentate patient presents in need of implant restorations to fill the gaps left from selected tooth removal, malignancy, or trauma, the process becomes more complicated. In a hospital setting, we certainly see more of the "nonroutine" cases for restoration.

The patient's expectations discovered during the interview must be taken into consideration when finalizing the treatment plan. The starting point for the patient and the final goal should be clearly understood by the dentist. To illustrate this, we can look at a lower denture wearer. Patients who have complete lower dentures soon after they loose their teeth usually have more residual alveolar ridge, and their dentures will function and be retained differently than patients who have been wearing dentures for many years. In Figure 5-7 we see a clear illustration of the changes of the mandible over time.

The resorption of the residual alveolar ridge is down and back. When a denture sits on the basal bone, there is limited stability and virtually no retention.

In this section I will use cases as examples of various treatment plan options for patients who present for implant therapy using small diameter implants.

Case Discussions

Let us begin the case discussions with a routine overdenture case. The cases presented in this chapter are representative of those found in our residency program as well as cases that present to a private practice. The incredible versatility of these implants allows a wide range of uses.

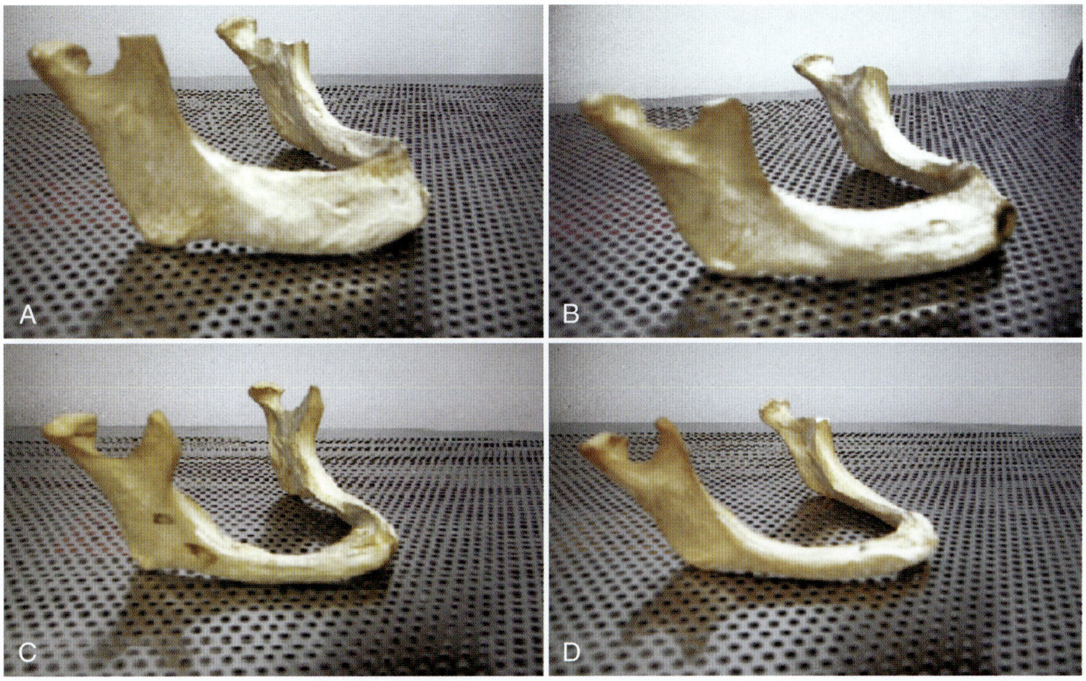

FIGURE 5-7. Atrophic changes in the mandible over time.

CASE DISCUSSION I

A 77-year-old man presents with a chief complaint of loose teeth. He claims during the interview that "I think I need full plates." After radiographs and complete diagnosis, it was determined that he did in fact need all of his teeth removed. His medical history included controlled hypertension and arthritis, with medications for each. He had no limitations other than walking slowly with a cane. From the radiographs, it was clear that lower denture retention would be an issue (Figure 5-8a). The option of MDIs was discussed and, after a complete informed consent, the case was scheduled.

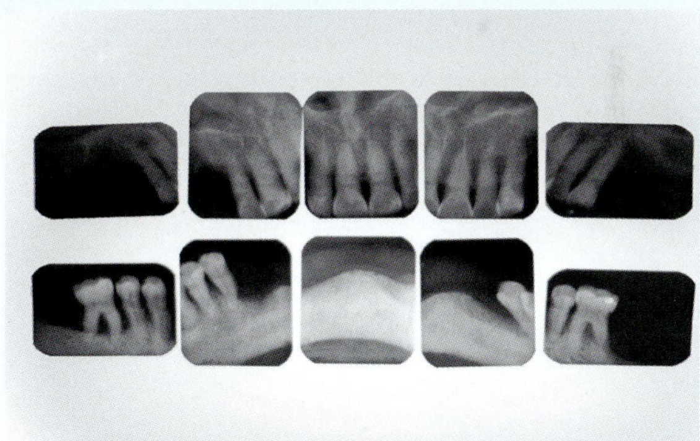

FIGURE 5-8a. Preoperative x-ray.

The patient's remaining teeth were extracted, and complete maxillary and mandibular dentures were fabricated. The patient wore the dentures for 2 weeks and was seen for adjustments during that time. He presented for the implant placement visit as directed. His medical history was again reviewed and no changes were noted. He also reported that the dentures were comfortable but loose. Local anesthesia was given. Bilateral mental blocks and local infiltrations were given using lidocaine 2%, 1:100,000 epinephrine (Figure 5-8b).

During the diagnosis and review of radiographs, it was clear that the patient had a significant buccal plate defect in the areas of the lower canines. It was elected to place three MDIs between these two defects. This would provide optimum retention and still allow him to remove the denture.

Continued

CASE DISCUSSION I—cont'd

After the surgical protocol, the sites were marked and the pilot hole was drilled to one third the length of the implant (Figure 5-8c).

The implant was then delivered to the site still attached to the plastic carrier (Figure 5-8d).

After the implant was engaged in bone, the carrier was changed for the finger driver. The implant was then advanced until it was tight with the finger driver. At this point, the finger driver was changed for the winged wrench driver, which provided much greater torque and allowed the implant to be taken to full length. In some cases, the winged wrench gets too tight to turn and the ratchet driver is used to completely seat the implant; there was no need for the ratchet in this case. The two most posterior implants were placed, and the center one was placed last (Figures 5-8e and 5-8f).

The denture was attached with metal housings and O-rings according the prescribed protocol.

A brief discussion of the number of implants needed is important. The "standard" number would be four implants placed between the canine sites. Most of our patients, however, do not

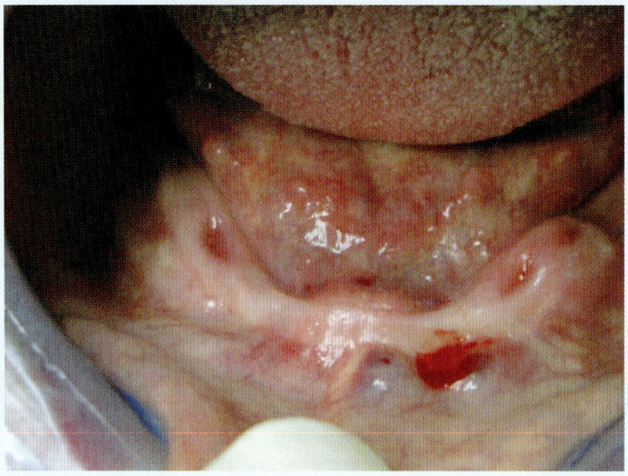

FIGURE 5-8b. Extractions healing and local given before MDI placement.

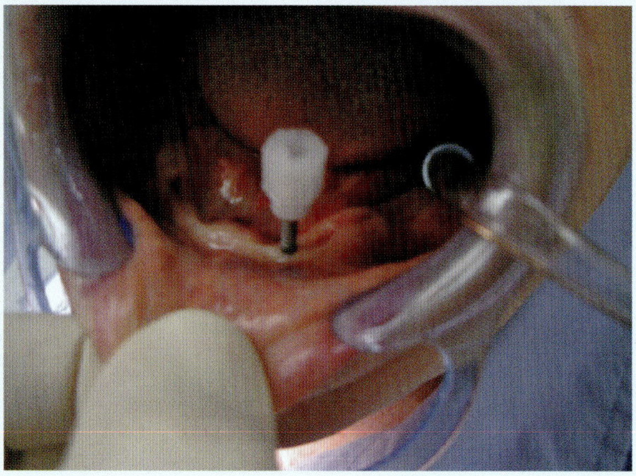

FIGURE 5-8d. MDI carried to site with plastic carrier.

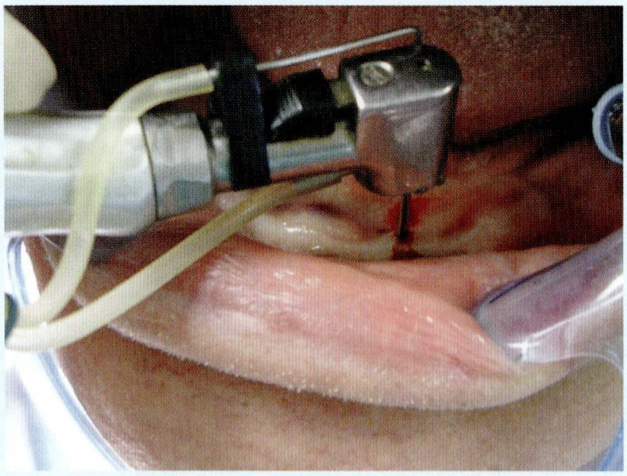

FIGURE 5-8c. Pilot "starter" opening.

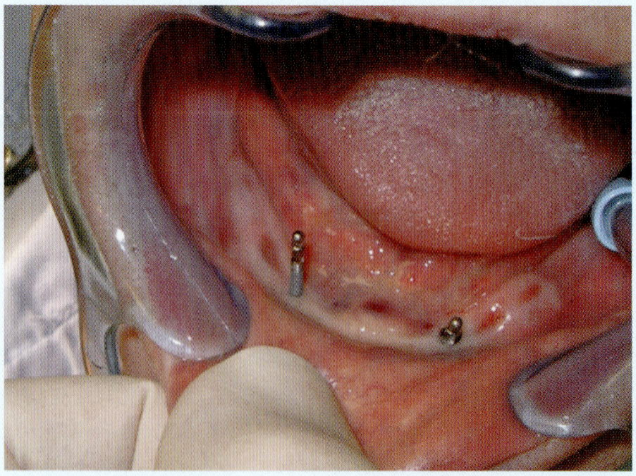

FIGURE 5-8e. Second implant going into place.

CASE DISCUSSION 1—cont'd

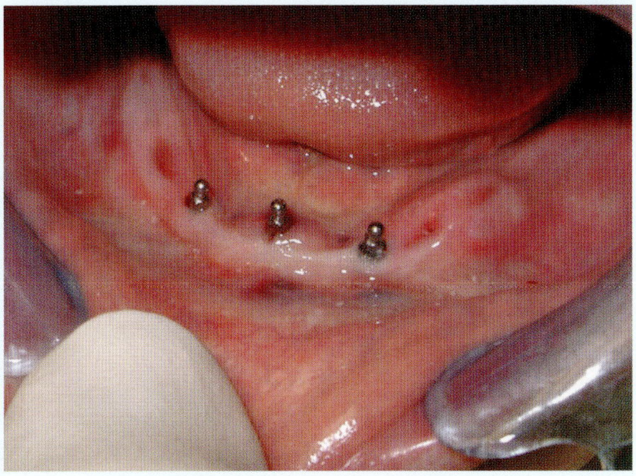

FIGURE 5-8f. Implants completed.

fit into the "standard" category. We have every intention of planning for four at the outset, but by the end of the patient's interview and complete diagnosis many mitigating circumstances come into play. In the previous case, we wanted to place four but two issues came up. The first was the buccal plate defects, which would not have prevented placement but made it more difficult, and the second was the patient's ability to remove the denture with the retention of four implants. With his arthritis, he had limited manual dexterity. We elected to go with three implants to still give him all the benefits.

Manual dexterity is a common complicating factor for good oral health habits (Figure 5-9). Often custom or specialized brushes are needed to help patients care for their remaining teeth and removable prosthetics.

Many patients seen in the clinic have no dental coverage or have coverage provided by the Department of Health. Many entitlement programs and managed care programs have limitations on the replacement of an existing denture. Situations are many in which patients with limited coverage or limited financial resources need to preserve their existing prosthesis even after loss of abutment teeth. The following two cases are just such situations.

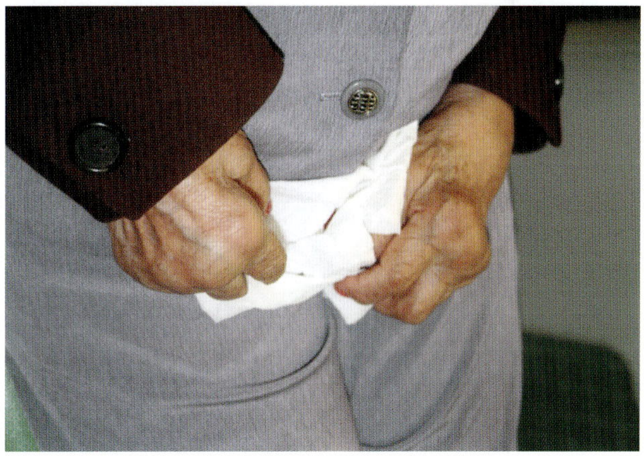

FIGURE 5-9. Arthritic hands making manipulation of prosthesis difficult.

CASE DISCUSSION 2

A woman in her sixties presented with a 15-year-old lower canine supported overdenture. The issue was that she lost one of the canines due to decay around the attachment. She had other teeth that were endodontically treated some time ago in hopes of using them later for attachments. These were decayed as well and needed extraction (Figures 5-10a and 5-10b). She was not eligible for a new denture for another 2 years. We elected to use two MDIs to replace the missing attachment tooth and used her existing lower. This plan saved her the expense of a new denture and still allowed her the quality of life of a supported denture. As a training program that treats a compromised population, we are able to provide the MDIs and a very reasonable fee.

Two MDIs were placed, one to replace the lower right canine and one in the center for added support. Figures 5-10c and 5-10d show the 2-week follow-up and the retrofitted denture. Due to the patient's minimal to flat ridge, we left a long-term soft reline in place even after attaching the O-rings.

Continued

CASE DISCUSSION 2—cont'd

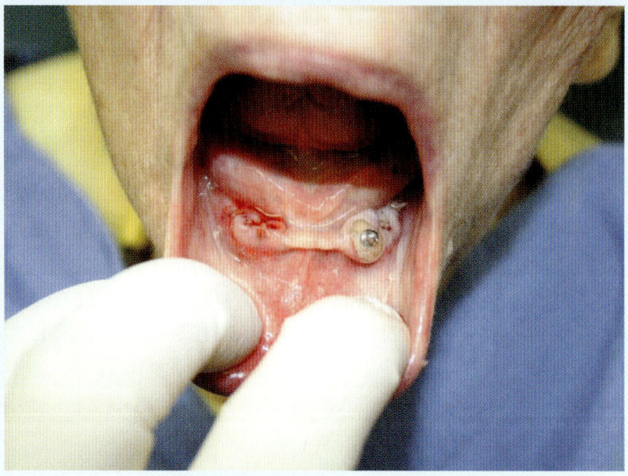

FIGURE 5-10a. Postextraction view.

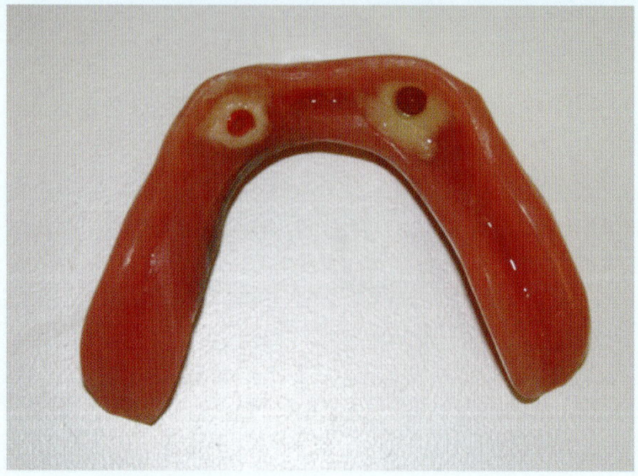

FIGURE 5-10b. Denture before modification.

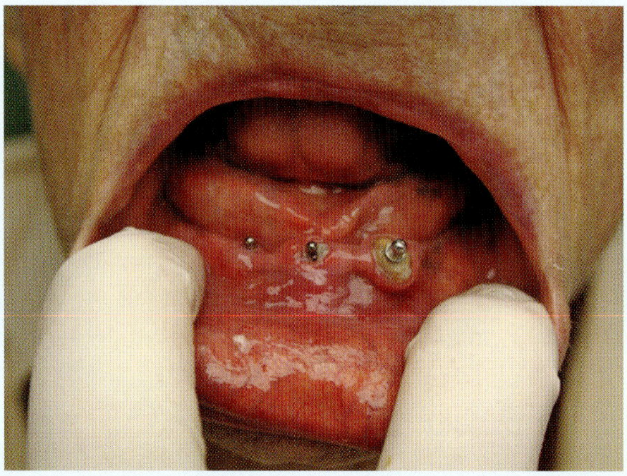

FIGURE 5-10c. At 2-week follow-up visit.

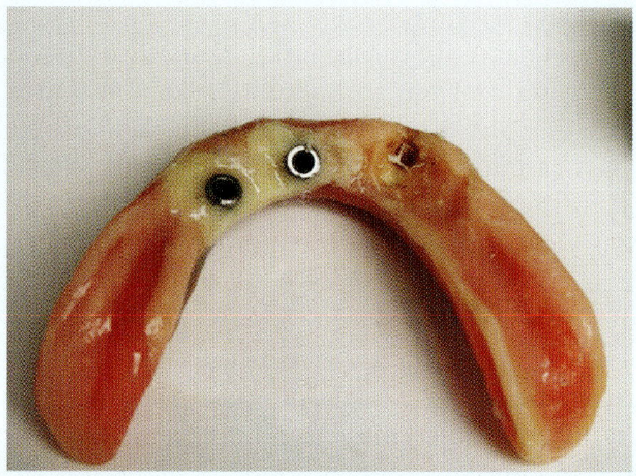

FIGURE 5-10d. Retrofitted denture to existing O-ball on teeth and new MDIs.

CASE DISCUSSION 3

A patient with an existing maxillary partial presented with broken abutment teeth on the right side (Figure 5-11a). The abutments on the left were stable, but even after adding teeth to the partial on the right, the retention was poor and it drooped. We elected to place MDIs to help retain the partial on the right, thus preserving the teeth on the left. His medical history was reviewed and the placement was scheduled.

Three MDIs were placed in the canine, first premolar, and between the first and second molar areas (Figure 5-11b).

The housings were placed and picked up (Figure 5-11c). The plan for the future of this partial was to place MDIs on the left in the same pattern when the teeth fail. This will allow the patient to function with the same prosthesis. After all six implants were in, a new prosthesis could be made.

CASE DISCUSSION 3—cont'd

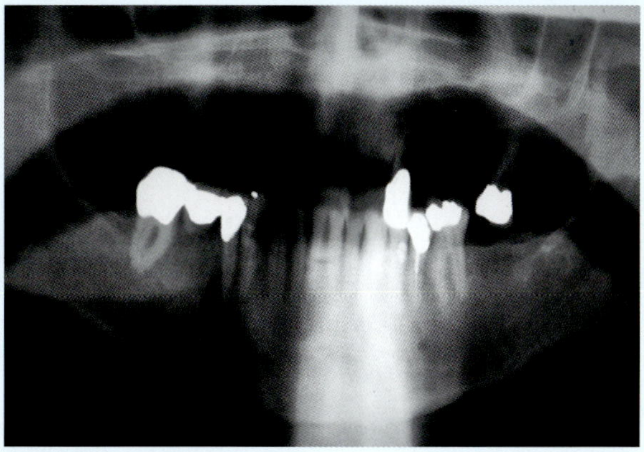

FIGURE 5-11a. Preoperative panoramic x-ray showing two remaining teeth on left as only support for partial denture.

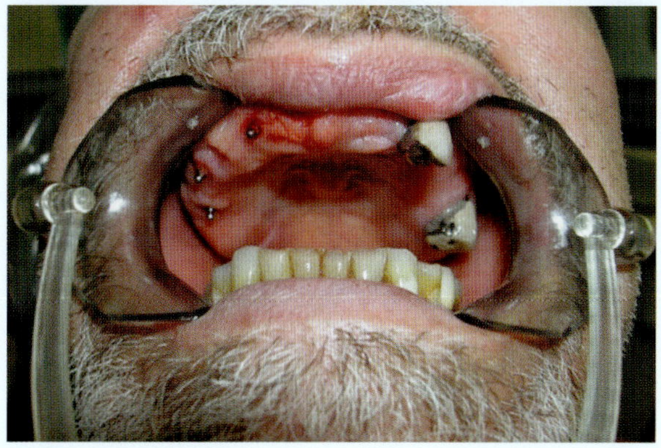

FIGURE 5-11b. Three maxillary MDIs in place.

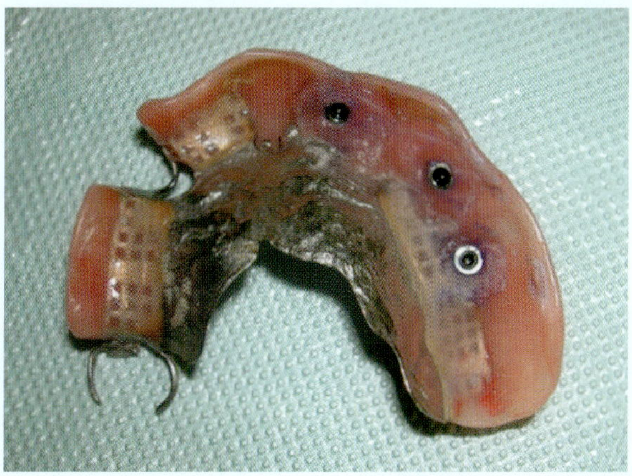

FIGURE 5-11c. Three housings picked up to retrofit denture.

CASE DISCUSSION 4

The next case involves a patient with an advanced cardiac history on multiple medications, including warfarin. The cardiac conditions were controlled with medications but at the advice of her cardiologist, extractions were to be avoided if possible.

In the past, patients on anticoagulant therapy presented a unique set of risks and management issues for even basic oral surgery. The current trend is to never discontinue the anticoagulants because it places the patient at greater risk for a clot during the subtherapeutic window. The safer way to manage patients is to perform the procedure as usual and mange the bleeding with localized techniques such as hemostatic agents, sutures, and even vasoconstrictors at the site.

The patient presented to our clinic with a fractured abutment to an all resin lower partial. The tooth had fractured below the gingival level almost to the osseous. A root canal was completed

Continued

CASE DISCUSSION 4—cont'd

to preserve the root and to avoid extraction. We elected to use MDIs to help retain the denture. After local infiltration using anesthetic with vasoconstrictor, pilot holes were made and the MDIs were delivered. Minimal bleeding was almost completely stopped when the implant was delivered to the site. The denture was then retrofitted to the housings (Figures 5-12a-d).

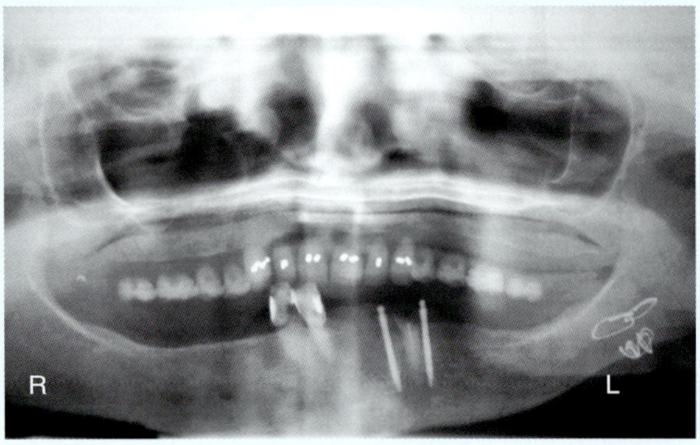

FIGURE 5-12a. Panoramic x-ray, postoperative placement.

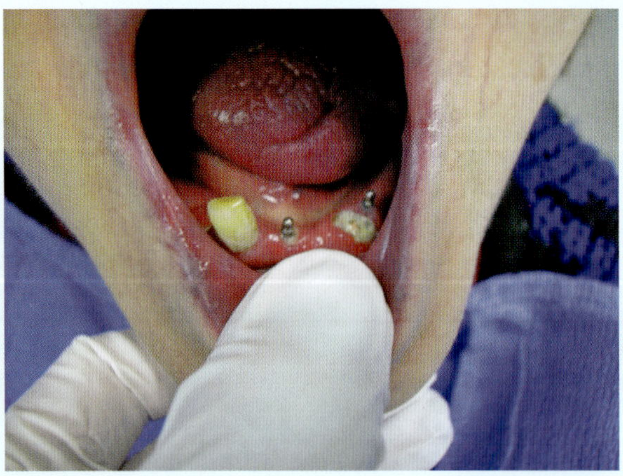

FIGURE 5-12b. Clinical view after placement.

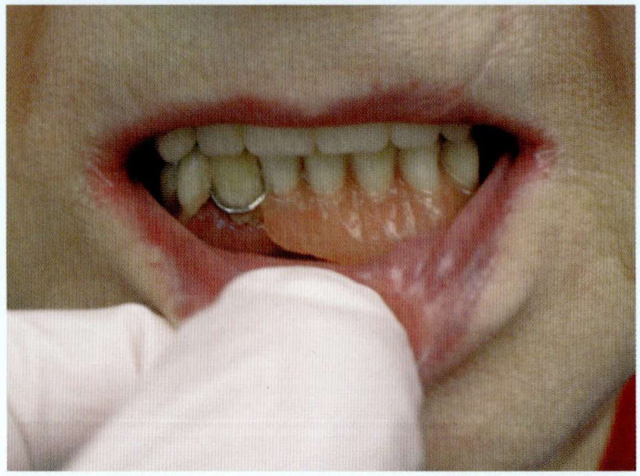

FIGURE 5-12c. Denture in place in occlusion.

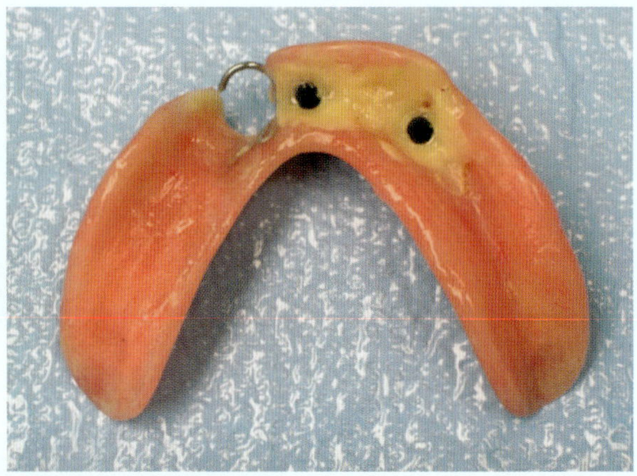

FIGURE 5-12d. Housings picked up to retrofit the denture.

CASE DISCUSSION 5 Fixed Restorations

The versatility and utility of small diameter, immediate load, nonsurgical implants cannot be appreciated until one uses them for a rapidly completed single tooth replacement in an esthetic zone. The following case of a middle-aged woman presenting with a missing lower left canine for some time illustrates this well. She had her lower left canine extracted after a failed root canal many years ago. She had a single tooth removable partial denture made, which she subsequently lost and has been without anything for that location for approximately 2 years (Figure 5-13a). She had no problem with the unesthetic space until her daughter decided to get married, and she would have to appear for pictures. She presented on a Wednesday stating "I need a tooth by this weekend."

Multiple other treatment modalities could provide the immediate esthetics needed, but all would compromise the function. A MDI would solve the esthetic and functional problems and fit the clinical situation. It seemed the canine was extracted and the buccal plate resorbed to some degree, leaving little width to place an implant (Figure 5-13b).

A MDI was placed and even with its small diameter it was a tight fit and required some interproximal reduction to allow the drivers to fit (Figures 5-13c to 5-13g). A plastic temporary was fabricated (Figure 5-13h), and the patient left the clinic with a tooth that filled the space and could fully function immediately. No other service could give the immediate gratification that the patient was seeking.

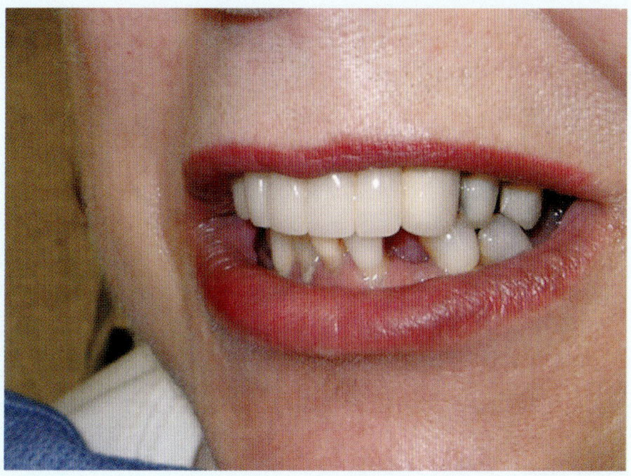

FIGURE 5-13a. Esthetic emergency

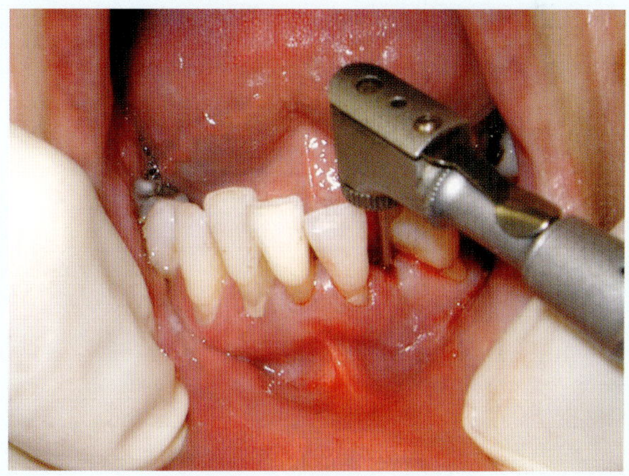

FIGURE 5-13c. Pilot hole.

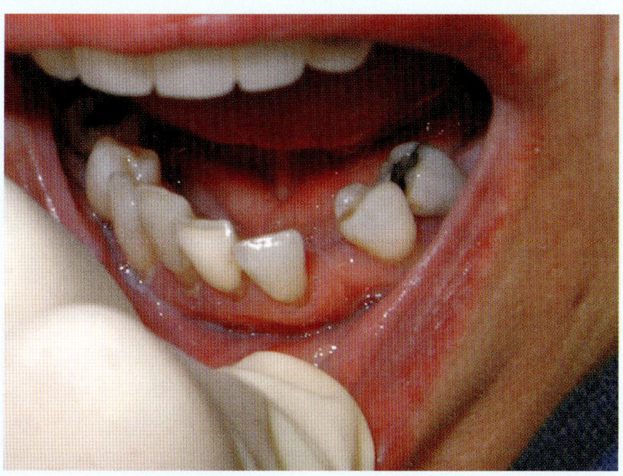

FIGURE 5-13b. Retracted intraoral view.

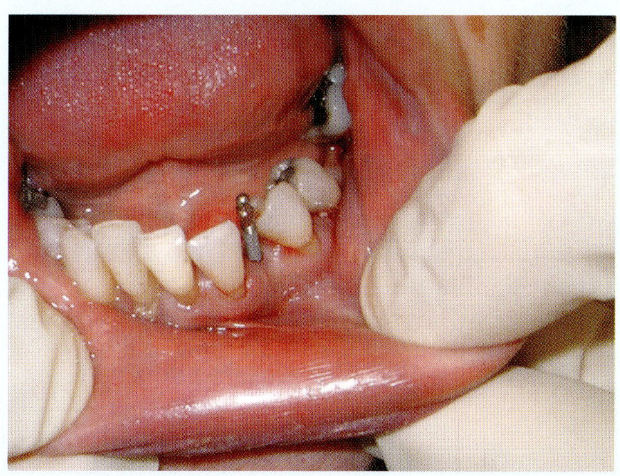

FIGURE 5-13d. MDI delivered to site.

Continued

CASE DISCUSSION 5 Fixed Restorations—cont'd

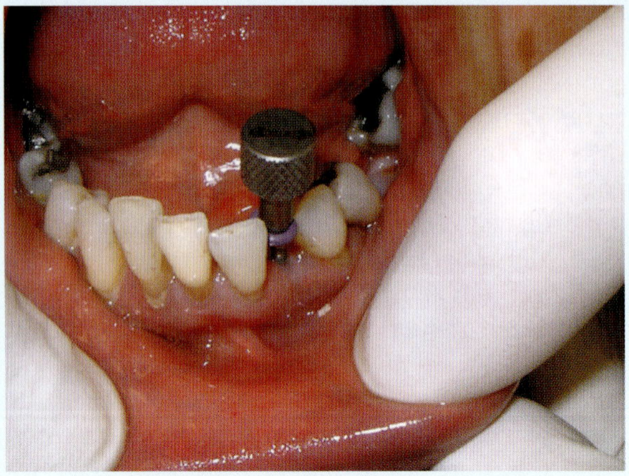

FIGURE 5-13e. MDI advanced into bone.

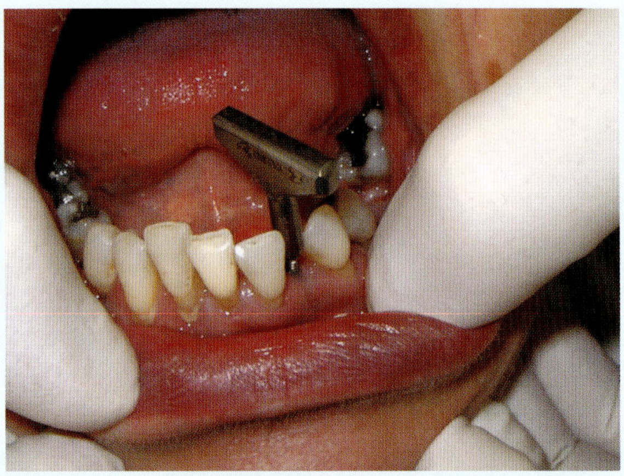

FIGURE 5-13f. MDI advanced to full depth.

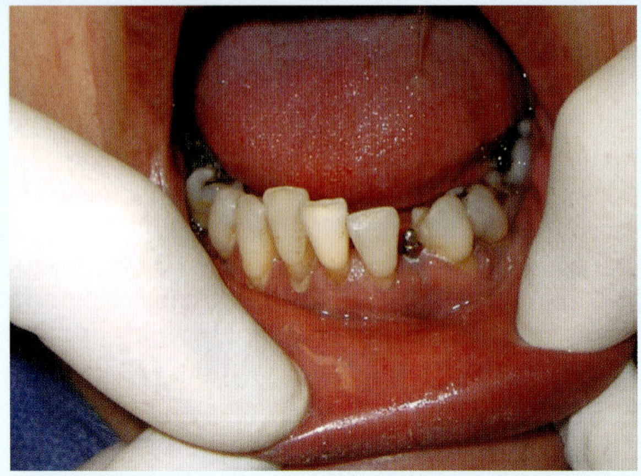

FIGURE 5-13g. MDI in place ready for restoration.

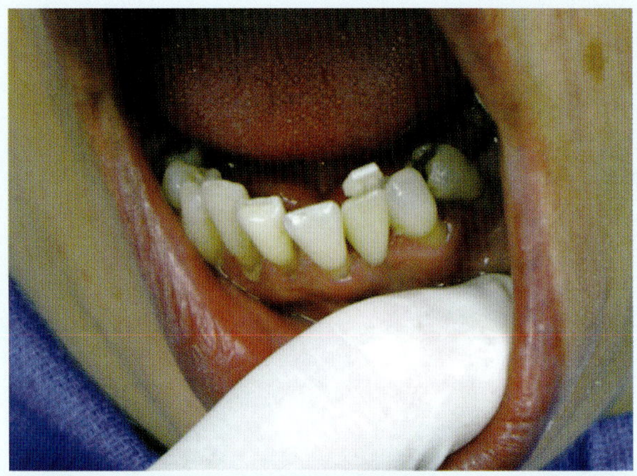

FIGURE 5-13h. Polycarbonate crown used to fabricate temporary restoration.

CASE DISCUSSION 6

We often find that a limitation to undergo conventional implant surgery is related simply to a patient's ability to sit in a routine dental setting. The next case is a 65-year-old woman whose medical history included multiple sclerosis (MS) and lung cancer in remission. She was confined to a motorized wheelchair. The majority of her care was done in her new wheelchair, which could tilt back to mimic the position of a dental chair, but before she had that wheelchair, moving her to a dental chair was required for anything more than minimal treatment. She had fractured the upper left first premolar (#12) and the remaining root segment was extracted (Figure 5-14a).

The patient desired a replacement. Due to MS, she could not sit in the dental chair for any length of time and, moreover, due to the advanced nature of the MS, she was prone to choking easily on fluids. After discussing her options, the preparation of a three-unit bridge was not advisable, and

CASE DISCUSSION 6—cont'd

a conventional implant was more surgery than she felt she could tolerate. It was decided to place a MSI. After 3 weeks of healing, she was scheduled for the procedure.

Under local anesthesia, the implant was placed under the standard minimally invasive nonsurgical protocol (Figure 5-14b).

A temporary crown was fabricated and cemented. The visit took 20 minutes and the patient was dismissed. The follow-up visit at which the impression for the final crown was taken took 20 minutes, and the delivery of the crown took 20 minutes. The patient had a fractured tooth replaced in 60 minutes of chair time over the course of 1 month without being moved from her wheelchair. Figures 5-14c and 5-14d show the 2-year and 4-year follow-up radiographs.

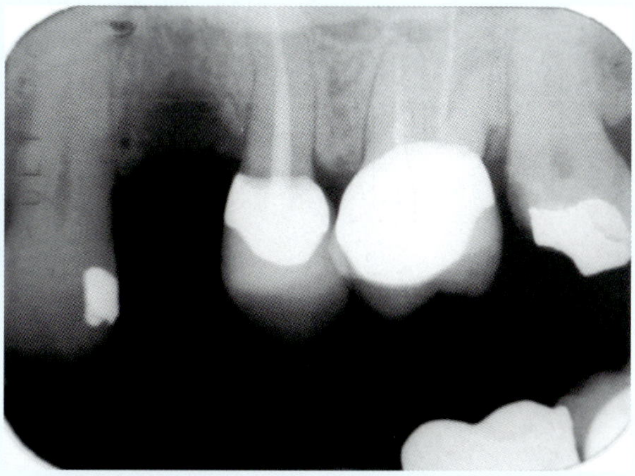

FIGURE 5-14a. Extraction of #12 healed.

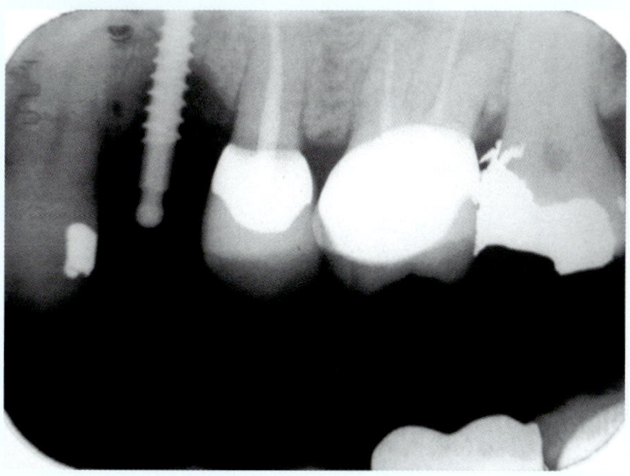

FIGURE 5-14b. MDI insertion.

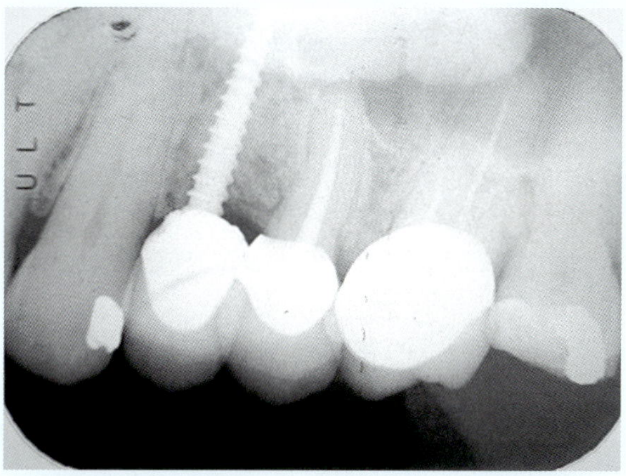

FIGURE 5-14c. Follow-up x-ray at 2 years.

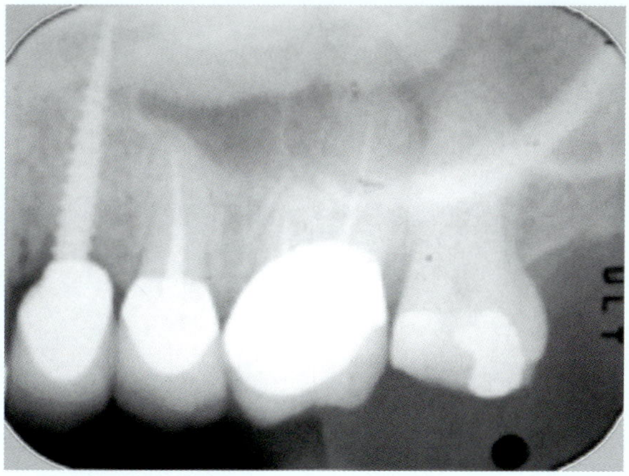

FIGURE 5-14d. Follow-up x-ray at 4 years.

Often, a case is limited by the lack of space required for a conventional implant. Small diameter implants are the fixture of choice in cases we refer to as salvage procedures. We often use MDIs to supplement conventional implants in areas where additional support is needed and even in cases of failing long-span bridges. The two cases that follow are illustrations of this point.

CASE DISCUSSION 7

The first is a very common patient presentation. Many patients have been involved with various implant restorations for many years and their panoramic x-ray looks like a teaching model for the various types of implants! This patient had a blade implant placed. Over the years the mesial aspect began to fail (Figure 5-15a). Over the years as other teeth in the quadrant failed, conventional root form implants were used to restore them. The blade showed no signs of mobility but developed occasional mucogingival infections.

Before periodontal surgery to degranulate and graft around the blade, it was decided that the mesial aspect needed additional support. There was not enough room between the blade and the root form implant for another conventional root form. A small diameter implant was selected to provide the needed support. A conventional flap was made and the blade implant exposed and the bony defect degranulated in preparation for bone grafting (Figure 5-15-b).

A MDI was placed in the site mesial to the blade, and the bridge was retrofitted and cemented (Figure 5-15c). In this case the MDI helped make a salvage procedure on the blade implant more successful by supporting the bridge and taking some occlusal load off the blade.

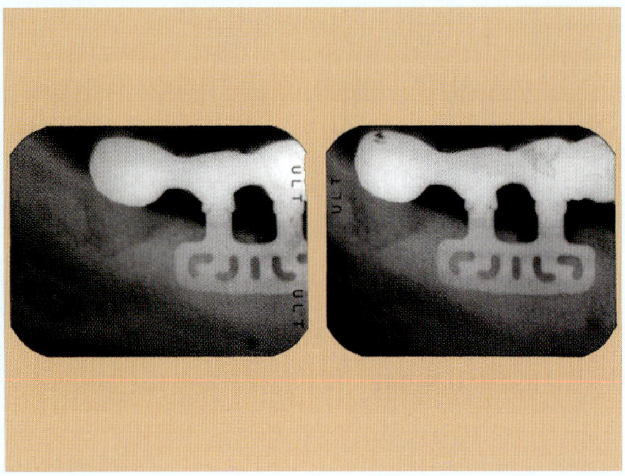

FIGURE 5-15a. Blade implant with bone loss on mesial aspect.

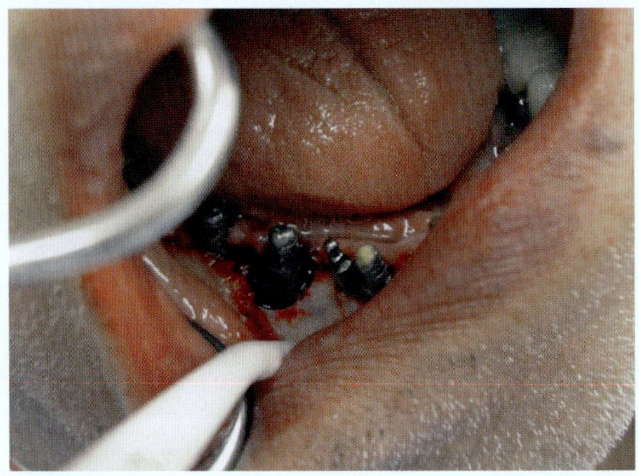

FIGURE 5-15b. Intraoperative view of bone defect around blade and MDI in place mesial to blade.

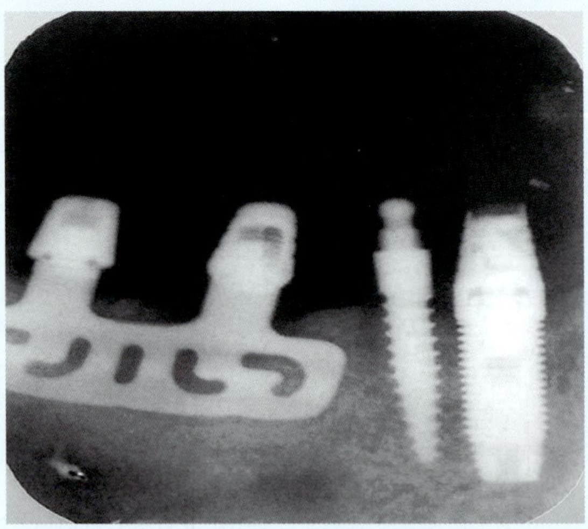

FIGURE 5-15c. Periapical of MDI.

CASE DISCUSSION 8

The next case is a true salvage procedure to save an implant supported fixed bridge that lost abutments due to decay (Figure 5-16a). The circumstances were not in favor of the patient getting more conventional implants and a new bridge, so we elected to use MDIs to support the bridge.

The bridge was removed and the roots were extracted. Holes were cut through the crowns to ensure that the implants would be placed at the proper angulations. Two implants were then placed, the bridge was recemented and the "access holes" were closed with composite (Figures 5-16b, c).

Figure 5-16d shows the 3-year clinical visit, retracted lip view. The soft tissue receded around the neck of one of the MDIs, but there was no mobility and no functional change. This salvage procedure saved the patient from the time and expense of a new fixed bridge. Figure 5-16e shows the smiling esthetics of the case 3 years after placement.

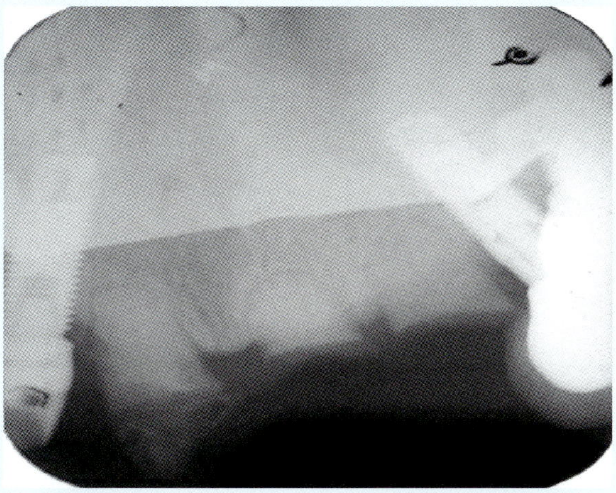

FIGURE 5-16a. Decayed abutment teeth.

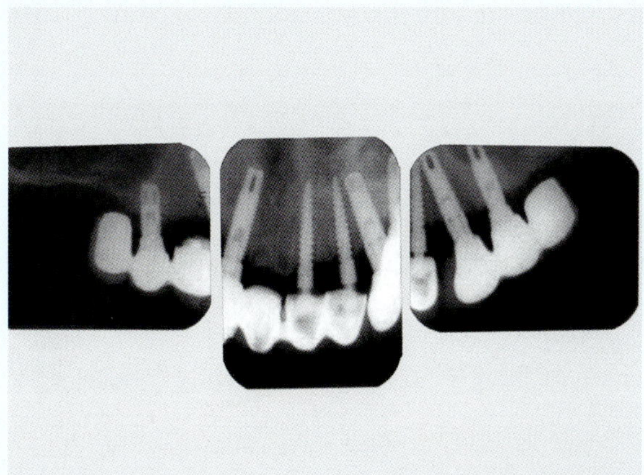

FIGURE 5-16c. X-rays after cementation.

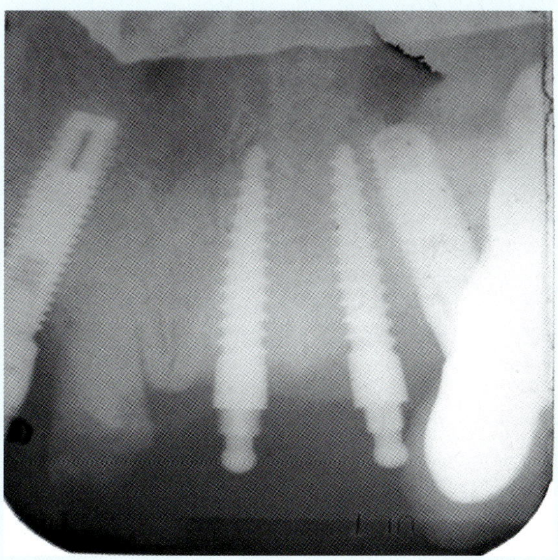

FIGURE 5-16b. Decayed teeth extracted and replaced with MDI.

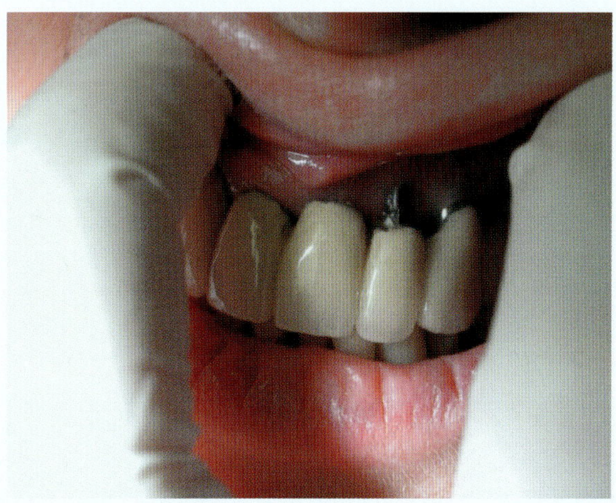

FIGURE 5-16d. Follow-up at 3 years, retracted view.

Continued

CASE DISCUSSION 8—cont'd

Often MDIs will be useful in all area of the mouth. The last case shows their use in the same patient for both fixed and removable prosthetics.

The patient wore a complete upper denture and was missing his lower front teeth for 5 years. He desired better denture retention and replacement of his missing lower anterior teeth.

He was not unhappy with his denture but wanted better retention. It was elected to place four implants in the maxilla with a sufficient anterior-posterior spread to give the denture better retention and better stability (Figure 5-16f). Four metal housings with O-rings were placed and picked up in the denture (Figure 5-16g).

The patient's lower anterior teeth were extracted due to periodontal disease approximately 5 years ago. Since then, the normal resorption pattern left a thin ridge, certainly not enough for conventional implants without ridge augmentation procedures. The MDIs were the best minimally invasive option. For financial reasons, the patient elected to have a lab processed temporary as his final restoration (Figures 5-16h, i).

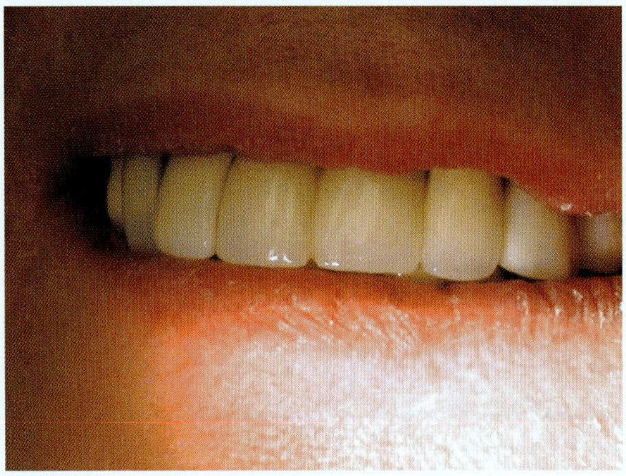

FIGURE 5-16e. Follow-up at 3 years, functional view.

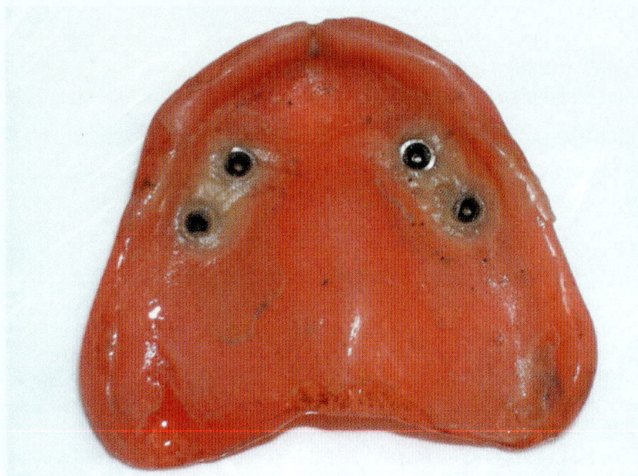

FIGURE 5-16g. Retrofitted denture with housings.

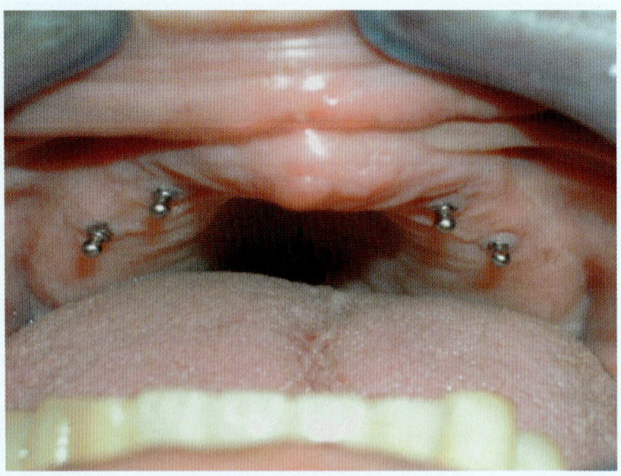

FIGURE 5-16f. MDIs in maxilla to retain denture.

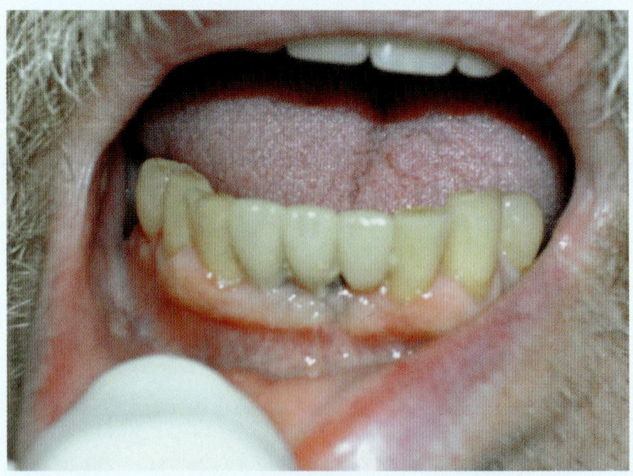

FIGURE 5-16h. Clinical retracted view of temporary in place.

CASE DISCUSSION 8—cont'd

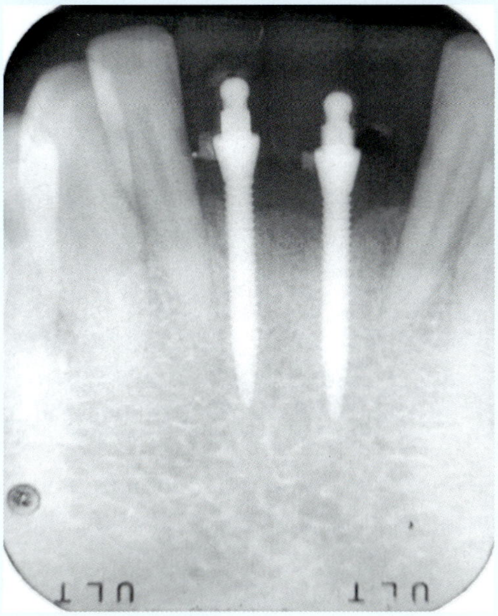

FIGURE 5-16i. Periapical of MDIs.

Everyday Problem-Solving with Mini Dental Implants: A Private Practitioner's General Practice Retrospective – Leonard R. Machi

If There is One Exception to a Rule then There is Proof that the Application of That Rule Must be Guided by Judgement

"Rules" in dentistry are rarely provable at the same level as mathematical proofs like "2 + 2 = 4" are. The science of dentistry is not nearly so developed. Too many variables exist, and so we rarely have exact answers, much less one right answer, to the problems patients need and desire us to solve for them.

Dentists must routinely rely both on their personal education (university and nonuniversity based) and all their experiential background to make judgments regarding proper patient care. At this time an organization called the "Dental Practice Based Research Network (website: http://www.dentalpbrn.org/home.asp) encourages dental practitioners in various ways to contribute data from their own practices about topics that university based research systems are not addressing or cannot address. As professionals it is the obligation of dentists to conscientiously broaden their educational and experiential backgrounds to make well-grounded, sound judgements concerning patient care.

Simply stated, clinical dentistry now and for any foreseeable future will require the use of professional judgment for even the most routine services provided. As the speed of development of new technologies increases and the introduction of new concepts expand the both the numbers and quality of options available for patient treatment it becomes more and more imperative for general dentists to investigate, study, and incorporate these advances appropriately into their practices.

Sendax mini dental implants (MDIs) warrant serious consideration for use in the general or for that matter any reconstructive or restorative based practice.

A Personal Pathway of Historical Experiential Evidence for Incorporating the Use of Sendax Mini Dental Implants into a General Practice

As previously stated, few if any "2 + 2 = 4" rules exist to confirm the particular desirability of using Sendax MDIs in every case for meeting any given patient's needs or desires. What is known at the "rule" level is that Sendax MDIs have FDA clearance to market to dentists for both short- and long-term use. This should usually be the starting point for most generalists to begin serious consideration of use of any noncustom implantable product's use.

This, coupled with the prospect of increasing patient treatment options, improving their outcomes, and my own personal experiential evidence, which included many similar implant placement protocols to those of the Sendax MDIs that have worked well for as long as 20 years for my own patients, led inevitably to the incorporation of Sendax MDIs into my own practice.

Several examples of similar successful protocols include:

1. Low/no heat generating hand instrumentation to place implants such as OMNI Implant hand held bone augers (Figure 5-17) eliminated bone heating while developing the implant osteotomy.
2. Dr. Hilt Tatum Jr. created the concept of bone expansion and developed instrumentation for it that requires little or no motorized drilling to create implant osteotomies (Figure 5-18). Frequently the implant itself acts the final expander. Also like the Sendax protocols, periods of rest during instrumentation are recommended to allow the bone to reshape itself without macrofracturing.
3. With the addition of increased availability and decreased costs for cross-sectional imaging to previous bone sounding techniques, flapless implant placement surgery has become more commonplace. Computer-aided sagittal and cross-sectional images show Sendax MDIs three-dimensional relationship to the maxillary bone and sinus (Figure 5-19).
4. MDIs have the strength to resist fracture under occlusal forces. There are a number of implant brands on the market that are 2 mm or less in diameter where they emerge at the bony crest of the ridge. I have experienced several cases of titanium endodontic stabilizers with diameters of

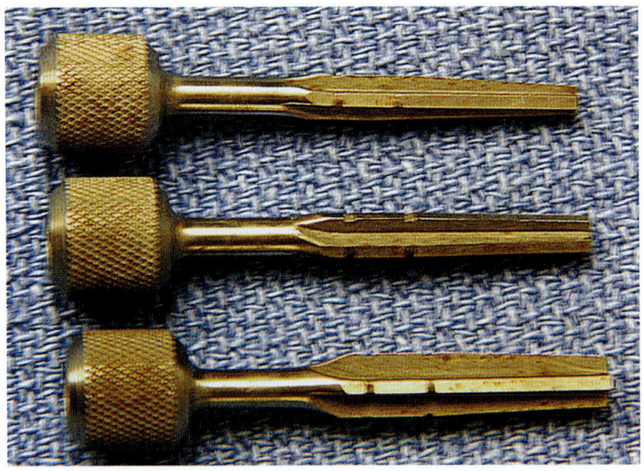

FIGURE 5-17. OMNI brand hand augers in 3.5, 4.0, 5.0 sizes. Note the deep grooves for harvesting bone without heat generation.

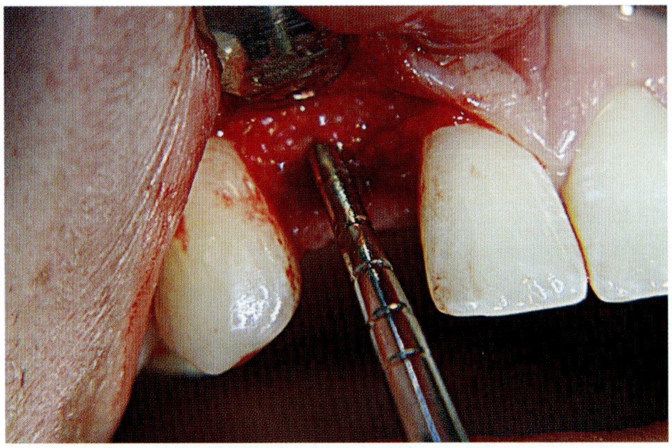

FIGURE 5-18. A 3.0 tapered bone spreader in place used to reshape and expand the patient's ridge width.

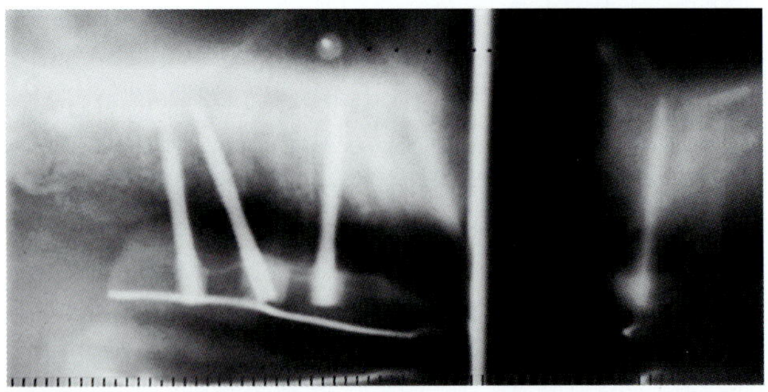

FIGURE 5-19. Postsurgical sagittal and cross-sectional images showing mini implant properly positioned in the bone to support a wire reinforced fixed acrylic prosthesis. Note the presence of a bone tack holding a membrane (not visible) of the adjacent bone graft.

2 mm or less that have successfully provided major support for a patient's prosthesis. Figure 5-20 shows an example of a 2.0-mm titanium endodontic stabilizer that was placed extending through a lower left cuspid to support a clip bar overdenture opposing natural dentition. After 2 years in function the stabilized cuspid was unrestorable due to recurrent decay and the tooth remains were removed; the 2-mm diameter endodontic stabilizer continued to function against fixed teeth without fracture, bone loss, or any other adverse response for 3 years more, after which time the office lost contact with the patient.

With the Sendax MDI data and personal experiential historical evidence, the question was no longer whether Sendax mini dental implants could work but how might they expand meeting patient needs, demands, and desires on a general practice in a safe and effective way.

A list of possible beneficial clinical uses and at least some patient risk factors should be considered before starting to clinically employ Sendax MDIs. The following list of factors is meant to help guide dentists considering incorporating MDIs into their own practices, but it is not to be considered a complete list, and the risk/benefit for each may vary between individual patients (not a "2 + 2 = 4" list).

Medical/Physical Factors

1. Straight forward/normal wound healing expected → complicated healing pattern expected.
2. Normal or controlled blood pressure → high/low pressure.
3. Negative history of stroke → history of stroke in the last 6 months.
4. Lack of drug or other allergy → serious allergies to drugs or materials that the patient might be exposed to during treatment.
5. No diabetes/well controlled diabetes → uncontrolled diabetes.
6. Healthy/no medications being taken or needed → medication limiting or preventing treatment.
7. Good tissue perfusion → poor tissue perfusion (i.e., cardiac pulmonary obstructive disease).
8. High vitality → low vitality.

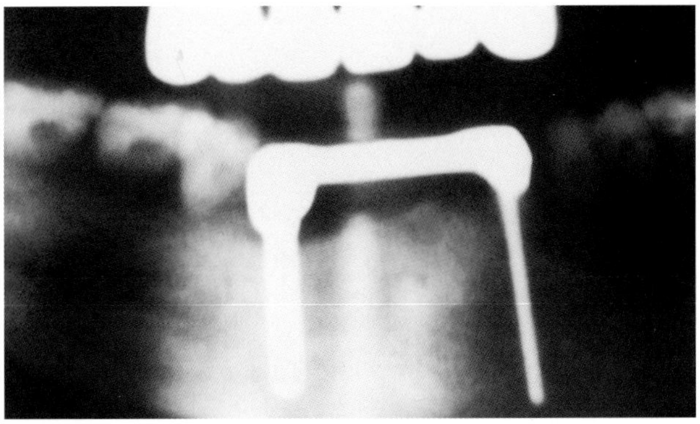

FIGURE 5-20. 3.25-mm diameter implant and a 2-mm diameter endodontic stabilizer supporting a bar overdenture. The cuspid supported by stabilizer decayed away leaving the stabilizer to act as a long-term "mini" implant.

Personality Factors

1. Easy going → demanding.
2. Adaptable → ridged.
3. Positive attitude → negative attitude.
4. Realistic attitude → unrealistic attitude.
5. High vitality → low vitality.

Dental Factors

1. Healthy bone and soft tissue → presence of bone and/or soft tissue infection.
2. No parafunctional jaw habits → extreme parafunctional jaw habits.
3. No tongue habits → severe tongue habits
4. Low biting forces → high biting forces.
5. Nonsmoking → heavy smoking.
6. No/low alcohol consumption → high alcohol consumption.
7. Treatment to oppose soft tissue supported teeth (i.e., denture) → treatment to oppose ridged teeth.
8. History of long-term success with implant therapy → history of failed implant therapy over a short term.
9. Location of fixed treatment to be in a cosmetic zone → location of implant to be in a noncosmetic zone.

Anatomical Factors

1. Implant location to be in basal bone → location to be in alveolar bone.
2. Implant location to be in high quality dense bone → location to be in low extremely porous poor quality bone.
3. Implant location to be in high quality bone with accessible cortical plates → implant location to be in nonaccessible/absent cortical plates.
4. More than adequate bone quantity available → less than adequate bone quantity available.

5. Long, narrow jawed with excellent anteroposterior (AP) spread → short, square jawed with insignificant AP spread.
6. Adequate attached gingival tissue → lack of attached gingival tissue.
7. No/low muscle pulls in treatment area → high strong muscle pulls present.

Therapy End Goals/Endpoints

1. Short term/provisional therapy → fixed long term endpoint therapy.
2. Removable treatment as endpoint therapy → fixed treatment as endpoint therapy.
3. Removable short-term treatment → removable long-term treatment.
4. Multiple implants with cross arch stabilization → single free standing implant therapy.
5. Traditional use for snap on overdenture or short-term fixed therapy → complex use of implant (i.e., orthodontic anchorage).
6. Retreatment of failed nonimplant case → retreatment of failed implant case.
7. Retreatment of failed traditional (nonimplant) dentistry → initial treatment of a straightforward concern of a patient (first time treatment).

Miscellaneous

1. Financially capable → financially limited.
2. Previously connected to the practice → new patient without connection.
3. Referred by a patient in the practice → referred through outside paid advertising.
4. Not cosmetically demanding → cosmetically driven.
5. Sufficient time available for treatment completion → limited time available (dentist's or patient's).
6. Reliable for keeping appointments → unreliable.
7. Reliable for following directions → unreliable.

A healthy patient with good bone quantity and quality with either short-term fixed partial arch treatment or full lower arch removable overdenture opposing an upper denture is rated as low risk; a medically compromised patient needing retreatment of failed implants with new implants is rated as high risk.

If the MDIs were to be the final treatment they were considered more risky, but if to be used provisionally less risky.

If patients had medical, physical, or other complicating factors, they were considered more risky; if medically normal and healthy without other complicating factors, they were considered less risky.

If patients had poor bone quality and were anatomically limited, they were considered more risky; but if they had high bone quality and adequate amounts of bone, they were rated less risky and so on.

Sendax MDI treatments were incorporated into the practice starting with low-risk, high-benefit treatments until our practice became experienced and comfortable with more complex MDI treatments. This is ongoing.

As is the case in all other areas of clinical practice, dentists must constantly sharpen their implant therapy skills to provide good professional judgment when offering modern, risk-managed treatments to meet the needs and desires of their patients.

Case Discussions

Here are some general practice cases of Sendax MDI uses.

CASE DISCUSSION 9 Complete Arch with Removable Treatment Endpoint Prosthetics

EXAMPLE

Maxillary and mandibular complete arch MDI retained over dentures endpoint treatment.

Patient history: A nonsmoking 68-year-old completely edentulous woman with an unremarkable medical/dental history. The patient had adequate anterior bone height and width for straightforward implant placement (Figures 5-21a, b).

Patient need: Improving retention of loose dentures to make more stable and comfortable in function.

Patient desire: Use implants to aid in long-term bone maintenance at a reasonable cost.

Endpoint treatment included placement of six maxillary and four mandibular Sendax MDIs (Figures 5-21c-e) and retrofitting the patient's current dentures.

CASE DISCUSSION 9 Complete Arch with Removable Treatment Endpoint Prosthetics—cont'd

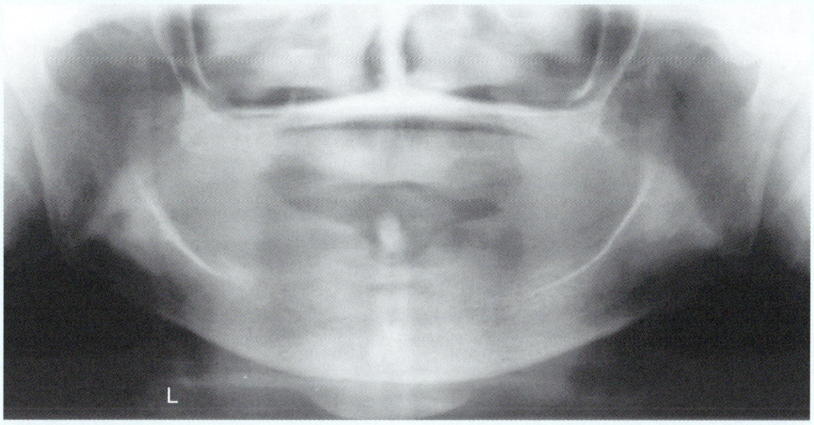

FIGURE 5-21a. Panoramic radiograph demonstrating adequate bone height.

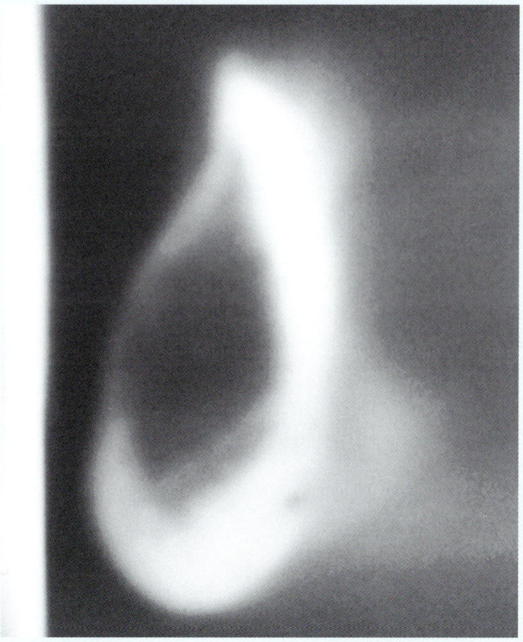

FIGURE 5-21b. Cross-sectional tomographic image showing adequate height and width for MDI placement in the area of the symphysis.

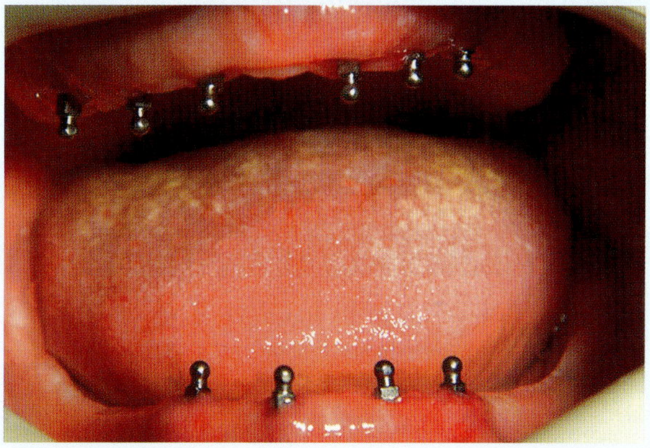

FIGURE 5-21c. Healthy attached gingival tissue surrounding the Sendax MDI at 6-month follow-up appointment.

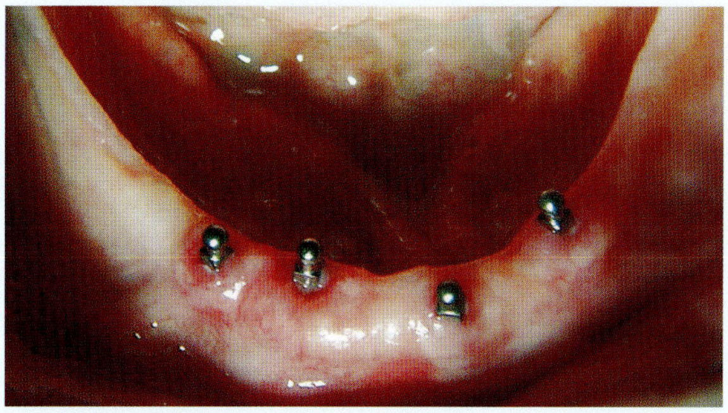

FIGURE 5-21d. Somewhat nonparallel/misaligned implants can function well and maintain a healthy bone and soft tissue state with O-rings retention.

Continued

CASE DISCUSSION 9 Complete Arch with Removable Treatment Endpoint Prosthetics—cont'd

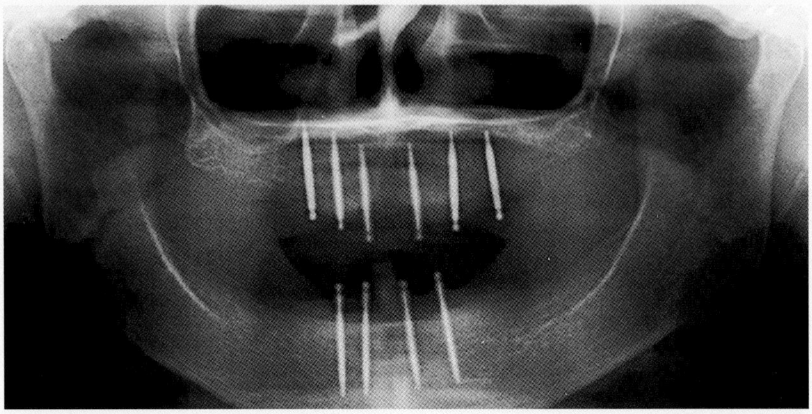

FIGURE 5-21e. Posttreatment panoramic radiograph showing typical placement of MDIs for upper and lower overdenture retention. Note that the maxillary implants are placed anterior to the maxillary sinuses, with the two most anterior implants placed lateral to the maxillary nerve and foramen. The mandibular implants are located in the symphysis area anterior to the mandibular nerve and foramen. All demonstrate bicortical stabilization for maximum osseoapposition support.

CASE DISCUSSION 10 Fixed Short Term

EXAMPLE 1

Complete arch short term.

Patient history: 45-year-old 275-lb man unable to eat normal diet with malocclusion, advanced periodontitis with tooth mobility, and severe gag reflex.

Patient need: Fixed upper and lower teeth.

Patient desire: Keep any teeth that are serviceable and cannot be without teeth during treatment (Figure 5-22a).

Phase I: Immediate maxillary fixed. Provisionalization with Sendax MDIs after upper teeth were

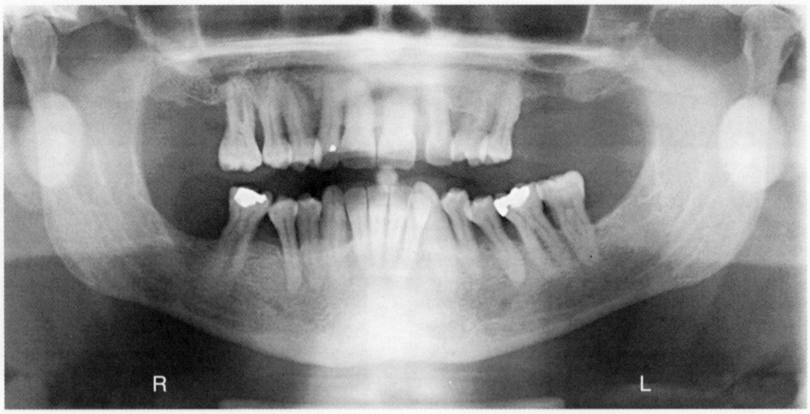

FIGURE 5-22a. Pretreatment panoramic radiograph. Note that in this case, unlike the mandible, no maxillary stable teeth are available to use as interim fixed treatment abutments.

CASE DISCUSSION 10 Fixed Short Term—cont'd

extracted from first molar to first molar, Placement of fixed mandibular provisional after crown preparations of the lower first molars (to be extracted in Phase III) and the three lower incisors (to be retained for endpoint treatment), Placement of mandibular endpoint implants where possible (Figure 5-22b).

Phase II: Maxillary implant placement after 6 months of healing. Note: Sendax MDIs continued functioning without problems against fixed lower teeth first during 6 months socket healing and then 6 months more while larger diameter maxillary implants were healing (Figure 5-22c).

Phase III: Included the removal of the two remaining mandibular molars. Placement of an implant in the lower left first molar socket, abutment connections, removal of the Sendax MDIs, and the fabrication of the final porcelain fused to metal prosthetics (Figure 5-22d).

EXAMPLE 2

Partial Arch Short Term

Patient history: 72-year-old man with medically controlled high blood pressure with failed upper right molars, bicuspids, and cuspid.

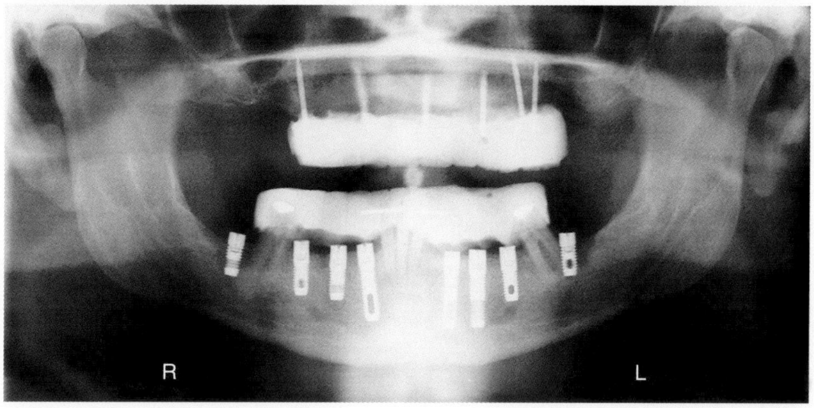

FIGURE 5-22b. Phase I 6-month healing period panoramic radiograph showing six Sendax MDIs supporting an acrylic fixed provisional bridge from first molar to first molar for the 6-months' socket healing for the maxillary sockets.

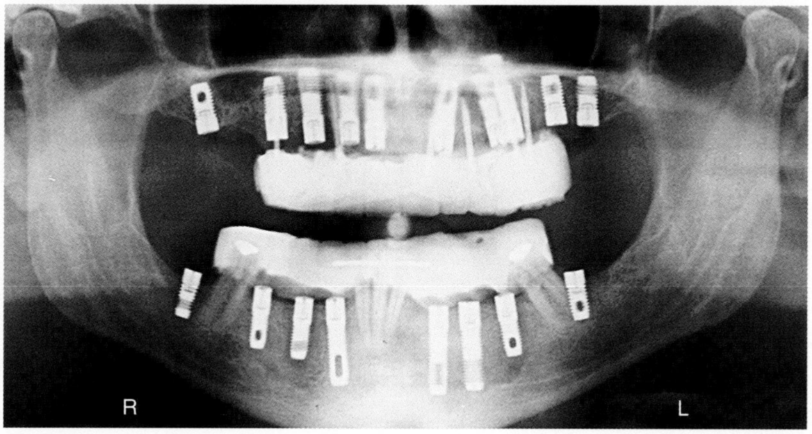

FIGURE 5-22c. After phase II intratreatment panoramic radiograph. Note the ability of Sendax MDIs to support fixed provisional teeth for more than 1 year without bone loss or discomfort, allowing for a smooth transition to a conventional implant prosthodontic support system for the full mouth reconstruction.

Continued

CASE DISCUSSION 10 Fixed Short Term—cont'd

Patient need: Fixed replacement to restore unilateral tooth loss soft tissue and bone defects and keep stress off remaining teeth (which are compromised) in the arch (Figure 5-23a).

Patient desire: Fixed teeth throughout treatment period. Patient does not wish teeth replaced past the first molar area.

Treatment included: Removal of failing teeth and placement of Sendax MDIs for immediate provisionalization (Figure 5-23b) along with socket grafts and placement of larger diameter implants (Figure 5-23c) to be used for endpoint treatment. In this case three Sendax MDIs were used for the provisional implants and an immediately loaded larger diameter implant. The positioning of two MDIs in buccal/lingual opposition enabled better treatment bridge stability and more room to position the endpoint implants.

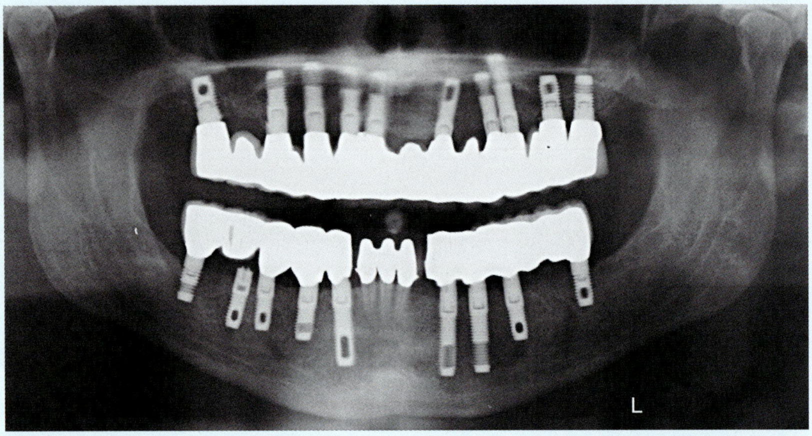

FIGURE 5-22d. Five-year follow-up endpoint treatment panoramic radiograph showing excellent long-term stability of the bone.

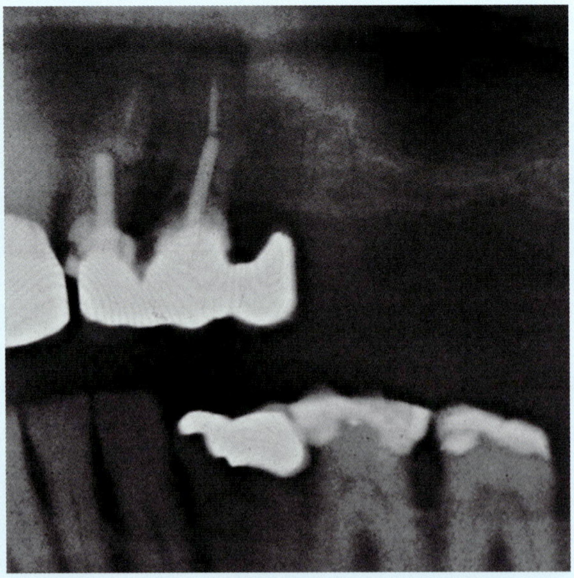

FIGURE 5-23a. Failing teeth in maxillary right quadrant. Note the periodontal defect between the cuspid and first bicuspid.

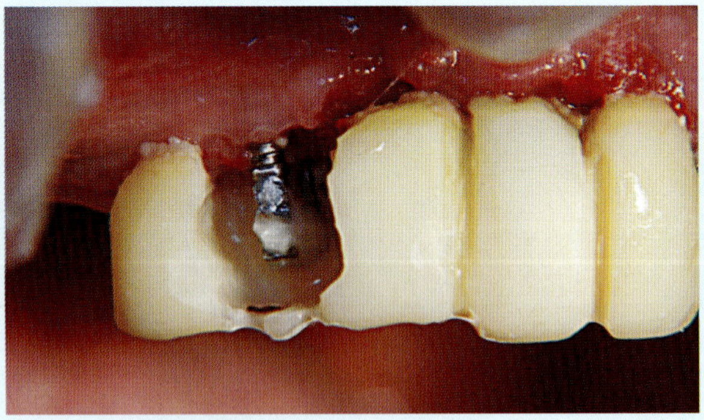

FIGURE 5-23b. Treatment in progress at removal of provisional acrylic bridge, which was freed by cutting the acrylic away. This had been permanently cemented on the Sendax MDIs to prevent any loosening.

CASE DISCUSSION 10 Fixed Short Term—cont'd

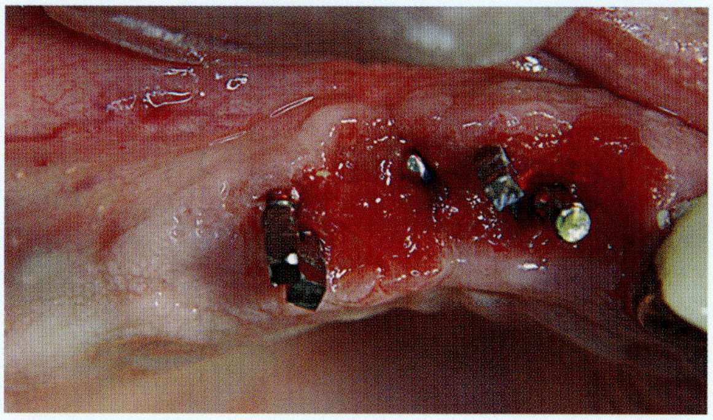

FIGURE 5-23c. Second stage surgery with both mini and regular sized implants. Note the buccal-lingual positions of the distal Sendax MDIs to improve support in Type III and IV bone and provide additional space for the endpoint implants for this patient.

CASE DISCUSSION 11 Fixed Long-Term Single Crown

Patient history: 28-year-old woman with unremarkable medical history with failing lower left lateral incisor primary and congenitally missing permanent successor with insufficient space to place an implant or construct a bridge with normal size pontics.

Patient need: Correction and stabilization of incisor area.

Patient desire: Fixed provisional porcelain veneer crown as soon as possible and fixed long-term implant supported free standing restoration.

Treatment included: Lower fixed orthodontics with open coil spring to create space for a 1.8 Sendax MDI placement (Figure 5-24a). The implant was immediately provisionalized with a composite crown bonded to adjacent teeth to stabilize the area see (Figure 5-24b). After 3 months a free standing porcelain veneer crown was constructed (Figure 5-24c).

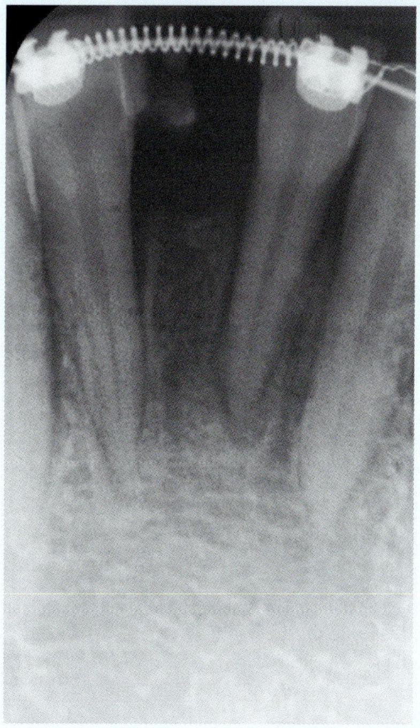

FIGURE 5-24a. Intratreatment periapical radiograph. Note the wider periodontal ligaments of the teeth adjacent to the edentulous space.

Continued

CASE DISCUSSION 11 Fixed Long-Term Single Crown—cont'd

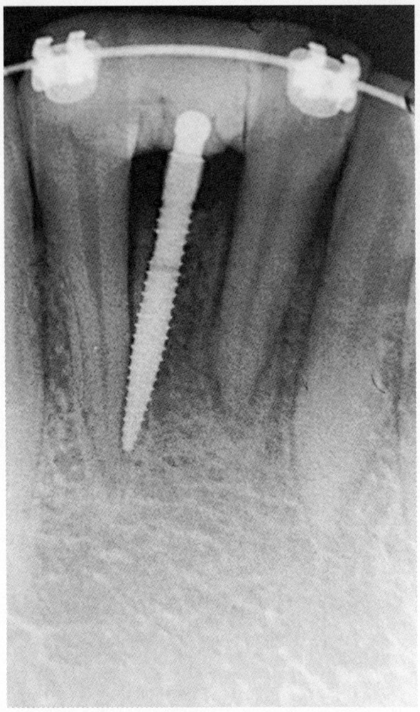

FIGURE 5-24b. Sendax 1.8-mm diameter implant in place with immediate composite provisional bonded to adjacent teeth to allow bone healing and solidification around the implant and adjacent teeth.

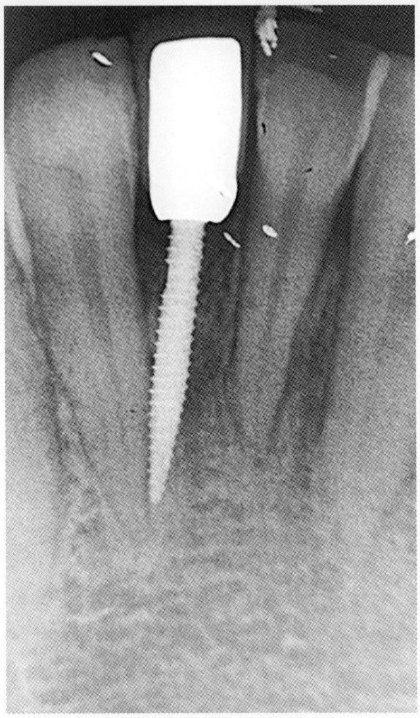

FIGURE 5-24c. Endpoint metal ceramic crown in place. Note the decreased periodontal ligament width.

CASE DISCUSSION 12 Fixed Long-Term Bridge Abutment

EXAMPLE 1

Anterior abutment.

Patient history: A 54-year-old 240-lb man, cigar and cigarette smoker with concurrent daily low dose aspirin and blood pressure controlled with medication.

Dental history: Included previous failure to adapt to removable partial denture, failing upper and lower dentition due to carries with moderate bony atrophy and periodontal disease (Figure 5-25a).

Patient need: Included rebuilding of deficient bone where needed to place sufficient implant support for fixed upper and lower restorations.

Patient desires: Included fixed interim treatment of approximately 1 year (during socket, implant and graft healing).

Interim treatment: Included removal of remaining teeth, bilateral subantral augmentation, placement of Sendax MDIs, and larger diameter implants (some with abutments to immediate load with the minis), and an acrylic prosthesis (Figure 5-25b).

Note: Use of Sendax MDI immediately loaded to share support of upper and lower provisional acrylic bridges with larger diameter implants and a natural tooth.

Endpoint treatment: Included keeping upper Sendax MDIs permanently to share support of the

CASE DISCUSSION 12 Fixed Long-Term Bridge Abutment—cont'd

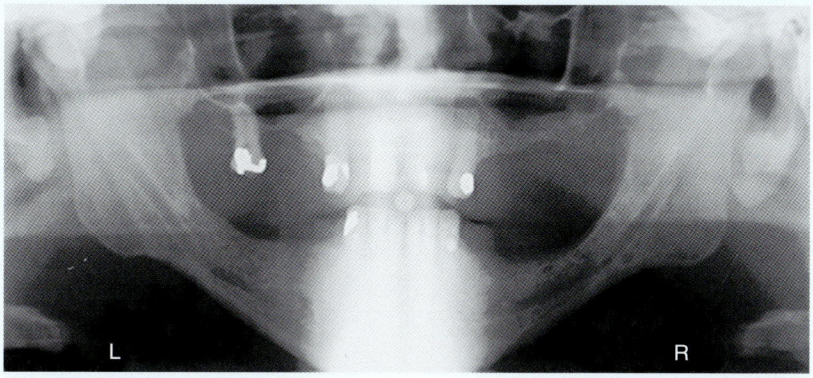

FIGURE 5-25a. Preoperative panoramic radiograph showing enlarged sinuses and atrophic mandibular bone.

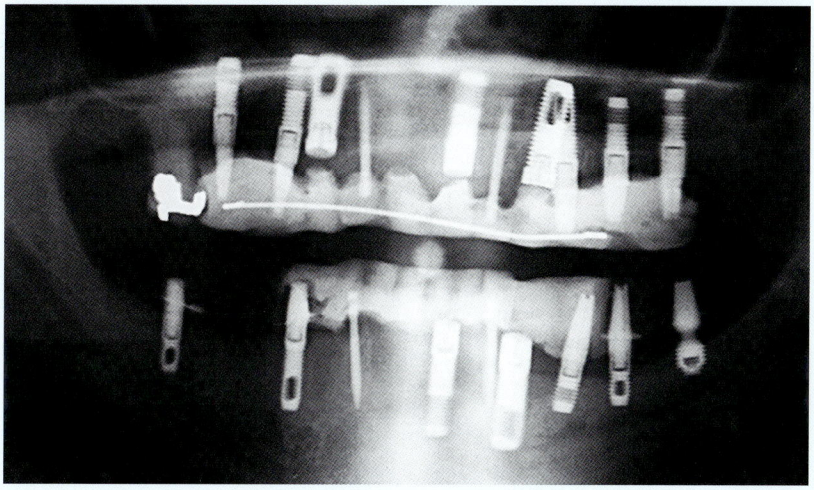

FIGURE 5-25b. Intratreatment panoramic radiograph showing Sendax MDIs and larger diameter implants supporting and immediately loaded provisional prosthesis. Note the broken opposing acrylic areas damaged by traumatic clenching.

final porcelain fused to metal fixed bridges. Also note that one Sendax MDI replacing an upper lateral incisor acted as a pier abutment for a bridge while the other acted to support a splinted crown (Figures 5-25c, d).

EXAMPLE 2

Posterior abutment: Fixed long term posterior bridge abutment.

Patient history: Postmenopausal woman, previous smoker, with an otherwise unremarkable medical history presented with failing teeth with some areas of atrophic bone due to advanced periodontal disease.

Patient need: Patient profession included public speaking requiring the ability to have fixed teeth during treatment to prevent excessive loss of personal income. The treatment of her dental needs was postponed for several years until an immediate fixed tooth solution was found.

Patient desire: Included complete fixed porcelain veneer crown and bridge as endpoint treatment (Figure 5-26a) showing continued loss of bone due to inability to originally treat patient chief complaint with immediate fixed teeth provisionals.

Intermediate treatment: Included removal of remaining teeth with immediate placement of Sendax 1.8-mm diameter MDIs in the maxilla

Continued

CASE DISCUSSION 12 Fixed Long-Term Bridge Abutment—cont'd

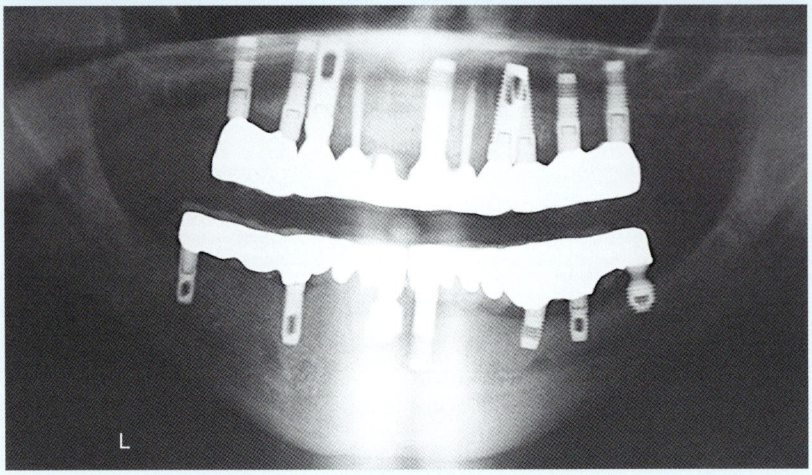

FIGURE 5-25c. Posttreatment panoramic radiograph showing use of Sendax MDIs as permanent anterior abutments. Note the upper right lateral MDI used as a splinted crown and the upper left mini implant acting as a pier abutment.

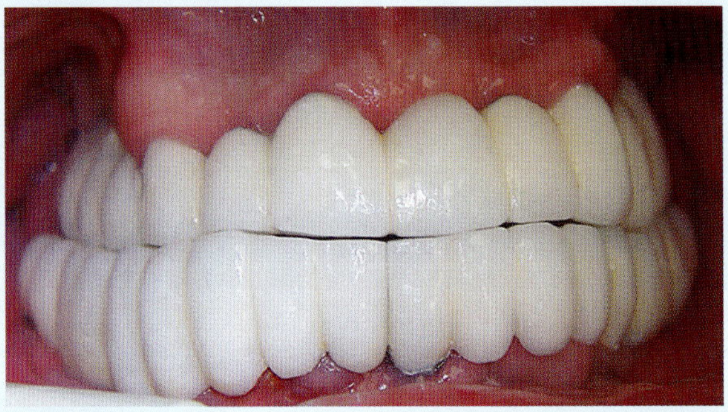

FIGURE 5-25d. Posttreatment photo showing the gingival architecture being maintained by using MDIs throughout the reconstructive process.

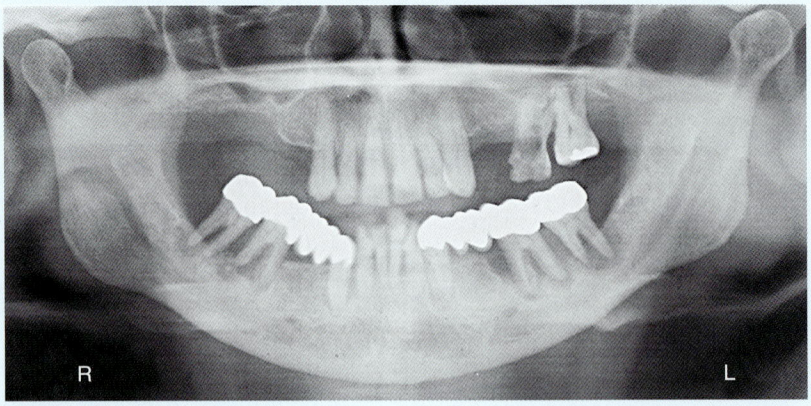

FIGURE 5-26a. Pretherapy panoramic radiograph. Note the extensive bone loss due to periodontal disease and overretention of failing teeth.

CASE DISCUSSION 12 Fixed Long-Term Bridge Abutment—cont'd

along with mandibular placement of both Sendax MDIs and larger diameter implants to support fully loaded fixed acrylic provisionals. Due to poor bone quality two MDIs were placed temporarily in the upper right second bicuspid area (Figure 5-26b). Later two of the MDIs were retained in the end-point prosthetics.

End treatment: Included placement of additional larger diameter implants and removal of the upper Sendax MDIs except for the lower left first bicuspid and one of the upper rights second bicuspid has buccal-lingual "doubled" MDIs (Figure 5-26c).

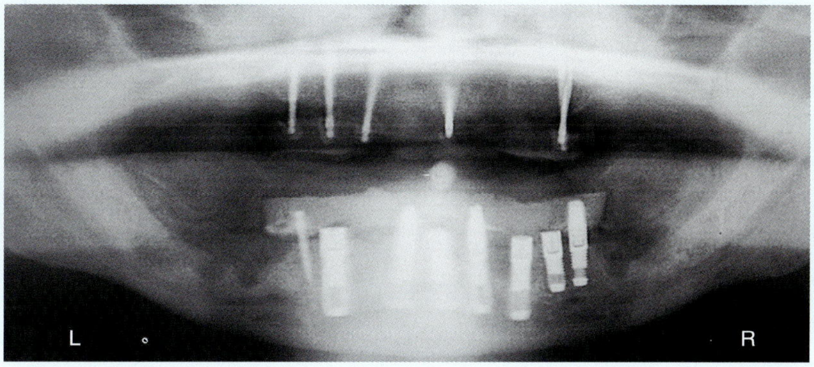

FIGURE 5-26b. Intratreatment panoramic radiograph. Note the presence of the single lower left Sendax MDI supporting the provisional, which, with one of two upper right bicuspid implants, were retained in the endpoint porcelain-veneer bridge restoration.

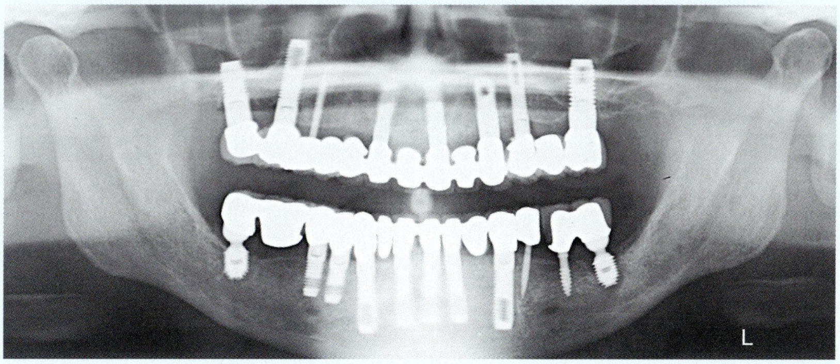

FIGURE 5-26c. Radiograph 5 years after treatment. Note the lower left Sendax MDI being used as the most distal bridge abutment to aid support, stability, and retention. Also note the remaining upper right second bicuspid mini implant being used as a pier abutment.

CASE DISCUSSION 13 Medically or Physically Compromised Patients: Complete Mandibular Overdenture

Patient history: An 86-year-old woman unable to wear her complete mandibular denture was unable to eat.

Medical history: Osteoporosis, cardiac disease, and limited ability for personal oral hygiene due to arthritis. Additionally, the patient's cardiologist recommended only flapless surgery immediately after clotting time tests at his office. Anatomically the patient had atrophic bone and bilateral dehiscence of the mandibular nerves (Figures 5-27a-c) and dysphasia from a denture-sore mouth.

Patient need: Stabilization of her lower denture with using a minimally invasive technique.

Patient desire: The ability to eat comfortably.

Pretreatment: Included blood tests at the patient's cardiologist office and bilateral tomographic imaging for guiding implant placement without flaps.

Patient treatment: Included flapless technique protocol for lower Sendax MDI placement under minimal infiltration local anesthesia. Due to the osteoporotic nature of the bone, four Sendax max thread design and one standard thread design

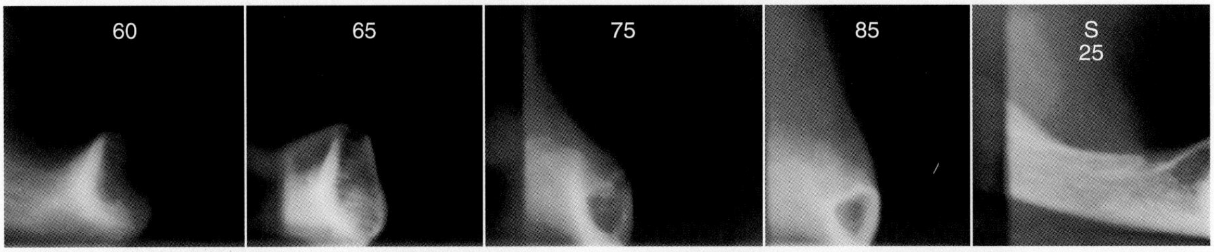

FIGURE 5-27a. Tomographic images of mandible cross-sectional and sagittal images. Note the dehiscence nerves slice (S25) and the resorbed posterior anatomy on the cross sections 65, 75, 85.

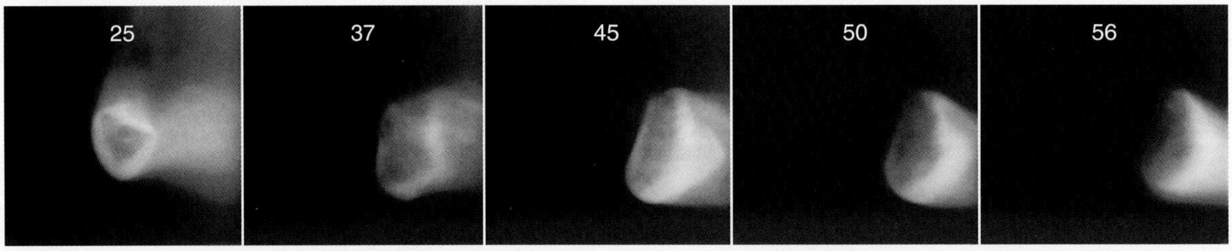

FIGURE 5-27b. Tomographic images of resorbed mandible. Note the pencil thin posterior image on cross section (25).

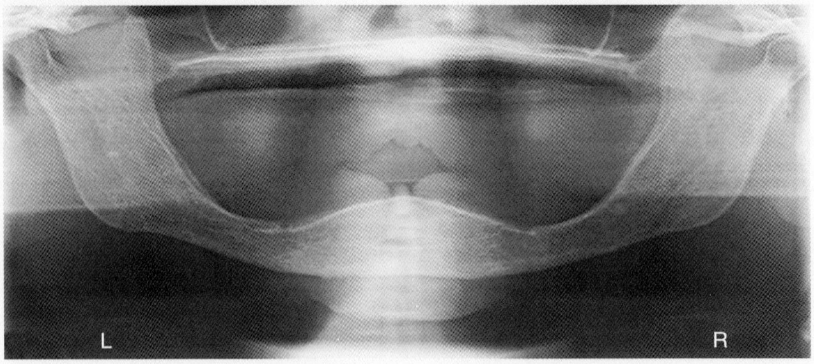

FIGURE 5-27c. Pretherapy panoramic radiograph. Note the generalized resorbed mandible with bilateral dehiscence mandibular nerves.

CASE DISCUSSION 13 Medically or Physically Compromised Patients: Complete Mandibular Overdenture—cont'd

implants were placed (Figures 5-27d,e). At the cardiologist's request the patient was to return for immediate follow-up. One week later this was followed by the fabrication of a new mandibular overdenture; 3-year follow-up showed healthy gingival and bony tissue (Figure 5-27f).

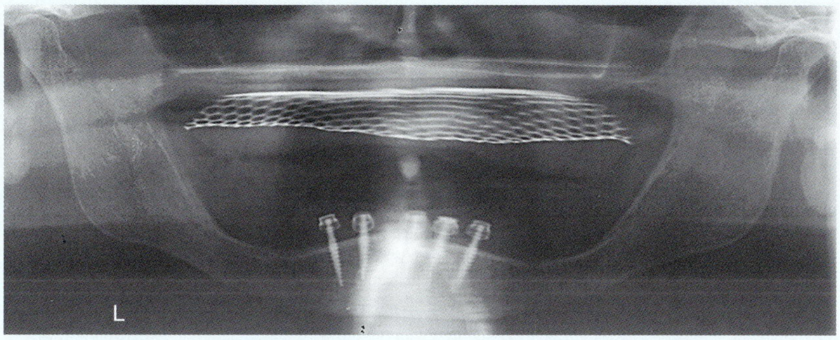

FIGURE 5-27d. Panoramic radiograph at 3-year follow-up. Note the lower denture with O-ring keepers fully seated in place.

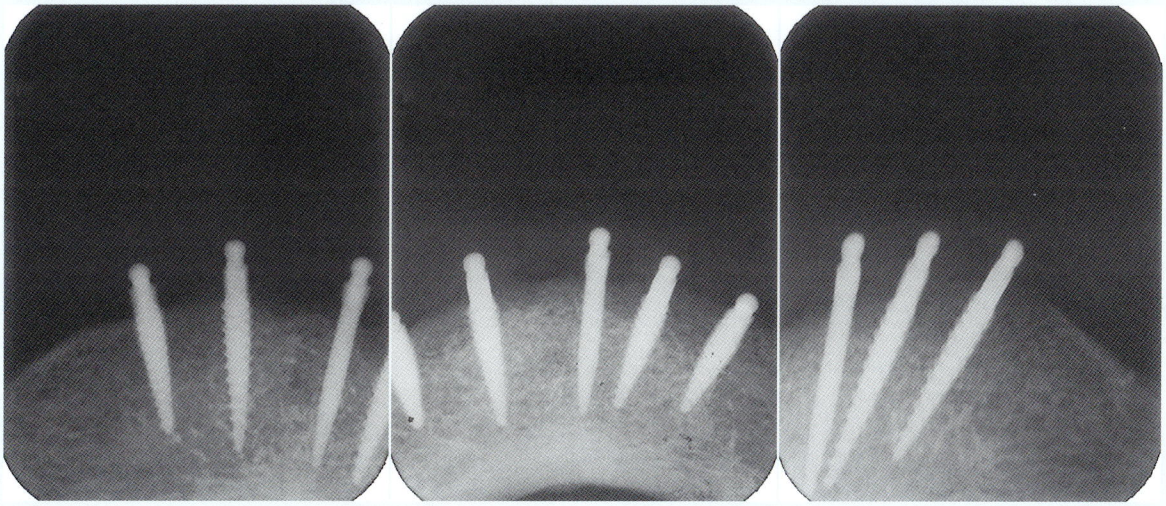

FIGURE 5-27e. Overlapping periapical radiographs at 3-year follow-up. Note the healthy bone level on all five Sendax MDIs. The middle implant is a standard mini while the other four are of the max thread design.

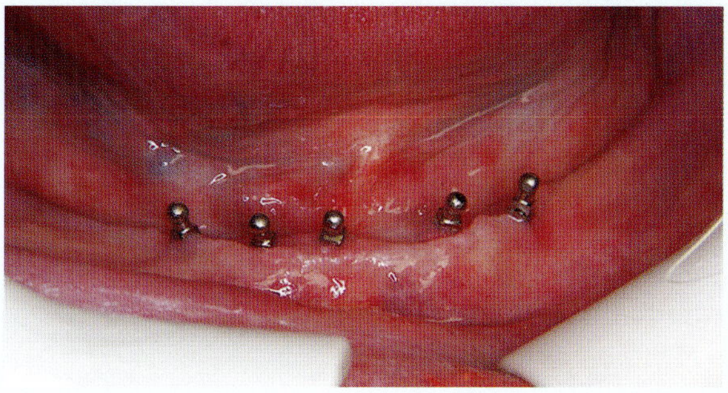

FIGURE 5-27f. End treatment photo 3 years later showing healthy tissue surrounding the Sendax MDIs.

CASE DISCUSSION 14 Orthodontic Anchorage

EXAMPLE 1

Orthodontic anchorage was used to reposition molar teeth while holding the adjacent tooth/teeth positions and minimizing the need for brackets and bands.

Patient history: 28-year-old woman with unremarkable medical history with missing lower right first molar, severely tipped lower right second and third molars with periodontal defect and rotated first bicuspid (Figure 5-28a).

Patient need: Correction of tipped molar malocclusion and correction of periodontal defect area lower left second molar.

Patient desire: Not wearing full arch orthodontic appliance and desires amalgams changed to cosmetic restorations.

Diagnosis: Tipped lower right second and third molars, rotated first bicuspid contributing to periodontal inflammation of molars, amalgam tattooing of the lower right bicuspids and first molar.

Treatment selected: Placing a 1.8-mm diameter Sendax MDI in remaining space between lower right second bicuspid and mesially inclined second molar (Figures 5-28b, c). Created occlusal clearance for the implant by removing the ball top (Figure 5-28d). The implant was bonded to the second

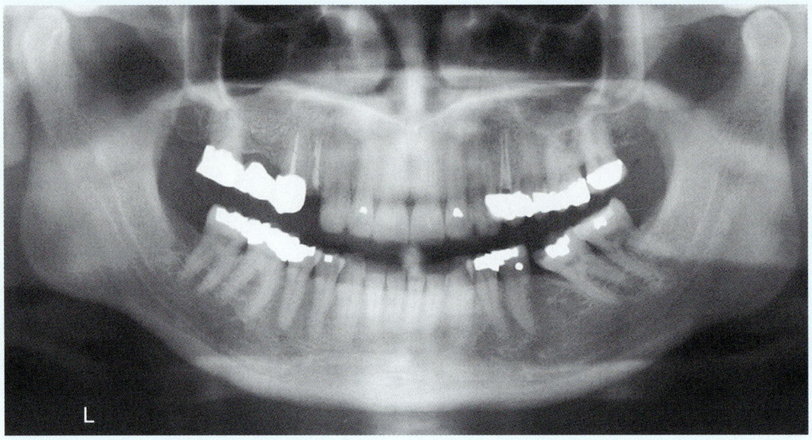

FIGURE 5-28a. Pretreatment panoramic radiograph showing missing lower right first molar with the second and third molars tipped into the space.

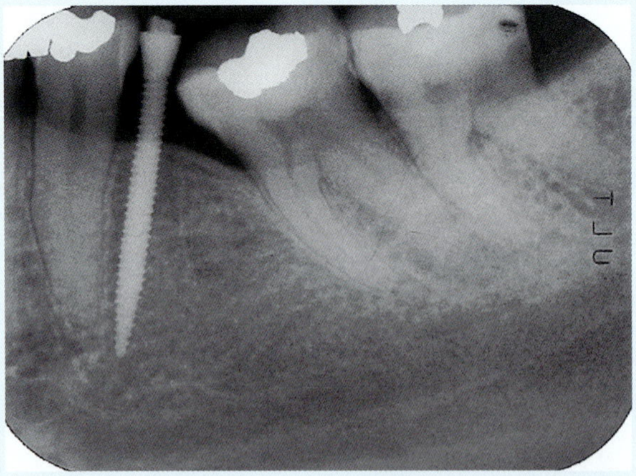

FIGURE 5-28b. Periapical radiograph of standard Sendax MDI in place for orthodontic anchorage. Note the lack of interproximal space for the implant to be fully seated and the ball portion removed for occlusal clearance.

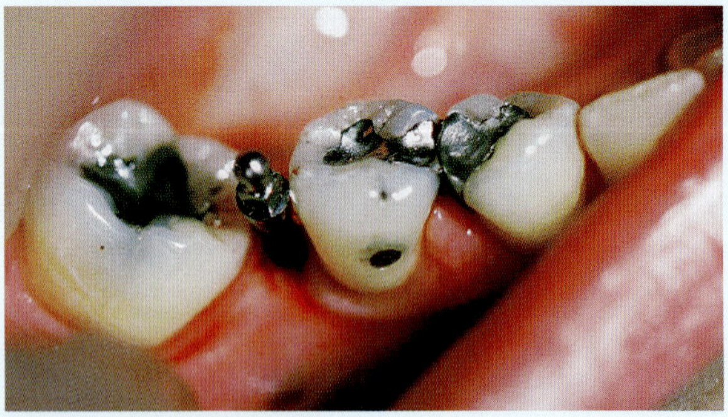

FIGURE 5-28c. MDI 1.8-mm diameter standard design in place for orthodontic anchorage.

CASE DISCUSSION 14 Orthodontic Anchorage—cont'd

bicuspid to prevent movement of the teeth anterior to the first molar space. Bonded brackets and molar band were placed only from lower right cuspid to lower right third molar. It was then safe to place an open coil spring to upright the molars. The rotation of the first bicuspid was accomplished by the arch wire itself with the bonded MDI preventing the second bicuspid from any movement (Figure 5-28e). After 3 months in which the molars were in the process of uprighting (Figure 5-28f), the mesial defect of lower right second molar was grafted with a mixture of irradiated bone (60%) and the beta form of tricalcium phosphate (40%) (Figures 5-28g-i).After 2 more months of retracting/closing the space (Figures 5-28j, k), the teeth were ready for final cosmetic restorations (Figure 5-28l).

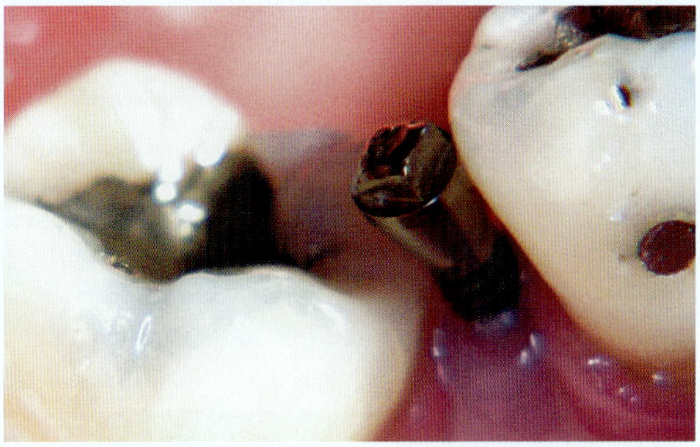

FIGURE 5-28d. Sendax 1.8-mm diameter with ball top removed for occlusal clearance and the square collar intact for later retrieval after the molar up righting competed.

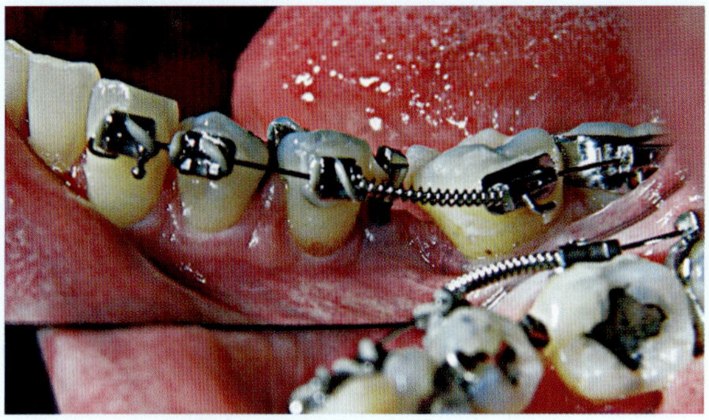

FIGURE 5-28f. Treatment in progress of uprighting and distally moving the molar. Note the space opening between the implant and molar but not between the bonded implant and bicuspid.

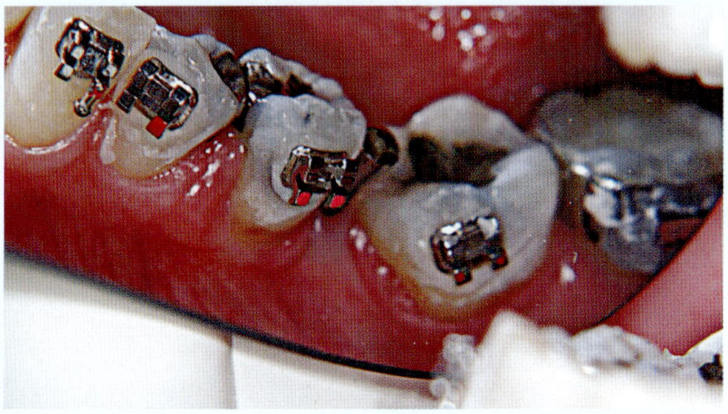

FIGURE 5-28e. The bonded and bracketed teeth. Note the severe angulation of the first molar with contact distally with the third molar requiring the anchorage by the Sendax MDI to be sufficient to upright and distally move the molar segment without causing anterior segment to advance facially. Also the first bicuspid required a rotation correction.

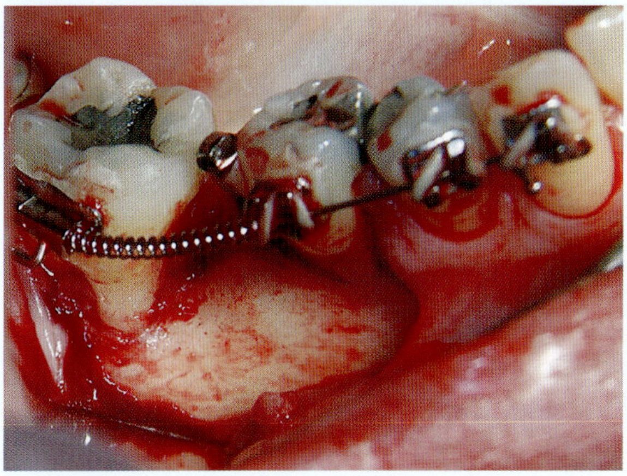

FIGURE 5-28g. Mesial bone defect before bone grafting at 3 months nearing the end of the uprighting/distal-moving phase of orthodontic treatment. Note that moving the molars forward to close the space before grafting could endanger the remaining integrity of the mesial root.

Continued

CASE DISCUSSION 14 Orthodontic Anchorage—cont'd

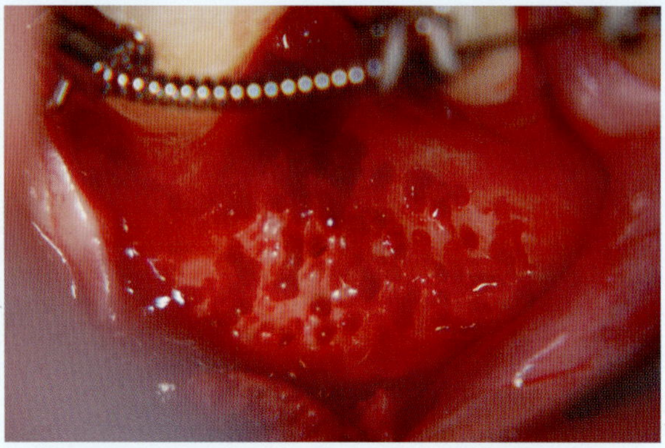

FIGURE 5-28h. Multiple bleeding points established in area to be grafted to weaken the cortical plate and promote new blood vessel growth into graft.

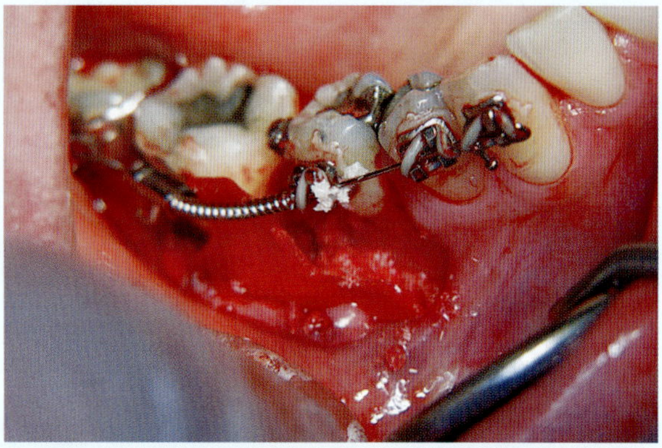

FIGURE 5-28i. Trimmed membrane in place to cover graft material over mesial root bony defect to improve potential for bony growth.

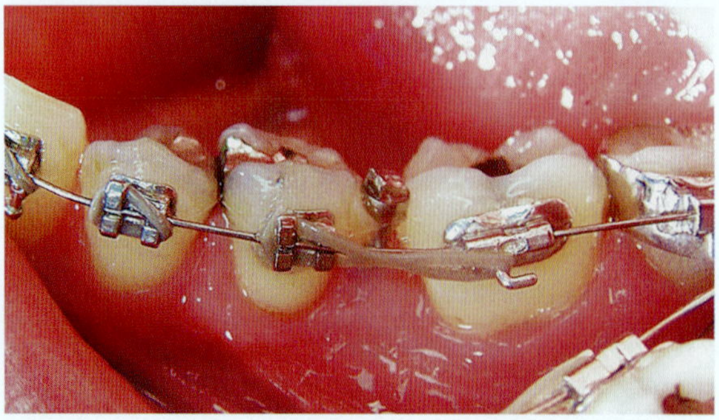

FIGURE 5-28j. Elastic chain placed to close the space after uprighting was completed. Note the correction of the rotated first bicuspid.

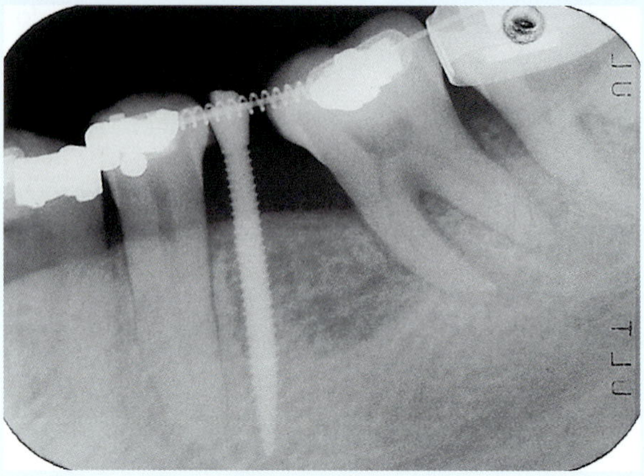

FIGURE 5-28k. Periapical radiograph showing uprighted and distally moved molars. Note the position in the bone of the Sendax standard thread MDI has remained stabile during the entire treatment.

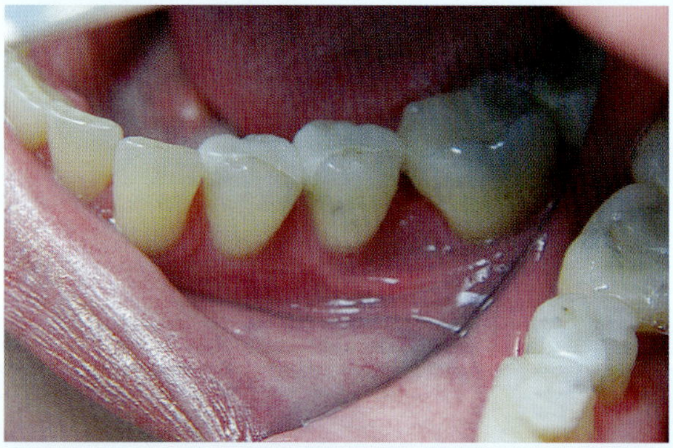

FIGURE 5-28l. Implant anchored orthodontic endpoint treatment (implant removed).

CASE DISCUSSION 15 Revision/Retreatment of Failed Implant Case

Patient history: A postmenopausal woman previously treated with implant supported fixed crown and bridge reported movement of the bridgework if pressed laterally. Upon examination a fracture of the metal substructure between the upper right cuspid and lateral incisor was detected (Figures 5-29a, b).

Patient treatment: Revision of the fractured implant porcelain bridge included removal of the three-unit fractured section with the molar dovetail from the Sendax MDI in the second premolar area. The cuspid pontic was hollowed out to create a receptacle for the additional MDI to be placed (Figure 5-29c). A Sendax MDI was placed into the abutment crown of the second premolar to act as a parallelism guide in conversion of the cuspid pontic into a MDI abutment crown and a pointed wire was fixated with composite in the cuspid receptacle (Figures 5-29d). The parallelism guide implant was removed, and the bridge was

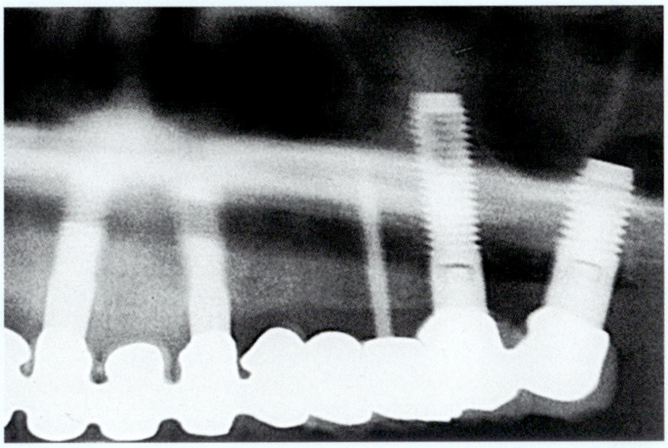

FIGURE 5-29a. Radiograph of implant bridge before fracture detection. Note the single Sendax MDI acting as a pier abutment in the second bicuspid area originally used in the fixed provisionals; the bone has remained stable.

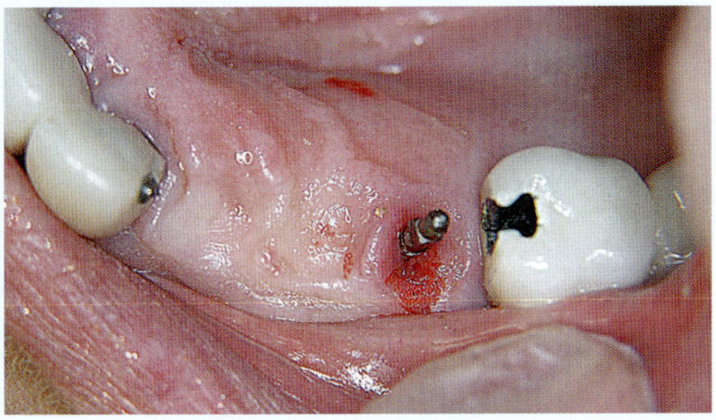

FIGURE 5-29b. Fractured metal on the distal of the lateral incisor. Note the fully functional Sendax MDI in the second bicuspid area and the mesial keyway/dovetail on the first molar.

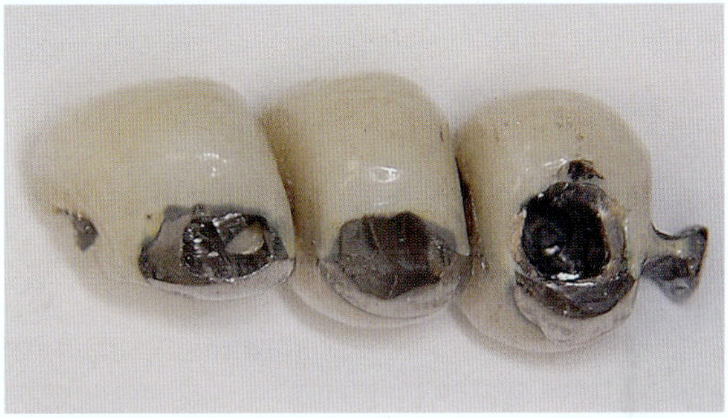

FIGURE 5-29c. Fractured section of the implant bridge with gingival metal removed to act as a receptor site for a Sendax MDI.

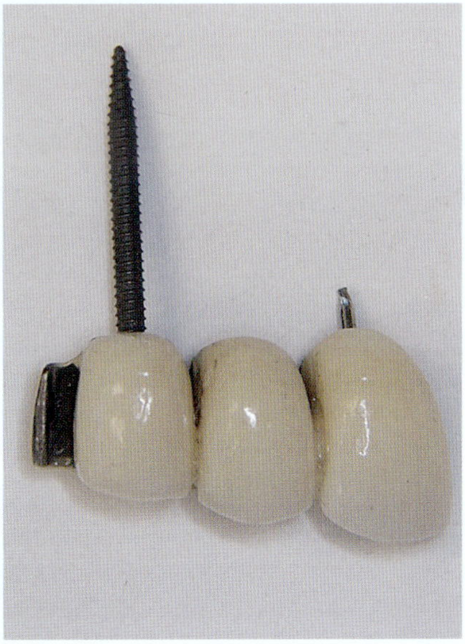

FIGURE 5-29d. Fractured implant bridge section with Sendax MDI in the second bicuspid retainer to act as a guide for converting the cuspid pontic to abutment retainer. A drill bit was ground to a point, sterilized, and placed in the bridges' new cuspid receptor to act as a tissue punch marker to locate the exact entry point for the additional MDI to be placed.

Continued

CASE DISCUSSION 15 Revision/Retreatment of Failed Implant Case—cont'd

reinserted to make a puncture point to act an exact location guide for the placement of a Sendax MDI in the cuspid location (Figure 5-29e). A Sendax MDI was placed at the exact location in the cuspid area and parallel to the bicuspid implant to allow immediate reseating and cementation of the original bridge. Follow-up at 6 months revealed healthy tissue and no mobility or drifting of the repaired bridge (Figure 5-29f). A radiograph revealed stable bone healing (Figure 5-29g).

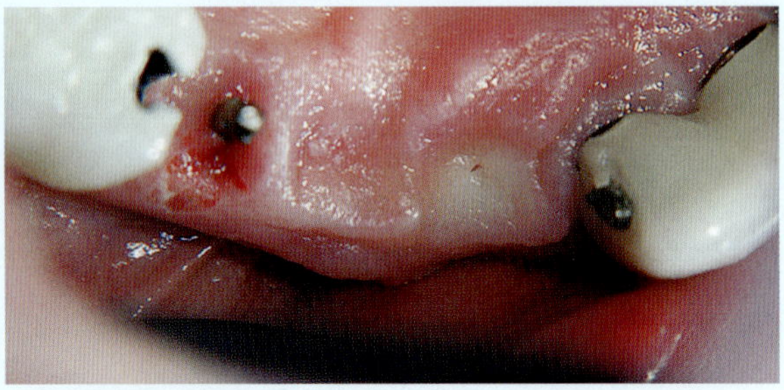

FIGURE 5-29e. Puncture point in cuspid area for exactly locating the entry point of the Sendax MDI to be placed as the new anterior support for the fractured bridge.

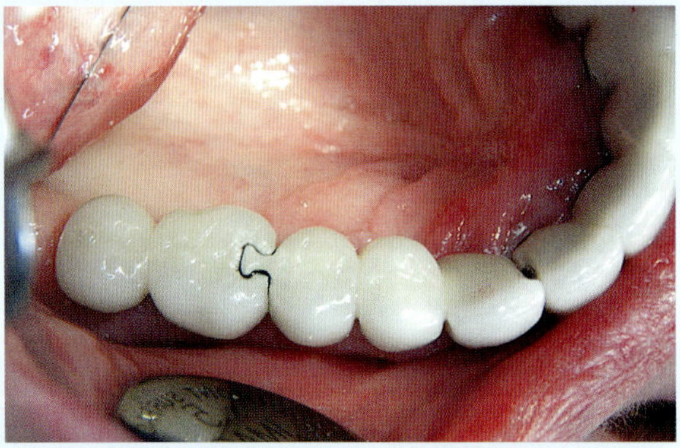

FIGURE 5-29f. Healthy tissue and no drifting of repaired bridge at 6-month follow-up.

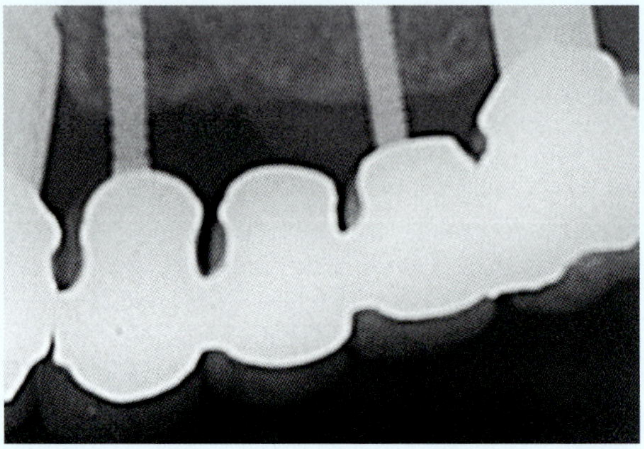

FIGURE 5-29g. Follow-up radiograph shows cortical crestal bone intact/stabile and good implant bone interface on all implants.

CASE DISCUSSION 16 Miscellaneous MDI Uses

EXAMPLE 1

Added support and retention for an otherwise cantilevered prosthesis. When bone is too narrow for placement of a terminal abutment and graft procedures and contraindicated Sendax MDI are useful in reducing occlusal load as well as aiding in retention against pull out forces of a fixed cantilevered prosthesis.

Patient history: A 65-year-old man with missing lower left molars and second bicuspid had three implants placed. The most anterior placed implant failed (Figure 5-30a).

Patient need: Replacement of failed implant.

Patient desire: No grafting procedures.

End treatment selected: After compromised healing, the patient did not wish bone grafting and

CASE DISCUSSION 16 Miscellaneous MDI Uses—cont'd

selected the Sendax MDI for replacement treatment. A Sendax standard thread design MDI was placed, and an immediate impression was made. Three splinted fixed gold crowns were fabricated and inserted 2 weeks later (Figures 5-30b, c), which avoided bone grafting and eliminated the potential adverse of a cantilevered pontic.

EXAMPLE 2

Repair of a fixed bridge with a vertically fractured distal abutment.

Patient history: An abscessed vertically fractured second molar bridge abutment (Figure 5-31a).

Patient medical history: In previous 2 years, multiple cancer surgeries and chemotherapy.

Patient need: Remove tooth and bridge to clear infection.

Patient desire: Replacement of the fixed bridge with fixed teeth.

Patient treatment: Included removal of the bridge and abscessed tooth, placing Sendax MDIs anterior to and posterior to the extraction site, adding core build up material to the emptied distal bridge abutment and immediately recementing the bridge (Figure 5-31b).

EXAMPLE 3

Long span fixed bridge retention improvement.

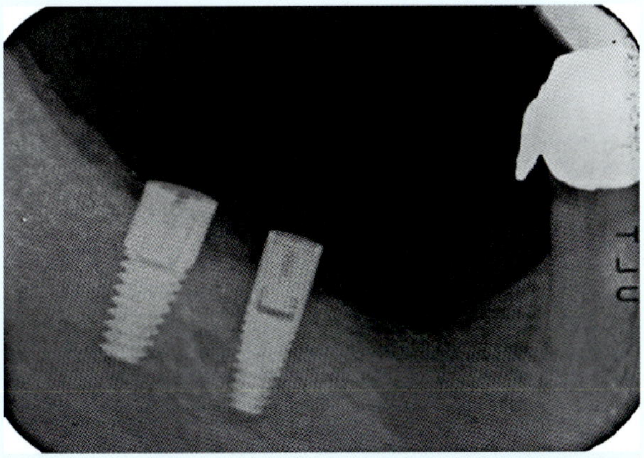

FIGURE 5-30a. Radiograph revealing compromised bone healing where failed implant was removed.

Patient history: Included a five-unit bridge that has repeatedly loosened due to insufficient retention (Figure 5-31c).

Patient need: Increased bridge retention.

Patient desire: Affordable solution.

Treatment: Included hollowing out the two central incisor pontics to accommodate two Sendax MDIs (Figure 5-31d). Local infiltration anesthetic was given and the two MDI osteotomies were

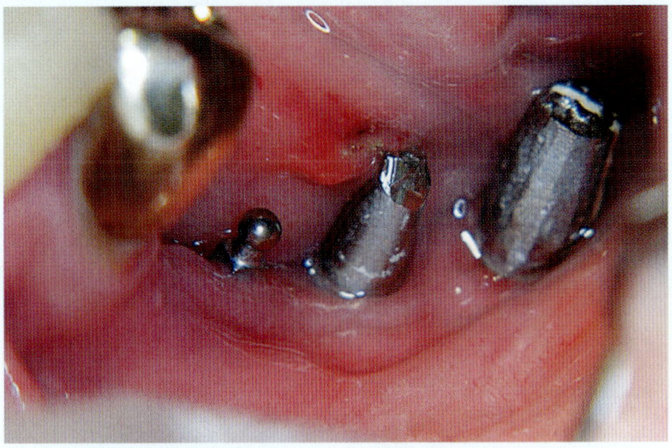

FIGURE 5-30b. Sendax MDI 2 weeks after placement at splinted crowns insertion appointment.

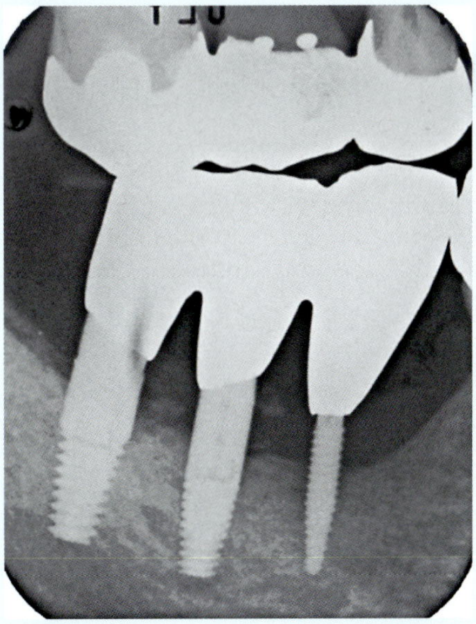

FIGURE 5-30c. Radiograph at 6-month follow-up appointment.

Continued

CASE DISCUSSION 16 Miscellaneous MDI Uses—cont'd

prepared through the bridge (Figure 5-31e). The bridge was removed and the location of the sites confirmed (Figure 5-31f). The bridge was recemented permanently (Figure 5-31g). Two minis were then inserted through the access holes in the bridge (Figures 5-31h, i). Dual cure core build-up material was placed in the voids of the access holes. After curing, the implants were shortened to within the bridge confines. Composite was placed over the build-up material and implants and polished (Figure 5-31j).

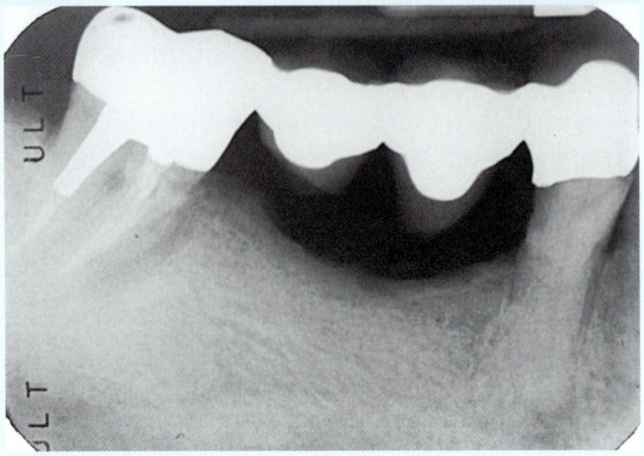

FIGURE 5-31a. Periapical radiograph showing vertically fractured root of molar abutments.

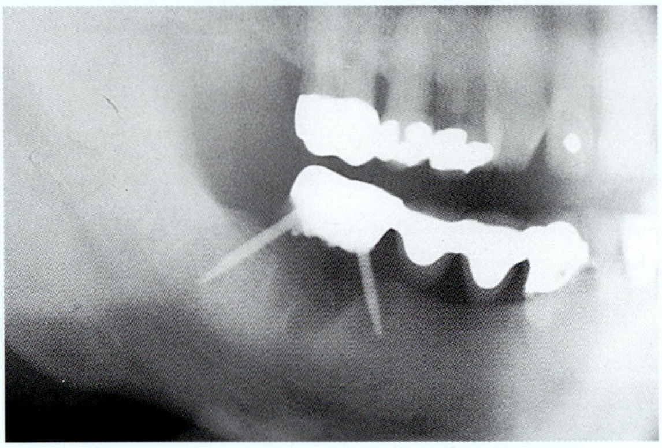

FIGURE 5-31b. Periapical radiograph showing positions of two Sendax MDIs that were placed in bone mesially and distally to the molar extraction site. Note the angulation of the implants to emerge underneath the original abutment crown.

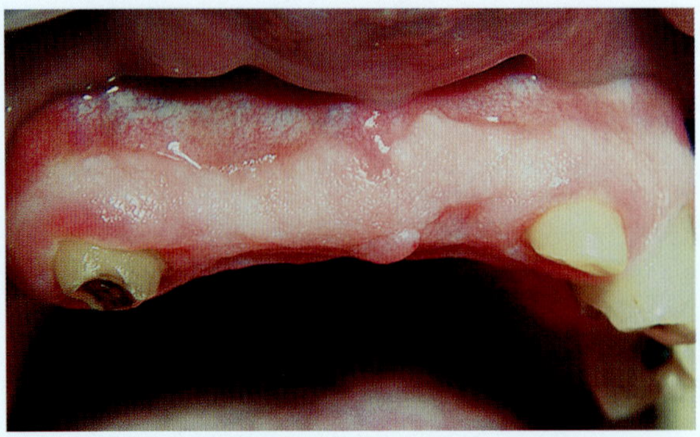

FIGURE 5-31c. Five-unit bridge with only short abutments for retention.

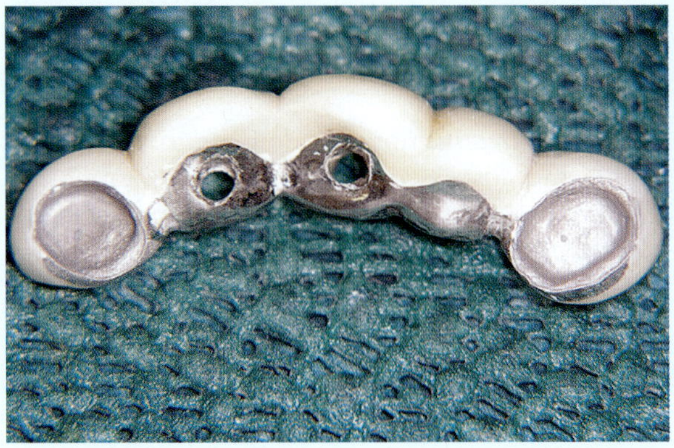

FIGURE 5-31d. Bridge has been ground through from gingival to lingual incisal areas of the central incisor pontics.

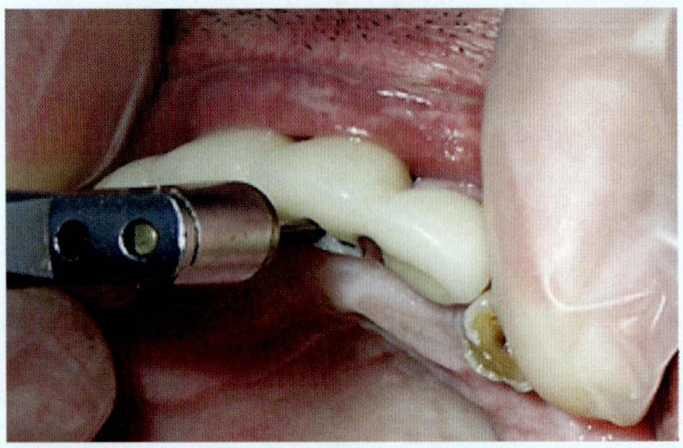

FIGURE 5-31e. Seated bridge acting as surgical guide for locating the exact pathway for the two Sendax MDIs to be placed ideally.

CASE DISCUSSION 16 Miscellaneous MDI Uses—cont'd

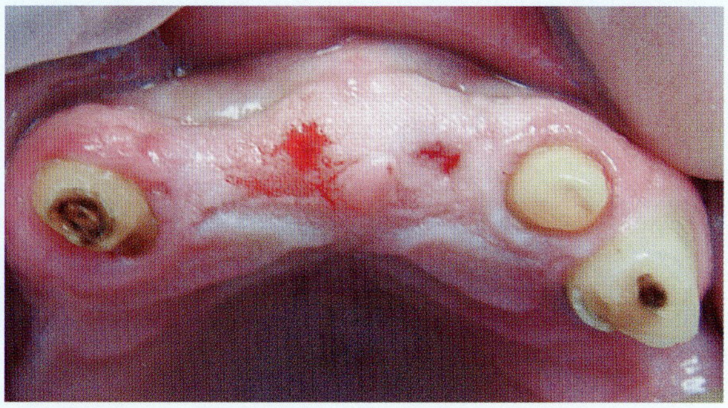

FIGURE 5-31f. Bleeding points verifying correct position of the two MDI insertion pathways.

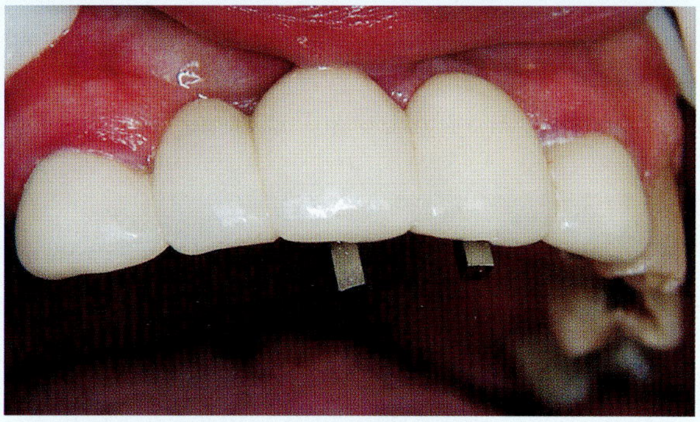

FIGURE 5-31i. Bridge with MDIs in place before core build-up material placed and the implants shortened to within the confines of the bridge.

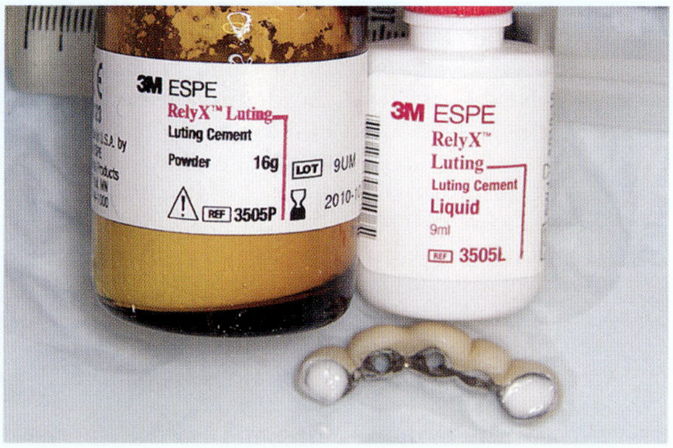

FIGURE 5-31g. Bridge filled with permanent cement for placement before the MDIs are inserted.

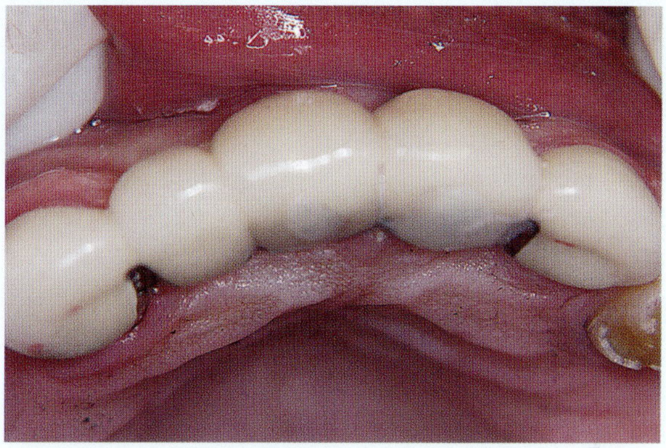

FIGURE 5-31j. Bridge in place after composite placed over core material and polished.

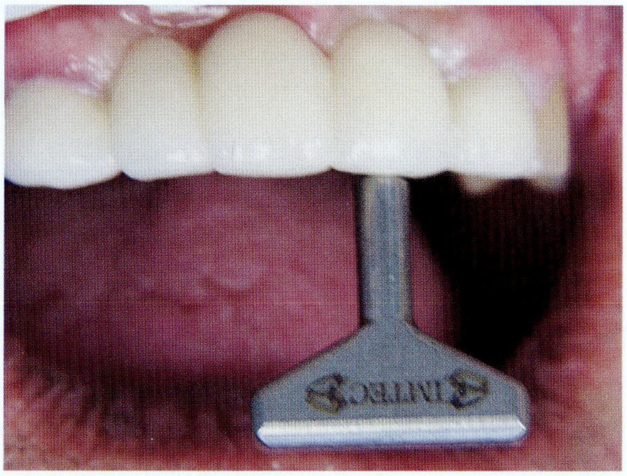

FIGURE 5-31h. Winged wrench used for final placement of the Sendax MDIs.

Summary

Because dentistry has few "2 + 2 = 4" rules, the incorporation of any new technology into one's practice requires judgment. Before making a judgment, the practitioner should use every available resource including past university board and all educational experiences (i.e., continuing education courses) and past experiential evidence that is relative to the potential for improvement of patient care. It has been said that implant therapy is a prosthetically driven discipline. To this I would add that patient's desires and demands drive the prosthetics. The dentist is responsible for a safe and efficacious ride for the patient passenger using all the resources available to aid them. Incorporating implant therapy into my practice over the last 25 years has been most satisfying professionally and economically. The addition of MDIs in the last 7 years has been the dessert.

MDI therapy is turbo charging the current implant evolution. Dentists are licensed to drive. Why ride? We're all in the race. Why be left behind?

P.S. Maybe even consider the fast lane. With discretion!

References

1. K Aitasalo - Acta Otolaryngol Suppl, 1986-ncbi.nlm.nih.gov. 1986;428:1–54. Bone tissue response to irradiation and treatment model of mandibular irradiation injury. An experimental and clinical study.
2. http://www.asahq.org/clinical/physicalstatus.htm
3. Atchison KA: *Journal of Dental Education*, 2002.
4. Christensen GJ: *Am Dent Assoc,* Vol 131, No 3, 359–361.
5. Degidi, Piattelli, and Carinci, Clinical Outcomes of Narrow diameter implants: a retrospective study of 510 Implants Journal of Periodontology 2005.
6. JB Epstein, M Robertson, S Emerton, N Phillips, P. Head & Neck, 2001-doi.wiley.com Page 1. Quality of Life and Oral Function in patients treated with Radiation for Head and neck Cancer
7. Harris J, Sengar D, Stewart T, Hyslop D: The effect of immunosuppressive chemotherapy on immune function in patients with malignant disease, *Cancer* 37(Suppl 2):1058–1069, 1976 Feb, ncbi.nlm.nih.gov. Cancer, 1976.
8. Lee, V. Frias, K. Lee, R. Wright Effect of implant size and shape on implant success rates: A literature review, *The Journal of Prosthetic Dentistry*, 94(4):377–381 J.
9. Misch: *Contemporary Implant Dentistry*, ed 2, 1999, Mosby.
10. Polizzi et al. 1999 Retrospective Evaluation of Mandibular incisor replacement with narrow diameter implants in the treatment of partially edentulous patients or in single tooth restorations.
11. Rhinelander FW: Circulation in bone. In Bourne G, editor: ed 2, *The Biochemistry and Physiology of Bone*, vol 2, New York, 1972, Academic Press. chap1.
12. Schomig A, Neumann FJ, Kastrati A, et al: A randomized comparison of antiplatelet and anticoagulant therapy after the placement of coronary-artery stents, *N Engl J Med* 334(17):1084–1089, 1996.
13. Vigolo, Givan: Clinical Outcomes of Narrow Diameter Implants, *Journal of Periodontology*, 2000.
14. Vigolo, et al: The impact of loads on standard diameter, narrow diameter, and mini implants: a cooperative laboratory study, *Clinical Oral Implants research*, 2004.
15. Zinsli, et al: Clinical Outcomes of Narrow Diameter Implants, *Journal of Periodontology*, 2004.

Chapter 6

MDI Solutions for the Medically Compromised Patient

HAROLD I. SUSSMAN   ARTHUR R. VOLKER

Outline

Treating patients in a long-term care facility for disabled and chronically ill patients presents many challenges to the restoring dentist. Because of multiple medical and physical conditions, hospitalized patients pose many additional risks and complications and may have interferences in the healing process. Patients cannot be treated in a conventional manner because they may have debilitating conditions, such as spinal and neurological deficiencies or be ventilator dependant. Scheduled appointments may have to be configured around a patient's medication regimens, such as anticoagulant therapy or chemotherapy. These hurdles have been remarkably overcome by the staff dental attendings and dental residents at our dental clinic facilities. In order to insure safety, pertinent blood tests are redone on the patient within 1 week of the scheduled surgery.

A medical assessment form (Figure 6-1) outlines the medical assessment protocol adhered to at Coler-Goldwater Hospital as a working guide to the strict guidelines in place at this clinical research facility.

Goldwater Hospital opened in 1939 as a long term care and rehabilitation hospital on Welfare Island, now renamed Roosevelt Island (Judith Berdy, Roosevelt Island Historian, personal communication). It is a municipal hospital operated by the New York City Health and Hospital Corporation serving all who need these special services. Goldwater Hospital merged with its sister hospital, Coler Memorial Hospital in 1996, forming the Coler-Goldwater Specialty Hospital and Nursing Facility, and has a total of 2000 beds between the two nearby campuses. The population of the hospital is divided between hospital beds and nursing home beds. A majority of the patient residents are long term and the hospital serves as their permanent home. The hospital has an extensive rehabilitation program for patients with traumatic injury and has the largest ventilator-dependent and ventilator-weaning unit in the country. Because it is both a nursing home and hospital, Coler-Goldwater offers many long-term services that an acute care facility would not.

The dental clinics contain 12 operatories that service the 2000 patients, with approximately 6000

Coler ♥Goldwater Specialty Hospital and Nursing Facility

DEPARTMENT OF DENTISTRY

☐ COLER ☐ GOLDWATER

MEDICAL CLEARANCE FOR ORAL SURGERY

DATE:	REQUESTED RESPONSE TIME:
	☐ 4 HOURS (Telephone call required)
TIME:	☐ 24 HOURS (Telephone call required)
	☐ ROUTINE

DENTIST

CLEARANCE REQUEST

Procedure(s) to be done: ______________________ Date scheduled: ______________________

______________________ Time scheduled: ______________________

ISSUES FOR REVIEW:

☐ Coagulation status ☐ Antibiotic prophylaxis ☐ Local anesthesia ☐ With epinephrine ☐ Other considerations (Specify.)

____

____

Name DDS/DMD ______ Signature ______ Code # ______ Date ______ Time ______

PHYSICIAN

CLEARANCE RESPONSE

1. Medical history summary: ______________________
2. Allergies: ______________________ 3. Bleeding history ______________________
4. Hemostasis status: ☐ Normal ☐ Abnormal, with recent labs, as indicated: Value Date

If ***abnormal****, due to:* ☐ Medical condition: ______________ ☐ PT ______ ______

☐ Medication ☐ Coumadin ☐ Heparin ☐ INR ______ ______

☐ Plavix ☐ ASA/NSAID ☐ PTT ______ ______

☐ Other: ______________ ☐ PLATELETS ______ ______

5. Antibiotic prophylaxis: *(AHA guidelines for indications and regimens for antibiotic prophylax is stated on back of this form.)*

☐ Not indicated

☐ Ordered for 1 hour prior to procedure, as scheduled above, as follows:

Medication: ______________ Dose: ________ Route: ________ Date: ________ Time: ________

6. Local anesthesia may be given as follows: ☐ With epinephrine ☐ With out epinephrine
7. Other considerations: ______________________

____

8. Clearance: ☐ **CLEARED** for procedure. (See progress notes.)

☐ **NOT CLEARED** for procedure at this time, because ______________________

____

(If NOT CLEARED, call dental department to discuss when and how indicated treatment can be provided.)

Name MD (Print) ______ Signature ______ Code # ______ Date ______ Time ______

NURSE

IMMEDIATELY PRIOR TO APPOINTMENT

Check one of the following boxes: ☐ Pre-operative antibiotics NOT given. ☐ Pre-operative antibiotics given as follows:

Medication: ______________ Dose: ________ Route: ________ Date: ________ Time: ________

Name RN (Print) ______ Signature ______ Code # ______

FIGURE 6-1. Medical assessment form.

visits per year. The staff includes 14 attending staff dentists, 4 dental hygienists, 9 dental assistants, 3 clerical staff, and 10 general dental residents, serving 1- to 2-year internships.

The many medical complications one may encounter have been dealt with in an article by English and Bohle.[15] However, because a number of our dental patients have diabetes, we shall expand on this condition.

Diabetes has long been thought to be a contraindication to implant placement. According to the Center for Disease Control's 2007 National Diabetes Fact Sheet,[10] approximately 23.6 million people in the United States will be diagnosed in their lifetime with diabetes, either type I or type II; 10.7% of adults age 20 years and older have diabetes, and the prevalence of diabetes in adults 60 years and older is 23.1%. Each year 1.6 million new cases of diabetes are diagnosed in adults 20 years or older. The distribution is almost equal between sexes; it appears in 11.2% of men (12 million people) and 10.2% of women (11.5 million people).

Among racial groups, the lowest prevalence is found among non-Hispanic Whites (6.6% of total non-Hispanic White population), with Asian Americans having a prevalence of 7.5%. The racial groups with the highest prevalence are Hispanics (10.4%) and non-Hispanic Blacks (11.8%). Currently insufficient data are available to wholly calculate prevalence rates of Native Americans, although normalized trends indicate that there is an even higher prevalence of diabetes than that found in non-Hispanic Blacks.

Patients at Coler-Goldwater Memorial Specialty Hospital and Nursing Facility are medically complex, often presenting with a medical diagnoses. The institution is a long-term care facility and some of the patients are transferred from local acute care hospitals. They may not have the financial resources to seek treatment or rehabilitation in a private setting. As such, some of the patients come to the hospital as either controlled or previously chronically uncontrolled diabetics.

The deleterious effects of diabetes on the body are numerous and well known. They include retinopathy, neuropathy, nephropathy, microvascular and macrovascular changes, polyuria, and polydipsia. Of interest to the dental clinician is the high incidence of periodontal disease found in those with diabetes.[36,38] This comorbidity may be a strong contributing factor to the edentulous nature of many patients.

BOX 6-1 Advantages of Using MDIs in a Hospital Setting

- Atraumatic surgery
- Most cases do not require the use of a scalpel or sutures
- Flapless surgery means no bone exposure
- Minimal bleeding
- Use of local anesthetic infiltration instead of bilateral mandibular blocks
- Simple insertion protocol to place implants
- Placement technique is critical, but easily mastered
- Few instruments required
- Inexpensive components
- Implants can be loaded immediately
- High degree of patient satisfaction
- Easy to maintain cleanliness of exposed ball tops
- No bone grafting or ridge augmentation required
- Ridge reduction to obtain increased crestal width via osseous reduction is avoided
- Reduced risk to medically compromised patients
- More likelihood of physician clearance to allow placing MDIs due to conservative insertion protocol
- MDIs, with their low ball-top profile, decrease the risk for lateral overloading forces
- Able to maintain the same vertical dimension of occlusion by using patient's preexisting denture

There are more than 200 edentulous patients at Coler-Goldwater or 10% of the general hospital population. Our residents fabricate approximately 120 complete dentures a year. Some patients had a comorbidity of diabetes. The overwhelming majority of them were type II and taking supplemental insulin.

The use and reliability of mini dental implants (MDI) have been shown to have a similar success rate to other implant systems. Bulard et al[8] and Shatkin et al[52] observed that for 3000 MDIs placed in the last 15 years, the survival rate was more than 92%. There are numerous advantages in using MDIs instead of standard implants for patients at the hospital. Box 6-1 lists the advantages of using MDIs.

Quality of Life

One of the benefits of using MDIs is the ability to increase the stability of dentures. This can present numerous advantages to patients with diabetes, including increased satisfaction and enhanced ability to masticate previously difficult-to-chew foods.

Patient Satisfaction

Studies have looked at patient satisfaction when using conventional versus implant-retained lower complete dentures. Edentulous seniors who received an implant-retained lower complete denture had a 36% higher satisfaction rating than those patients who were given a conventional lower complete denture.[56] Awad et al[3] had demonstrated similar satisfaction data for middle-age adults with implant retained dentures. These trends have also been reported among those with diabetes (age range not specified) who have been given an implant-retained mandibular complete denture.[31]

Improved Nutritional Uptake

Significant anthropometric improvements have been observed in patients utilizing implant-retained mandibular complete dentures compared with conventional complete dentures.[41] Geertman et al[19] have also reported similar results. Additionally, patients given an implant-retained lower complete denture were more able to chew hard foods than those with a conventional complete denture.[43] Similar results were observed in those with diabetes who had received an implant-retained mandibular complete denture versus a conventional complete denture.[32]

Effect of Diabetes on Implant Morbidity

The chronic effects of high glucose and subsequent accumulated glycosylation end products from diabetes result in reactions that can affect the success rate of implant stability and retention. These negative effects include a reduction in the quantity and quality of collagen, laminin, and osteocalcin.[30] Additionally, bone healing and remodeling is impaired in the presence of diabetes mellitus, most likely due to a decrease in insulin and insulin-like growth factor-I (IGF-I) levels and increased levels of advanced glycosylation end products such as HbA1c and proinflammatory cytokines. The result is decreased bone density and increased turnover rate and bone loss. However, diabetes has not been proven to be an absolute contraindication for implant success and osseointegration; Morris et al[42] found 93% success in patients without diabetes and 92% in patients with type II diabetes in a 3-year time period.

Another important consideration is the effect of bone-to-implant contact for implants placed in recipients with diabetes. Early implant failures have been shown to result from a lack of an intimate bone-to-implant contact.[16] However, bone-to-implant contact can be maintained in animal models with chemically induced diabetes, although the bone was found to be less mature.[9,21,33] Long term prognosis studies have shown that bone-to-implant contact deceased with time in rats with uncontrolled diabetes, but rats with controlled diabetes had maintained osseointegration.[35,45,53]

Note that the animal models used in these studies were designed to mimic uncontrolled type I diabetes in that pancreatic beta cells were chemically destroyed. When similar models were given insulin, an increase in trabecular bone volume and a sustained bone-to-implant contact were observed.[40,53,55] Similar findings were reported in a study by Goodman and Hori[22] in which bone formation was decreased in rats with diabetes. When these animals were given insulin, bone growth rates were similar to control animals. Fiorellini et al[18] observed that supplemental insulin did increase bone volume around implants, although bone-to-implant contact was not improved.

To date, few animal studies have examined the effect of implant osseointegration in type II diabetes. Using Otsuka Long-Evans Tokushima Fatty rats, a modified type II diabetes animal model, Hasegawa et al[26] observed that early bone volume around implants were lower in tibial cortical bone yet roughly the same in marrow areas against control rats. Casap et al[9] reported similar findings, although no differences in implant osseointegration for diabetes and control models were observed. The rats with diabetes in both studies were not given supplemental insulin. Additionally, lower bone-to-implant contact was seen in rats with diabetes than that of the control group in both studies. It was further seen that there were chondrocyte-like cells within the bone, although hematopoietic and adipose cells had also been observed.[47] Hasegawa et al[26] note, however, that such a result would not occur in human subjects because the mandible does not have chondrogenic capability, only osteogenic capability.

Healing appears to be most critical in the first month after surgery because impaired bone maturation has been observed in animals with diabetes. Studies demonstrate a disorganization of trabecular woven bone at the implant-bone interface in those with diabetes within this time frame.[5,9] Chondrocyte-like cells instead of osteocytes were also observed at the implant-bone interface in animal models with uncontrolled diabetes.[53]

Additionally, the accumulation of advanced glycosylation end products from chronically elevated glucose levels and affiliated receptors on large size proteins, lipoproteins, and lipids have been implicated in a number of factors that contribute to unsuccessful implant therapy and periodontal disease.[37,36] Advanced glycosylation end products have been shown to inhibit osteoblast function,[51] reduce wound healing,[27] and reduce osseointegration of implants to bone.[45]

Considerations for the Treatment of Patients with Diabetes

Box 6-2 contains a list of considerations when treating a patient with diabetes.

Implant failure rates in patients with diabetes can be comparable to patients with diabetes if plasma glucose is close to normal.[7,17] This may be particularly true for controlled type II diabetes.[2,1] Furthermore, patients with type I diabetes show less bone mineral density and may be more prone to bone loss than those with type II. Therefore patients with controlled type II diabetes may be better candidates for MDI placement.[48,57]

Patients with type 2 diabetes may also need a longer course of antibiotics (7 to 10 days versus 3 days for patients without diabetes), although no effect was seen between antibiotic usage and early implant failures.[2,50]

Additionally, a clinician may wish to review the patient's glycated hemoglobin (HbA1c) levels, which is an indicator of glycemic control. Normal levels are < 6.0%. In uncontrolled diabetes it is defined as > 10%. However, there has been some debate over the appropriate blood markers used to determine glycemia and coordinate the suitable course and timing of treatment. HbA1c levels measure glycemia from the preceding 2 to 3 months, whereas plasma glucose levels measure moment-to-moment glucose levels.[30] Dowell et al[14] did not find significance between HbA1c levels and implant success in type II diabetes; however, future research must be done to best determine the more clinically significant parameter for dental implant outcomes.

BOX 6-2 Therapeutic Considerations for the Treatment of Patients with Diabetes

1. May want patients with type I and type II to supplement with insulin, even if type II is controlled by diet and/or controlled by oral hypoglycemics
2. May want to increase course of antibiotics
3. Patients with type I diabetes:
   a. Have less bone density than type II
   b. Exhibit more bone loss than type II
   c. Take longer to heal than type II
   d. Are associated with more delayed bone repair around implants than type II
4. May not want to give NSAIDS to patients with diabetes postoperatively due to antiproliferative effects that can delay healing
5. Select an appropriate indicator of glycemic control (glycated hemoglobin [HbA1c] versus plasma glucose)
6. Immediate load versus delayed load
7. Patients with diabetes may be more prone to periimplantitis than those without diabetes

Another topic of concern is the utilization of immediate load verses delayed loading of dental implants. It has been suggested that the practitioner delay loading, although Balshi et al[4] found via resonance frequency analysis, which measures the in vivo stability of an endosseous implant, that an immediate load protocol is feasible and had shown implant survival in a patient with controlled type II diabetes. Although metabolic and histologic differences were seen in the healing diabetic bone, particularly in the first 30 days, osseointegration and survival were seen to rival that without the presence of diabetes. The key to the protocol is that the interim provisional restoration must not be disturbed for the critical first 30 days after implant placement.[5,59] Following this protocol, we have not had any placed MDIs fail to integrate in the past several years at our hospital.

Patients with diabetes have been observed to have impaired wound healing.[13,49] This can be attributed to a number of factors including decreased macrophage number,[39] reduced collagenase,[28] and reduced fibroblast proliferation.[6,23] Additionally, it has been observed in animal models that impaired wound healing in diabetes has been co-related with a decrease in tissue factor.[11]

The use of insulin has been shown to aid in wound healing because it has an antiapoptotic effect.[12] Rai et al[49] reported an increase in apoptosis in uncontrolled diabetes as well as an increase in apoptosis for patients with diabetes taking oral hypoglycemics versus those taking insulin. Other factors that may be employed in the future to enhance wound healing include epidermal growth factor and IGF-1. Epidermal growth factor, normally found in large quantities in salivary glands, aids in wound healing.[25] It is decreased in diabetes, both type I and II.[44,46] IGF-1, produced in the liver, has been shown to be anabolic, increasing osteoblastic activity, which can enhance osseointegration.[20,58]

Because most MDI placements do not require the use of a surgical flap and use a smaller diameter fixture, it is anticipated that wound healing for patients with diabetes will proceed with less sequelae than would have been seen with conventional standard implant placements, provided proper protocol is followed.

Sendax Mini Dental Implant (MDI)

Many edentulous patients have loose or unstable mandibular denture prostheses, making it difficult for them to masticate properly or comfortably. The new standard of care for edentulous patients at New York University College of Dentistry is an implant-supported lower overdenture. The usual placement of two 4-mm wide fixtures in the mandibular cuspid regions requires open flap surgery. However, many of our patients, even with adequate ridge width, are medically compromised and cannot undergo standard implant surgery.

MDIs were introduced into the dental armamentarium of the hospital in the year 2000. The major use in the general population for MDIs is where the crest of the edentulous ridge is only 4 to 6mm wide, which would be too narrow (without bone grafts or osteoplasty) for the normal 4-mm wide implant fixtures. MDI placement is significantly less invasive than conventional implant placement. MDIs have enabled us to provide increased dental function, comfort, and esthetics plus self-confidence and esteem to our population of patients.

MDIs are typically placed, according to the Sendax insertion protocol, straight through the overlying gingival tissues into the underlying alveolar bone without the need of a surgical incision and flap. The surgical procedure involves infiltration of some local anesthesia and drilling a 1.1-mm wide by 6-mm deep pilot starter hole into the bone for each implant to be placed. The average time for dental residents to insert four MDIs is usually an hour. The surgery is practically bloodless because the width of the MDI is at least 1.8 mm, which completely obturates the 1.1-mm pilot hole. The implant company states that loading of the implants can be at the same visit as insertion, but we find it more prudent to have the patient return in 4 weeks to place the metal housings in the overlying denture intaglio. In the interim, a groove is channeled through the underside of the denture, creating a trough to clear the exposed ball tops of the inserted MDIs. Soft-cure liner is placed into the opening of this channel and will provide transitional denture stabilization for the patient.

This technique makes for shorter individual dental appointments and allows the operator to place the metal housings in the proper position within the denture intaglio. The patient is not anesthetized for this visit and will more likely give a proper centric occlusal bite. At the 1-month follow-up visit, the implants are tested for initial integration, and, if stable, the soft liner is removed and the metal housings are inserted using hard self-cure acrylic. Sometimes metal housings are not loaded if they are not in proper alignment or would impart too much retention for the patient to manage. The metal housings that now engage the exposed MDI O-ball tops convey to the denture the anticipated stable retention that is desirable.

When the first MDIs were placed, some of our patients were incapable of mastering the skills necessary for removal and insertion of their dental prosthesis. The cause was usually poor manual dexterity, as with severe arthritis and hand tremors. The difficulty arose from the fact that there was off-angle alignment of the MDI fixtures that were placed. This was overcome by designing a dental drill guide, the patented Sussman Implant Guide (SIG) (Salvin Dental Specialties, Inc., Charlotte, NC). It allowed for MDI fixtures to be placed exactly 10 mm apart, parallel to each other, and perpendicular to the dental ridge. In

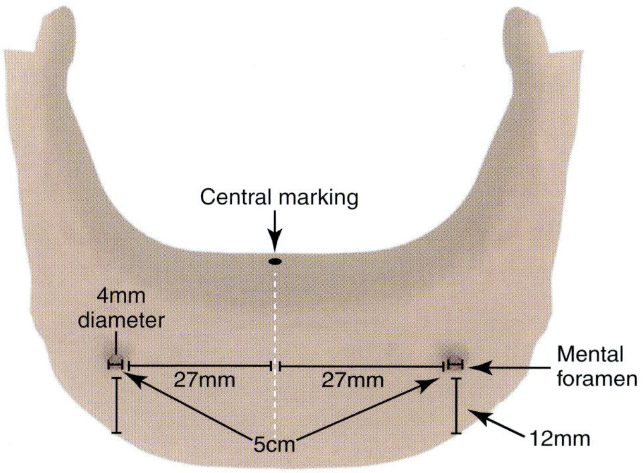

FIGURE 6-2. Diagram of mandible. Note that mental foramina are approximately 27 mm from the midline.

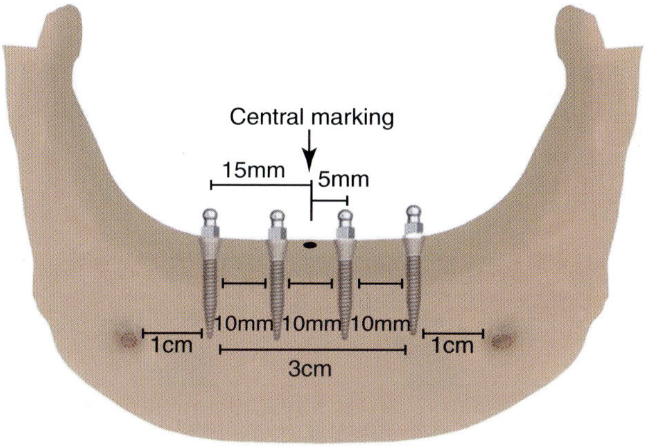

FIGURE 6-3. Diagram of placement positions of four MDIs using the Sussman Implant Guide (SIG).

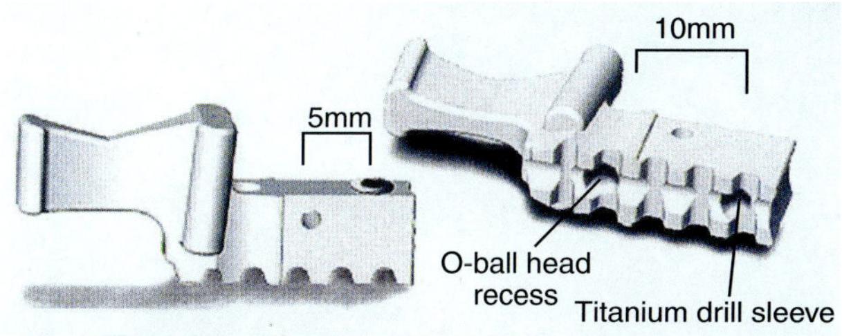

FIGURE 6-4. SIG device with its components labeled.

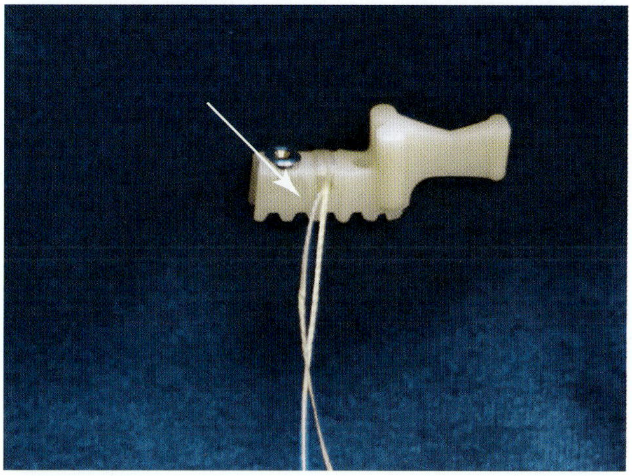

FIGURE 6-5. The dental floss is inserted through the side opening, 5 mm from either aperture.

so doing, a straight path was created for the patient, making it easier to master the insertion and removal techniques. It was first demonstrated and published with the insertion of three MDIs.[54]

The protocol for inserting MDIs with the aid of the SIG eliminates the need for finding the indentation of the mental foramina and marking their location on the buccal side of the mandible and then on the ridge crest directly above the site, which was the original method of Dr. Charles English.[15]

The method used at Coler-Goldwater Hospital by the dental residents is based on actual mandibular anatomy[24] (Figure 6-2). When four MDIs are placed using the SIG device, the fixtures will be spaced evenly along a 3-cm arc (Figure 6-3) The components of the SIG device are shown in Figure 6-4. The SIG consists of an anterior titanium ring that is 1.5 mm in diameter to allow for a 1.1-mm twist drill to pass through (see Figure 6-4). The center of the body of the SIG has a side 1-mm opening to allow for dental floss to be inserted at a point 5 mm from the ring opening. The floss serves as a safety feature to prevent accidental swallowing of the device and as a measuring line to be placed over the central marking point (Figure 6-5). The handle of the SIG is directed in a horizontal direction backwards to give increased stability to its usage. There is a 2.5-mm O-ball head recess at a point 10 mm from the ring opening, directly below the anterior guard handle. There is also a 4-mm sweeping concavity below the handle to allow for the device to pass over previously inserted MDIs with their exposed O-ball heads. In addition, the body of the SIG has basal serrations to prevent slippage over gingival tissues. Note that this technique utilizes the placement of the fixtures directly into and through the overlying crestal gingiva. The first intraoral step is for the operator to mark the center of the mandibular crest with an indelible tissue marker (Figure 6-6). This can best

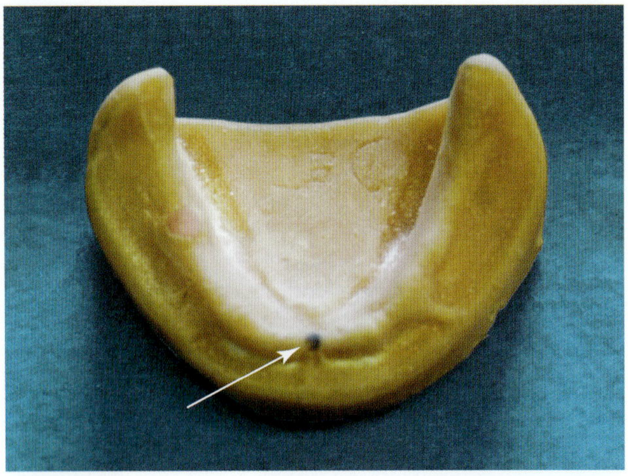

FIGURE 6-6. Central marking made on the mandibular crest.

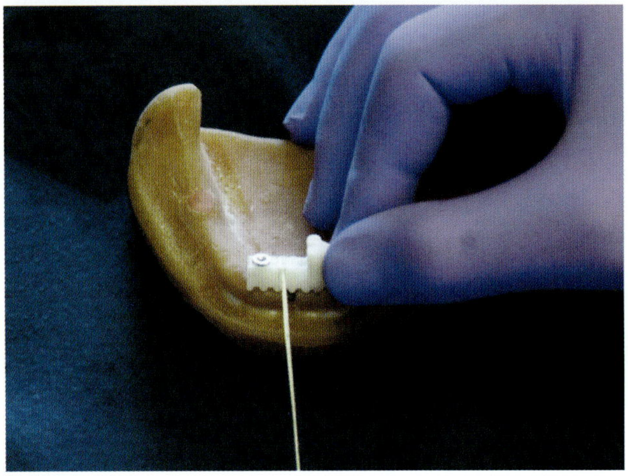

FIGURE 6-7. SIG device placed on top of the mandible with dental floss over central point.

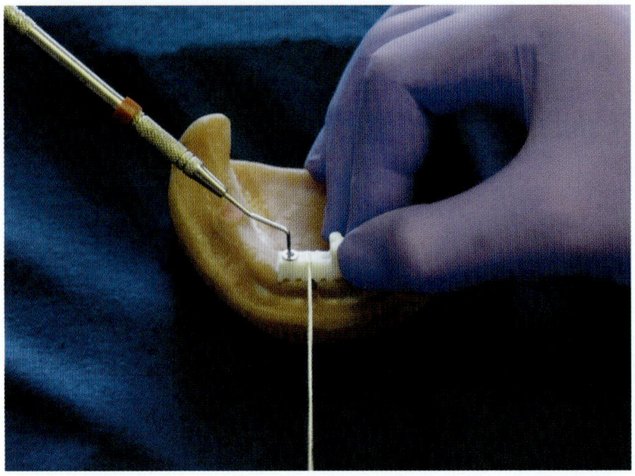

FIGURE 6-8. Periodontal probe inserted through the 1.3-mm anterior titanium ring to "sound" for bone to corroborate proper positioning.

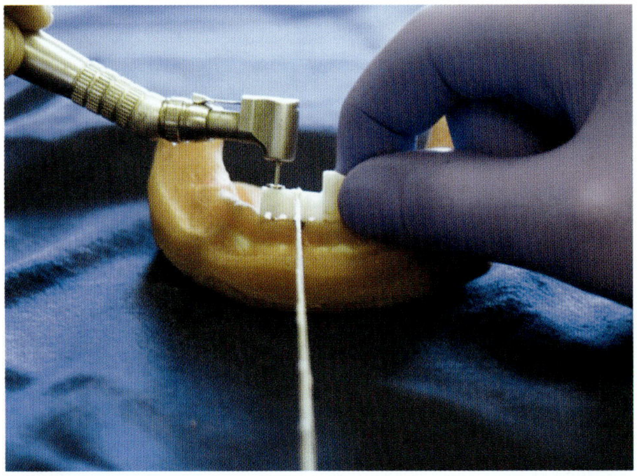

FIGURE 6-9. Side view of 1.1-mm twist drill inserted through the titanium ring to create a 6-mm deep "pilot starting hole."

be found by locating the labial or lingual frenum or with a line down from the tip of nose using a ruler or floss. The next step is to place the SIG over the mandibular anterior crest with the dental floss draped over the central mark (Figure 6-7). The next step, which is critical, is to "sound" for the bone crest by placing a periodontal probe through the titanium ring (Figure 6-8). The 1.1-mm twist drill, which has been inserted in a surgical handpiece, is then used at approximately 1200 rpm, along with a saline coolant, to create a 6-mm "pilot starter hole" through the crest of bone (Figure 6-9). The SIG device will only allow the bur to penetrate 6 mm into bone, which is the proper depth according to the MDI protocol (Sendax, personal communication; Figure 6-10). The MDI is then hand inserted into the mandible to a point where the square neck below the O-ball is approximately 1 mm subgingival (Figure 6-11). This will obviate the necessity for placing plastic block-out shims before metal housing insertion in the denture intaglio. The SIG device handle is then placed over the exposed O-ball head of the first MDI, in a direction to pass over the central marking point, to locate the second MDI site (Figure 6-12). The second MDI will be inserted 10 mm from the first MDI and parallel to it (Figure 6-13). The SIG device is then placed over the second MDI exposed O-ball head, and the bone for the third site is "sounded" (Figure 6-14). After the third MDI is inserted, the SIG is then placed over the first MDI O-ball head to locate the fourth MDI

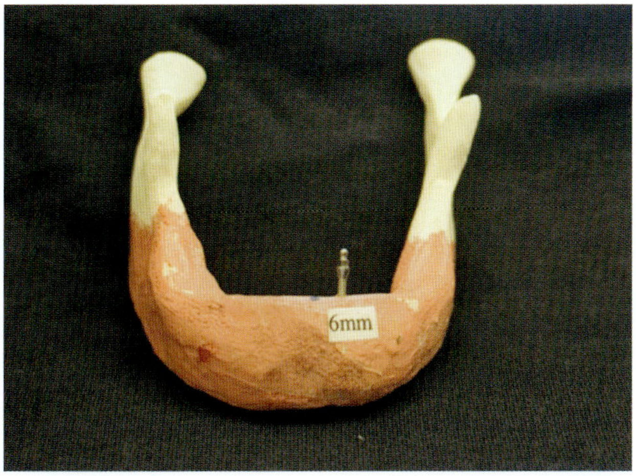

FIGURE 6-10. MDI placed into the initial starter hole to a depth of 6 mm.

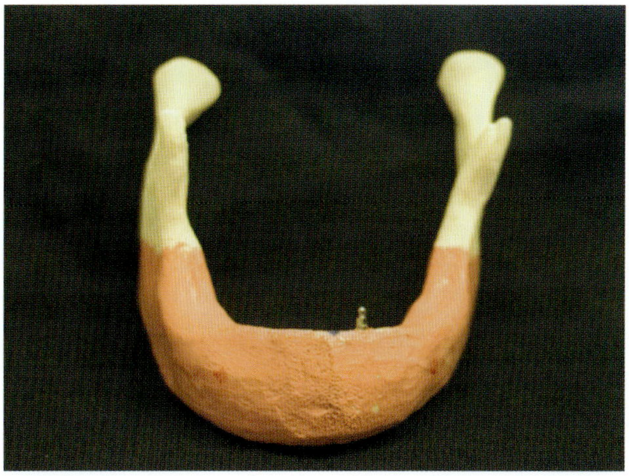

FIGURE 6-11. First MDI placed into the mandible to a point where square top below O-ball is 1 mm subgingival.

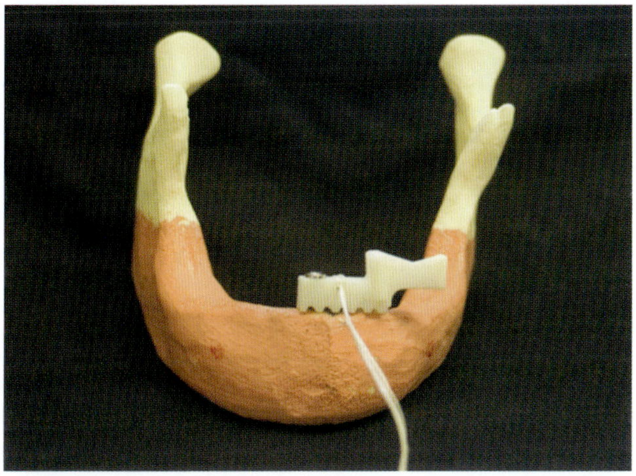

FIGURE 6-12. SIG device with handle placed with O-ball recess over exposed O-ball top.

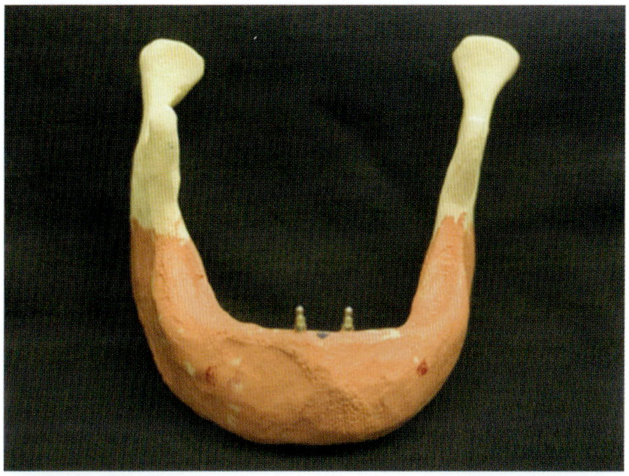

FIGURE 6-13. Second MDI in place perpendicular to ridge, 10 mm from first MDI, and parallel to it.

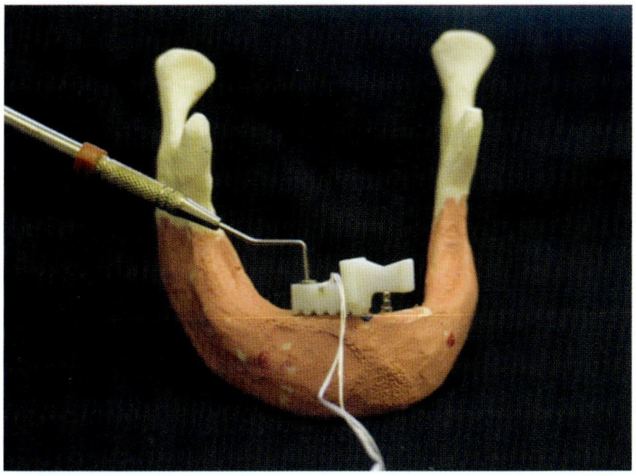

FIGURE 6-14. SIG device positioned over second exposed MDI O-ball top to prepare for the third MDI placement.

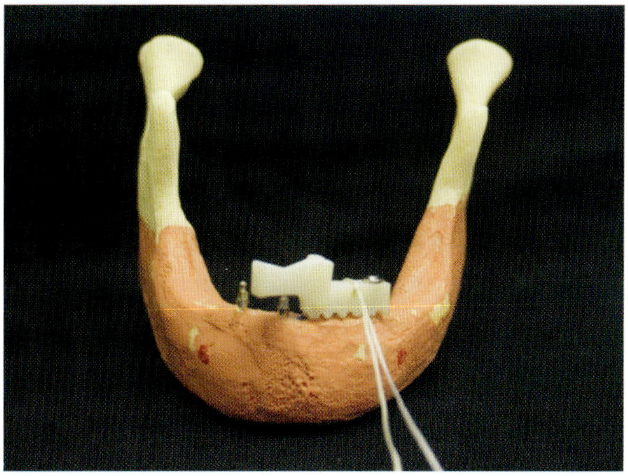

FIGURE 6-15. SIG device handle placed over exposed O-ball top of #1 fixture to drill pilot starter hole for #4 MDI.

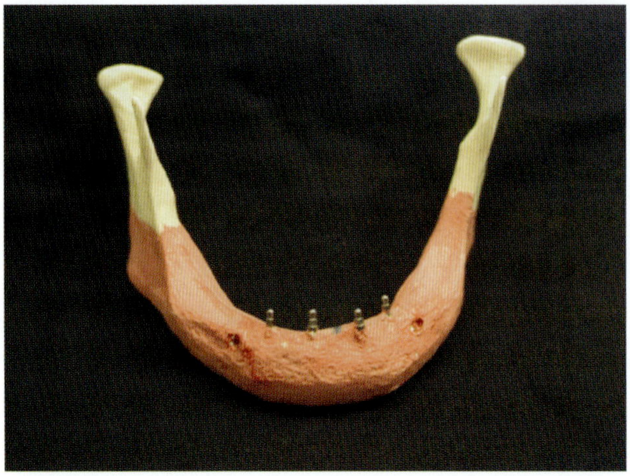

FIGURE 6-16. Four MDIs placed in anterior mandible. They are 10 mm apart, perpendicular to the bone crest, and parallel to each other. In addition, the terminal implants are at a safe 10 mm from the mental foramina.

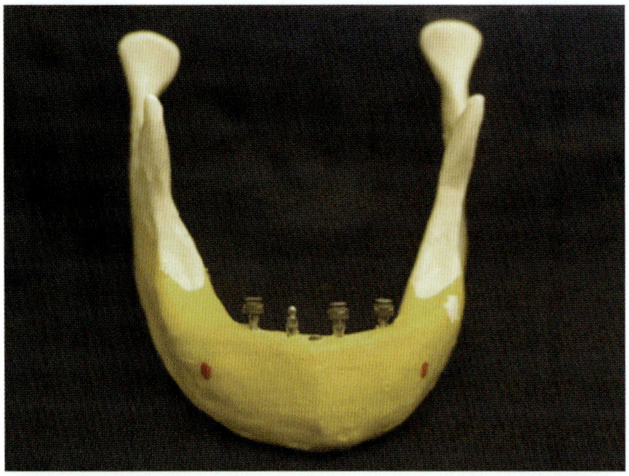

FIGURE 6-17. Metal housings will be incorporated into the overlying denture intaglio.

site (Figure 6-15). When all four MDIs have been inserted, they should be 10 mm apart, perpendicular to the bony ridge, parallel to each other, and at a safe distance from the mental foramina (Figure 6-16). Metal housings will then be placed over the O-ball tops at 30 days after insertion according to our hospital protocol (Figure 6-17). The metal housings are fixed into the denture intaglio with hard self-curing acrylic (Figure 6-18).

Box 6-3 lists the ten benefits of using the SIG device.

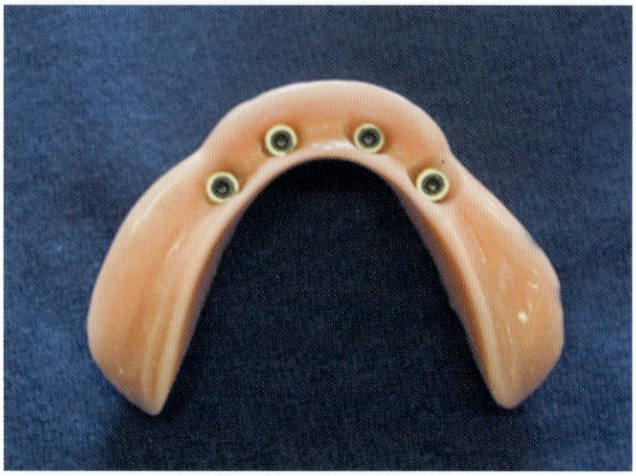

FIGURE 6-18. Metal housings secured in denture base with hard-curing acrylic.

BOX 6-3 Benefits of Using the Sussman Implant Guide (SIG) Device

1. Proper site selection of 5 mm from the midline on either side
2. Proper 6-mm limited depth penetration of the 1.1-mm spiral twist drill into bone
3. Perpendicular insertion of MDI from ridge crest into body of mandible
4. Proper spacing 10 mm apart to allow room for metal housings
5. Parallelism of implants to enable the patient to easily remove and insert denture prosthesis
6. Safe placement of implant fixtures to ensure adequate distance from mental foramina to prevent lip paresthesia
7. Low cost of purchase of SIG device
8. Simplicity of one-piece design of SIG device
9. Easy to master and use the SIG device
10. SIG device is made out of hard plastic with a titanium ring and can be sterilized for re-use with patients

CASE DISCUSSION I

A patient with type II diabetes, insulin-dependent, blind and nonambulatory. In addition to having a flat mandibular ridge that was in line with the floor of the mouth, below the mylohyoid, his sublingual plica overlapped the ridge. Figures 6-19a-h show the placement of four MDIs in the mandible. Figure 6-19i shows a trough drilled into the denture base for self-cure soft liner material, which we use for initial stabilization for 1 month. Figure 6-19j shows the O-ball indentations, equally spaced, in the soft reline material. Note that when the metal housings are placed after 30 days, the parallelism of the MDIs allows the rubber gaskets in the metal housings to last for more than 2 years. When the MDIs are not inserted parallel, the rubber O-rings last only 4 to 6 months before needing replacement.

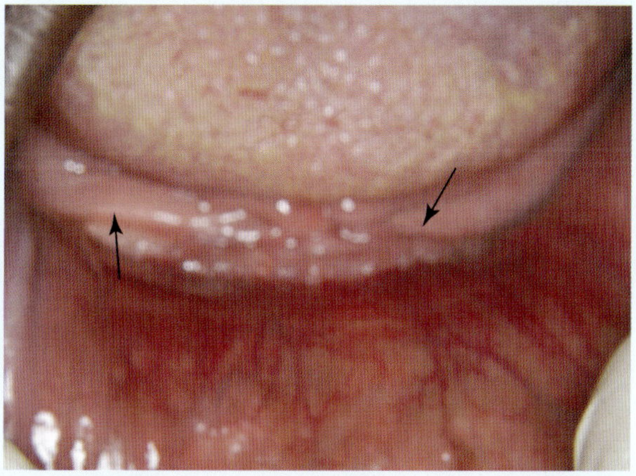

FIGURE 6-19a. Sublingual plica overlying alveolar ridge.

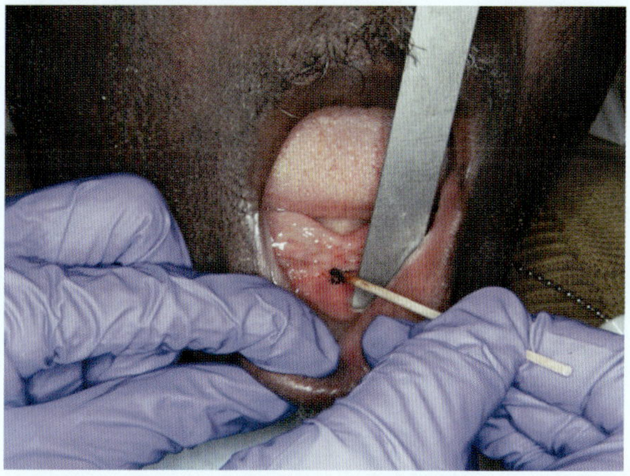

FIGURE 6-19b. A straight-edge ruler is used from tip of nose.

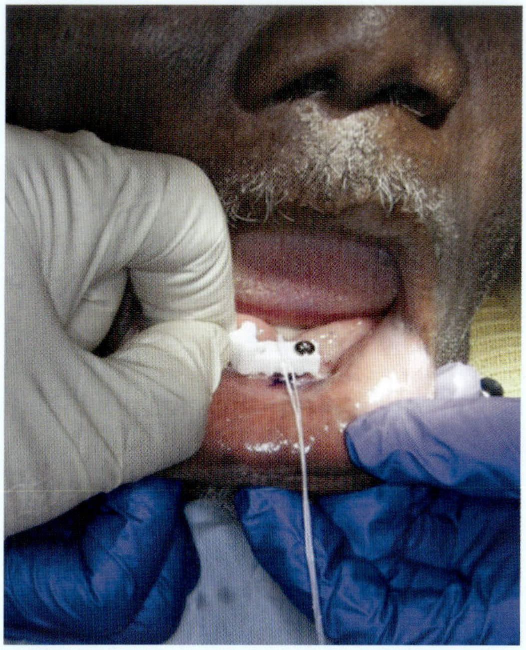

FIGURE 6-19c. Dental floss in SIG device over central marking.

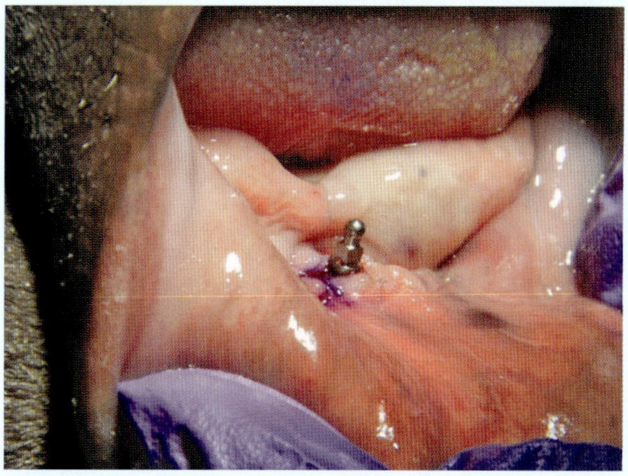

FIGURE 6-19d. First implant seated to square hub.

CASE DISCUSSION 1—cont'd

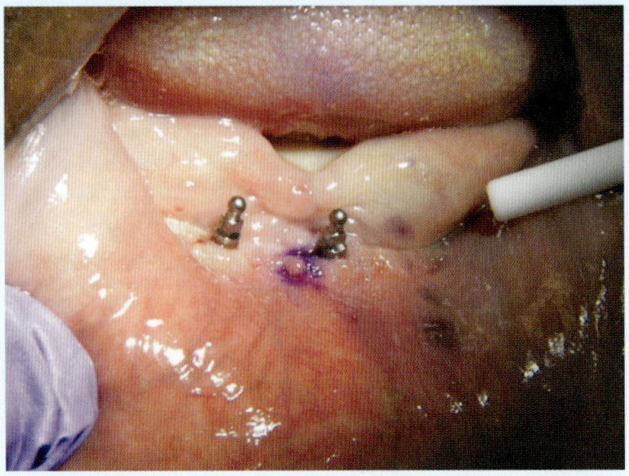

FIGURE 6-19e. First two MDIs are 10 mm apart and parallel.

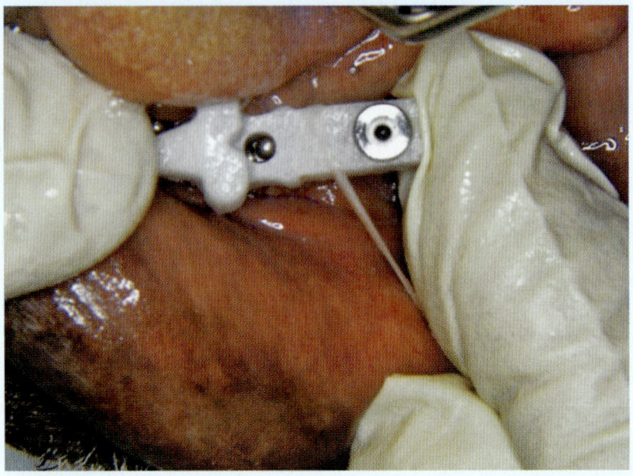

FIGURE 6-19f. SIG device over first MDI ball top to drill third pilot hole.

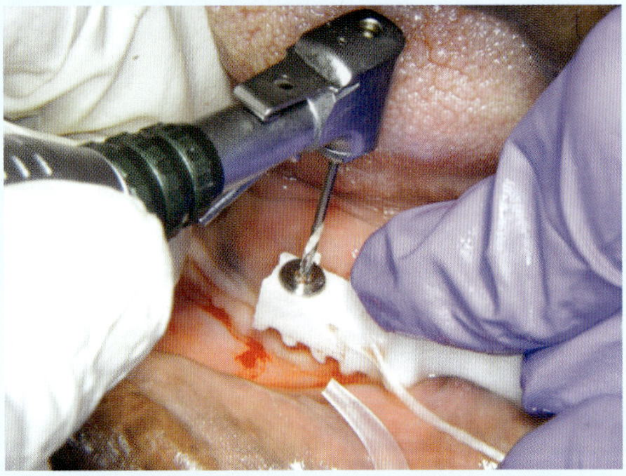

FIGURE 6-19g. Note the bone chips in the spiral drill flutes.

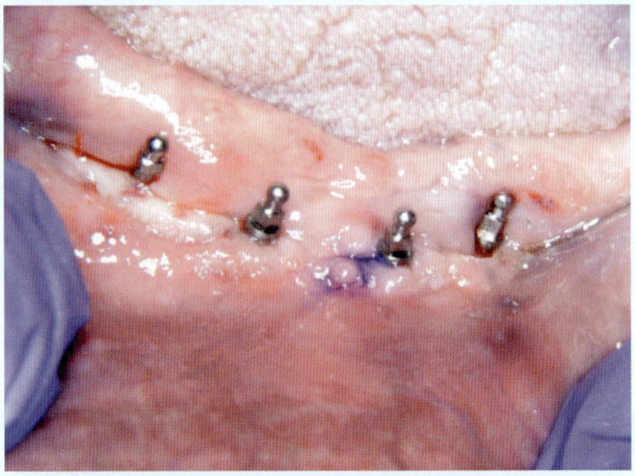

FIGURE 6-19h. Four MDIs in position, all 10 mm apart and parallel to each other.

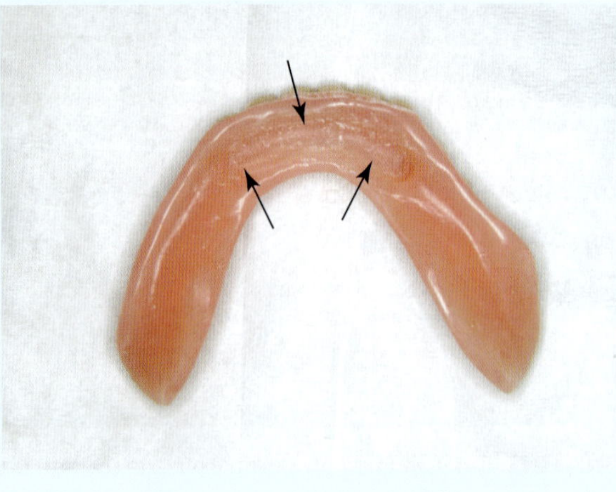

FIGURE 6-19i. Acrylic drilled out of denture intaglio.

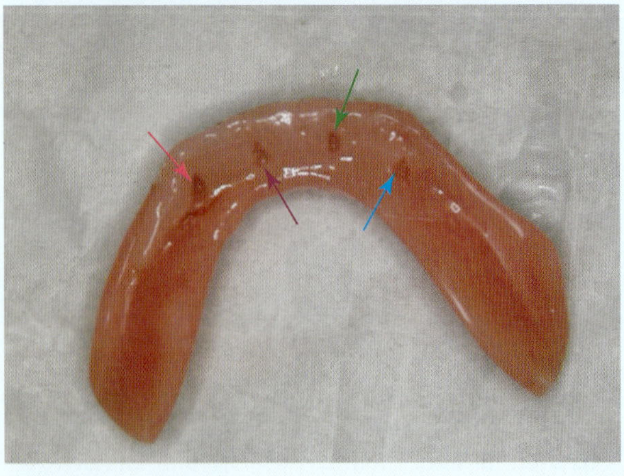

FIGURE 6-19j. O-ball indentations, equally spaced, in the soft reline material.

Chapter 7

An Oral and Maxillofacial Surgeon's Role in Advanced MDI Therapeutics

Engineering Assisted Surgery™, MDIs in Functional Reconstructive Surgery Within Great Britain and New Zealand Venues

NINIAN SPENCELEY PECKITT

Outline

Engineering Assisted Surgery™ (EAS) Medical Art and Surgical Craft

Successful clinical interventions rely heavily on human qualities of the clinician and an association with inaccurate replication and transfer of the treatment plans into patients in three dimensions. Clinical outcomes must vary as a consequence of the inconsistencies related to planning, human, and therapeutic trauma variables. Healthcare modernization has not as yet mirrored what was achieved in the 1960s by the manufacturing industry, which achieved modernization of management, service delivery, standardization of quality, reduction in human error, and improved ergonomics, by the *rapid assimilation* of *state of the art* technology and automation.

Engineering Assisted Surgery™ (EAS) may be defined as "the application of industrial and engineering systems to healthcare delivery"[15] with respect to existing interventions and new and evolving surgical procedures and includes:

- Identification of and appropriate industrial input in healthcare modernization programs at a global level;
- Facilitation of transfer of industrial and engineering solutions to healthcare;
- Bringing industrial concepts of service, management, and delivery into healthcare;
- Improved diagnosis and replicable 3D planning for all medical and surgical specialities;
- Customized medical devices (e.g., tissue engineering, implants, custom jigs);
- Reduction in intervention trauma with appropriate use of available resources;
- A universal improvement of quality and standardization of outcome;
- Facilitation of audit with demonstrated significant reduction in cost and intervention;
- Improved ergonomics and reduction in waiting lists;
- Minimizing the cost of disability for the nation;
- Reduction in medical negligence litigation.

EAS heralds new gold standards in the provision of global healthcare with an improvement in efficiency, quality, and outcome, already seen in other industries, and promotes the concept of ***best practice.*** The value of an industrial contribution to healthcare modernization has been now recognized. However, such a process can only be effectively implemented within an EAS center of excellence and in partnership with concomitant reforms in healthcare management and delivery, without which healthcare modernization will be ineffective. EAS provides an evidence-based and efficacious industrial model on which to build a modernized National Health Service (NHS) and requires utmost priority within the modernization process.

Logistical Considerations

Reconstructive surgery traditionally involves long* complex procedures, which often involve the

*Surgical procedures as long as 12 to 18 hours are not uncommon and involve multiple surgical teams.

harvesting of complex composite free flaps from a second surgical site and microvascular techniques. The dentition is reconstructed using osseointegrated titanium implants in multistaged procedures.

If a functional result can be achieved by means other than additional reconstructive surgical trauma, parameters associated with major surgical procedures such as perioperative mortality, morbidity, and overall rehabilitation may be favorably influenced.

Functional Reconstruction

Functional reconstruction—i.e., accurate replication of volume, contour, and function of hard and soft tissues—is impossible to achieve with living donor tissue, especially in those cases involving replication of complex osseous anatomy.

Mini Dental Implants

The introduction of Dr. Victor Sendax's concept of a mini dental implant (MDI) system[17,18,19,20,21] has produced a major impact in tissue engineering techniques employed in otolaryngology/head and neck surgery, craniomaxillofacial surgery, and oral and maxillofacial reconstructive surgery.

Definition of MDI

In UK MDI training workshops, Peckitt defines MDIs with the following characteristics:

- Implant: titanium alloy or other implantable material
- Implant dimensions (< 2.5 mm in diameter)
- Fused abutment (for additional strength)
- Atraumatic placement (minimal surgery)

Indications for the Use of MDIs

Medical Considerations

Minimal surgery is needed in nearly all patient groups. MDIs have advantages for patient groups in which minimal surgical trauma is an added advantage or quite simply mandatory. MDI placement is often flapless, predictable, and quick. This offers advantages to medically compromised patients (e.g., patients with stable anticoagulation and antiplatelet medication regimens) and those undergoing major reconstructive maxillofacial surgery (Figure 7-1).

The knife edged alveolar ridge may require direct exposure for access and trimming of the alveolar crest. However, this can often be achieved with direct exposure and with minimal tissue reflection, which is of distinct benefit to medically compromised patients.

Surgical Considerations

Five-year survival rates for patients with advanced squamous cell carcinoma of the oral cavity are poor and have not improved significantly in the past 30 years.[1,13] Current treatment modalities are:

- Multidisciplinary;
- Complex and multistaged;
- Multimodal, involving complex composite surgery, radiotherapy, and possible chemotherapy;
- Associated with significant perioperative morbidity:
    - From the donor site;
    - From the recipient site;
    - From radiotherapy;
    - From chemotherapy;
- Associated with significant perioperative mortality as a function of the metabolic response to major surgical trauma.

Although there have been significant advances in free flap tissue transfer, especially in the reconstruction of the hemimandible and anterior mandible, the introduction of techniques such as the free fibula flap has an association with both donor and recipient site morbidity, cumulating in the disaster of flap loss and loss of the patient (Figure 7-2).

Patients with oral cancer are commonly debilitated and are more likely to have higher American Joint Committee on Cancer (AJCC) fitness scores.[3]

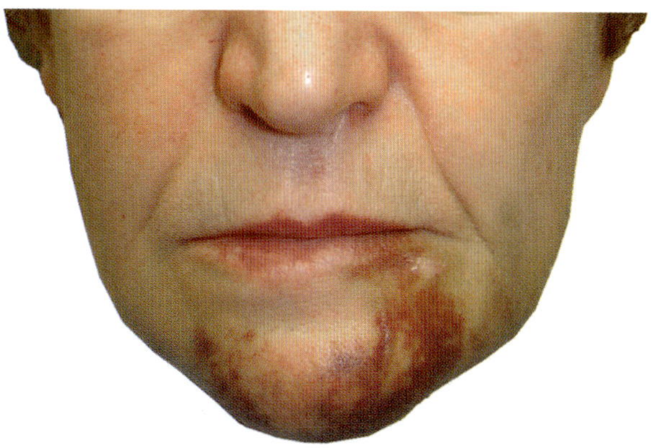

FIGURE 7-1. Hematoma after flap surgery and placement of four standard endosseous dental implants in the anterior mandible for the provision of an overdenture.

The implications are that this group of patients is more likely to succumb to the consequences of major surgery. Therefore offering patients treatment options involving reduced surgical trauma has distinct advantages (Table 7-1).

Moreover, major surgical treatment modalities are costly to the purchasers of healthcare, and if neither cure nor adequate palliation can be achieved at reasonable cost, the value of such treatment protocols requires reappraisal.[22]

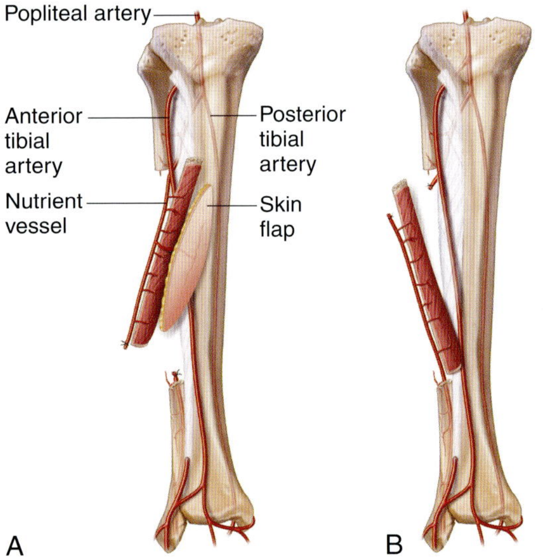

FIGURE 7-2. Anatomy of Free Fibula Flap.
A free fibula flap is commonly used in the reconstruction of the anterior mandible and body of mandible on the premise that vascularized bone maintains its volume and contour.

TABLE 7-1

AJCC Fitness Scores

AJCC (H) Performance Scale	Definition
H0	Normal activity
H1	Symptomatic and ambulatory
H2	Ambulatory > 50% of time Occasionally needs assistance
H3	Ambulatory < 50% of time Nursing care required
H4	Bedridden May need hospitalization

Logistical Issues

The low cost of MDIs is of special interest to state healthcare systems providing complex composite reconstructive head and neck cancer services. With modern planning techniques, MDI placement is possible at the time of resection and reconstruction with presurgical manufacture of the dental prosthesis. As we shall see, treatment is even possible without the use of flap surgery. This further improves the efficiency of the treatment modality, making treatment possible in a single surgical procedure. The financial implications of this scenario are profound for the patient whose surgery is simplified, for the provider with reduced demand for resources, and for the purchaser with significant reduction in cost (Table 7-2).

Indications: MDI Implants in Oral Rehabilitation?

- For stabilization of any overdenture system
  - Anterior Mandible
  - Posterior Mandible
  - Maxilla
- Overdenture
- Obturator
  - Craniofacial applications
- Obturator

Anatomical Considerations

Atrophic Ridges

Ridge Height. It is traditionally advocated that the longest implant should be used. This may pose problems in patients with postresection trismus, and it is advocated that implants should be placed at the time of the resection or reconstruction to overcome this problem. This will facilitate MDI location in patients with additional screws and plates for osteosynthesis.

Although it has been suggested that MDI implants should not be used as a transmandibular system, it is our experience that penetration of the inferior mandibular border results in no problems. This

TABLE 7-2

Oral Cancer Surgery Costs

Type of Surgery	Annual Cost
Reconstructive surgery	£18,125,000 ($28, 206,078)
Engineering assisted surgery™	£10,537,875 ($16,399,014)
Savings	£7,587,125 ($11,807,064)

method permits the placement of larger diameter implants down to the lower border of the mandible with an increased surface area for osseointegration. Currently the role of the denser cortex at the lower border is undetermined; however, it is likely that this will enhance the osseointegration process.

Any protruding sharp MDI tips may be smoothed as required before wound closure.

Ridge Width. MDIs readily meet the challenge of compromised ridge width, obviating the need for bone grafting, ridge splitting, and other additional techniques that complicate otherwise fairly simple treatment plans.

Immediate Loading. Immediate loading only appears to be an issue in bone of poor density; 10% of implants may be expected to fail in the maxilla under normal immediate loading conditions, but it has been noted that total implant failure has been documented in the maxilla in patients with good bone density (Misch Grade 1 to 2) and who have natural opposing dental dentition. Immediate loading of MDIs in this situation is contraindicated and methods of shielding the implants are discussed later in this chapter.

Factors Influencing Functional Dentition

The 1998 Adult Dental Health Survey (Oral Health)[26] in the United Kingdom documented that a minimum of 21 teeth are required for functioning dentition (Figure 7-3).

In a base sample size of 923 adults with dental prostheses, speaking difficulties (9%), eating difficulties (37%), and other problems (16%) were recorded. An overall incidence of prosthetic problems was documented in 40% of patients sampled (Tables 7-3 to 7-6).

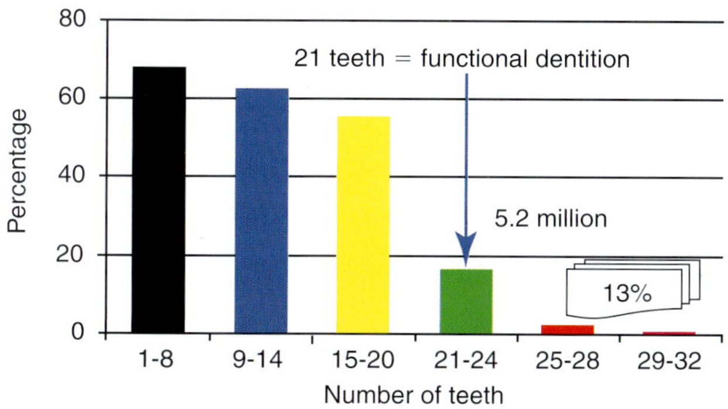

FIGURE 7-3. Proportion of dentate adults who have partial dentures by the number of natural teeth.

TABLE 7-3

Problems with Speaking with Dentures

Problem with Speaking	Percentage
Loose denture/slips when talking	4%
Alters or slurs speech	3%
Other speaking problems	2%
No problems	93%

Data modified from Adult Dental Health Survey Oral Health in the United Kingdom 1998. Office for National Statistics; London: The Stationery Office.

TABLE 7-4

Problems with Eating with Dentures

Problems with Eating	Percentage
Food sticks under denture plate	12%
Loose/denture/slips when eating	9%
Hurts gums	8%
Cannot chew or bite well	5%
Other eating problems	3%
No problems	74%

36% of patients have eating difficulties.
Data modified from Adult Dental Health Survey Oral Health in the United Kingdom 1998. Office for National Statistics; London: The Stationery Office.

TABLE 7-5

Other Denture Problems

Other Denture Problems	Percentage
Loose dentures	5%
Gets ulcers	3%
Sore gum/plate rubs gums	3%
Denture worn down	1%
Other denture problem	4%
No problems	84%

16% of patients have other denture problems.
Data modified from Adult Dental Health Survey Oral Health in the United Kingdom 1998. Office for National Statistics; London: The Stationery Office.

TABLE 7-6

Prosthetic Outcomes

Prosthetic Outcome	Percentage
Prosthetic problems (incidents)	40%
No problems	60%

Data modified from Adult Dental Health Survey Oral Health in the United Kingdom 1998. Office for National Statistics; London: The Stationery Office.

The implications of this survey imply that conventional prosthetic practice is delivering a quality of service with a 40% complication rate in the United Kingdom, and current primary treatment options require reappraisal in the light of recent technical advances in the sphere of MDI dentistry.

Because stability of the lower denture is now so effective with inexpensive MDIs and outcomes so superior (compared with the tissue-borne full lower denture prosthesis, which is indicated only if dental implant placement is contraindicated), Peckitt now advocates that the MDI-retained lower overdenture is now the primary denture treatment option.[22]

MDIs and Complex Maxillofacial Reconstruction

If we consider the 40% prosthetic complication rate for routine edentulous cases, it is clear that more complex cases will present greater problems for the prosthetician, and it is advocated that a simple reliable cost effect system is required. Peckitt argues that MDIs fulfill many of the requirements:

- Simple fused abutment system
- Simple instrumentation
- MDI max system is particularly useful in less dense bone
- Immediate loading possible in mandible
- Concomitant placement at time of resection and reconstruction
- Placement without flap surgery
- Presurgical fabrication of prosthesis
- Single staged technique
- Effective in maxilla, mandible, and craniofacial regions
- Able to be used in curative procedures
- Especially useful in palliative procedures and associated issues related to the cost of effective palliation
- Postoperative irradiation may be given
- Implant loss is readily retrievable, often without bone grafting
- Low cost of implant System

Contraindications to the Use of MDIs

There are few, but include:

Medical
- Psychiatric disease
- Chronic facial pain syndromes
- History of infected endocarditis
- Rheumatic fever

Rheumatic fever is not necessarily a contraindication; some cases may be deemed low risk. Treatment should be carried out in conjunction with a cardiology opinion. Echocardiography is a useful investigation in the assessment of risk.

Surgical
- Severe jaw atrophy (bone height)
- Grade 4 bone density (not necessarily)
- Heavy occlusion that cannot be relieved
- Gross dental sepsis
- Immediate tooth replacement after extraction may present problems

Peckitt has demonstrated the successful use of MDI implants in severe maxillary atrophy[16] and in grade 4 bone density in conjunction with bone grafting and platelet rich plasma techniques,[12] with stability at 9 years.

Management of the Complex Reconstruction Case

History

- Congenital
- Acquired
- Growth disorder
  - Trauma

Medical Status

- The patient must be declared medically fit for surgical component.
- A detailed medical examination is mandatory.

Surgical

- Biopsy (confirmational diagnosis)
- Clinical photography
- CT, MRI scan planning
  - Head and neck
  - Chest
  - Abdomen
- Anatomical biomodeling
- Multidisciplinary treatment planning
- Tumor staging
- Treatment options
  - Excision for local clearance
  - Neck dissection
  - Adjuvant therapy
    - Radiotherapy
    - Chemotherapy
- Curative versus palliative treatment options

Dental

Dental considerations are of prime importance in achieving a satisfactory functional and esthetic result.

- A thorough dental examination is required for every patient.
- Teeth with poor prognosis must be identified and excluded from the treatment plan.
- If radiotherapy is planned, teeth in the immediate radiation field should be extracted.
- Adequate bone width is required.

Examination

- Sepsis
- Periodontal status
- Occlusion

Investigations

- OPT / lat chin / PA bone density
- I.D. nerve / sinus status
- Implant sites / selection / templates
- Study models / crown bridge
- Putty jig / suck down splint / drill guide
- CT scan for biomodel manufacture mandatory for complex orofacial or panfacial reconstructions

Prosthetic Evaluation

- Existing or conversion
- New prosthesis

What are Current Treatment Modalities and How do They Work?

Treatment planning involves clinical assessment, stabilization, and investigation using noninvasive and invasive techniques. Historically case planning implied a total reliance on the skills and performance of the clinician. In some cases resuscitation and emergency interventions are required to preserve life; in such cases secondary interventions are carried out to complete the treatment plan.

When the timing of an intervention and clinical stability permits planning as a single intervention, this is traditionally two dimensional (2D) with existing imaging technology that is commonly available. The treatment plan must then be replicated and translated into a three- dimensional (3D) patient. These protocols must have an association with a compromised outcome as a function of inaccuracy of plan translation, and it is to be noted that such comparable practice has been abandoned by other industries that have since demonstrated an improvement.

EAS concepts may be used in conjunction with the planning and facilitation of established interventions (i.e., current practice), new surgical procedures and medical devices (in particular MDIs), and customized medical devices.

The Art and Craft of Clinical Practice

Clinical practice has traditionally and *proudly* been regarded as an art or craft acquired through apprenticeship. However, the reliance on human performance does not lend itself to efficiency and homogeneity of outcome and has been superseded in industry by new reverse engineering planning technology, rapid prototyping, automation, and standardization of the production processes.

Although dental casts of the teeth and jaws have been used successfully for many years in treatment planning, recently new advances in engineering technology have made EAS possible for sister specialties. These advances include:

- The discovery of osseointegration;
- Transmucosal or transcutaneous implant systems (in particular the MDI concept of Dr. Victor Sendax);
- New (bio)engineering materials;
- Advanced computer technology;
- Computer assisted diagnosis, design, and manufacture;
- Rapid prototyping, reverse engineering, and biomodel manufacture;
- New manufacturing processes;
- Customized templates, jigs, and implants;
- Applications in customized tissue engineering.

These developments herald the introduction of new gold standards in healthcare, with an improvement in efficiency and quality already seen in other industries.

Successful Outcome

The parameters of successful outcome are often arbitrary and based on current practice, which does not necessarily portray the best outcome possible and does not take into account recent developments especially in the field of EAS. Best practice is a complex function of many parameters in relation to accepted national standards of outcome. In the United Kingdom, crucial data are not freely available or have not been documented; for many parameters, no national standards have been agreed upon. This has an adverse effect on clinical audit, evidence-based practice, and clinical governance issues.

Performance data related to other aspects of best practice throughout the healthcare industry is deficient, but if one considers the model of quality improvement in the manufacturing industry after advances in computer technology and adoption of automated processes, it is likely that poor performance indicators are related to human factors.

Medical Negligence

EAS technology provides the opportunity for presentation of hard copy evidence for cases of personal injury. The use of anatomical biomodels may protect both the patient and clinician in medical negligence cases. The use of EAS techniques is likely to reduce the incidence of litigation related to human error. The current annual cost of the United Kingdom's NHS related medicolegal litigation runs at £7billion (USD $10.9 billion)/annum. If a 14% reduction in the cost of medical negligence litigation could be achieved by the adoption of EAS technology as the gold standard of duty of care, this would result in a saving of £1billion (USD $1.5 billion)/annum in the United Kingdom.

Applications of EAS in Healthcare

Let us therefore examine the effects of EAS on the delivery of healthcare on the available evidence.

Oral Cancer

The Logistics of MDIs in Orofacial Reconstruction

Each year in the United Kingdom there are more than 2500 new cases of oral cancer[14,15,24] (approximately 1% of all cancer registrations) with an annual mortality of approximately 1400 compared with 1339 deaths from cervical cancer in 1995. Some evidence shows that oral cancer is becoming more common in women and younger patients in the United Kingdom and other countries. Oral cancer is twice as common in men.

Although the incidence of oral cancer was static in the 1980s, now signs show a rising incidence. Four patients die of this disease every day in the United Kingdom.[4]

In the 1960s 15% of patients presented with T3 or T4 tumors; this increased to 28% in the 1980s, which implies that in England and Wales approximately 724 patients presented in 1991 with disease that would probably have been treated with complex composite free flap techniques in the United Kingdom.

In the United States in 2005, new cases of cancer of the oral cavity and pharynx were estimated at 29,370, with an estimated annual mortality of 7320[2] (Table 7-7).

Lymph Node Status and Survival

In a series of 2550 cases of epidermoid carcinoma of the oral cavity and oropharynx, Spiro et al[25] observed a 14% reduction in 5-year survival—from 51% for the clinically negative neck (cN0) to 37% if only one node was histologically diagnosed positive for metastatic tumor,. If multiple unilat-

TABLE 7-7

American Cancer Society Oral Cancer Estimates
New Cases and Mortality (2005)

	Estimated New Cases			Estimated Deaths		
	Both Sexes	Men	Women	Both Sexes	Men	Women
Oral cavity and pharynx	29,370	19,100	10,270	7320	4910	2410
Tongue	7660	5050	2610	1730	1120	610
Mouth	10,070	5370	4700	1890	1100	790
Pharynx	8590	6520	2070	2130	1490	640
Other	3050	2160	890	1570	1200	370

Data from American Cancer Society.

eral nodes were histologically positive, the 5-year survival was reduced to 24% (i.e., the survival rate was nearly halved). For histologically involved bilateral nodes, the 5-year survival dropped to 5%. This series of patients roughly numbers the new cases that would be expected to present annually in the United Kingdom.

If it is accepted that the majority of deaths in oral cancer are related to local recurrence or direct extension of disease rather than from distant metastasis, it would appear that current treatment modalities are failing in their palliative aims, most commonly within the first 2 years of treatment.

National Cancer Statistics (United Kingdom)[7]

In the United Kingdom in 2005, 4926 persons were diagnosed with an oral cancer. Across countries, the highest incidence for both male and female patients is in Scotland.

In 2006 there were nearly 1700 deaths from oral cancer in the United Kingdom.

The overall age-standardized mortality rate has remained fairly stable between 1971 and 2006 at approximately 3.5 and 1.4 per 100,000 for male and female patients, respectively.

As with the incidence trends, the all-ages oral cancer mortality figure masks the variation in age-specific trends. Mortality rates have more than halved since the 1970s for men in their 70s and 80s. On the contrary, for men in their 40s, 50s, and 60s there has been a small but steady increase. For younger men the rate has remained stable.

The mortality in oral cancer is to be considered in context with epidemiologic data for all cancer registrations and associated mortality in the United Kingdom. The cost to the nation in terms of overall patient mortality is that 62% of patients will die from the disease.

Head and Neck Surgery: Cost of Treatment[15]

Complex Composite Free Flap Techniques

In 1993 at the British Association of Oral and Maxillofacial Surgeons meeting in Cardiff, Lavery estimated the true cost of microvascular free flap transfer at £25,000 (USD $38,900) per oral cancer case.

Average Costs of Treatment: One Live Patient at 2 years

The average cost of a 2-year survival episode is documented at £85,000 (USD $132,000) for patients treated with complex composite microvascular techniques (assuming a 70% 2-year mortality rate at £25,000 (USD $38,900) per case in line with Lavery's estimation). In a pilot study of seven patients with cancer treated in Doncaster Royal Infirmary with customized titanium implants,[15] zero mortality was recorded at 4.5 years at a cost of £14,535 (USD $22,600) per case episode for those patients treated 1994 to 1996.

Complex composite microvascular flap reconstructive techniques are reserved for patients with advanced disease, the majority of which affect the mandible. If the percentage of cases presenting as T3/T4 cases of 28% is accepted, approximately 725 microvascular oral reconstruction episodes per year are carried out in the United Kingdom, at an annual cost of £18,125,000 (USD $28,206,000) (assuming the estimated cost of £25,000 (USD $38,9000) per episode has remained unchanged since 1993).[15]

The cost of free flap surgery in New Zealand has been estimated at NZ $60,000 to NZ $80,000 per case intervention (Izzard: 2007 Auckland Head and Neck Cancer Centre) (Table 7-8).

Simplification of treatment plans incorporating (EAS techniques has demonstrated a reduction in cost (see Table 7-2) of treatment to £14,535 (USD $22,600) per surgical intervention and, in comparison, the national annual total cost of treatment would be £10,537,875 (USD $16,399,000) for this

TABLE 7-8

Cost Comparison: Composite Free Flap Transfer Versus Engineering Assisted Surgery (EAS)

Composite Free Flap Transfer	EAS
£25,000 (USD $38,900)/case	£14,535 (USD $22,600)/case (7 patients)
70% expected mortality @ 2 years	0% mortality @ 4 years
Average cost: 2 year survival £85,000 (USD $132,000)	Average cost: 2 year survival £14,535 (USD $22,600)

Data from Peckitt: EAS Costs 1994-1996. Doncaster Royal Infirmary, United Kingdom, www.maxfac.com/costsavings.html.

option, an annual saving to the nation of £7,587,125 (USD $11,807,000) plus an associated improvement in long-term overall mortality figures and statistical significance even on a small sample size.

Research and Development

The palliative care of patients with head and neck cancer is discussed by Lovel,[11] who quotes Stjernsward: "No further research is required; the knowledge of what needs to be done exists. The single most useful thing that we can do is to make sure that every patient benefits from that knowledge."

However, *"If surgical treatment is a component of such palliation, it is argued that there is still much to learn"* (Peckitt).[15]

Treatment Planning: Huge Cost Savings with Biomodels

For the management of complex reconstruction and trauma cases, savings are higher per unit case as a function of the consequences of reduced surgical trauma. Savings of £30,000 (USD $46,685) per case intervention are possible[1] with projections of reduced operating times, less dependency on critical care facilities, earlier discharge from hospital, and enhanced rehabilitation.

EAS: Discussion

New developments in engineering, used for the first time in oral and maxillofacial surgery,[15,22] permit the manufacture of accurate anatomical biomodels of the skeleton from CT scans, using a variety of reverse engineering methods. Biomodels have been used in treatment planning and the design and manufacture of customized titanium implants for the single staged reconstruction of the orofacial region using very simple cost effective interventions. These may carried out without surgery from a second surgical site and obviate the necessity for complex flap surgery.

In our experience, the Sendax MDI system has a pivotal role in complex orofacial reconstruction within the context of EAS. The system is a great example of EAS thinking.

We now have a treatment option that permits endosseous stabilization of a prosthetic device:

- With the advantages of a flapless technique and minimal trauma;
- In cases of compromised osseous width and/or bone volume;
- As a single staged or immediate technique;
- At low cost;
- To produce an excellent quality of prosthetic retention and palliation;
- With simple and economical salvage in the event of implant loss.

Moreover, the Sendax MDI system can be used in conjunction with anatomical biomodels and custom drill guides for precision placement. We have also used the MDI O-ring system in conjunction with customized implant manufacture where conventional MDI placement has been impossible, and we have used this method to replace the whole maxilla and midface in a surgery time of 1.5 hours and with patient discharge at 20 hours (i.e., same-day surgery).

With EAS planning techniques and relatively atraumatic surgical protocols, a single staged orofacial reconstruction, including the dentition, is now possible in most cases, obviating the need for multistaged and increasingly expensive treatment options for patients with a guarded prognosis.

The use of the Sendax MDI system has been so successful in head and neck reconstructive surgery practice in New Zealand that it is rapidly becoming the implant system of choice for this group of patients.

Within oral and maxillofacial surgery, EAS has special relevance in the planning and treatment of complex trauma, facial deformity, craniofacial/skull base surgery, and reconstructive surgery.

Applications are possible in many surgical disciplines, especially orthopaedic trauma, treatment of deformity, and orthopaedic implants, including customized joint replacement. EAS technology permits the design and manufacture of customized implants to an accuracy not before possible. Applications pertaining to medicolegal practice, the demonstration of personal injury, and audit of outcomes, herald new standards in duty of care, and there are applications in high-risk procedures in which precision is of primary importance (e.g., in spinal surgery, where surgical precision could be improved with position and cutting jigs).

As this technology is development and mastered, reappraisal of the principles of surgery in general are warranted, especially in relation to the incredible accuracy that is possible using these techniques and the potential of the elimination of operator error.

Resource Implications

In oral and maxillofacial surgery, there are important resource implications relating to the utilization of:

- Single surgical teams;
- Short simple operations; single site and/or single staged surgery;
- Reduced surgical trauma;
- Reduction in the use of donor sites and their morbidity if flaps are not used;
- Projections of reduced morbidity; projections of reduced perioperative mortality;
- Reduction in use of critical care facilities;
- Projections of reduction in hospitalization times;
- Reduction in cost of surgical episodes.

It is advocated that:

- Surgical planning is facilitated;
- Nonmutilating reconstructions are possible;
- Excellent esthetics and immediate dental rehabilitation is possible;
- Tumor recurrence is not possible in the titanium prosthesis;
- Intraoral wound breakdown is not related to failure of the technique;
- Implants can be salvaged in the presence of complications that would have resulted in total loss of alternative surgical methods of reconstruction:
- Conventional surgery can still be employed in cases of implant failure;

The introduction of this technology has far reaching implications for surgery in general, and further development and research is advocated with respect to:

- Implant biotechnology and design;
- Treatment planning and protocols;
- Morbidity and mortality studies;
- Hospitalization and rehabilitation times;
- Quality outcomes and cost savings.

Indications For EAS

EAS has relevance to many specialties, especially maxillofacial surgery and orthopaedics:

- To promote the accuracy of planning and delivery of surgical treatment plans.
- To facilitate the transfer of the surgical plan from biomodel to patient.
- To replicate bone resection cuts exactly at operation with customized cutting jigs.
- To accurately determine positions of the bones with position jigs.
- To eliminate operator error.
- To facilitate single stage reconstructive surgery.
- To facilitate single site surgery.
- To reduce surgical trauma.
- To reduce the dependency on postoperative critical care.
- To guarantee quality of outcome related to technique.
- To facilitate audit of outcomes.
- To promote the principles of clinical effectiveness and governance.

Projections of Cost Savings in Clinical Practice

It is likely that cost savings and enhanced outcome illustrated in oral and maxillofacial reconstructive surgery will be mirrored in other specialties, especially in orthopedics; in the United Kingdom the logistics of major trauma management and their outcomes have been reassessed.[5]

Large cost savings related to the introduction of EAS techniques and potential improvement in outcome are possible and have already been documented in maxillofacial surgery related to:

- Accuracy of diagnosis;
- Treatment planning;
- Translation of plan to patient;
- Reduction in surgical trauma and operating time;
- Overall reduction in cost;
- Promotion of rehabilitation and earlier return to employment.

Application of EAS to the Healthcare Industry

Conventional techniques related to the successful outcome of clinical intervention rely heavily on human qualities of the clinician. Although many interventions are carried out with no planning in advance or with planning only possible during the intervention, other cases are planned in advance using composite systems, often involving 2D radiographs and computer generated scans, which do not permit the accurate replication and transfer of the plan into the 3D patient.

The consequences of this modus operandi are that interventions rely heavily on (variable) human ability, performance, and a complex and expensive resource network, which is inefficiently used. The quality of outcome must vary as a consequence of the inconsistencies related to planning variables, the human variable, the degree of clinical trauma required to achieve the outcome.

EAS: Oral and Maxillofacial Surgery Model

In maxillofacial surgery, EAS techniques have been shown to facilitate:

- Accuracy of diagnosis and treatment planning;
- Translation of a 3D plan into a 3D patient;
- Reduction in surgical trauma and operating time;
- Accuracy in existing interventions;
- Treatment previously thought impossible using established interventions;
- The creation of new procedures that simplify treatment;
- The conversion of staged multiple interventions into a single intervention;
- Overall reduction in cost;
- Promotion of normal esthetics and functional rehabilitation;
- Earlier return to employment;
- Facilitation of clinical audit.

MDIs and Mandibular Reconstruction

It has long been known within the sphere of dental surgery that the oral cavity has the ability to heal by secondary intention without complication, even in the environment of hostile sepsis. Postextraction sockets illustrate this "par excellence" and yet this innate gift is ill recognized by those providing reconstructive services within this hostile oral environment. This situation has led to the generation and propagation of myths and guidelines on the requirements for oral healing that have in reality no basis in fact or experience (Figure 7-4).

It would appear that vascularized bone irrespective of periosteal cover has the ability to encourage reepithelialization within 7 to 10 days in the oral and nasal cavities.

Reepithelialization produces an attached mucosa that is relatively immobile compared with the surrounding reflected mucosa tissue. This tissue provides an excellent epithelial cuff around implant abutments and gives a superior outcome than epithelial cuffs associated with relatively bulky intraoral flaps, especially free flaps.

This implies that flaps are not required to effect oral mucosa closure and regeneration, in the same way that a flap is not required to close a tooth socket after extraction. This contention is supported by our experience in the management of:

- Degloving injuries of the lips;
- Orthognathic surgery, especially maxillary bone grafting following Le Fort I downfracture: In this scenario nasal mucosa does not break down even though the maxillary graft is initially avascular;
- Orbital reconstruction (bone graft): In this scenario, exposure of the graft to the maxillary sinus does not result in infection and loss of graft;

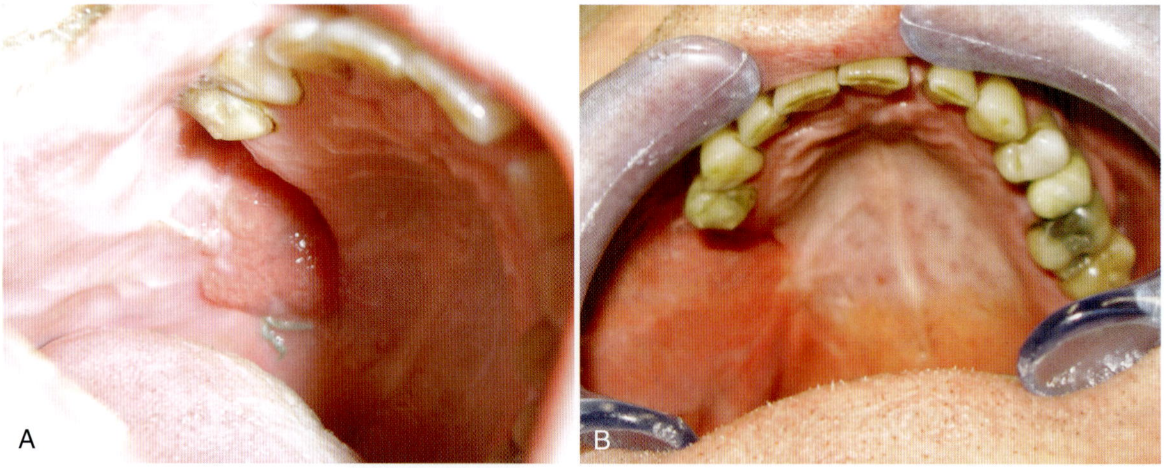

FIGURE 7-4. **A,** 2 weeks after alveolar resection for squamous cell carcinoma of the gingiva. **B,** 3 months after alveolar resection.

- Similarly, sinus lift surgery in cases where the schneiderian membrane is breached does not invariably result in the loss of graft;
- The use of deepithelialized flaps in reconstructive surgery.

The routine use of flaps for bone cover in the oral cavity must be questioned.

It is advocated that the use of intraoral flapless reconstruction techniques prevents the development of the so-called "Burger Syndrome" in which bulky patty-sized intraoral flaps prevent the effective oral rehabilitation so often impossible in these cases and yet necessary for the maintenance of an adequate quality of life. This is especially important in palliative cases, where outcomes often do not always represent an improvement of morbidity.

The introduction of EAS planning techniques in conjunction with the Sendax MDI system greatly simplifies orofacial reconstruction, making single staged reconstruction possible for most patients.

This has major effects on:

- Informed consent;
- Single staged treatment plans;
- Presurgical fabrication of prostheses;
- Early outcome aesthetics;
- Affect on patient;
- Affect on family;
- Reduction of surgical trauma;
- Reduction in morbidity;
- Reduction in cost of treatment;
- Enhanced rehabilitation.

Anterior Rim Sparing Mandibulectomy

The basis of this procedure is that the lingual periosteum acts as a barrier for tumor invasion from the floor of the mouth and gingiva; the edentulous mandible is invaded through the superior aspect of alveolar crest. The tumor invades the mandible as far as the inferior dental canal and then spreads in an anteroposterior direction along the inferior dental canal but rarely below it. Therefore a localized mandibulectomy, sparing the lower mandibular border, may result in tumor clearance.

In a nonatrophic or dentate case, marginal resection of the hemi/anterior mandible and the assessment of residual alveolar height will determine the feasibility of the use of MDIs.

The concept using of the Sendax MDI system to stabilize an immediate overdenture at the time of marginal mandibulectomy has its origin in the use of the system for stabilizing an immediate lower dental prosthesis after a lower dental clearance.

In end-stage periodontal disease, the alveolar bone has often resorbed to the degree that very little alveolectomy is required to trim the bone to the level of the tooth apices. After this task has been performed, MDIs can be simply placed, and gingival margins appropriately trimmed and sutured for healing by primary intention around the emerging implant abutments. A localizing hard resin impression is straightforward, and this is now the method of choice for stabilizing the full lower immediate removable dental prosthesis.

The procedure is simple, reliable, and well tolerated by patients. The outcome is a positive life changing experience for patients, who otherwise would be condemned to a lifestyle of unstable prosthetic dentistry.

In marginal mandibulectomy, the dental clearance is carried out, only this time with an oscillating saw and the dental clearance concomitantly with the jaw resection.

CASE DISCUSSION 1 Marginal Mandibulectomy and Concomitant Reconstruction of the Dentition with an MDI Technique

An 82-year-old woman presented with a well differentiated squamous cell carcinoma of the gingiva.

Past Medical History: Poorly controlled hypertension (Figures 7-5 and 7-6).

TREATMENT PLANNING

The patient was staged at the local multidisciplinary treatment planning head and neck clinic using panoramic dental radiographs and CT scanning, which confirmed staging stage cT2cN0M0.

Selected treatment option: Marginal mandibulectomy without neck dissection.

EAS surgical plan: Resection mapping (Figure 7-7).

CASE DISCUSSION 1 Marginal Mandibulectomy and Concomitant Reconstruction of the Dentition with an MDI Technique—cont'd

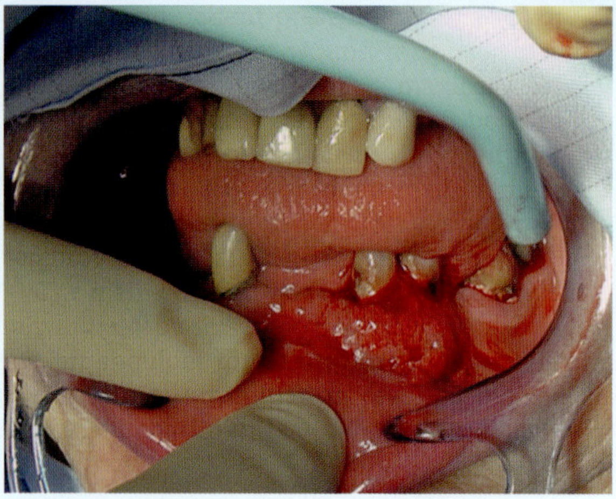

FIGURE 7-5. Oral squamous cell carcinoma: marginal mandibulectomy with MDI placement.

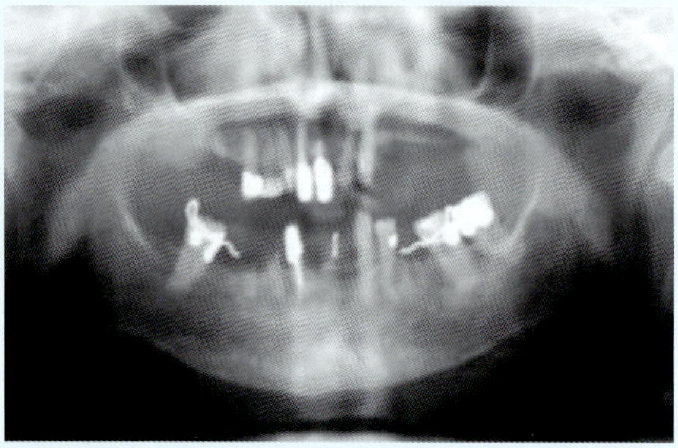

FIGURE 7-6. Panoramic x-ray showing the preservation of mental nerves.

The margins of the tumor were estimated and marked on the panoramic x-ray. A symmetrical resection margin was planned:

1. To produce a smooth homogeneous ridge for the denture base;
2. To facilitate the mirror image location of the MDIs on the contralateral side;
3. To produce bilateral mirroring of the vertical position of the abutment head in the horizontal plane;
4. To prevent potential rocking of the implant due to asymmetrical abutment positioning;
5. To prevent asymmetrical reattachment of mentalis.

The planned resection preserved the mental foramina bilaterally and the innervations of the lower lip.

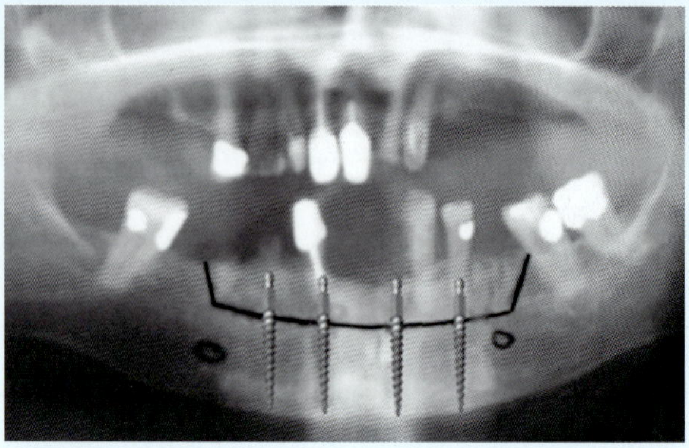

FIGURE 7-7. Gingival Carcinoma 25 to 28; Staging: T2N0M0.

This plan simulates that of a conventional lower dental clearance with immediate stabilization of a prefabricated overdenture. MDI templates have been copied and pasted using Adobe Photoshop software. Note:

- The symmetrical resection for implant placement along a horizontal plane;
- Preservation of the mental nerves;
- Implants permitted to pierce the lower border of the mandible;
- Bevelled resection proximally.

The dimensions of the residual mandible were calculated and templates used to select the correct length of MDI for each osteotomy site.

Impressions were taken for the construction of an immediate overdenture with replication of the vertical dimension of the preexisting occlusion.

SURGERY

Surgery was performed under general anaesthesia via nasal intubation and additional infiltration with citanest and octapressin in view of the history of hypertension.

The tumor was resected with a transoral approach without a lip split and without any external skin incisions.

Sagittal and reciprocating saws were used to make the required osteotomy, and the tumor was excised with clear margins. The resection margin involved the mucosa extending into the floor of mouth and the inside of the lower lip (Figure 7-8).

RECONSTRUCTION

The posterior margins of the marginal mandibulectomy were smoothed and four Sendax MDI Max collared implants were placed in the positions 28, 26, 23 and 44 using the thumb wrench

CASE DISCUSSION 1 Marginal Mandibulectomy and Concomitant Reconstruction of the Dentition with an MDI Technique—cont'd

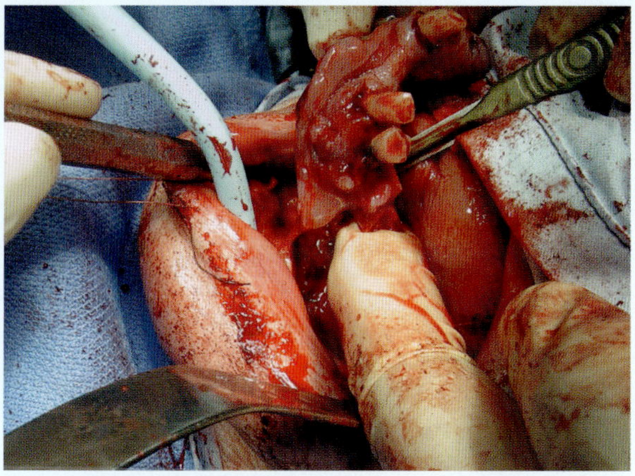

FIGURE 7-8. Tumor delivery.

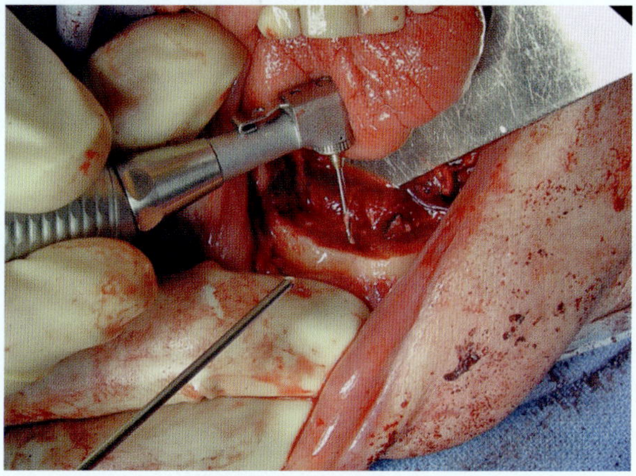

FIGURE 7-9. Pilot hole.

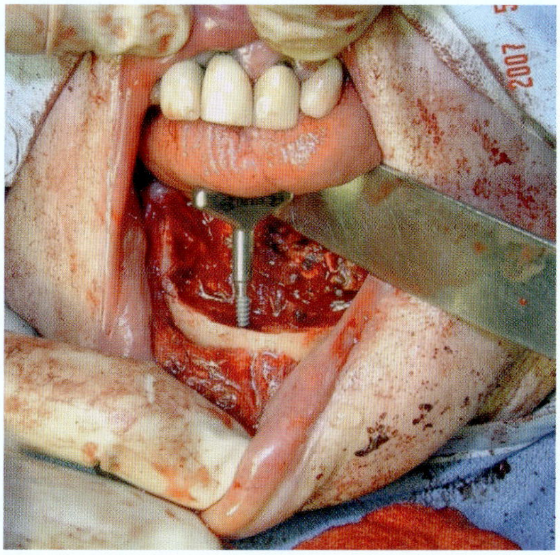

FIGURE 7-10. Thumb wrench.

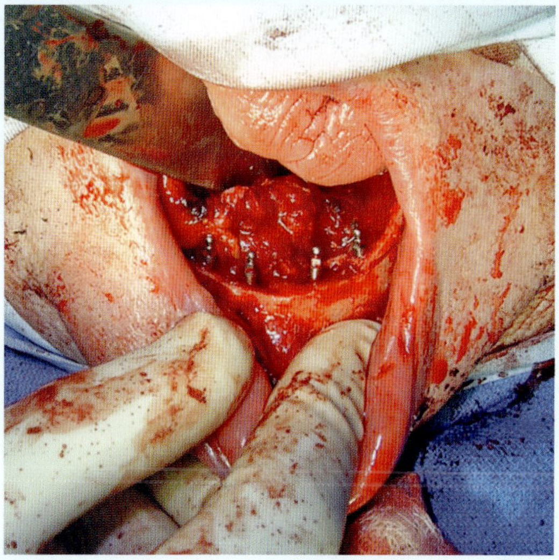

FIGURE 7-11. Four MDI Max have been placed preserving the innervation to the lower lip.

(Figures 7-9 to 7-11). Note the height of the abutments above the resection margin, just extending into the screw thread area.

CLOSURE

Two Vicryl sutures were placed in the floor of the mouth to close sublingual tissues across the midline between the plica fimbriata. The floor of mouth was not closed and the osseous denture base was not closed with soft tissue.

REBASING IMPRESSION

Four impression shims were trimmed and placed over the ball abutments. Standard housings were placed over the abutments and the overdenture (Figures 7-12 and 7-13).

The lower denture was rebased to fit into the osseous denture base area. Additional resin material was added, and muscle trimming was performed to determine the extension specifically of the labial flange (Figure 7-14).

The resection margin produced such a large void that a complete pack of hard pickup resin was required for rebasing the immediate denture (Figure 7-15).

The overdenture was removed with shims and trimmed for final insertion (Figures 7-16 to 7-18).

A mentalis strapping with adhesive tape was placed across the chin area to encourage apposition of tissues with the mentum and reattachment of mentalis.

CASE DISCUSSION I Marginal Mandibulectomy and Concomitant Reconstruction of the Dentition with an MDI Technique—cont'd

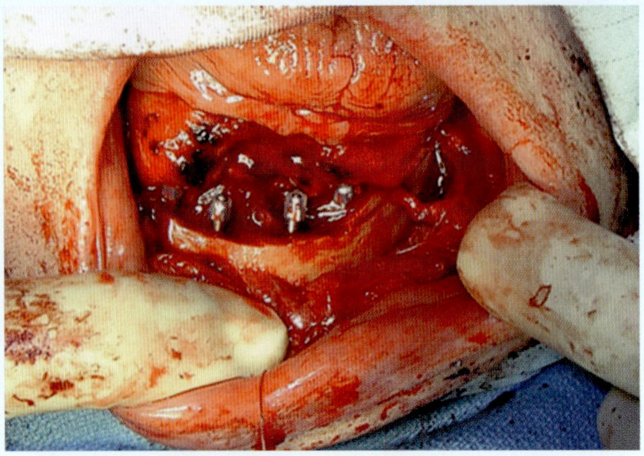

FIGURE 7-12. Shims.

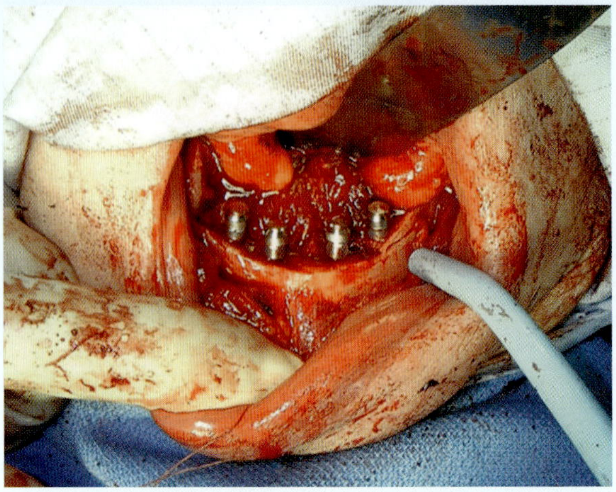

FIGURE 7-13. Housings.

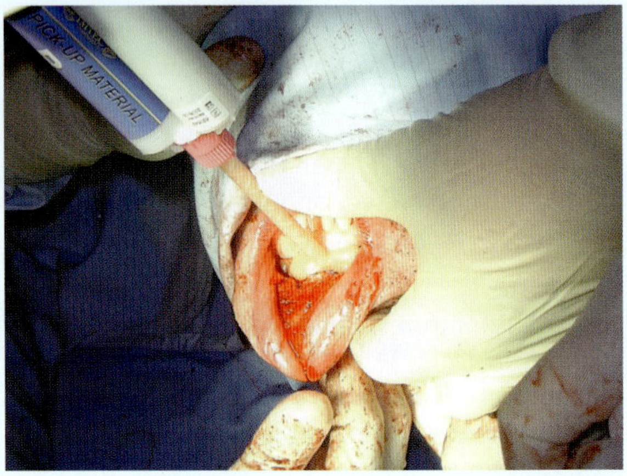

FIGURE 7-14. A whole gun full of hard pickup was required to extend the denture base into the resection bed. Dental laboratories are advised to overextend the denture base accordingly.

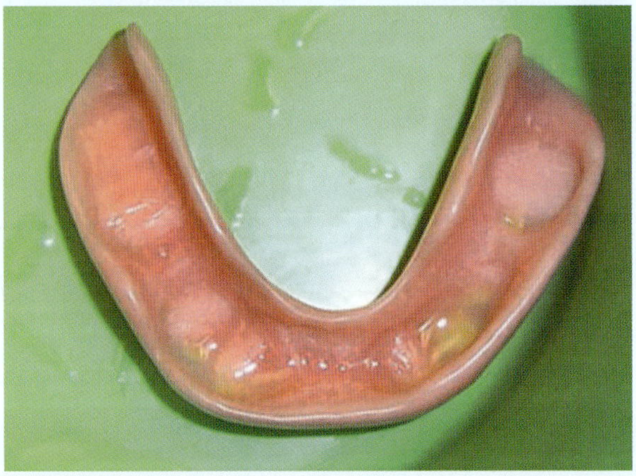

FIGURE 7-15. Prefabricated prosthesis. (Courtesy Ashley Hughes, Broadway Dental Laboratory, Palmerston North, Manawatu-Wanganui, New Zealand.)

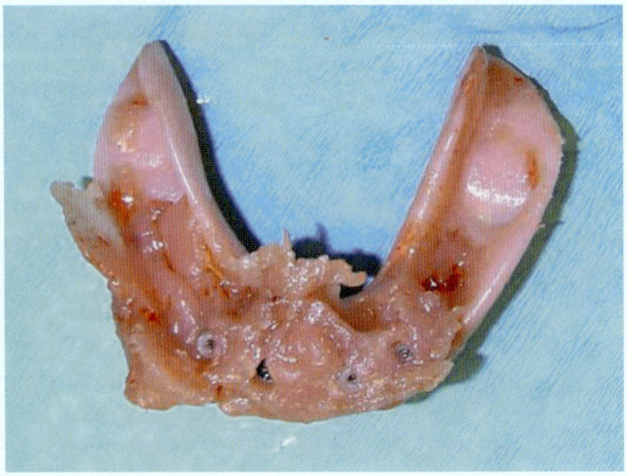

FIGURE 7-16. Relined overdenture.

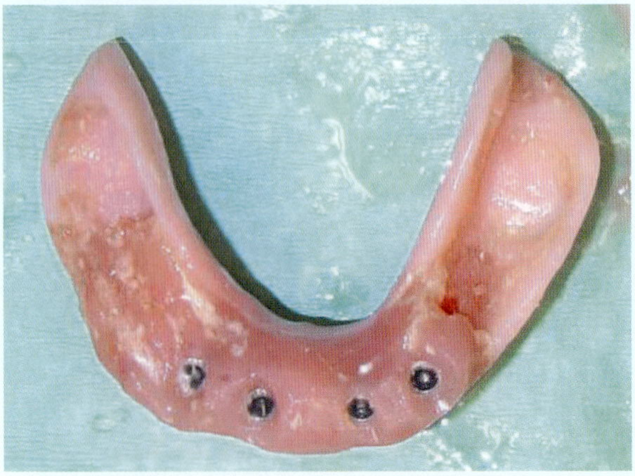

FIGURE 7-17. Overdenture flash removal.

CASE DISCUSSION 1 Marginal Mandibulectomy and Concomitant Reconstruction of the Dentition with an MDI Technique—cont'd

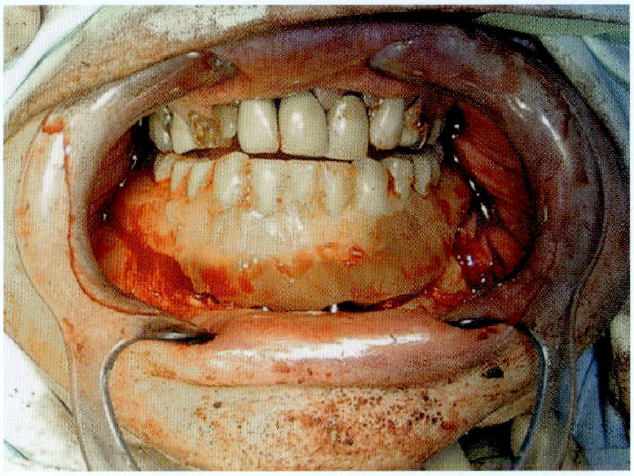

FIGURE 7-18. Placement of overdenture directly on alveolus and adjustment of occlusion.

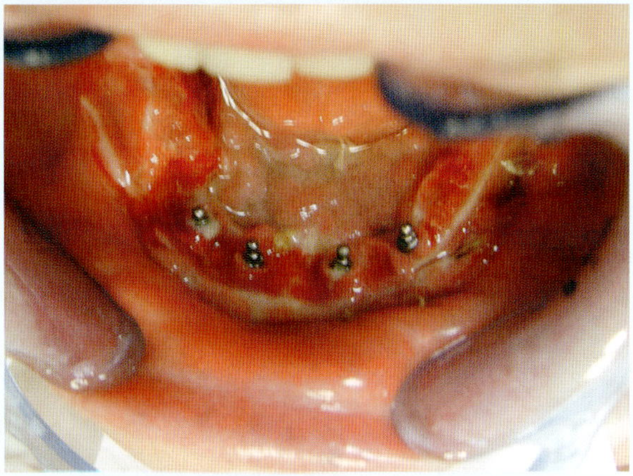

FIGURE 7-19. Overdenture removal 13 days. Note complete reepithelialization.

Surgery time was 1.5 hours.

The patient underwent this procedure:

- Without lip split or external incisions;
- Without tracheostomy;
- Without admission to a high dependency unit;
- Without admission to an intensive care unit;
- Without perioperative complication.

The patient made an uneventful recovery, required very little analgesia, and was discharged at 5 days.

OUTCOME

The overdenture was removed at 13 days to reveal complete reepithelialization of the osseous denture base area. The chin and lower lip had gained its attachment with competent lips (Figure 7-19). The outcome at 33 days is illustrated in Figures 7-20 to 7-22.

COMPLICATIONS

After a 3-month period of alveolar resorption, a new overdenture was required. Tissue encroachment occurred primarily from the buccal side as the mentalis and lip reattachment matured. Eventually the abutments became completely covered by regenerated oral mucosa (Figure 7-23). Attempts to remove this tissue by localized electrocautery failed to produce a lasting result and tissue advancement recurred.

A decision was made to carry out an anterior mandibular sulcoplasty under general anaesthesia. After curettage of regenerated attached mucosa from the neoalveolar crest, the exposure of the abutments was reduced and there was no sign of any screw threads. This implied osseous migration up the fixture (Figures 7-24 and 7-25).

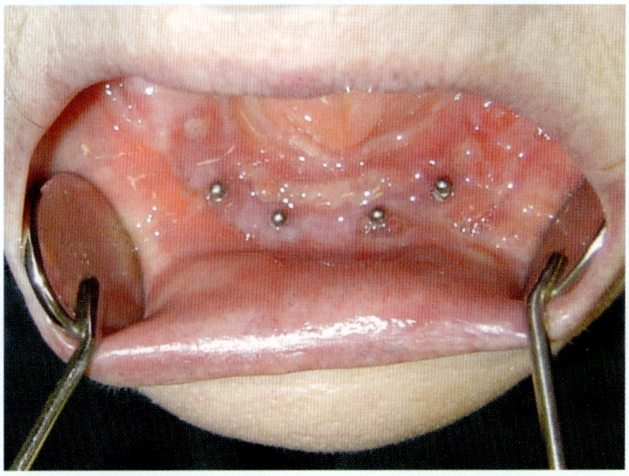

FIGURE 7-20. 33 days post surgery.

The floor of mouth and labial sulcus were repositioned with four circummandibular 4/0 nylon sutures placed using a transcutaneous awl technique. Shims and housings were placed over the implants and a hard resin stent was made to fit over the alveolus. No skin grafting techniques were employed.

Postoperative oral feeding was immediately instigated and supplemented with Fortisip. The

CASE DISCUSSION I Marginal Mandibulectomy and Concomitant Reconstruction of the Dentition with an MDI Technique—cont'd

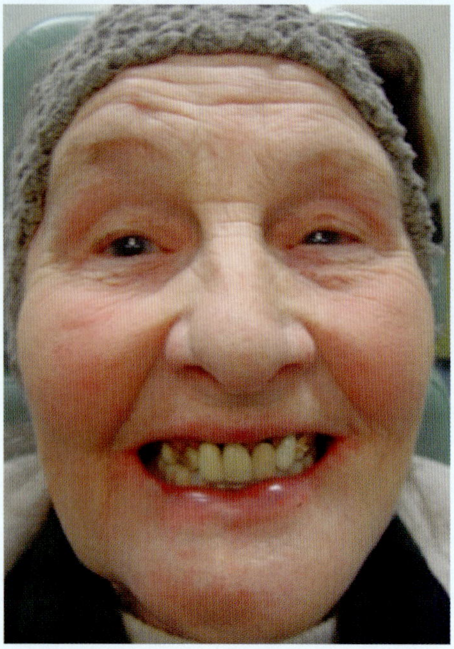

FIGURE 7-21. Initial outcome.
- Surgery in 1.5 hrs
- Flapless technique
- No lip split
- No tracheostomy
- No intensive care and no special nursing
- Discharge after 5 days

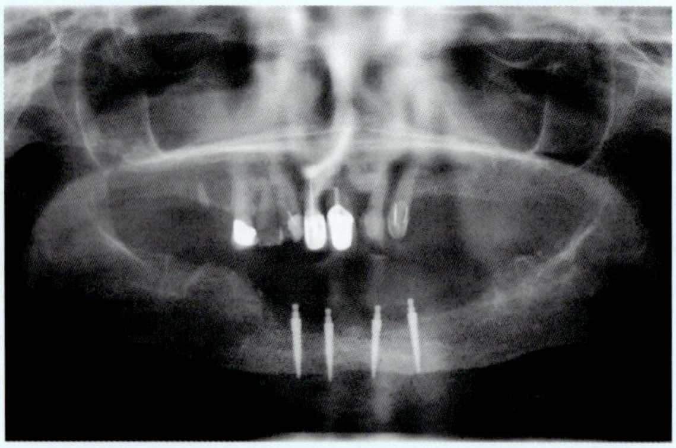

FIGURE 7-22. Outcome, panoramic x-ray.

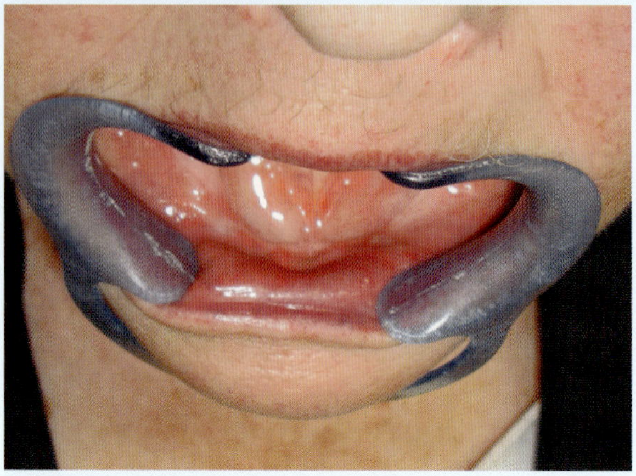

FIGURE 7-23. Reattachment of mentalis and lower lip with coverage of implants. Attempt to treat locally with electrosurgery failed to prevent regrowth of tissue. Patient underwent sulcoplasty.

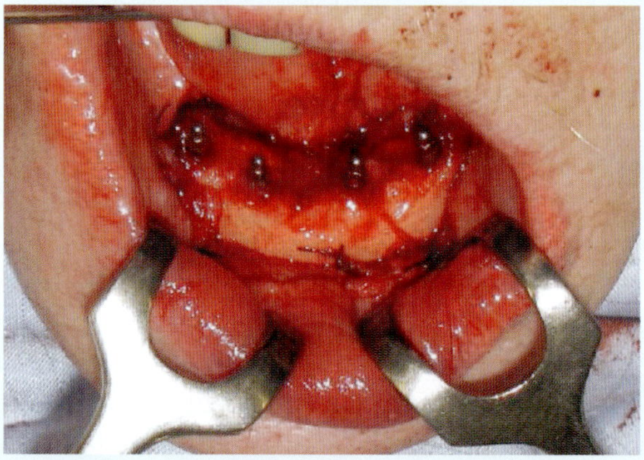

FIGURE 7-24. After lower anterior sulcoplasty. No skin grafting, Nylon circummandibular sutures retained. Sulcoplasty covered with stent.

CASE DISCUSSION I Marginal Mandibulectomy and Concomitant Reconstruction of the Dentition with an MDI Technique—cont'd

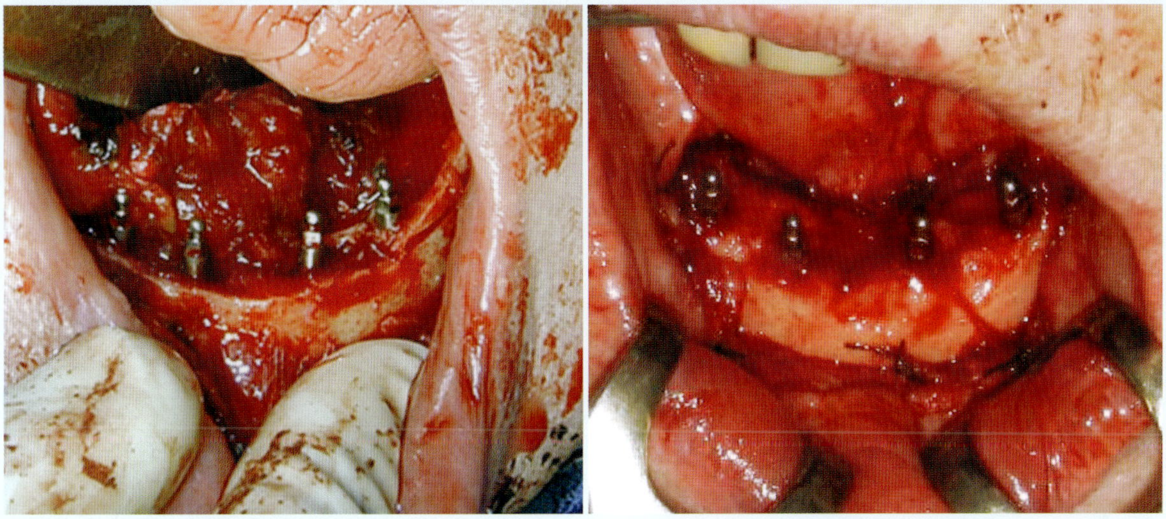

FIGURE 7-25. Alveolar osseous migration and MDIs. Note that the alveolar bone has migrated up the collars of all MDIs placed. This is in part responsible for implant coverage by soft tissue. Implants should be ideally placed with ball abutments located just below the normal occlusal plane in the edentulous maxilla. The development of MDIs with longer collars would solve the problem and make sulcoplasty unnecessary. Until this implant is developed a limited lower anterior sulcoplasty is advocated at the time of resection.

patient was instructed in oral hygiene methods, particularly oral irrigation with a 20-mL syringe.

She was discharged at 3 days and reviewed at 2 weeks.

A labial sulcus was created and this altered the resting position of the lower lip. The existing lower denture was used in a rebasing technique to make a new lower overdenture using the stent as the foundation for the base plate (Figures 7-26 to 7-32).

Rubber O rings provided such good retention that it was necessary to remove them from stent housings to facilitate wax bite block removal after bite registration. This action produced an error of location of the finished prosthesis requiring relocation of housings in the traditional manner with a locating resin impression.

Dr. Victor Sendax advises that O rings may be trimmed with a high speed bur to facilitate removal of the prosthesis: "If a moderately tapered diamond drill in a standard handpiece is used at medium speed (with or without water spray) and moved quickly in and out, just enough of the inner diameter of the rubber 'O ring(s)' in the prosthesis can be stripped so that a much easier fitting 'O ring' attachment(s) results. Once a minimal facility has been developed with this process, custom modification of the fit of 'O rings' can be obtained in a few seconds. This readily solves one of the most elusive variables in this system."

Although the required vertical dimension of the face did not alter, repositioning of the lower lip occurred as a consequence of sulcoplasty, making lip incompetence an issue with the preexisting facial height. This lip incompetence was partly addressed by significant reduction of facial height by dropping the lower occlusal plane.

FINAL OUTCOME

The patient was very pleased with the outcome in terms of:

1. Minimal surgery;
2. No second donor surgical site;
3. Esthetics;
4. Quality of speech (unchanged);
5. Prosthetic retention (excellent);
6. Mastication (unchanged);
7. Maintenance of lip sensation;
8. Stable reconstruction 17 months after surgery.

CRITIQUE

Although an excellent outcome was initially obtained before sulcoplasty, revision was required

CASE DISCUSSION I Marginal Mandibulectomy and Concomitant Reconstruction of the Dentition with an MDI Technique—cont'd

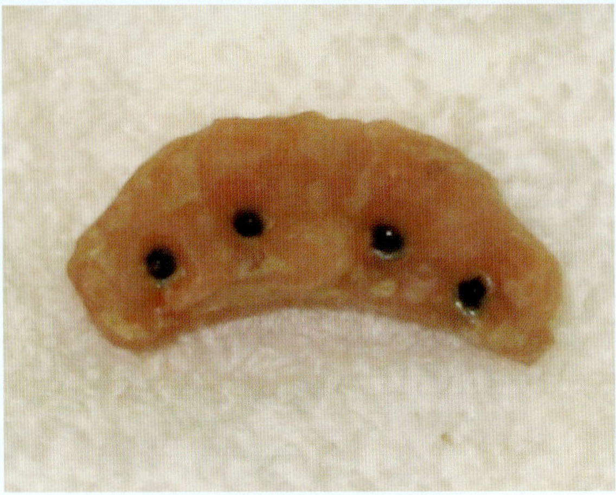

FIGURE 7-26. MDI stent.

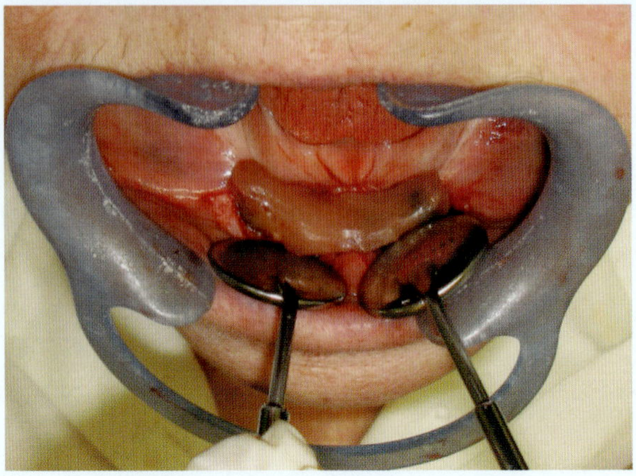

FIGURE 7-27. Sulcoplasty stent in situ.

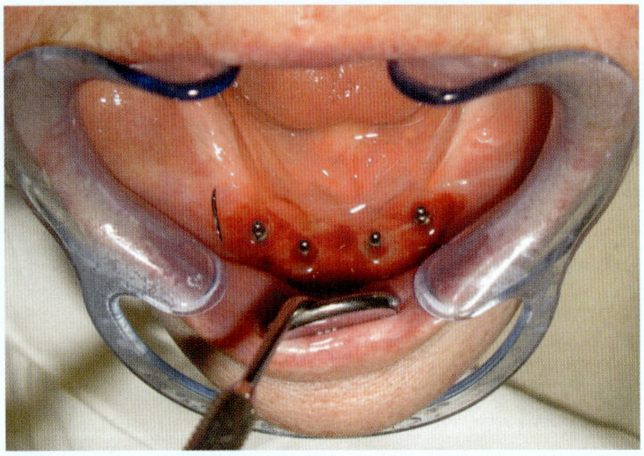

FIGURE 7-28. 2 weeks after lower anterior sulcoplasty. No skin grafting, nylon circummandibular sutures retained.

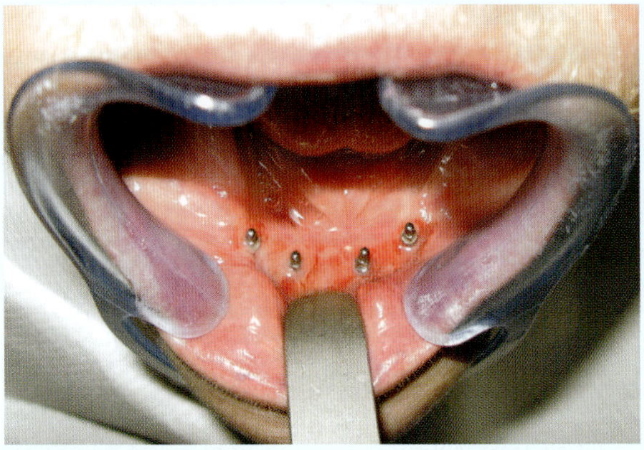

FIGURE 7-29. Sulcoplasty outcome at 1 month. Note complete reepithelialization without skin grafting of flaps.

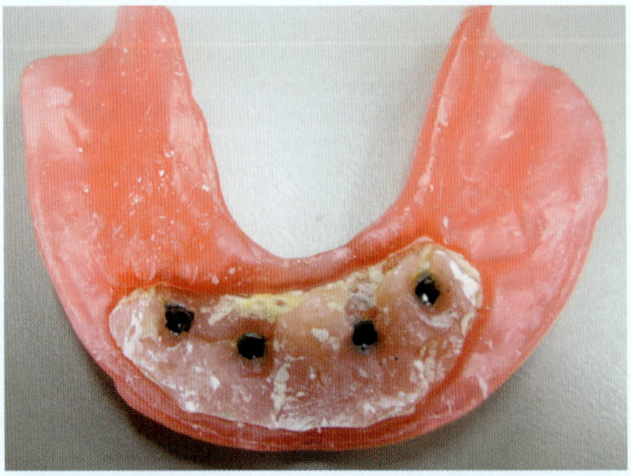

FIGURE 7-30. Bite block with stent baseplate. O rings make removal of the bite block difficult without its disintegration. Attempts to facilitate removal by omitting the O rings from the housings led to problems with final location of the prosthesis. If this technique is to be used, O rings should not be removed from the housings during occlusal registration.

CASE DISCUSSION I Marginal Mandibulectomy and Concomitant Reconstruction of the Dentition with an MDI Technique—cont'd

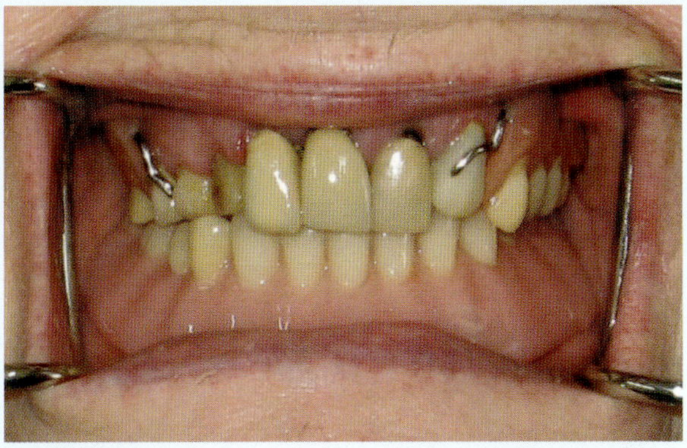

FIGURE 7-31. Sulcoplasty final prosthesis. (Upper prosthesis courtesy of Dr. Phillip Marshal BDS Director of Dental Surgery, MidCentral Health District Health Board, New Zealand. Lower overdenture courtesy of Leslie - Broadway Dental Laboratory Palamerston North)

due to an unanticipated migration of lip attachment, which could not be prevented by the prosthesis.

It is not known at this time whether the placement of a mucosal graft or skin graft over the alveolus could have prevented this event, and further evaluation of these technique modifications are warranted.

Another issue is whether sulcoplasty should have been done at the time of tumor resection and whether alternative fixation methods can be employed to reduce the tendency to lip incompetence after this procedure, such as transmandibular fixation of the sulcus with sutures passing horizontally through the mandible rather than circummandibular sutures that pull the attachments almost to the lower border.

Finally the problem of soft tissue migration and implant coverage could be addressed by MDIs with a longer collar, permitting placement of the ball abutment just below the occlusal plane. This is probably the best solution.

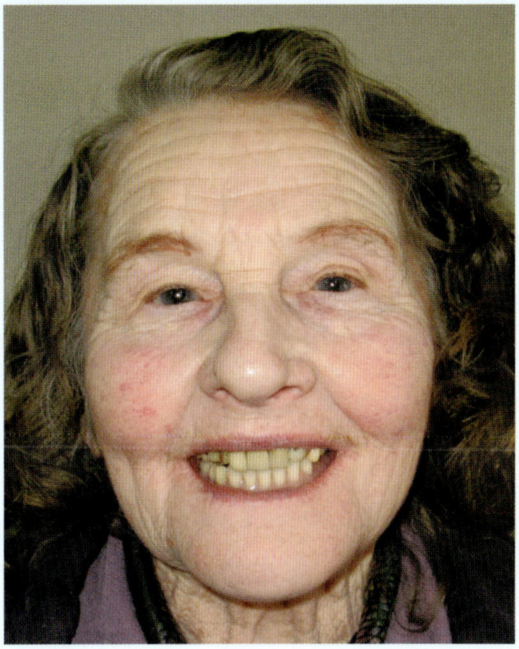

FIGURE 7-32. Sulcoplasty outcome. Normal (unchanged) speech, normal swallowing, normal mastication.

COST OF TREATMENT (NEW ZEALAND DOLLARS)

Implant system / pickup kit	$1145
Denture (laboratory costs)	$ 450
Theatre $3k/hr	$4500
Inpatient @ $500/day	$2500
Total	**$8595 (New Zealand)**

This is to be compared with $80,000 (New Zealand) for a free flap tissue transfer (Izzard Auckland Head and Neck Centre 2007).

CASE DISCUSSION 2 The Management of Major Facial Trauma with a Combined EAS/MDI Technique

A 64-year-old patient presented with a history of a 30-year old gunshot wound to the face, which had been reconstructed with a maxillary obturator and an iliac crest graft to the left body of the mandible. Soft tissue repair to the mentum with a deltopectoral flap was performed. Some years after the injury, the patient lost his sight after a cerebrovascular episode.

The main concern was of incompetent lips and salivary escape so severe that he wore a towel on his left shoulder to soak up the moisture (Figure 7-33). Clinical examination revealed the following dental charting:

Maxilla: 15 14 2
Mandible: 20* 21 28 *root

Teeth 21 and 28 showed excessive wear and were the shape of chisels. A maxillary obturator was present replacing teeth 13, 12, 11, 10, 9, 8, 7, 6, 5, 4 and 3.

The critical clinical decision in this case was related to mandibular dental clearance and maintenance of the residual mandibular dentition. The patient's choice was to maintain the dentition that would afford some degree of occlusion in the event of implant failure (Figures 7-34 to 7-36)

An anatomical biomodel was manufactured with fused deposition modelling technology from CT scans that illustrated:

1. Loss of the central portion of the lower midface;
2. Nasal collapse with twisting of the nasal bones to the left;
3. Malunion of a midface fracture at the Le Fort II level in the region of the lower orbital rims;
4. Overclosure of the mandible;
5. A short left-sided iliac crest graft, which had been placed backwards and upside down so that the curve around the vertical axis, normally associated with the position of the canine tooth as the body of the mandible swings medially to run into the mentum, was located in the region of the molar tooth (implying that the hip was taken from the incorrect side);
6. Medial swing of the right ramus related to a bony union with the short mandibular bone graft;

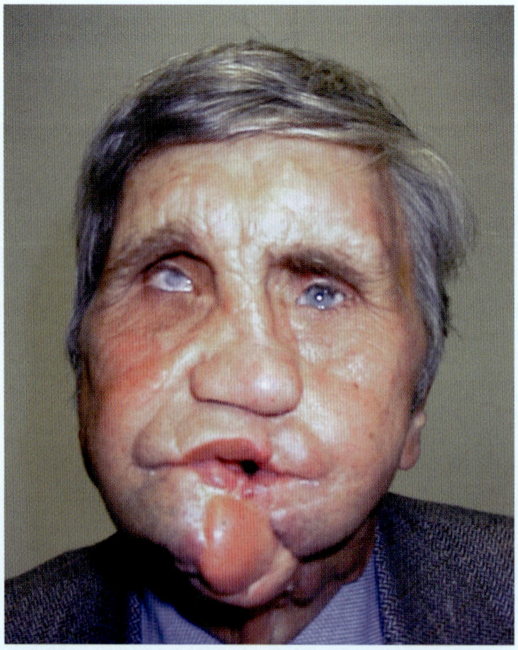

FIGURE 7-33. Gunshot injury occurred 30 years previously. Note midface collapse, lip incompetence.

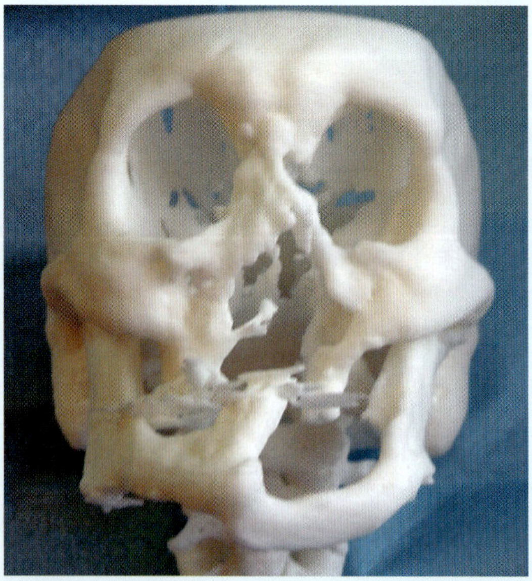

FIGURE 7-34. An anatomical biomodel was manufactured from CT scans using a fused deposition modelling (FDM) technique, a rapid prototyping or rapid manufacturing technology commonly used within CAD/CAM and engineering design.

CASE DISCUSSION 2 The Management of Major Facial Trauma with a Combined EAS/MDI Technique—cont'd

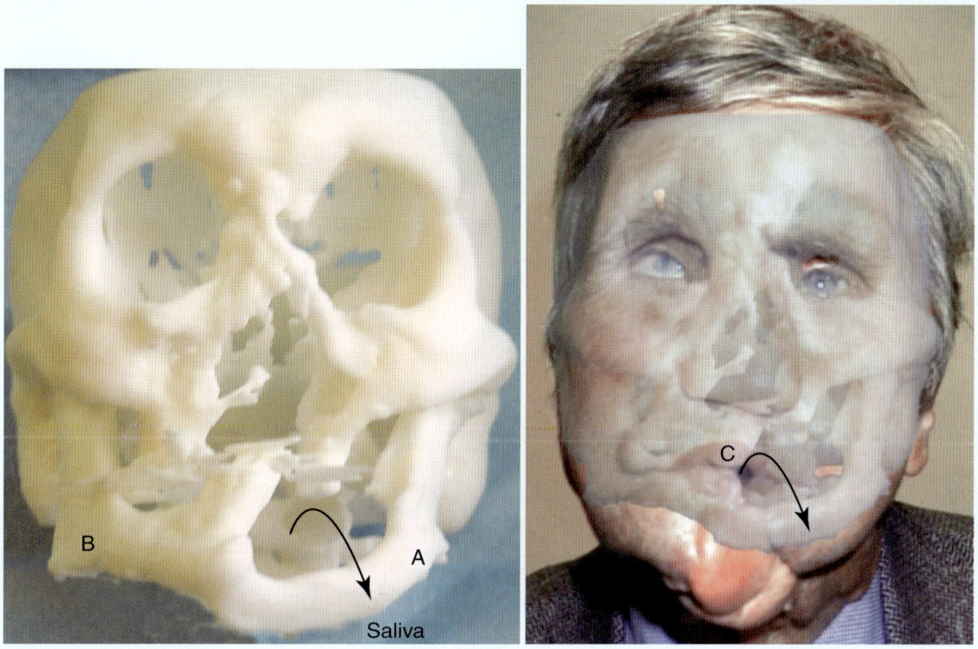

FIGURE 7-35. Using digital imaging software the face can be layered over the skull for hard and soft tissue analysis in a process defined as *photomorphanalysis*. In this case, the bone from the left iliac crest has been taken and used to reconstruct hemimandible, and the iliac crest angulation normally reserved for the canine area is seen to be placed more posteriorly, near the angle of the mandible **(A).** In modern practice the iliac crest would be taken from the contralateral (right) side to prevent this problem. The graft is too short in length and the right ramus has swung medially **(B).** There is a malunion with the mandibular remnant producing a bucket handle deformity. This has lowered the floor of mouth by 2.5 cm and adversely affected the reattachments of the orbicularis oris muscle, so that lip incompetence is produced **(C),** just to the left of the midline. This analysis explains precisely the anatomical basis of the presenting features of salivary escape (*arrows*) and defines treatment logistics with great precision.

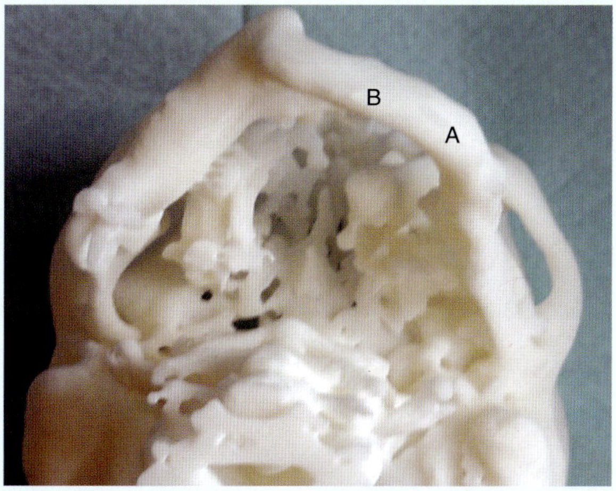

FIGURE 7-36. In the submentovertex view, the significance of correct placement of the iliac crest angulation **(A)** is readily appreciated. The body of the mandible **(B)** is incorrectly angulated and normal aesthetics cannot be achieved.

7. Bucket handle displacement of the mandibular graft, which brings the alveolar crest to the same horizontal plane of the floor of mouth, and lowers the attachment of musculature—producing incompetence of the perioral seal and promoting the egress of saliva.

The relationships of the hard and soft tissue were confirmed using a photomorphanalysis technique[15] in which biomodel and clinical images are layered with approximately 50% transparency so that the relationships of the hard and soft tissues can be analyzed together.

In this case the bucket handle malunion of the iliac crest graft was responsible for the production of a labial notch that channeled the saliva to the left. The situation was aggravated by the inability to wear a lower denture.

CASE DISCUSSION 2 The Management of Major Facial Trauma with a Combined EAS/MDI Technique—cont'd

TREATMENT PLAN: OBJECTIVES

The treatment plan in this case was directed at the presenting complaint in the mandible:

1. To elevate the alveolus and floor of mouth on the grafted side and promote lip seal and competence;
2. To restore a functioning mandibular dentition:
   a. To enhance salivary retention;
   b. To improve mastication;
   c. To enhance overall quality of life;
3. To achieve the above outcomes without recourse to major surgery.

BIOMODEL ANALYSIS

A custom cutting jig was manufactured to carry out a precision body osteotomy at an angle of precisely 8 degrees, an angle that combined with an anterior osteotomy permitted rotation and elevation of the osteotomized graft along its axis with a vertical impaction to raise the alveolus by 2.5 cm (Figures 7-37 to 7-39).

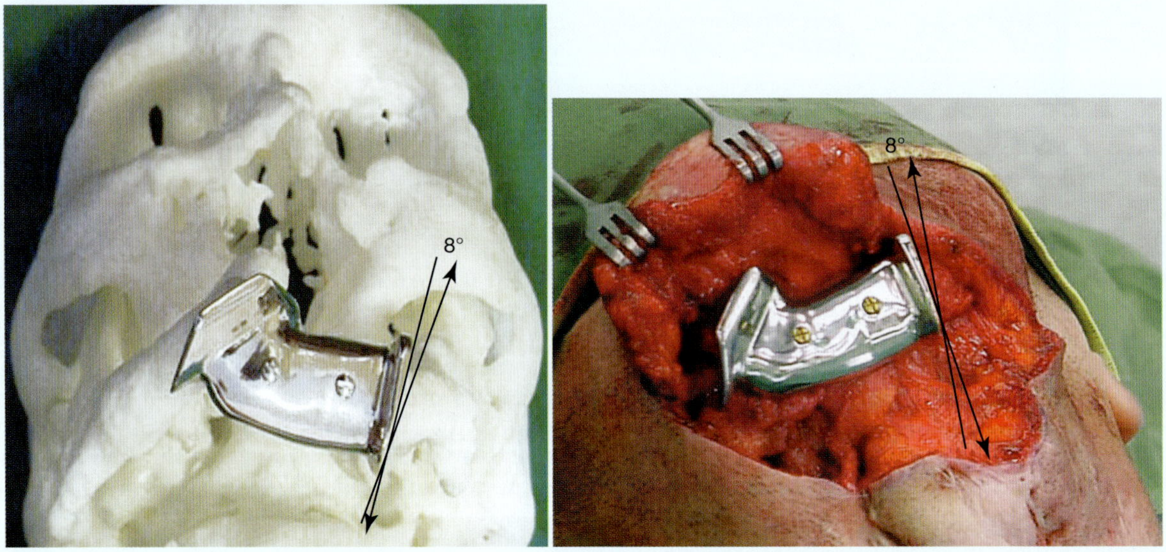

FIGURE 7-37. A precision osteotomy cut was designed using a customized cutting jig with an angled proximal cutting flange. This was designed for use with a reciprocating saw to excise a wedge of bone at a precise 8-degree angle with the apex. Combined with an anterior osteotomy, this frees up the bucket handled segment, which can be repositioned with a slight rotation to elevate the floor of mouth by 2.5 cm.

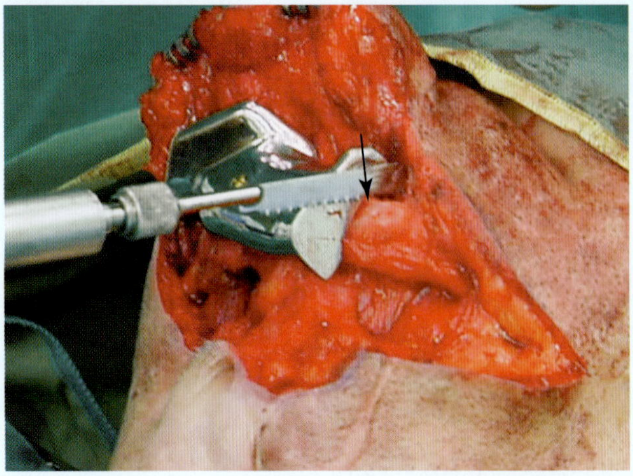

FIGURE 7-38. The anterior wedge resection cut is made from the top of the flange in an inferior direction. The cutting jig is used to start the osteotomy cut at the correct angle.

CASE DISCUSSION 2 The Management of Major Facial Trauma with a Combined EAS/MDI Technique—cont'd

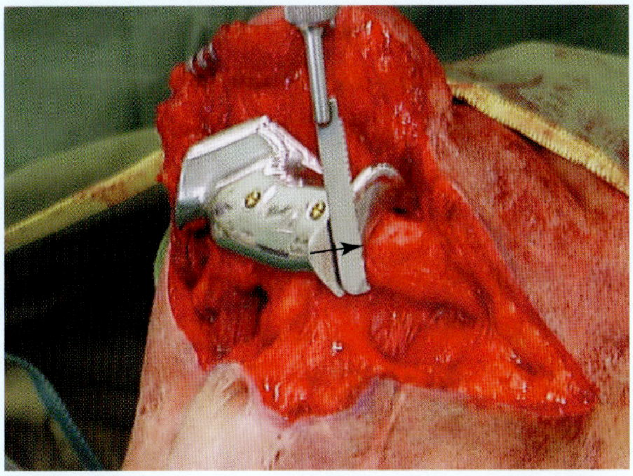

FIGURE 7-39. The posterior cut is made from the bottom of the flange in a superior direction to complete the wedge resection at an angle of 8 degrees.

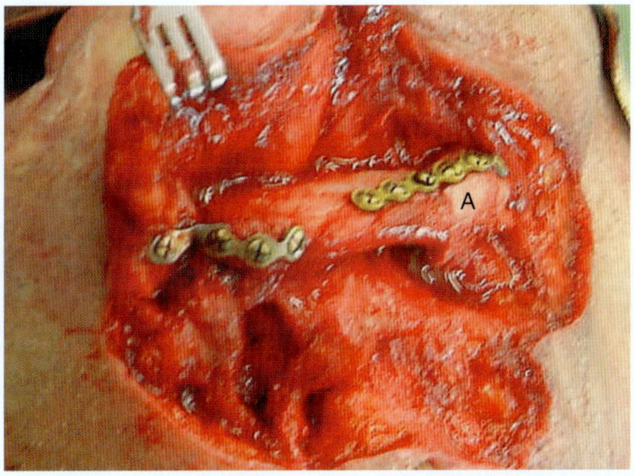

FIGURE 7-40. Completed osteotomy with miniplate osteosynthesis. Note the accuracy of bone apposition in relation to the posterior osteotomy cut **(A)**. Fixation Synthes 2.0-mm titanium bone plates.

The angle of cut was made possible by the construction of the angled cutting flange located on the posterior aspect of the cutting jig, which was screwed to the graft during the procedure. A saw cut on the posterior flange made from a superior to inferior direction met with a saw cut from an inferior to superior direction to create a wedge of the required angle. This permitted bone-to-bone contact for primary bony union and obviated the requirement for major surgery.

SURGERY

The planned osteotomy was carried out under general anaesthesia in a 1.5-hour procedure with an external approach through old scars. Fixation was achieved with miniplates and 2.0-mm screw fixation for osteosynthesis. The patient made an uneventful recovery (Figures 7-40 to 7-42).

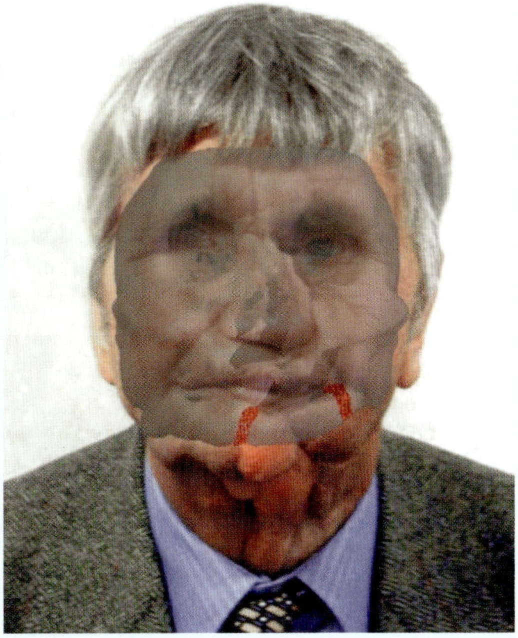

FIGURE 7-41. Elevation of bucket handled malunion and lip competence.

CASE DISCUSSION 2 The Management of Major Facial Trauma with a Combined EAS/MDI Technique—cont'd

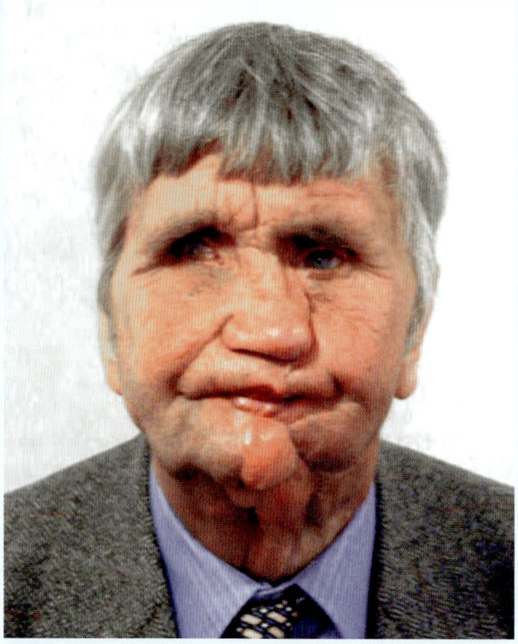

FIGURE 7-42. Lip competence has been achieved with EAS planning and simplified surgery.

MDI RECONSTRUCTION OF THE DENTITION

Reconstruction was carried out as a second staged procedure under local anaesthesia (Figures 7-43 to 7-46). Placement of implants was facilitated by a palatal dehiscence that counteracted mild trismus. Use of the 20* root for MDI cementation as an endodontic post was not possible, and the root was surgically removed.

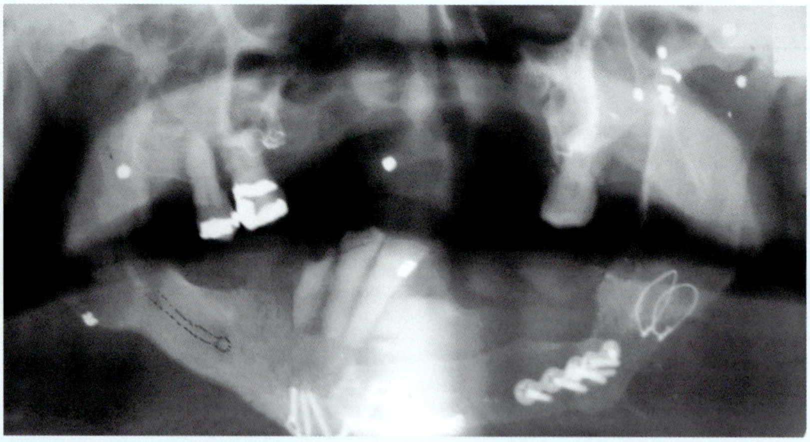

FIGURE 7-43. The panoramic x-ray of the osteotomized segment shows good positioning of the graft with elimination of the bucket handle deformity. Note the presence of multiple shotgun pellets.

CASE DISCUSSION 2 The Management of Major Facial Trauma with a Combined EAS/MDI Technique—cont'd

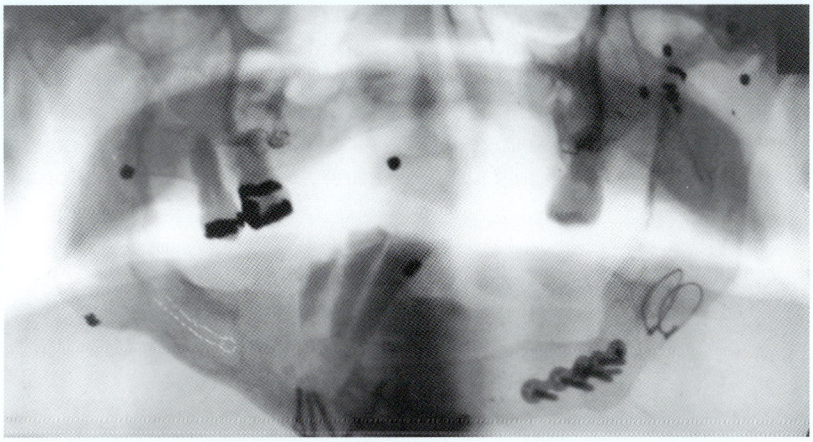

FIGURE 7-44. Image manipulation is a useful technique to enhance surgical anatomy. In this example, image inversion enhances to positioning of the bone screws and plates and is very useful in defining the alveolus in the maxilla.

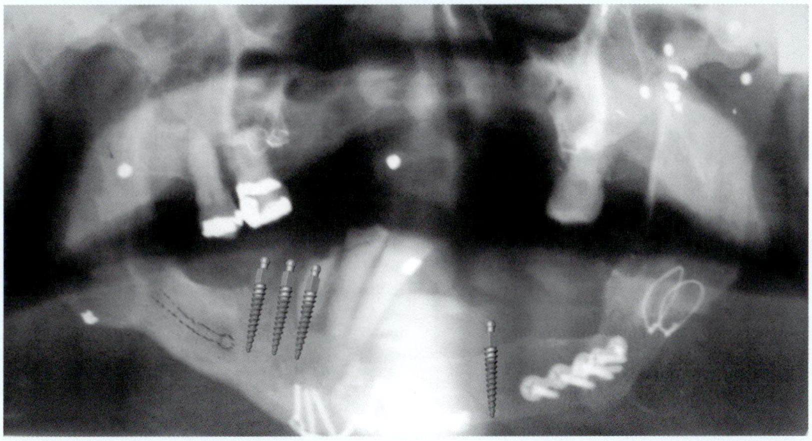

FIGURE 7-45. Plan: 18-mm MDI Max placement. Implants were placed 6 months after osteotomy surgery. The patient declined the option of a full lower dental clearance in case of implant failure. An attempt to cement a MDI down the root of 45 failed because of lateral root perforation. The root was extracted. Three 18-mm MDI Max were placed in the lower right mandible; only one 18-mm MDI Max could be placed in the iliac crest graft in view of the bone plates and screws. There was a degree of trismus and placement of long MDIs was only possible because a palatal defect was present. Note that placement of MDIs are facilitated if they are placed under general anaesthetic at the time of reconstructive surgery.

CASE DISCUSSION 2 The Management of Major Facial Trauma with a Combined EAS/MDI Technique—cont'd

Three MDI Max 13-mm implants were placed in the body of the right mandible. To avoid the miniplate screws used for osteosynthesis, the placement of only one MDI Max 13-mm implant was possible in the left side in the iliac crest graft area (Figures 7-47 to 7-49).

OUTCOME

The floor of mouth was elevated by the planned 2.5 cm and perioral seal was obtained. The patient abandoned the use of the towel (Figures 7-50 to 7-53). The patient commented about the overdenture, "It is extremely comfortable. I can bite hard

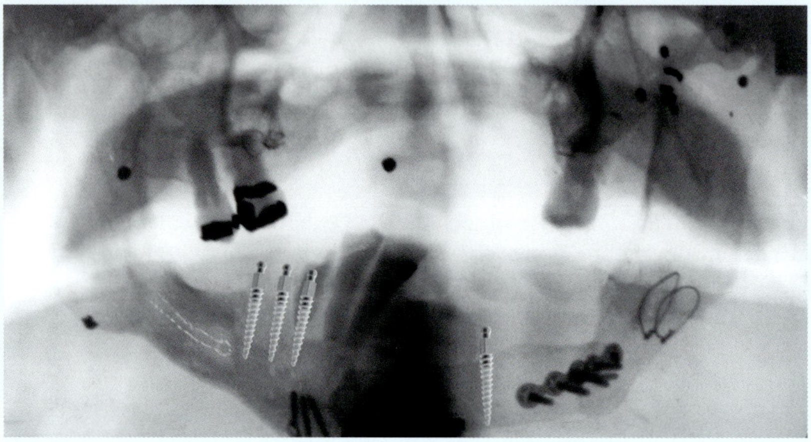

FIGURE 7-46. Panoramic x-ray, image inversion.

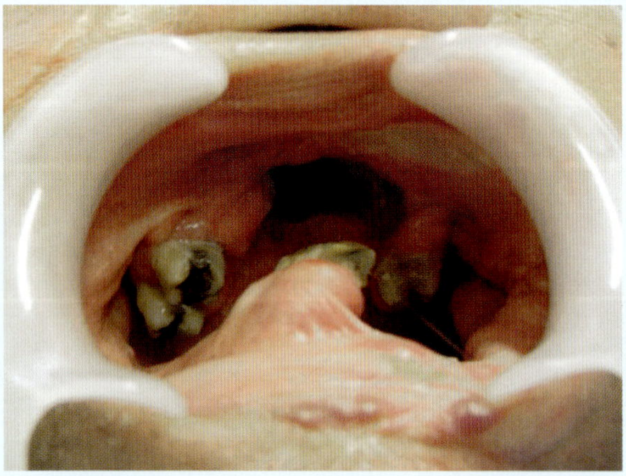

FIGURE 7-47. Reconstruction of mandibular dentition. Note the palatal dehiscence, absent premaxilla and chisel-like mandibular teeth.

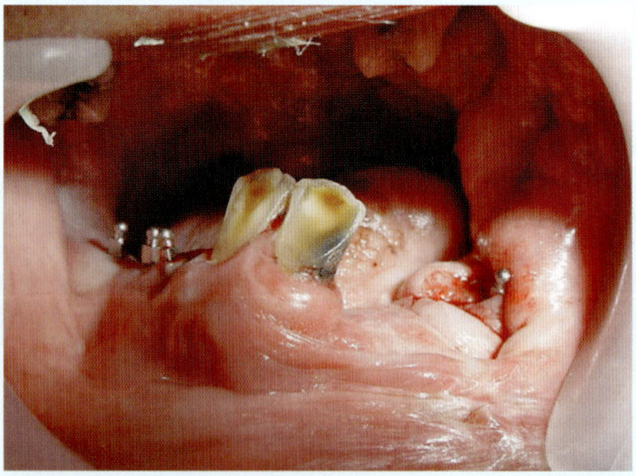

FIGURE 7-48. Placement of four 18-mm MDI Max. Note the thickness of the flap covering the iliac crest graft. (Courtesy Andrews Dental, Clay Cross, Derbyshire, United Kingdom.)

CASE DISCUSSION 2 The Management of Major Facial Trauma with a Combined EAS/MDI Technique—cont'd

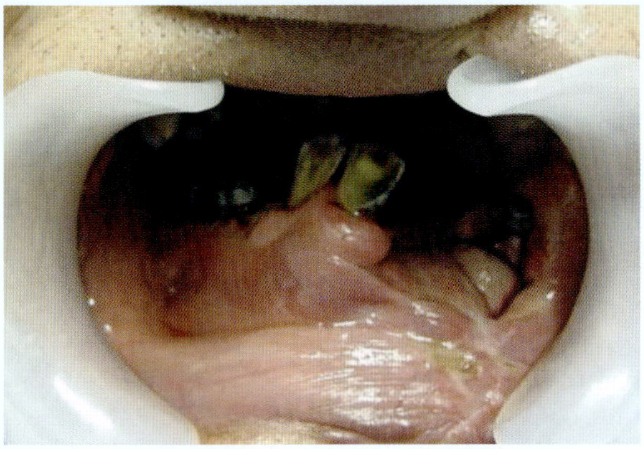

FIGURE 7-49. Placement of shims and housings.

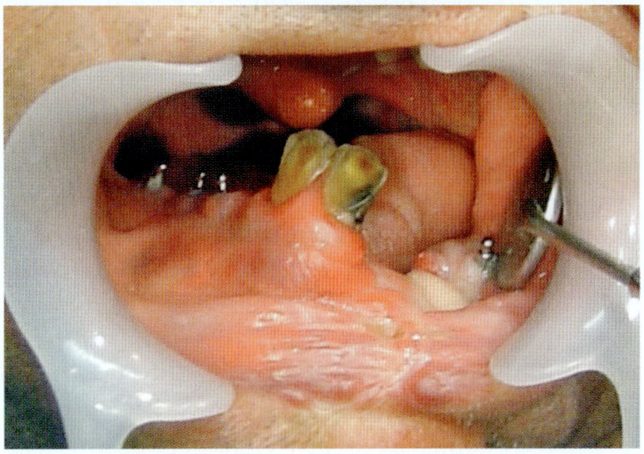

FIGURE 7-50. MDI placement outcome.

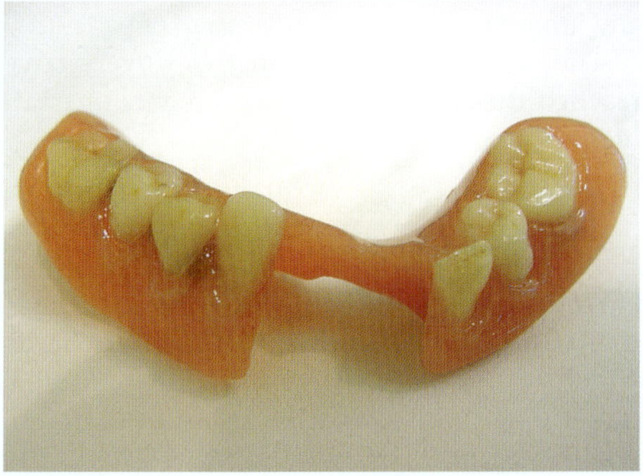

FIGURE 7-51. Overdenture. (Courtesy Ben Swindell of Crown Ceramics Codnor, United Kingdom.)

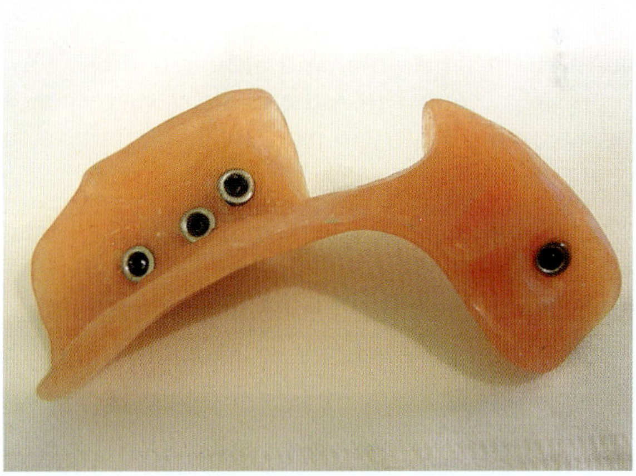

FIGURE 7-52. Overdenture.

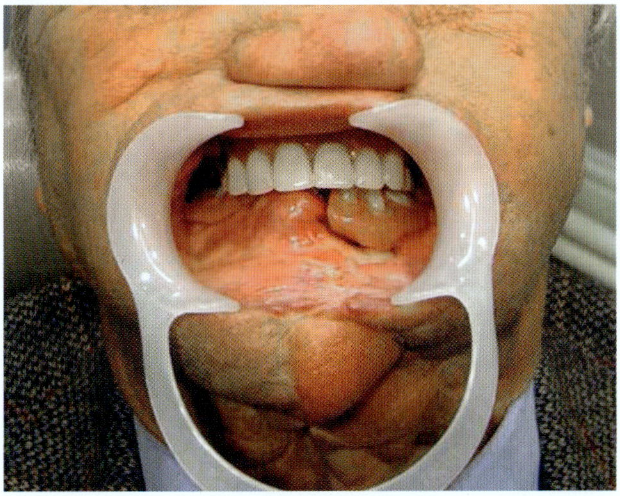

FIGURE 7-53. Outcome. Salivary escape eliminated completely with combined approach of mandibular osteotomy and MDI-retained overdenture. Denture stability and retention was excellent. Speech was enhanced; Mastication: patient can eat "anything" including nuts; a life transforming solution; stable outcome at 5 years; new O rings required at 5 years.

CASE DISCUSSION 2 The Management of Major Facial Trauma with a Combined EAS/MDI Technique—cont'd

on any type of hard food and it is easy to put in and easy to remove." The reconstruction is stable at 10 years and has transformed the quality of life for this patient.

DISCUSSION

This case illustrates the challenges of facial reconstruction after major trauma and how the quality of life is adversely and severely affected by compromised anatomy contour after attempted reconstruction with bone grafts and pedicled flaps. This situation has improved with the advent of free tissue transfer, but the anatomical anomalies of microvascular reconstruction persist into the 21st century, especially in cases of skeletal defect.

There is no doubt that accurate reconstruction of the jaws and dentition is essential for an aesthetic facial profile, and although these concepts are accepted in esthetic facial surgery and orthognathic surgery in particular, they appear to be ignored in cases of facial reconstruction after trauma or tumor ablation. In other words, clinicians have one set of standards for patients with esthetic issues and another for patients with tumors, which is simply wrong and unacceptable.

Through EAS, the technology exists to plan these cases with esthetic parameters and values, and the author advocates that significant skeletal deformity is no longer acceptable.

The use of the ingenious and inexpensive implant Sendax MDI system makes the case that routine comprehensive oral rehabilitation is achievable, and modern treatment plans need to take these developments into consideration if we are to prevent patient mutilation, maintain quality of life, and improve palliation for this group of patients.

The concepts of reconstructive surgery have reached the stage where reassessments of treatment protocols are required.

Reconstruction of the Midface

Tissue Engineering: Maxillary Atrophy

We have been able to demonstrate successful regeneration of the upper jaw using EAS planning and MDI techniques. Maxillary atrophy[16] occurs in patients after an upper dental clearance, and historically it has been an extremely difficult problem to solve, often involving major surgery, not without risk for many patients.

Patients with maxillary atrophy have a significant disability that significantly impairs the quality of life. Upper dentures become extremely loose to the extent that they cannot be worn—not even with the use of denture fixative. The condition may be initiated by the rocking motion of an upper denture in a patient with missing lower posterior teeth and who does not wear an occlusion-balancing lower denture. This rocking motion is produced by the lower anterior incisor teeth, which bite only into the front upper denture. The underlying bone cannot withstand this trauma—and disappears.

The management of this condition has been revolutionized by EAS planning, tissue engineering, and the use of MDI techniques. Safer treatment options are now possible without recourse to major surgery, or even hospitalization, and management can now be undertaken in the dental office under local anaesthesia.

After upper jaw regeneration, upper dentures can be made and stabilized with dental implants, without palatal cover, greatly enhancing the quality of life for patients. The cost of this treatment modality is very much reduced, making these treatment options more accessible for patients.

CASE DISCUSSION 3 Maxillary Atrophy

A 62–year-old woman with a 20-year history of inability to wear upper denture presents with severe maxillary atrophy (Figures 7-54, 7-55).

TREATMENT PLAN: GUIDED BONE REGENERATION

- Bio-Oss and demineralized bone matrix graft material
- Platelet rich plasma

PROCEDURES

- Bilateral maxillary sinus lifts
- Bilateral nasal floor lifts
- Alveolar augmentation to increase width
- MDI stabilization of upper dental prosthesis

PLATELET RICH PLASMA

Platelets are rich in:

- Chemical messengers, and
- Growth factors.

These factors increase:

- Cell mitosis;
- Chemotaxis associated with healing;
- The differentiation of cells associated with tissue formation and wound healing;
- Promotion of enhanced healing and regeneration of bone and soft tissue;
- The growth of *soft tissue* in the reconstruction of defects;
- The growth of *bone* in the reconstruction of defect;
- Bone trabecular density by 15% to 30%, which is equivalent to increasing bone density by one Misch grade;
- Acceleration of bone maturation by 2 months;
- Earlier placement of implants.[16,12]

SURGERY

Surgery was performed under local anaesthesia in a dental office setting under local anaesthesia, without sedation, and was well tolerated by this patient (Figures 7-56 to 7-62). Intravenous sedation is an option, but it was not required in this case.

Bio-Oss and human banked bone grafts (demineralized bone matrix) were mixed with platelet rich

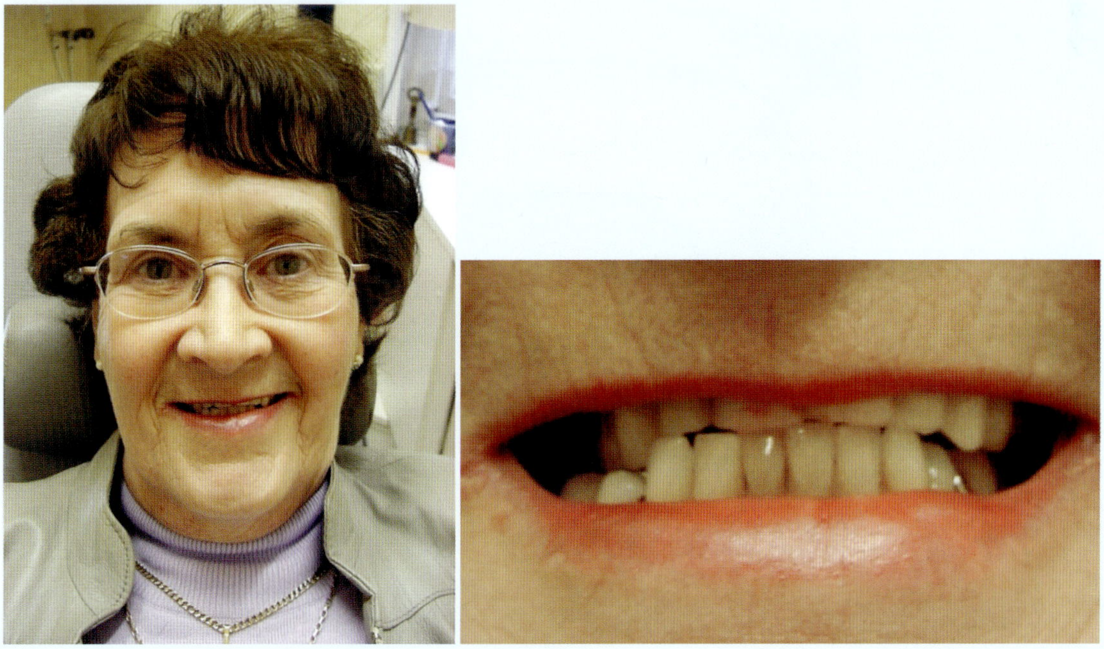

FIGURE 7-54. Maxillary atrophy. Note the collapse of the midface with poor lip support; cross bite 20, 22, 24, 23 with bone loss at 20; pronounced nasolabial folds.

CASE DISCUSSION 3 Maxillary Atrophy—cont'd

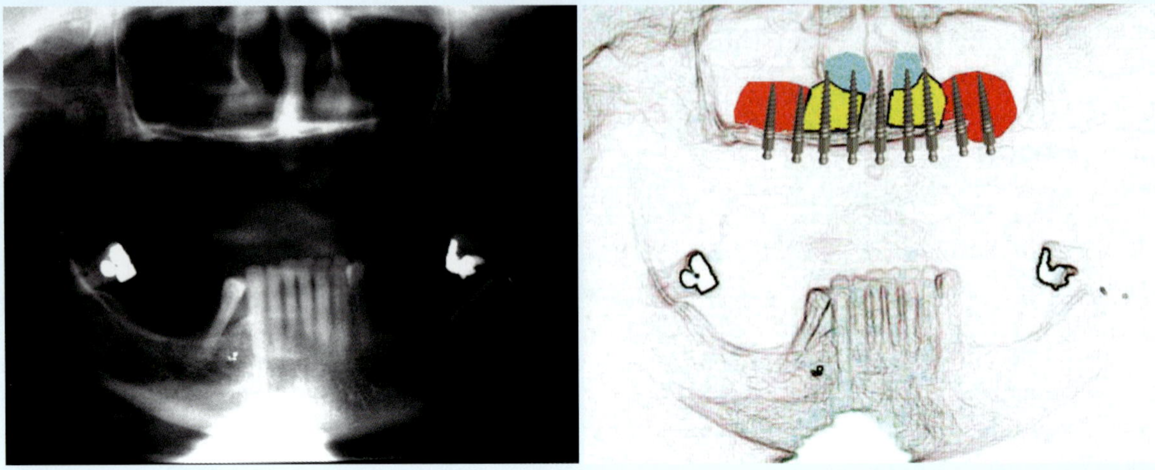

FIGURE 7-55. The panoramic x-ray confirms profound maxillary atrophy and advanced periodontal disease in the mandibular dentition. The treatment plan provided for the insertion of 9 maxillary implants into the grafted area. If 33% of these were lost, the remaining 6 implants would permit the retention of a palateless maxillary overdenture. A lower dental clearance was planned as a secondary procedure at the patient's request. An animated gif file was made that demonstrated the placement of bone grafts and successive placement of implants. This may be viewed at www.maxfac.com.

Key:

- Sinus lift *(red)*
- Nasal floor lift *(turquoise)*
- Anterior alveolar augmentation—width *(yellow)*

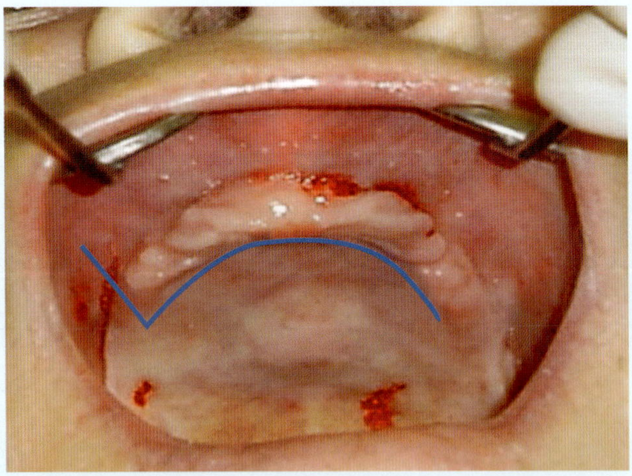

FIGURE 7-56. Defensive incision. To reduce the risk for an oroantral fistula, a triangular flap was raised with the relieving incision based over alveolar bone rather than the underlying Schneiderian membrane in the upper left quadrant. Note how the incision is based on the palatal side of the maxilla on alveolar bone. (Courtesy Andrews Dental, Cray Cross, Derbyshire, United Kingdom.)

CASE DISCUSSION 3 Maxillary Atrophy—cont'd

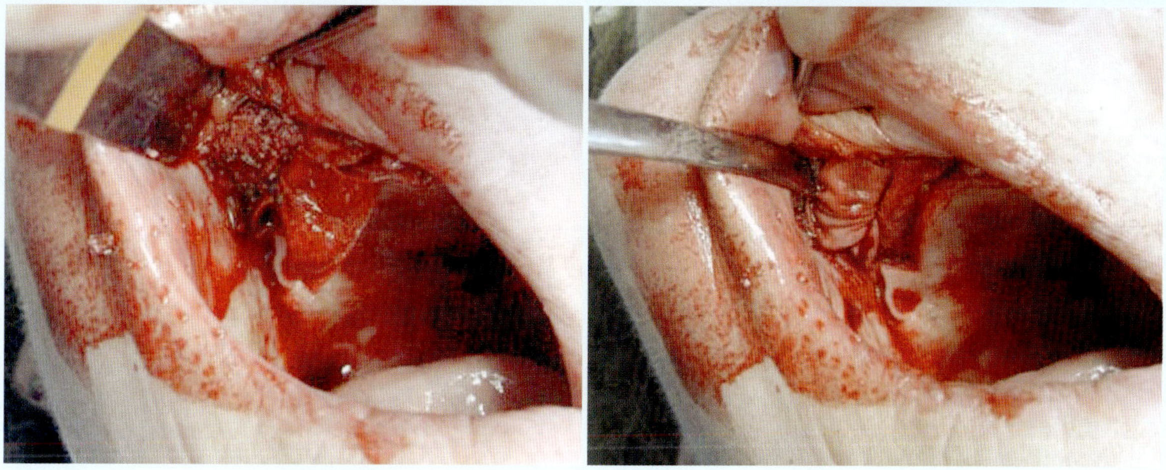

Bio-oss block Collagen membrane

FIGURE 7-57. Bilateral tearing on elevation of Schneiderian membranes occurred on elevation from floor of sinus. A Bio-Oss block graft and collagen membrane were soaked in platelet rich plasma. The membrane wrapped around graft like envelope and wedged into floor of sinus.

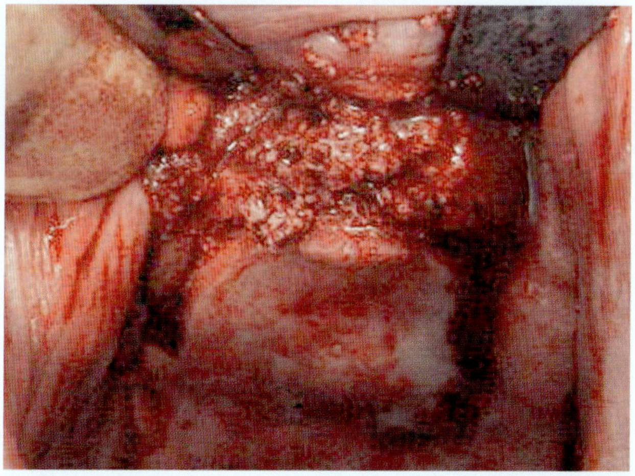

FIGURE 7-58. Additional Bio-Oss block grafting was mixed with platelet rich plasma (PRP) and placed in nasal floor bilaterally. Anterior alveolus augmented with DBM bone putty mixed with a platelet poor plasma membrane (PPP).

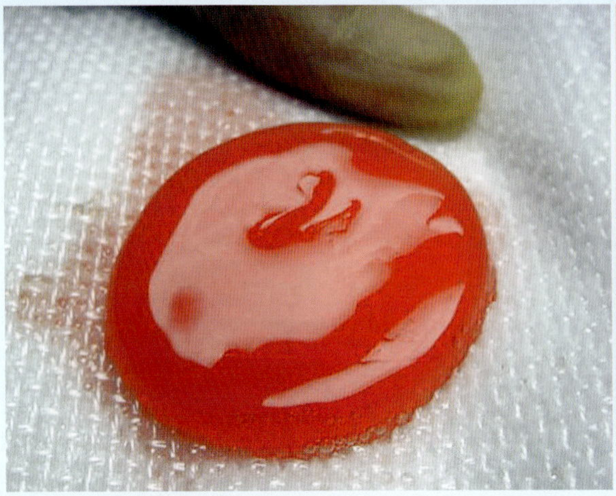

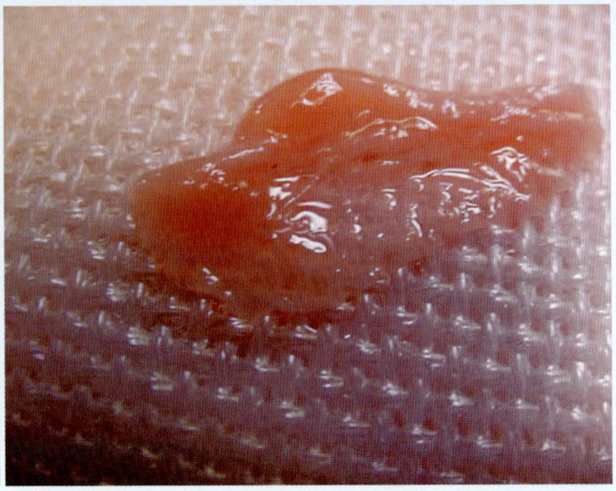

FIGURE 7-59. Platelet poor plasma was manipulated and compressed to form a biological membrane to cover the anterior alveolus.

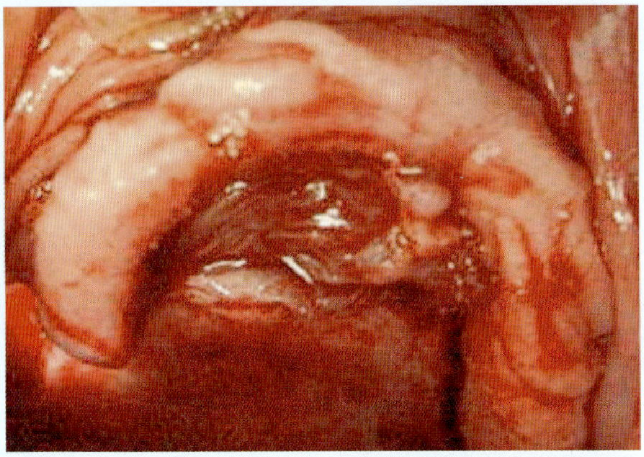

FIGURE 7-60. Platelet poor plasma membrane.

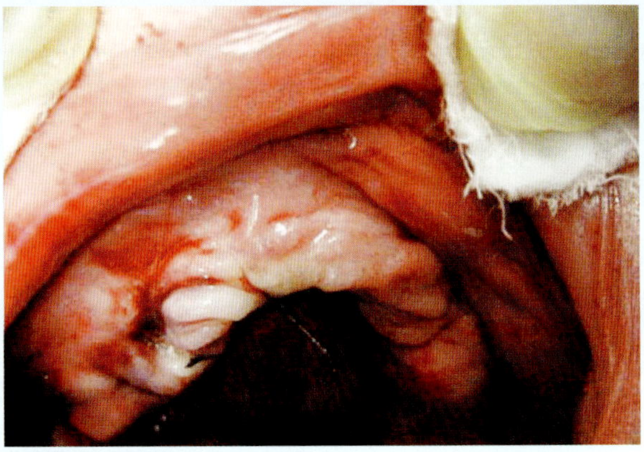

FIGURE 7-61. Wound closure was achieved with multiple subperiosteal relieving buccal incisions.

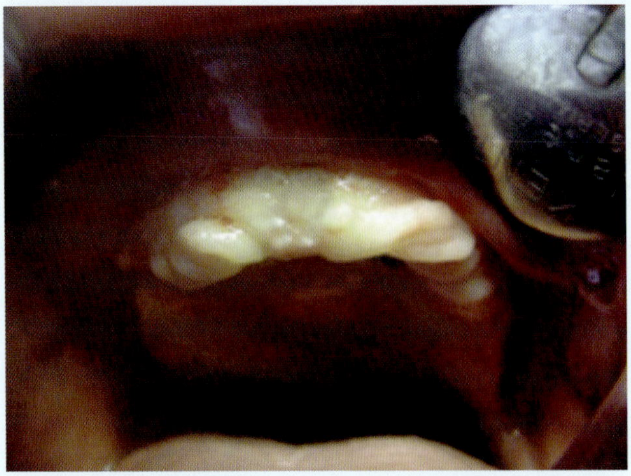

FIGURE 7-62. Transitional stabilization was performed at 3 weeks, with placement of a standard titanium 10-mm MDI Max through the anterior nasal spine or nasal septum (i.e., not a stainless steel transitional implant). Good quality of bone is encountered in the region of the anterior nasal spine, even in atrophic cases, and this is useful anchorage for the implant. Note the improvement of maxillary ridge form and that healing with primary intention has been achieved with the platelet rich plasma technique.

plasma (SmartPrep System). Grafts were covered with resorbable collagen membranes to prevent the unwanted ingress of soft tissue into the grafted area. In this case, an additional biologic membrane was created using platelet poor plasma (see Figures 7-59 and 7-60).

The surgery time was 1.5 hours. This technique obviates the need for hospital admission and major surgery and is a major advance.

TRANSITIONAL STABILIZATION

Transitional stabilization (Figures 7-63 to 7-66) was achieved at 3 weeks after grafting with a single 10-mm MDI Max placed in the anterior nasal spine (after discussion of the case with Victor Sendax). This provided *remarkable* transitional stabilization of the upper prosthesis. Although this implant became loose in a 3-month period, it still maintained its function of excellent stabilization

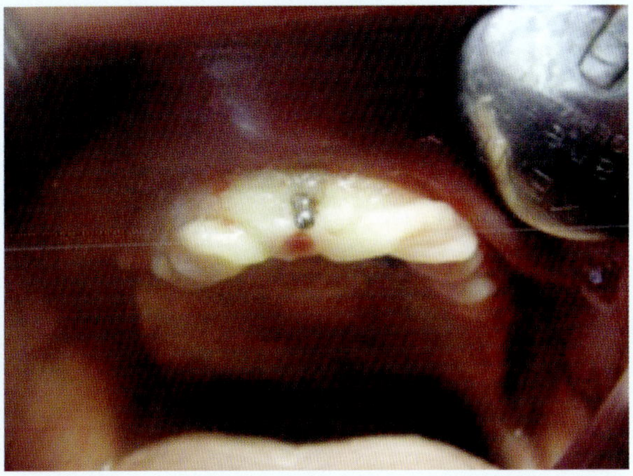

FIGURE 7-63. Transitional stabilization was performed at 3 weeks. The MDI was placed through the bone at the base of the anterior nasal spine or nasal septum.

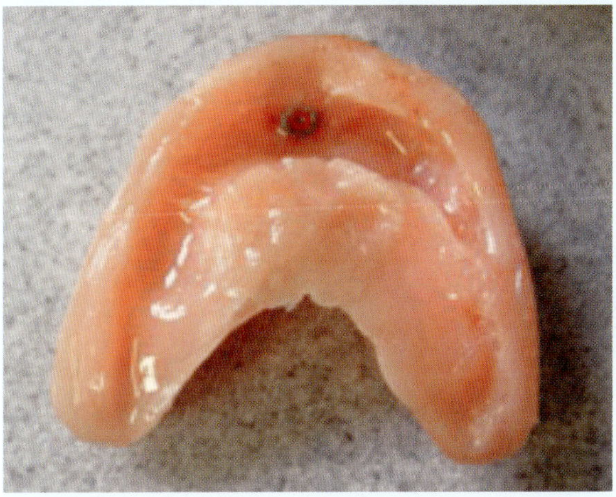

FIGURE 7-65. The upper denture was relined with soft resin in an attempt to reduce loading of the transitional implant.

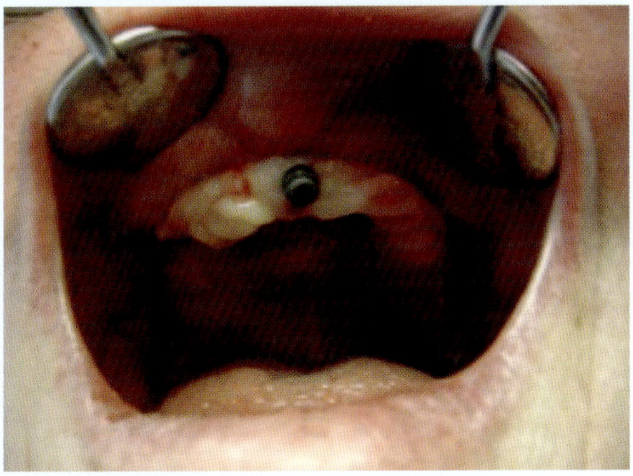

FIGURE 7-64. The shim and housing have been placed awaiting the pickup impression with soft resin.

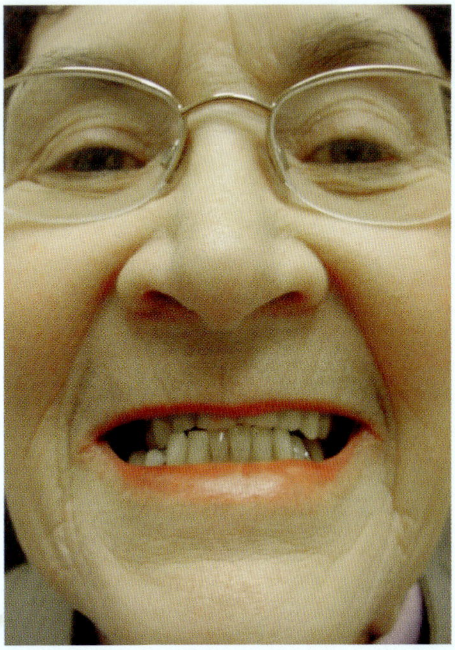

FIGURE 7-66. Excellent retention was obtained with this method of using the MDI as a transitional implant. The patient stated that the denture was more stable than it had been for 20 years. This in itself is a life changing event.

CASE DISCUSSION 3 Maxillary Atrophy—cont'd

of the upper denture for a period of 6 months. Radiographs show that the implant lost its attachment to bone, but the clinical image shows that the implant, although submerged, was functioning without any evidence of periimplantitis (Figures 7-67 to 7-69).

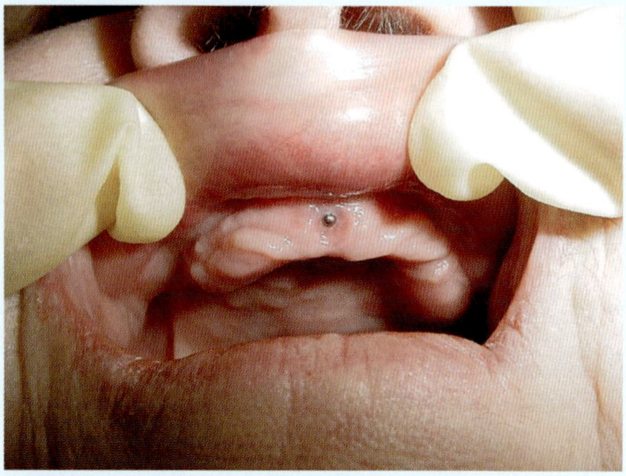

FIGURE 7-67. Outcome at 6 months. Functional stabilization of the overdenture has been maintained at 6 months despite the absence of osseointegration, submergence of the MDI implant, and mobility of the MDI. There appeared to be an element of soft tissue integration rather than osseointegration. The soft tissues were adherent to the implant screw threads. A heavy edge-to-edge occlusion (see Figure 7-54) contributes to the submergence of the transitional implant in the anterior nasal spine. A more stable transitional outcome might have resulted if a lower dental clearance had been employed at the time of bone grafting. The patient was not in favor of this option until the success of the MDI system had been demonstrated.

DENTURE CONVERSION AND STABILIZATION AT 6 MONTHS

Six long Sendax MDI Max 18-mm units were placed in the grafted area in positions 14, 13, 12, 10, 6, 5 and 4 with immediate loading. Excellent denture stabilization was immediately achieved.

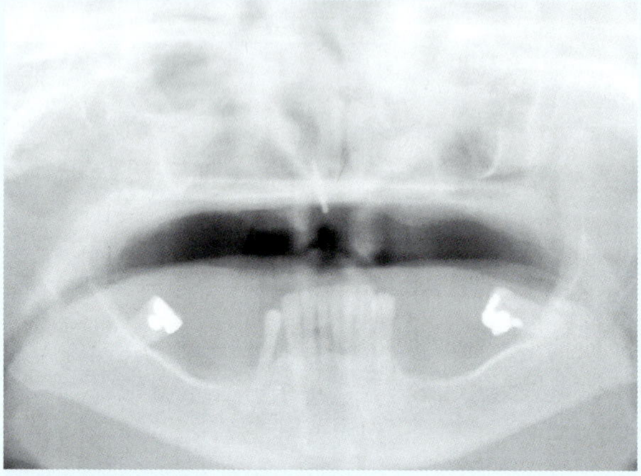

FIGURE 7-68. Outcome: panoramic x-ray at 6 months. The MDI Max slipped position and its apex projected to the right of the nasal septum, into the floor of nose. Despite this, the implant functioned well in retaining the overdenture. A lower dental clearance and provision of F/F dentures with a balanced occlusion may have prevented this complication; however, in another completely edentulous case, transitional stabilization of the upper overdenture using the same technique failed and the MDI was lost. In this case, no soft tissue integration was observed. It is advocated that the quality of bone at the base of the anterior nasal spine is crucial in the success of this transitional technique.

CASE DISCUSSION 3 Maxillary Atrophy—cont'd

In a 3-month period, the MDIs at positions 12, 10 and 6 were lost and were simply replaced without significant increase in overall cost (Figures 7-70 to 7-74). A lower clearance was carried out at 6 months with stabilization of an immediate lower denture (Figure 7-75). An upper overdenture was made without palatal cover. The esthetic outcomes are presented in Figures 7-76 and 7-77. Note the remarkable facial rejuvenation achieved with this technique.

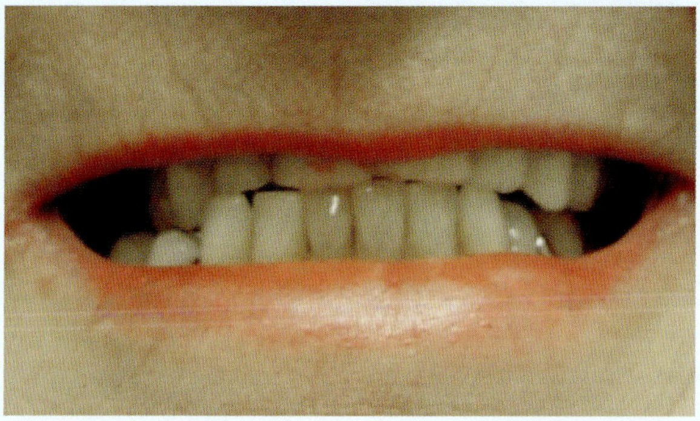

FIGURE 7-69. A heavy edge-to-edge occlusion contributes to the submergence of the transitional implant in the anterior nasal spine. A more stable transitional outcome might have resulted if a lower dental clearance had been employed at the time of bone grafting. The patient was not in favor of this option until the success of the MDI system had been demonstrated.

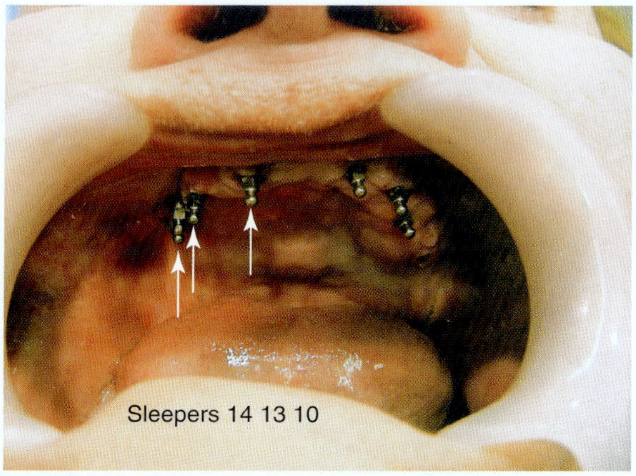

FIGURE 7-70. Outcome at 6 months. Placement of seven 18-mm MDI Max at positions 14, 13, 12, 10, 6, 5, and 4 with immediate loading. Three MDIs were lost and were replaced in 12, 10, and 6 positions at 3 months.

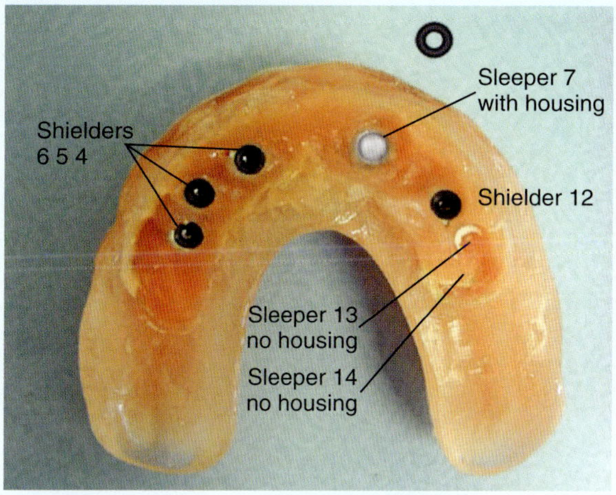

FIGURE 7-71. After loss of implants at 13. 10, 6 at 3 months after grafting the concept of shielding and sleeping implants was adopted. Replacement 18-mm MDI Max were placed into areas 10 and 12 adjacent to the area of implant loss. The quality of bone appeared to have become denser with more resistance to placement with the thumb wrench and was graded at D2. Implants at 13 and 14 appeared to have grade 1 mobility, and a decision was made to sleep all implants except 12 for 3 months. On the left side, a replacement 18-mm MDI Max was placed in the 6 area into bone estimated as Misch grade 2 and loaded as a potential sacrificial implant with the aim of achieving the maximum degree of osseointegration in the upper right quadrant. Shielders 12, 6, 5 and 4 are located in the areas of greatest bone density (Misch D2) and protect three unloaded sleepers at 10, 13 and 14 in areas of bone density estimated at Misch D3 on clinical placement of the implants.

CASE DISCUSSION 3 Maxillary Atrophy—cont'd

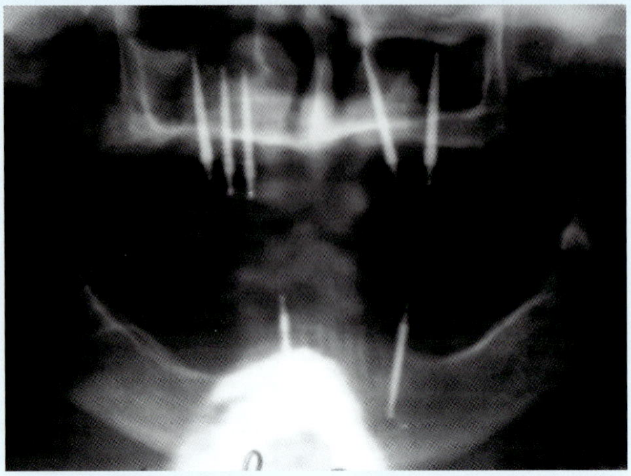

FIGURE 7-72. Outcome at 9 months. Surviving implants at 14, 13, 11, 5 and 4. Lower immediate overdenture has been fitted over two MDIs. Note the loss of the shielder implant at 6 and buccally placed sleeper at 13. Another 18-mm MDI was placed in 6 area.

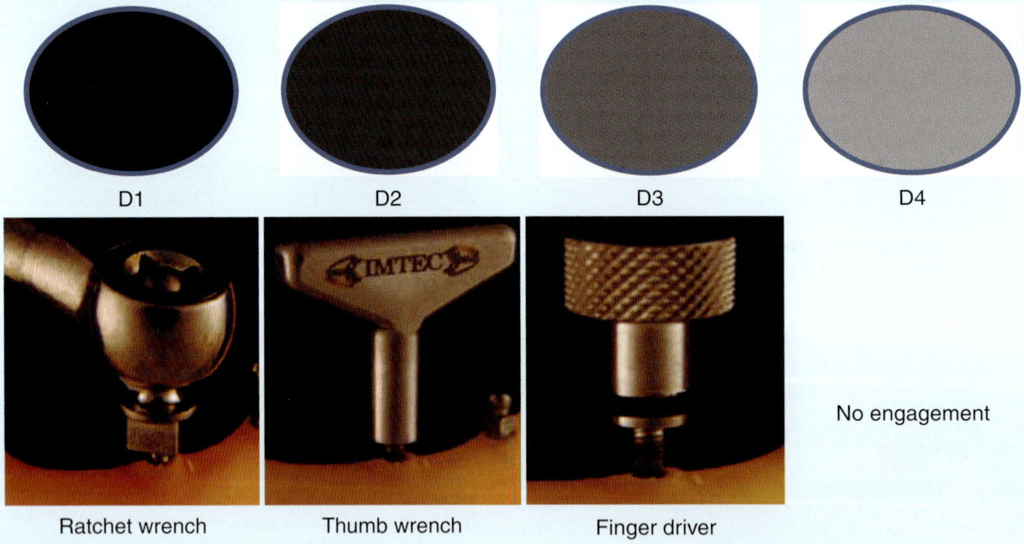

FIGURE 7-73. Clinical estimation of Misch grading of bone density. As a rule of thumb, Misch bone density may be approximated with the following guidelines:
D1: Implant placement required use of ratchet wrench (note risk of implant fracture)
D2: Implant placement may be placed with the thumb wrench
D3: Implant placement may be achieved with the finger driver
D4: No implant engagement with bone

CASE DISCUSSION 3 Maxillary Atrophy—cont'd

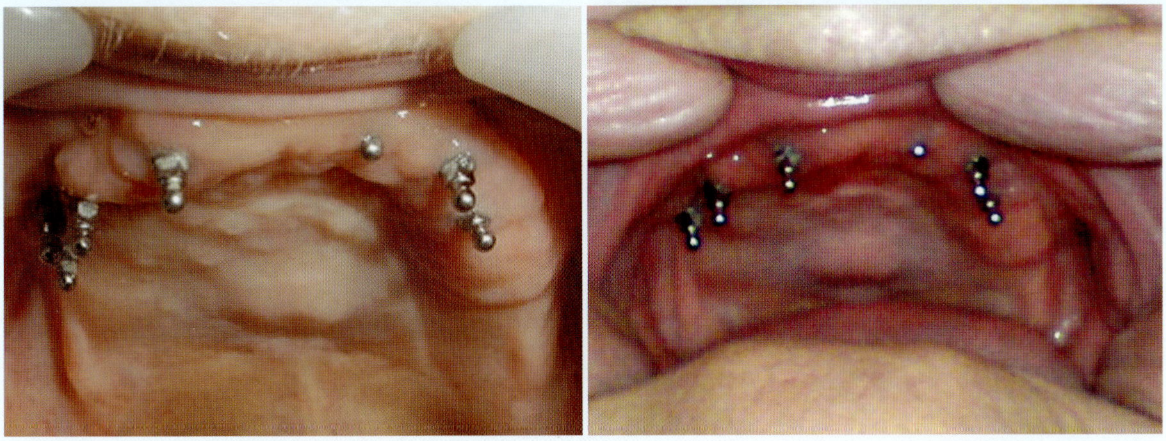

FIGURE 7-74. Outcome at 2 years with 18-mm MDI Max. At 5 years, osseointegration of MDIs is maintained in positions 14, 12, 11, 6 and 5. Implant 13 was lost and the sacrificial shielder at 6 is submerging, but despite this at 5 years 6 was firm and not mobile. It appeared to be making a contribution to the overdenture retention despite a progressive submergence, but was lost within 10 years. Sleepers 10 and 14 have been retained and have osseointegrated despite signs of mobility within the first 3 months. The patient is functioning on six 18-mm MDI with a palateless maxillary overdenture.

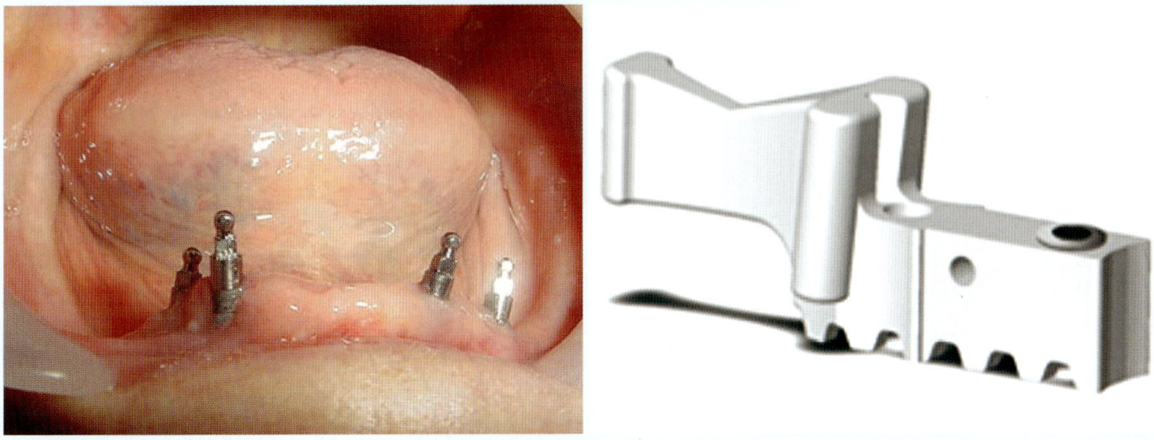

FIGURE 7-75. MDIs at 22 and 27 have been supplemented with two additional MDIs in positions 22 and 28. Irregular ridge shape and placement at the time of a lower clearance made implant alignment difficult in this case. Nevertheless the implants successfully delivered excellent denture retention by virtue of the O ball and O ring system. The use of Dr. Harold Sussman's SIG drill guide is recommended for the placement of MDIs because malalignment of the implants may result in repetitive excessive lateral forces on insertion and removal of the prosthesis and long-term failure of osseointegration. All mandibular implants were functioning at 10 years.

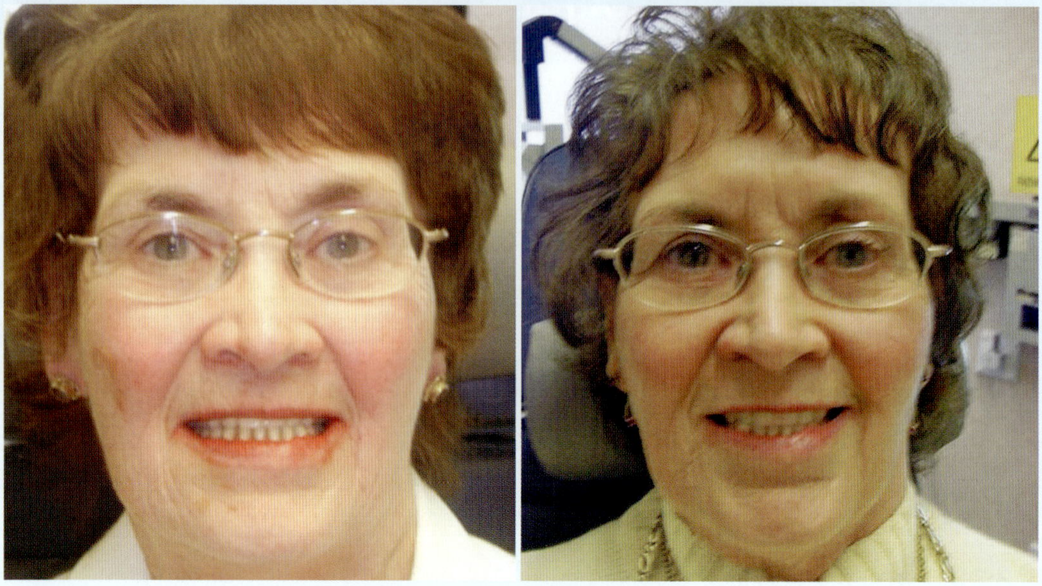

9 months 2 years

FIGURE 7-76. Esthetic outcomes at 9 months and 2 years. Note the remarkable facial rejuvenation that has occurred and been maintained with this technique.

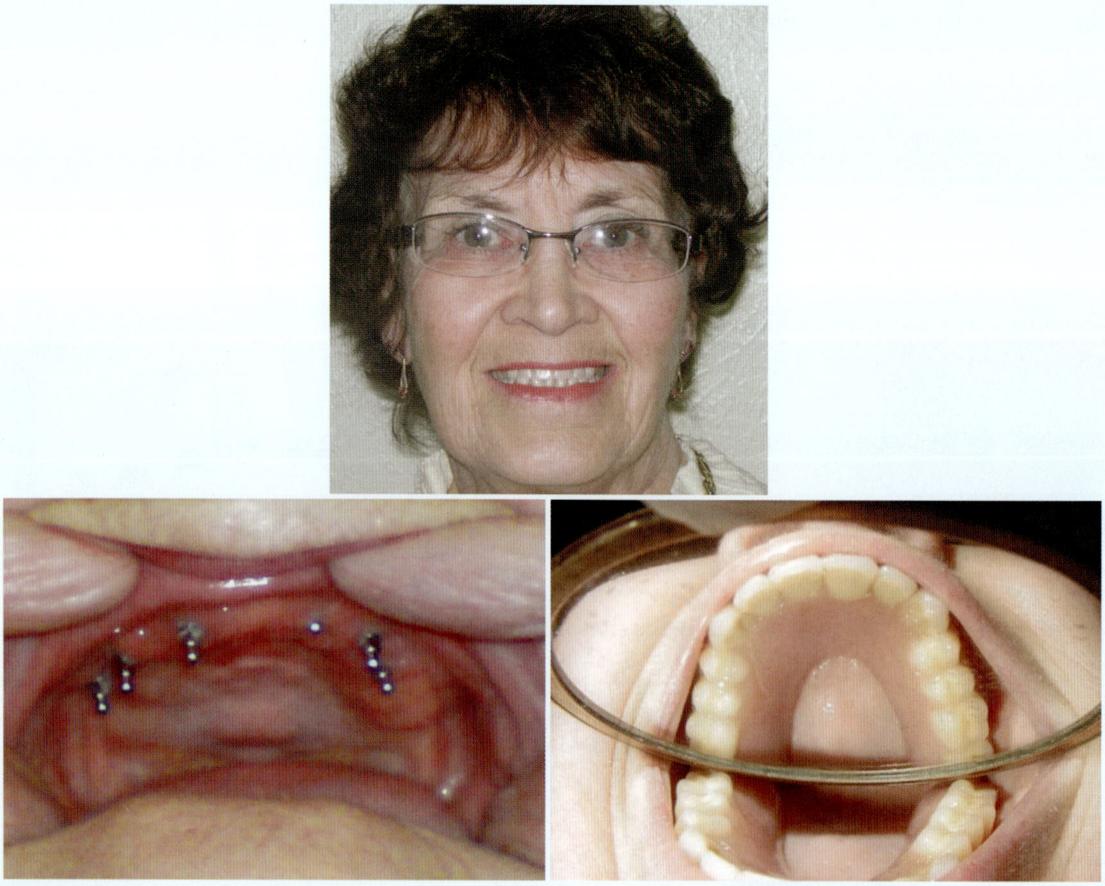

FIGURE 7-77. At 5 years the patient reports no further problems with the implants. Five MDI Max are functioning. Implant 7 is submerged and asymptomatic and was retained at the patient's request. All mandibular implants are functioning. Overdenture retention is excellent and speech quality is enhanced. Swallowing, mastication, taste, and thermal recognition in the mouth are within normal limits with this palateless prosthetic option.

CASE DISCUSSION 3 Maxillary Atrophy—cont'd

This was achieved without recourse to soft tissue enhancement of any kind, without redraping the soft tissues through rhytidectomy, and illustrates the importance of the restoration of maxillary bone volume, teeth positioning, lip support, and restoration of the vertical dimension—all achieved by grafting and MDI-retained overdenture. This treatment option facilitates the regeneration of facial harmony.

There is improvement in muscle tone, better exposure of the upper incisor teeth, and filling out of the nasolabial folds. This outcome would not have been possible with a single tooth implant treatment plan unless combined with major jaw advancement osteotomy surgery, which still would have provided an inferior rejuvenation effect.

Outcome at 2 years confirmed osseointegration of 5 of the 6 MDI Max implants in the maxilla. It is unclear whether the one submerging implant has subsequently osseointegrated. The upper palateless denture had superb retention. In the mandible all four 18-mm MDIs have integrated retaining a full lower overdenture. This outcome was maintained at 5 years.

The procedure was a life-changing event for the patient, whose quality of life was enhanced beyond her expectations.

DISCUSSION

This case illustrates how MDIs can be used in conjunction with advanced tissue engineering techniques to reconstruct the atrophic maxilla, one of most technically demanding reconstructions in oral and maxillofacial surgery.

Complications related to failure of osseointegration and implant loss in the maxilla may be associated with:

- Potential premature placement of the implants into the bone graft (at 6 months);
- Premature loading of MDIs in grafted bone that has undergone insufficient remodelling;
- Early excessive loading of MDIs by the mandibular dentition rather than reduced occlusal loading of a tissue borne prosthesis;
- Increased occlusal loading of maxillary MDIs by a natural mandibular dentition rather than reduced occlusal loading of a tissue borne prosthesis;
- Inadequate bone density of the grafted site for MDI placement.

CASE DISCUSSION 4 Maxillary Atrophy

In a second case of maxillary atrophy (completely edentulous in the mandibular arch), using the same tissue engineering technique all MDI implants were all lost in the maxilla.[13] CT scans and SimPlant 9 analysis indicated that the quality of bone was of Misch grade D1 in the periapical area, Misch D2 in the alveolar crestal area, and Misch D3 in the middle third of the alveolar crest. An unexpected finding was a retained fragment of a fractured MDI in an area of periapical bone with a designated density of Misch D2 (Figures 7-78 to 7-81).

This implies that although the density of bone was adequate for implant placement, the problem lies in the elasticity of the grafted area.

HOOKE'S LAW OF ELASTICITY

Stated simply, an elastic body stretches (strain) in proportion to the force (stress) on it. Mathematically, the formula is as follows:

$$F = kx$$

where:

F = force,
k = proportional constant, and
x = distance of stretching.

YOUNG'S MODULUS

When any substance is subjected to stress it is deformed by that stress. If it recovers its original dimensions when the stress ceases, it is termed "elastic,"

CASE DISCUSSION 4 Maxillary Atrophy—cont'd

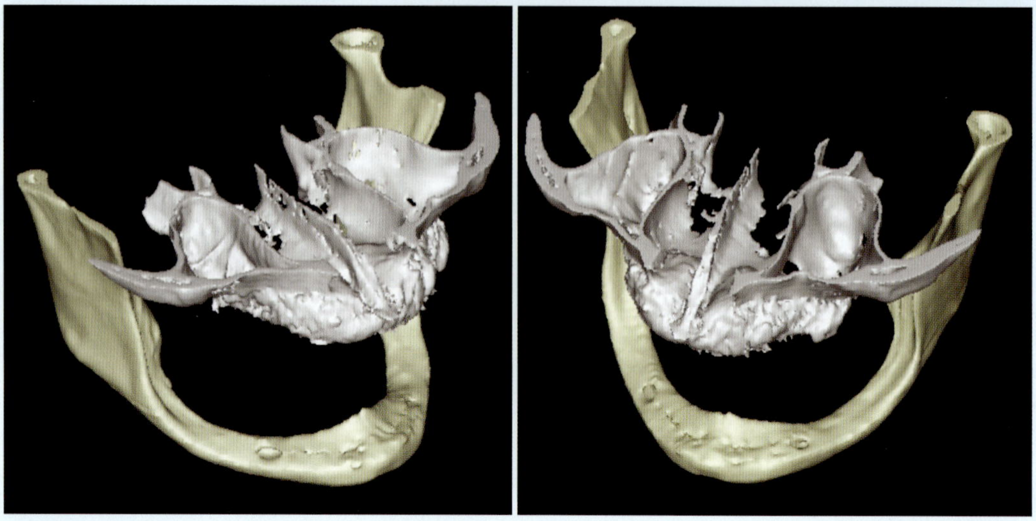

FIGURE 7-78. Maxillary Atrophy Case 2: The grafted maxilla. Bilateral sinus lifts have been carried out with bilateral nasal floor lifts and anterior alveolar augmentation to increase alveolar width. Bio-Oss platelet rich plasma (SmartPrep System). Bone density is excellent. Despite this outcome and placement of six MDI Max at 6 months in the maxilla, all implants were ultimately lost. CT scans were taken and used to analyze bone quality and the potential reasons for implant failure.

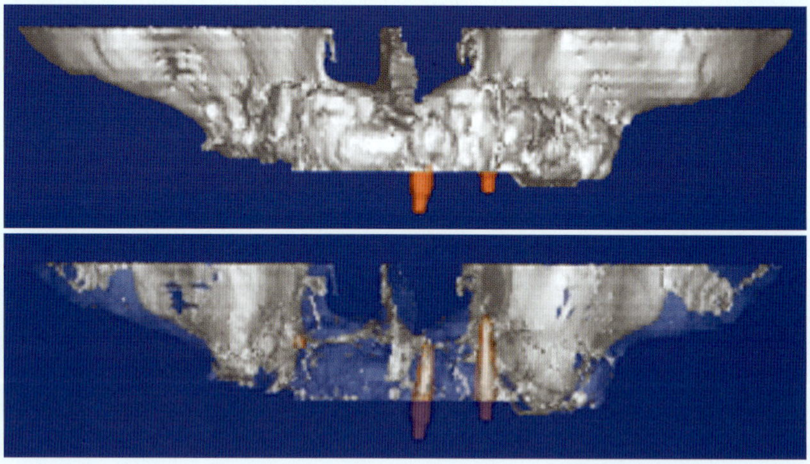

FIGURE 7-79. Maxillary Atrophy Case 2: The grafted maxilla is illustrated with SimPlant 9 Software after the loss of four MDIs. The two remaining implants are mobile. With transparent mode the fractured tip of the MDI in apical area of 11 is visible.

whereas if the deformation persists in whole or in part it is termed "inelastic" or "plastic."

Young's modulus, *E*, can be calculated by dividing the tensile stress by the tensile strain:

$$E = \frac{\text{tensile stress}}{\text{tensile strain}} = \frac{\sigma}{\varepsilon} = \frac{F/A_0}{\Delta L/L_0} = \frac{FL_0}{A_0 \Delta L}$$

where:

E = Young's modulus (modulus of elasticity),

F = force applied to the object,

A_0 = original cross-sectional area through which the force is applied,

ΔL = amount by which the length of the object changes, and

L_0 = original length of the object.

For any elastic substance, there is an upper limit of stress, namely *the elastic limit*, beyond which

CASE DISCUSSION 4 Maxillary Atrophy—cont'd

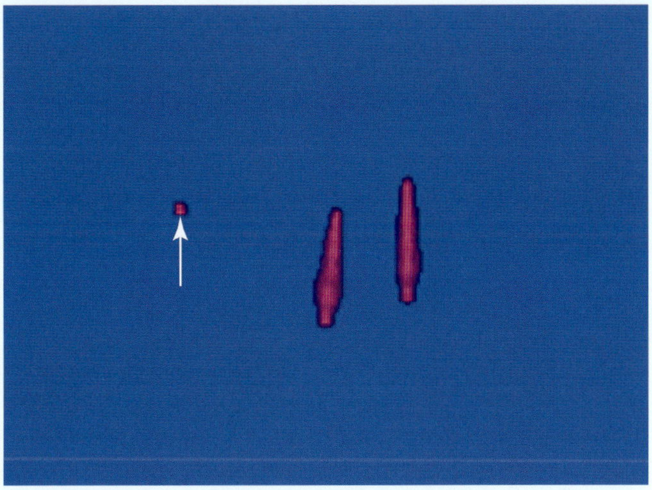

FIGURE 7-80. Maxillary Atrophy Case 2: The fractured apex of a MDI is identified. The implant has osseointegrated in the coronal and apical thirds representing Misch D2 and D1 bone, respectively. The fractured apex has been retained in Misch D1 bone. Osseointegration has not occurred in the mid third of the implant corresponding to Misch D3.

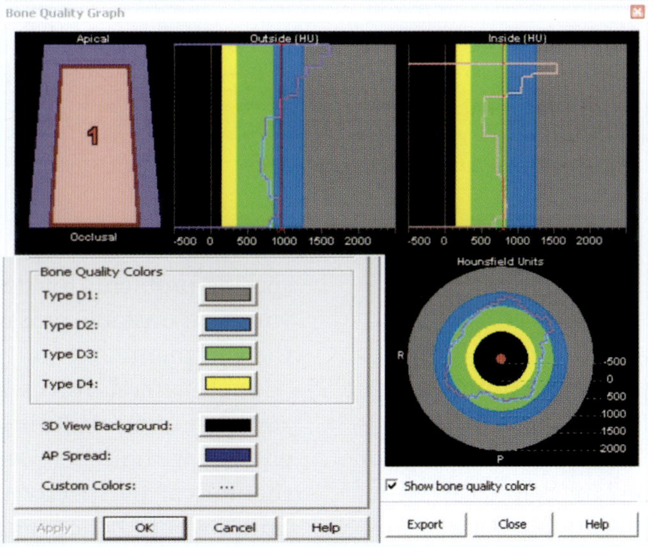

FIGURE 7-81. Maxillary Atrophy Case 2: SimPlant 9 bone quality graph mode with corresponding Misch grading. Misch D1 bone is identified in the apical area (*gray*). A small amount of Misch D2 is identified in the coronal region (*blue*). The remainder is Misch D3 (mid third).

the property of elasticity is lost. The extent of the deformation caused by a given intensity of stress varies in different elastic substances. In the case of tensile stress the extensibility is usually expressed inversely by the constant known as Young's modulus (E). Thus under a given tensile stress a piece of rubber will extend more than a piece of steel of the same dimensions, and therefore the value of Young's modulus for rubber is lower than that for steel.

Although Young's modulus is thus defined in terms of tensile strength, it is also closely related to the flexibility of a body when it is subjected to a bending stress, so that a low value of Young's modulus is associated with comparatively flexible substances and vice versa. For this reason the

CASE DISCUSSION 4 Maxillary Atrophy—cont'd

modulus is frequently used as an inverse index of both the extensibility and the flexibility of materials, and its value for bone from various sources has been determined by many authors.

In our second case of maxillary atrophy, the value of Young's modulus must have increased in association with the increased bone density, which was confirmed by CT scans and SimPlant analysis. This led to a concentration of stress forces in the apical third of the MDI, the point of fracture. This situation is contrary to finite element analysis studies in other dental implant systems in ungrafted bone sites where stress concentration occurs in the neck of the implant system.

A possible explanation of this difference in stress concentration of grafted versus ungrafted cases is related to the location of greatest bone density. CT scans confirmed that the densest bone is found in the periapical areas in our grafted case using tissue engineering techniques and platelet rich plasma impregnated graft material. An increase in Young's modulus is to be expected and with it a concentration of stress in the area leading to MDI fracture in the periapical area.

Possible solutions to this problem are:

- To place shorter implants into the grafted areas;

It is to be noted that we placed 18-mm implants into Misch grade 1 bone, and this may be in part responsible for implant fracture and loss. This was in line with MDI case planning protocols and recommendations of placing the longest implant possible into bone.

- To rest maxillary implants (sleeping phase) after placement in an unloaded state.

Sleeping MDIs may promote osseointegration and bony remodelling. However, if there is a relative deficiency of collagen in grade Misch D1 bone, potential issues with Young's modulus may not be addressed to prevent implant fracture. However, we have only documented implant fracture in one MDI. The majority of failures were in MDIs that failed to osseointegrate.

Our failed case of MDIs in the atrophic maxilla was retrieved using a standard endosseous implant system as a two staged technique, and the patient outcome was stable at 5 years.

Sleeping MDIs

Although MDI osseointegration success is estimated at > 95% in the mandible, an estimated 10% of implants are lost in the ungrafted maxilla. It is postulated that this is in relation to immediate or premature loading of the implant before osseointegration has taken place (see Figures 7-70 and 7-71).

Empirical attempts to rest implants have been undertaken with:

- Soft lining;
- Removal of "O rings";
- Removal of housings and relief of the denture base in the housing area;
- Preferential or sacrificial loading (Peckitt).

Implants best resist occlusal forces along their long axes, and the immediate loading of implants along their long axes permits the development of osseointegration. Lateral forces appear to adversely affect the osseointegration process; this creates specific problems for the case of an overdenture in which an unstable prosthesis moves laterally against the abutment.

Such lateral forces could be reduced by the addition of a soft lining and removal of "O rings" with or without removal of the housings. From a theoretical perspective, Young's modulus of soft lining would be low and dissipate any build up of stress around the implant. The prosthesis would become more tissue borne than implant borne. However, it is critical to eliminate any lateral prosthetic movement against the implant abutment during function; such movement may cause macro movements, failure to osseointegrate, and implant loss.

An option favored by Peckitt is to use key *shielding implants* to stabilize a soft lined and primarily tissue borne prosthesis during the sleeping phase. These implants act as sacrificial lambs for their sleeping sisters that are shielded (especially from lateral forces) during the osseointegration period.

It is advocated that shielding implants:

- Provide prosthetic stability and good retention;
- Shield sleeping implants for which the O rings and housings have been removed with relief of the denture base in the housing area so that no lateral forces can be applied to the implant;
- Be used in the definitive overdenture prosthesis if they survive;
- Be removed if they fail or be replaced as the clinical situation demands.

Shielders are not transitional implants; they are employed long term if they survive. The low cost of MDIs and the simplicity of placement lends itself particularly to this option. The mechanics of the protocol makes sense in that this is the only method with MDIs that will shield sleeping implants from disruptive lateral functional forces.

Occlusion is critical in all implant cases but especially so in the sleeping phase. Patients are the best witnesses of inadvertent loading of a sleeper, and clinicians must be diligent if they are to achieve success in these complex cases.

It would appear that potentially failing implants can be salvaged with this method.

Although we have demonstrated that the cost effective reconstruction of the atrophic maxilla is possible with the MDI system, further research in this area is warranted to define protocols and guidelines for the management of such cases, especially with respect to:

1. Optimum bone grafting techniques;
2. Timing of implant placement;
3. Transitional stabilization;
4. Loading protocols;
5. Concepts of shielding and sleeping;
6. Clinical trial designs.

CASE DISCUSSION 5 Customized Hybrid Implant Systems

A 50-year-old man underwent midface resection of a sarcomatous carcinoma and received postoperative radiotherapy. Posterior maxillary teeth were retained to facilitate retention of a maxillary obturator, and the patient was tumor free at 4 years (Figures 7-82 and 7-83).

TREATMENT PLANNING

The patient was deemed unsuitable for placement conventional osseointegrated implants because:

1. There was insufficient bone volume for placement;
2. The use of zygomatic endosseous implants on their own could not deliver the required denture base and retention;
3. The placement of MDIs, similarly, was not possible because the available bone could not even accommodate the width of this implant system;
4. The option of advanced complex composite free flap transfer was an option but increased the risk for failure, especially in view of the history of postoperative radiotherapy. This option would have significantly added to the cost of treatment, and free flap surgery often compromises midface esthetics, especially the dental esthetics. In particular there is an inability to recreate optimum crown and gingival exposure in the dental aesthetic zone with replication of the Golden Ratio Φ. This has a profound and adverse effect on dental esthetics.

THE GOLDEN RATIO Φ

The Golden Ration[9,10] is a mathematical ratio of 1.618:1 that seems to appear recurrently in beautiful things in nature as well as in other things that are seen as "beautiful." The number **1.618** was designated Φ (Phi) by Mark Barr, an American mathematician in 1909. It is the first Greek letter in the name of Phidias, the Greek sculptor who lived around 450 BC.

The crucial importance of these ratios to the planning of midface reconstruction and dentition is shown in Figures 7-84 to 7-86.

IMPLANT DESIGN

The cantilevered maxillary implant described by Peckitt[22] offers a potential and simple solution for the reconstruction of this defect. The issues related to implant design are as follows:

1. Radiotherapy fields;
2. Viability of osteosynthesis in the areas adjacent to the resection margins;
3. An inability to secure adequate skeletal fixation medially may have an effect on

CASE DISCUSSION 5 Customized Hybrid Implant Systems—cont'd

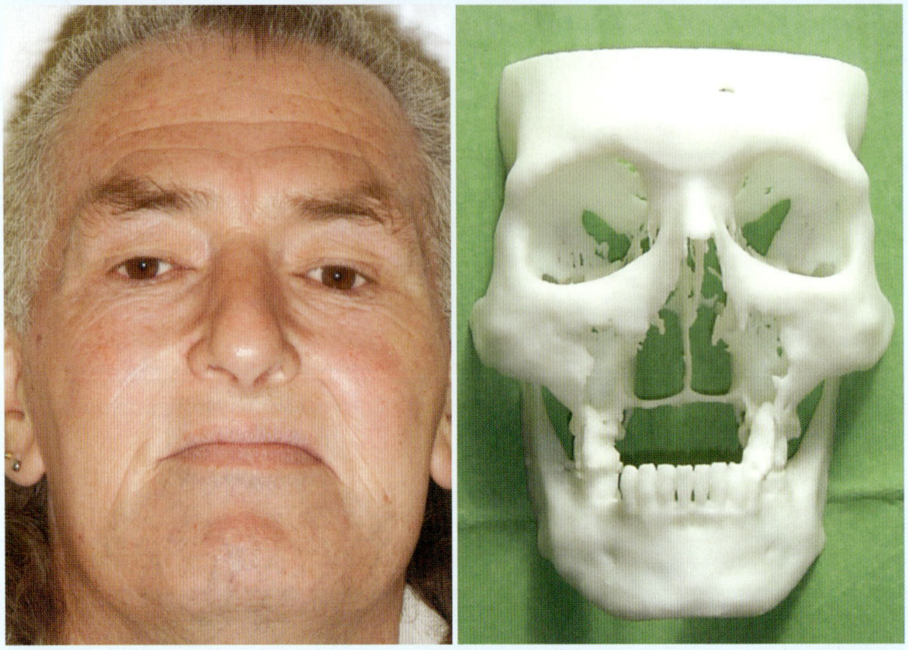

FIGURE 7-82. Customized hybrid implant systems: the cantilevered maxillary implant. Note the collapse of the midface and upper lip. His posterior maxillary teeth are retained by granulation tissue only. He wears a maxillary obturator the retention of which has been lost as the periodontal condition has deteriorated.

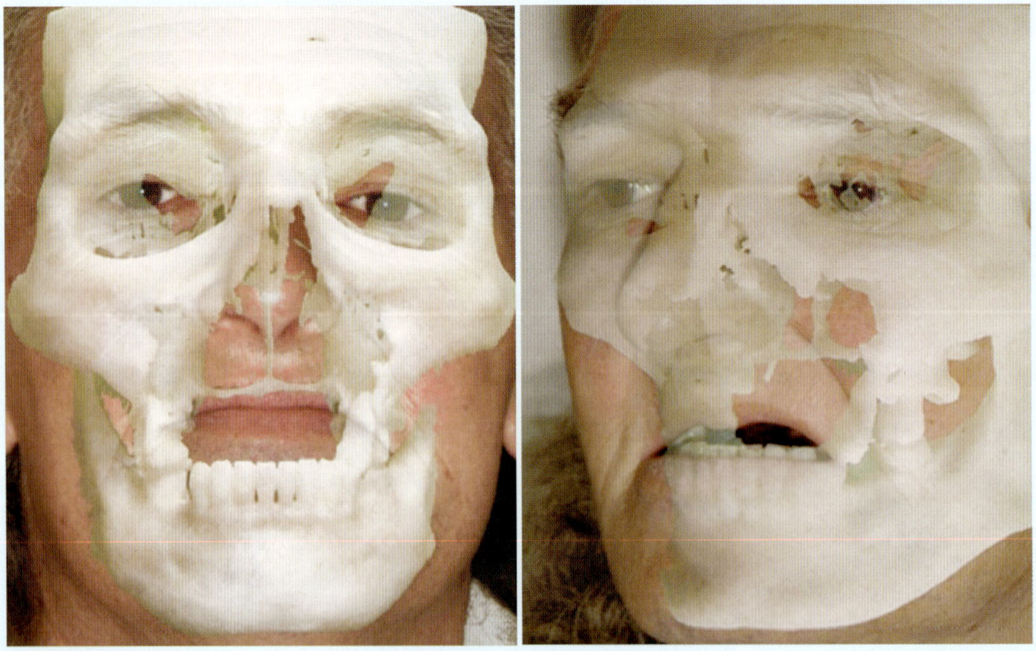

FIGURE 7-83. The relationships between the hard and soft tissues are clearly demonstrated as an adjunct to EAS treatment planning.

CASE DISCUSSION 5 Customized Hybrid Implant Systems—cont'd

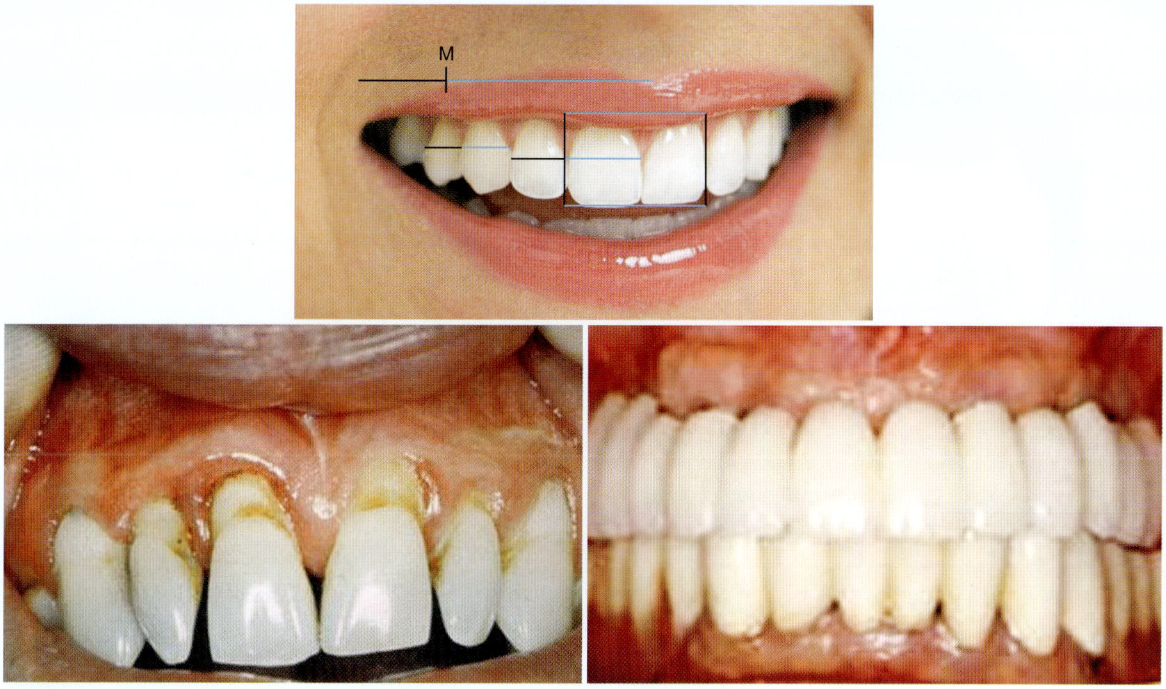

FIGURE 7-84. The ratios in the esthetic face are complex and summarized in the perioral area.
Absent golden ratio Φ**:** The effect on dental esthetics is clearly visible in periodontal disease and the reconstruction of the edentulous maxilla with individual implant retained teeth.
Key:
Black = 1 unit.
Blue = 1.618 units.
M = Midpoint of the crown of 12.

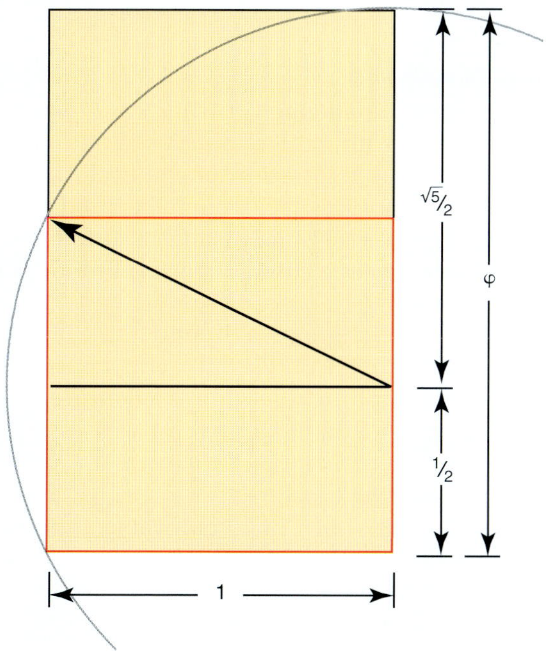

FIGURE 7-85. Construction of a golden rectangle:
1. Construct a unit square *(red)*.
2. Draw a line from the midpoint of one side to an opposite corner.
3. Use that line as the radius to draw an arc that defines the long dimension of the rectangle.
   Length of face / width of face;
   Distance between the lips and where the eyebrows meet / length of nose;
   Length of face / distance between tip of jaw and where the eyebrows meet;
   Length of mouth / width of nose;
   Width of nose / distance between nostrils;
   Distance between pupils / distance between eyebrows.

CASE DISCUSSION 5 Customized Hybrid Implant Systems—cont'd

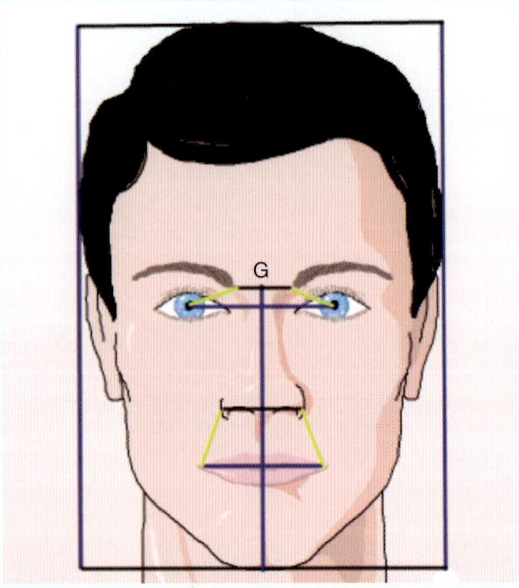

FIGURE 7-86. Facial harmony.
1. Glabella/ lips / lips / menton
2. Interpupillary distance / medial canthal distance
3. Glabella/ lips / length of nose
4. Intercommisural distance / intermalar distance
5. Intermalar distance / width columella

In the case of midface reconstruction the crucial issues are related to replication of normal:
- Anterior upper facial height (glabella / anterior nasal spine)
- Anterior lower facial height (anterior nasal spine / menton) - prevention of overclosure of the mandible
- Intermalar width, which increased after resection of the pyriform aperture of the nose
- Exposure of the maxillary incisor tooth in repose (3 mm)

The required golden proportions for facial harmony cannot be created by reconstructive surgery alone and require prosthetic expertise.

the long-term stability of certain implant system designs. A solution to this problem might be to make a cantilevered implant with osteosynthesis positioned some distance away from the defect and to cantilever an armature across the defect, thus avoiding skeletal fixation and osteosynthesis in the region of irradiated bone.

Although the implant might be placed via incisions over the zygomatic buttresses, this would involve more stripping of tissues in the area for medial entry into the oronasal defect.

4. Closure of the oronasal defect may be achieved in two ways:
   a. By a conventional custom implant supported obturator. A scaffolding design would permit easy inspection of the nasal cavity and facilitate the management of any recurrence, but it adds to the complexity of manufacture.
   b. The implant itself could obturate the defect and provide a stable base for a dental prosthesis that could be fixed or removable. A titanium obturator with a precision fit could be designed to be removable and form a solid platform on which to reconstruct the dentition. A removable design would facilitate oral hygiene of the oronasal cavity. However, such a design would increase the cost, and the availability of nasendoscopy could be argued to obviate the requirement for more complex designs. As a general rule the simplest designs are the best options, and a titanium diaphragm obturator and overdenture attachment system was the method chosen. This would be the most simple system and would need to be relined on the table with the extraction of the posterior maxillary teeth.

CASE PLANNING

The greatest challenge of this case was to fabricate an implant retained obturator and simultaneous restoration of the occlusion so that a functioning device could be fitted at the time of surgery. The solution was as follows:

1. Construction of a fused deposition model for case planning;
2. CAD-CAM design of a hybrid Cantilevered Maxillary Implant® (Peckitt) with removable titanium diaphragm serving as a denture base;
3. Rapid product manufacture[23] of a customized titanium implant—CAD to metal to reduce manufacturing costs;
4. Manufacture of a removable palatal diaphragm with CAD/CAM 5 axis CNC milling technology;

CASE DISCUSSION 5 Customized Hybrid Implant Systems—cont'd

5. Dental and occlusal rehabilitation using the current obturator as a template;
6. A spare removable obturator to be provided in this treatment plan;
7. Bilateral mandibular bounded saddle areas were to be reconstructed MDIs and two removable MiniDentures® (Peckitt)[15] to reduce costs.

The first stage was to determine the vertical dimensions of the face and the dental occlusion (Figures 7-87 and 7-88).

IMPLANT MANUFACTURE

A Cantilevered Maxillary Implant (Computer-Gen Implants Ltd, New Zealand) and its customized hybrid variation (worldwide rights

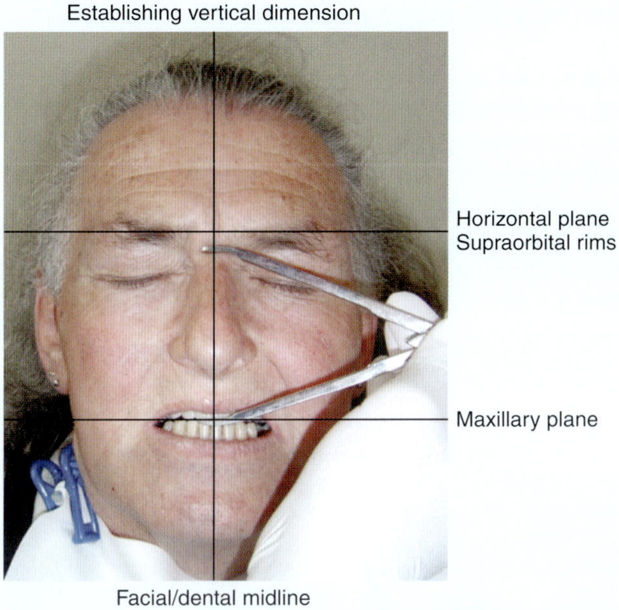

FIGURE 7-87. EAS planning: estimation of the anterior facial height and exposure of the incisor teeth. Exposure of the upper incisor teeth is the crucial measurement for good midface esthetics. Estimated from soft tissue nasion to the incisal tip so that 3 mm of upper incisor tooth is exposed in lip repose and teeth gently in occlusion.

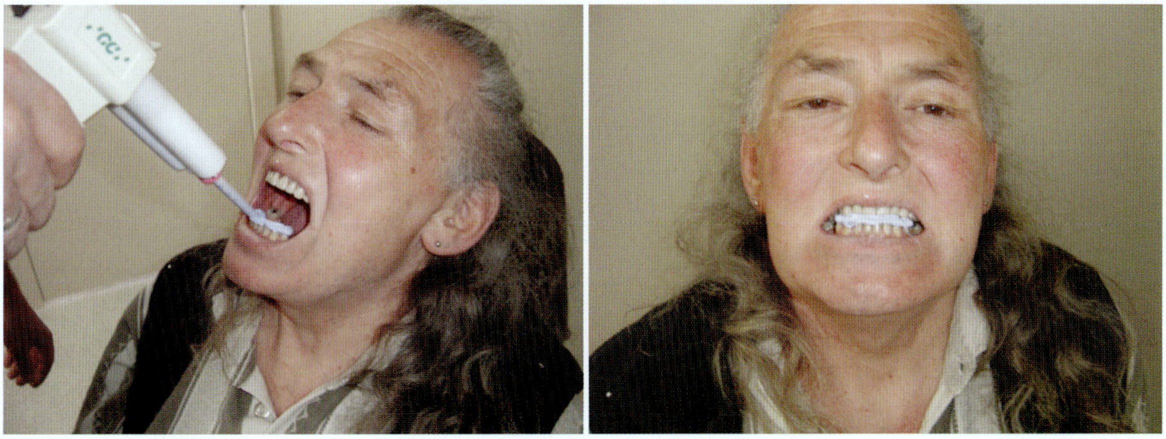

FIGURE 7-88. Occlusal registration.

CASE DISCUSSION 5 Customized Hybrid Implant Systems—cont'd

pending) has been manufactured using rapid product manufacturing technology.[9] The implant is grown using a 3D printing system from medical grade titanium powder, which is melted with an electron beam. The implant system incorporates MDIs O rings for overdenture retention.

The path of implant insertion is crucial in these cases and determines the surgical approach. (Figures 7-89 to 7-95). Surgery was performed under general anaesthesia with nasal intubation in 1.5 hours.

After the extraction of the remaining maxillary dentition, sockets were prepared with a denture finishing bur to remove any interferences to the path of insertion. A buccal flap was raised using a horizontal incision in the buccal segments as far posteriorly as the first molar tooth. This permits access to the zygomas without entering the temporal extension of the buccal fat pad. The mucosal tissue around the titanium pyriform fossa was deepithelialized.

In this case, the implant was designed to fit inside the molar alveolar remnants. Osteosynthesis screw fixation was with 2.0-mm maxillofacial titanium screws in the zygomatic flanges and 1.5-mm screws in the nasal flanges.

Two screw holes towards the neck of the skeletal fixation flange were left without screws. This permitted soft tissue attachment to the bone of the zygoma and assisted in the formation of a soft tissue cuff that isolated the potential tissue space around the flange from the oral cavity.

Other potential variations to enhance soft tissue adherence to the screw flanges include placement of bone grafts and the use of bone morphogenetic protein delivery systems. Bone morphogenetic protein is angiogenic and until safety is established its use is contraindicated at the time of benign and malignant tumor resection because it may theoretically influence the development of local recurrence from microscopic tumor remnants.

Cantilevered maxillary implant

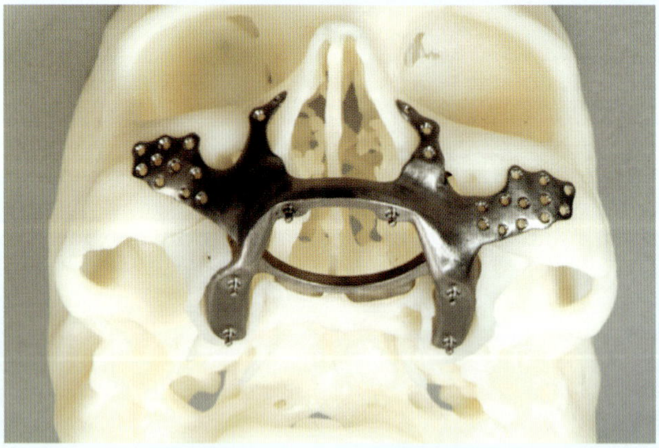

CAD/metal manufacturing (EBM)

FIGURE 7-89. Six holes in the implant suprastructure receive a 1.5-degree tapered locking ball head abutment. These abutments are tapped into the docking holes to produce a cold weld. Thus the abutments can be located without screw fixation and without recourse to titanium welding. Furthermore the possibility exists to replace and these abutments by their removal with dental forceps. (Courtesy Massey University Centre of Engineering Assisted Surgery, ComputerGen Implants Ltd [Ninian Peckitt Implant concept, design and choice of manufacture]; ENZTEC Ltd,*New Zealand [CAD/CAM and implant finishing], Medical Modeling Inc., United States [EBM manufacture].)
(*Enztec Ltd withdrew from the EAS Programme in 2008.)

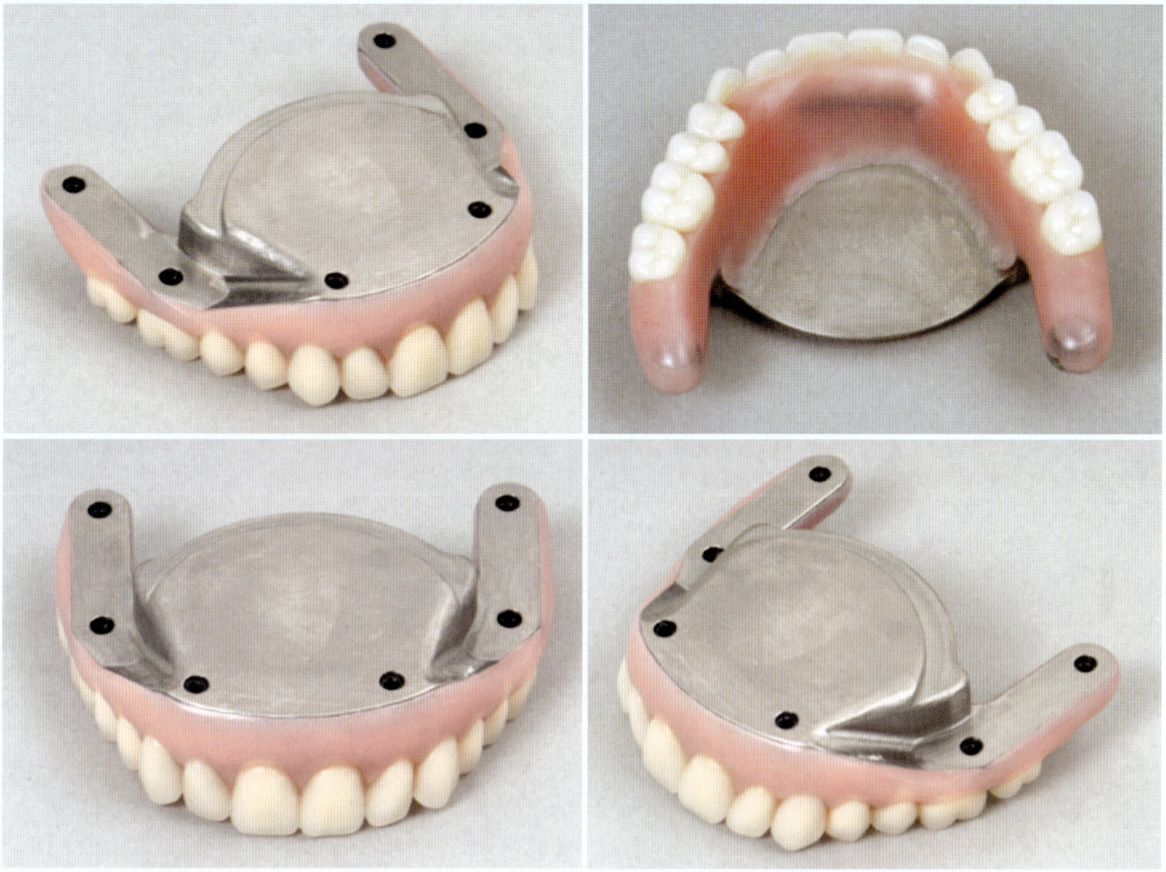

FIGURE 7-90. Six MDI O rings are placed into the housing recesses machined into the denture base.

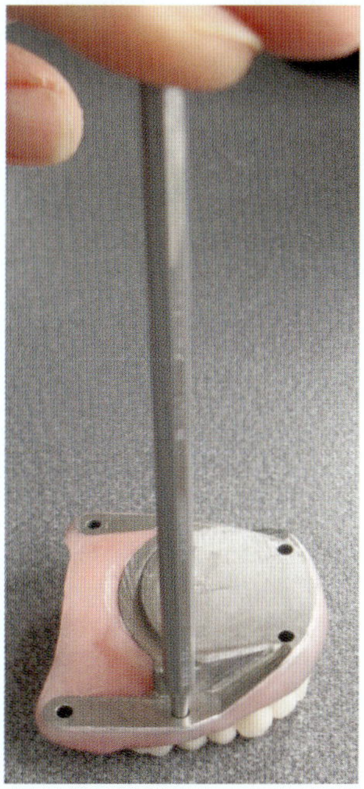

FIGURE 7-91. MDI O rings are placed into the housing recess using a specially adapted instrument.

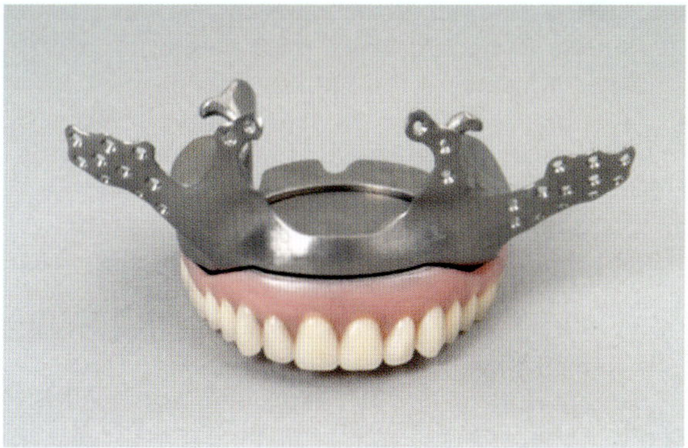

FIGURE 7-92. The assembled implant system (anterior aspect).

CASE DISCUSSION 5 Customized Hybrid Implant Systems—cont'd

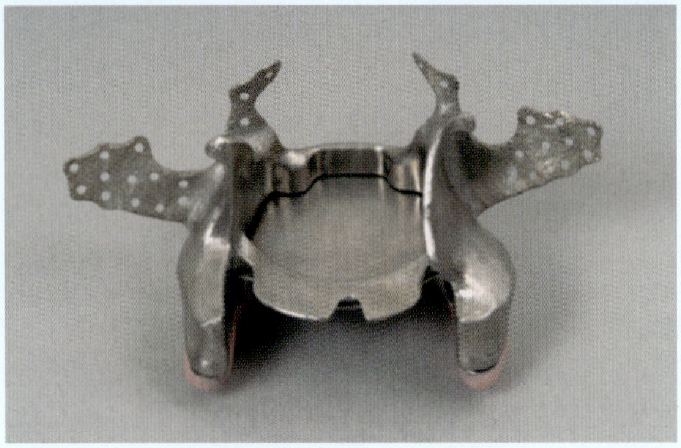

FIGURE 7-93. Assembled implant (posterior aspect).

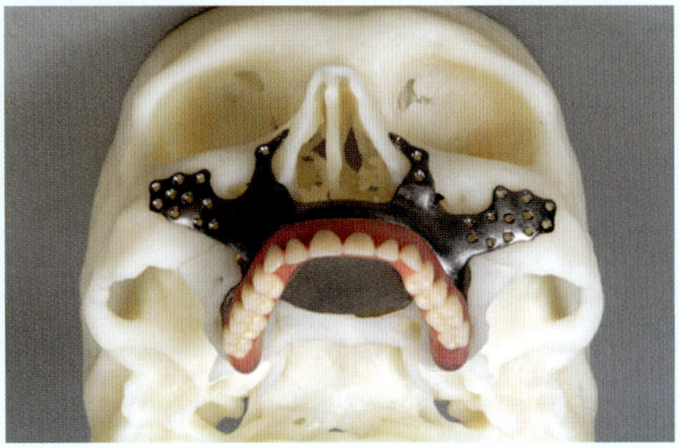

FIGURE 7-94. Biomodel planning is crucial in:
- Implant design and prototype manufacture;
- Determination of the path of insertion, which must be compatible with the surgical approach;
- Presurgical manufacture of the definitive dental prosthesis, which is possible with this approach;
- The design and manufacture of the implant system, which is the responsibility of the supervising clinician and not the engineer;
- A close working relationship, which is essential between clinicians and the engineering team.

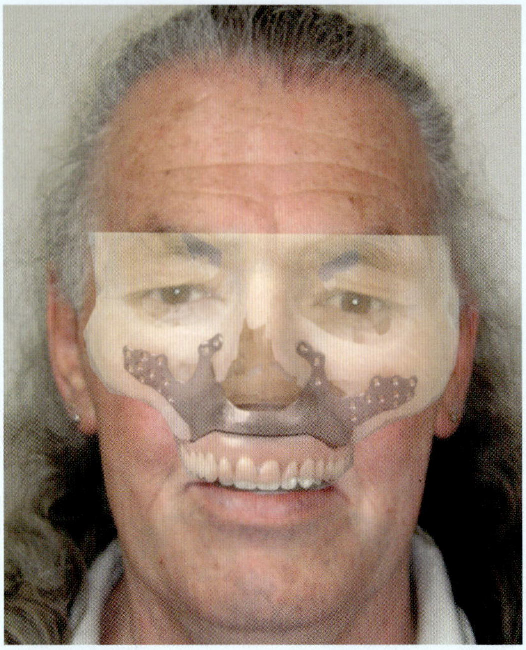

FIGURE 7-95. A computer prediction is used to check the anatomical relationships between the hard and soft tissues and the customized implant. (Courtesy ComputerGen Implants Ltd, New Zealand.)

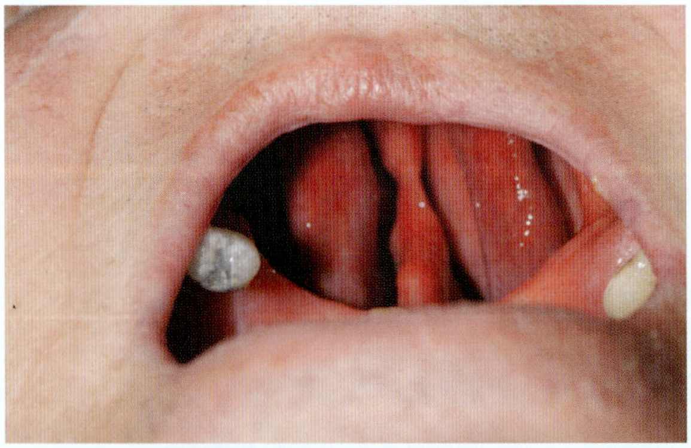

FIGURE 7-96. Intraoral defect.

No soft tissue coverage of the implant was employed with this technique (Figures 7-96 to 7-98).

OUTCOME

The clinical outcome was remarkable, with restoration of normal aesthetics, phonation, swallowing, and absolute stability of the prosthesis. The MDI O rings produced such excellent overdenture retention to the implant that a screwdriver device was later manufactured to remove the overdenture from the mouth.

CASE DISCUSSION 5 Customized Hybrid Implant Systems—cont'd

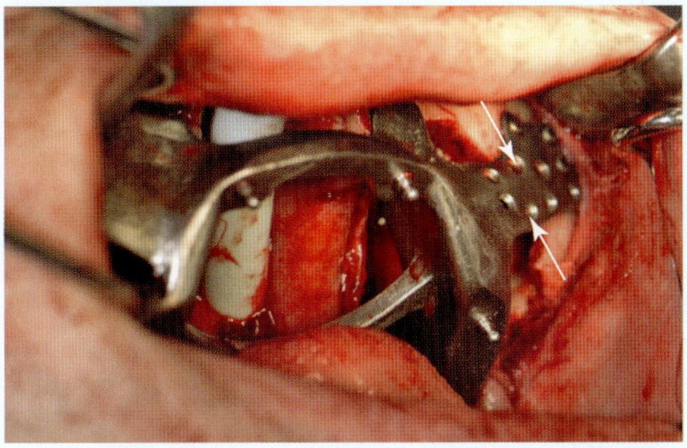

FIGURE 7-97. After the extraction of the remaining maxillary dentition, sockets are prepared with a denture finishing bur. A buccal flap is raised using a horizontal incision in the buccal segments as far posteriorly as the first molar tooth. This permits access to the zygomas without entering the temporal extension of the buccal fat pad. The mucosal tissue around the titanium pyriform fossa is deepithelialized. In this case, the implant is designed to fit inside the alveolar remnant. Screw fixation is with 2.0-mm maxillofacial titanium screws in the zygomatic flanges and 1.5-mm screws in the nasal flanges. Two screw holes towards the neck of the skeletal fixation flange are left without screws. This permits soft tissue attachment to the bone of the zygoma and assists in the formation of a soft tissue cuff, which isolates the potential tissue space around the flange from the oral cavity. Other variations to enhance soft tissue adherence to the screw flanges include:

- Placement of bone grafts;
- The use of bone morphogenetic protein delivery systems.*

(*Bone morphogenetic protein is angiogenic and until safety is established its use is contraindicated at the time of benign and malignant tumor resection because it may theoretically influence the development of local recurrence from microscopic tumor remnants.)

The patient was discharged at **20 hours** with minimum swelling. This is the first reported case of midface reconstruction (including the dentition) being performed as a same-day outpatient procedure (Figures 7-99 to 7-103).

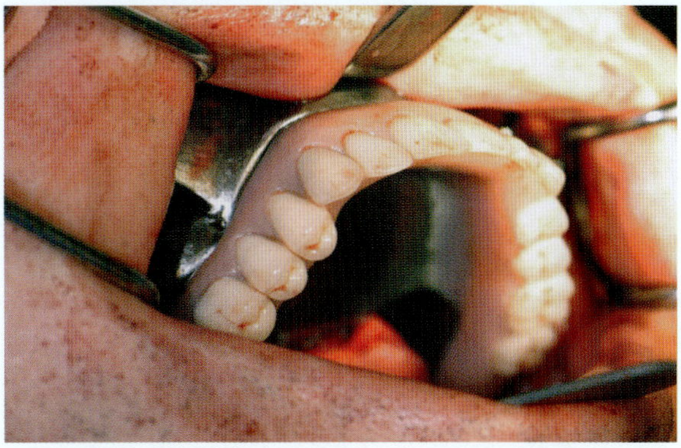

FIGURE 7-98. Perioperative assembly.

The patient was placed on a course of oral amoxicillin clavulanate (Augmentin) and nonsteroidal antiinflammatory analgesics and tutored in issues related to oral hygiene and the use of dilute chlorhexidine mouthwashes and oral hygiene sponges. Pain was experienced in the region of the anterior border of the soft palate. Otherwise he made an uneventful recovery.

The overdenture was removed from the mouth at 3 weeks after the operation when tenderness was subsiding using a cement spatula as a lever between the implant and the overdenture. This was cleaned free of old debris and blood clot, and the oronasal cavity was gently irrigated with diluted chlorhexidine. This produced significant tenderness in the region of the soft palate on the left side where bony interferences had been removed. We adopted a regimen of using benzydamine spray before oral hygiene measures, which helped significantly.

In the next month, the anterior border of the soft palate was seen to retract away from the post dam bar of the implant in relation to the left side of the soft palate where bony interfaces had been trimmed to create the path of insertion. As the tissue retracted, mild nasal escape developed on phonation. This matter was addressed with a simple rebasing of the obturator with cold cure acrylic resin.

CASE DISCUSSION 5 Customized Hybrid Implant Systems—cont'd

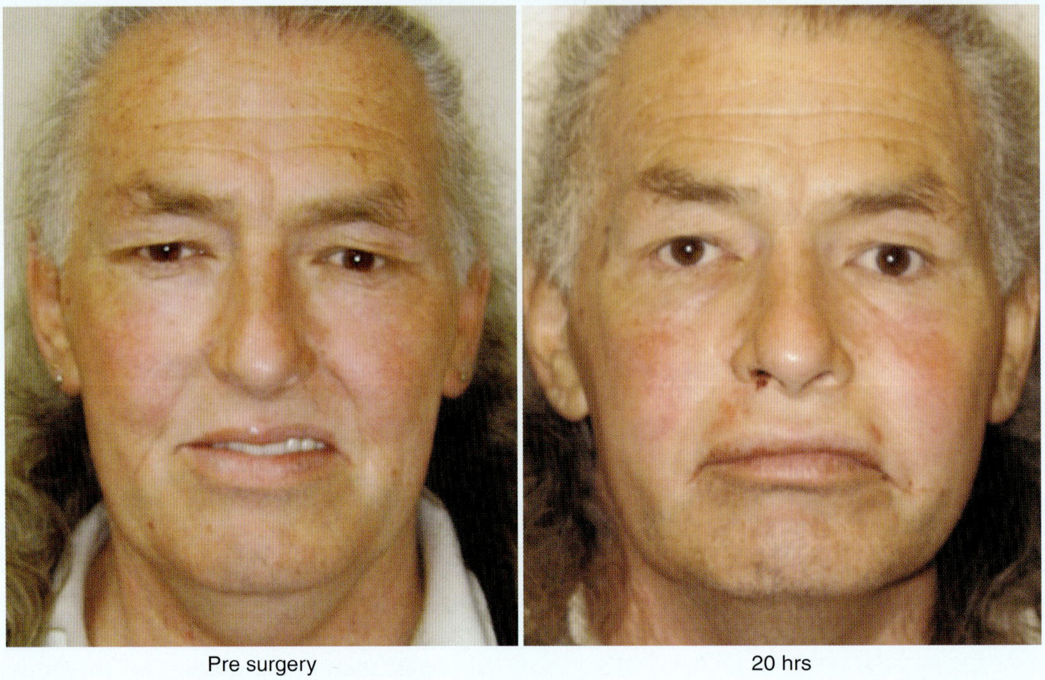

FIGURE 7-99. Outcome at 20 hours. The anterior facial height is normal. A criticism is that there is a deficiency of exposure of the upper incisor teeth in repose. This was later corrected with a denture modification.

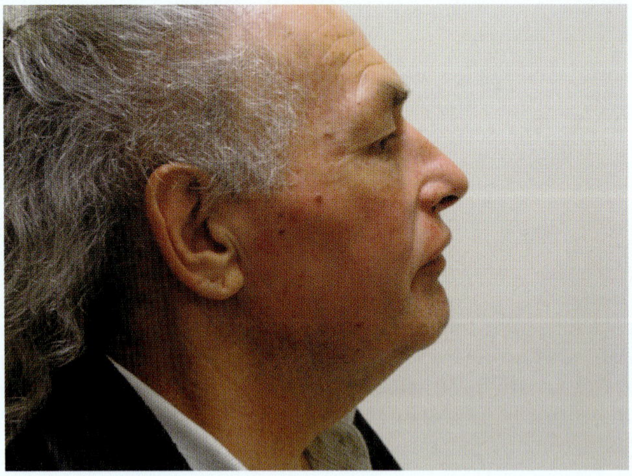

FIGURE 7-100. Outcome at 20 hours. The anterior facial height is normal. Good lip support.

CASE DISCUSSION 5 Customized Hybrid Implant Systems—cont'd

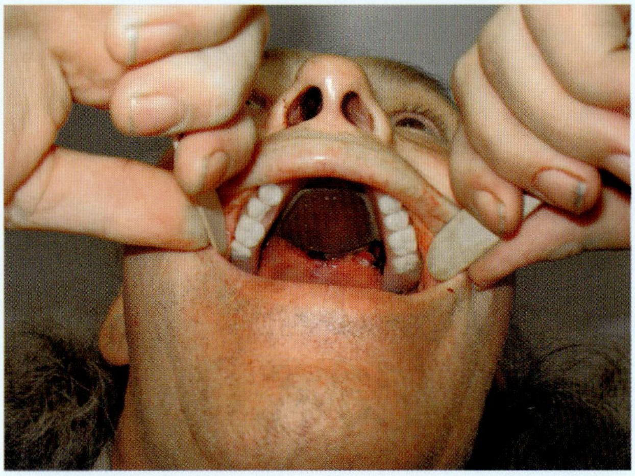

FIGURE 7-101. The implant was designed so that the titanium post dam flange would be enveloped by soft tissue on the oral and nasal aspects, and a horizontal incision was made along the anterior aspect of the soft palate remnant to accommodate the titanium post dam. The soft tissue is seen to retract from this area as a consequence, and it is suggested that the post dam should be placed on the nasal side of the soft palate and extended for 1 to 1.5 cm to prevent this problem. In this case, removal of a bony undercut in the medial wall of the left posterior maxillary sinus was required to seat the implant. This was anticipated at the time of implant design. An oronasal fistula resulted, producing mild nasal escape on phonation. This was later obturated by incorporating a resin extension of the denture base on to the palatal aspect.

The patient was discharged at 20 hours on amoxicillin clavulanate (Augmentin) and ibuprofen analgesia. Normal oral feeding was instigated and the patient instructed in oral hygiene. The denture was not removed for 3 weeks for inspection and oral debridement. Denture retention was excellent; a device was constructed to assist in its removal.

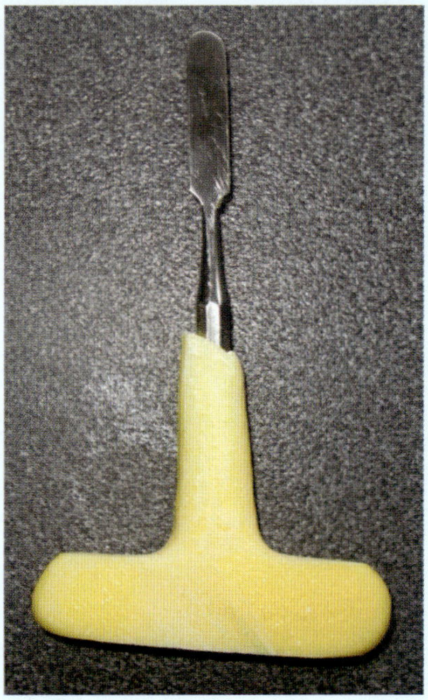

FIGURE 7-102. The instrument has been adapted from a cement spatula and is used to remove the upper overdenture.

CASE DISCUSSION 5 Customized Hybrid Implant Systems—cont'd

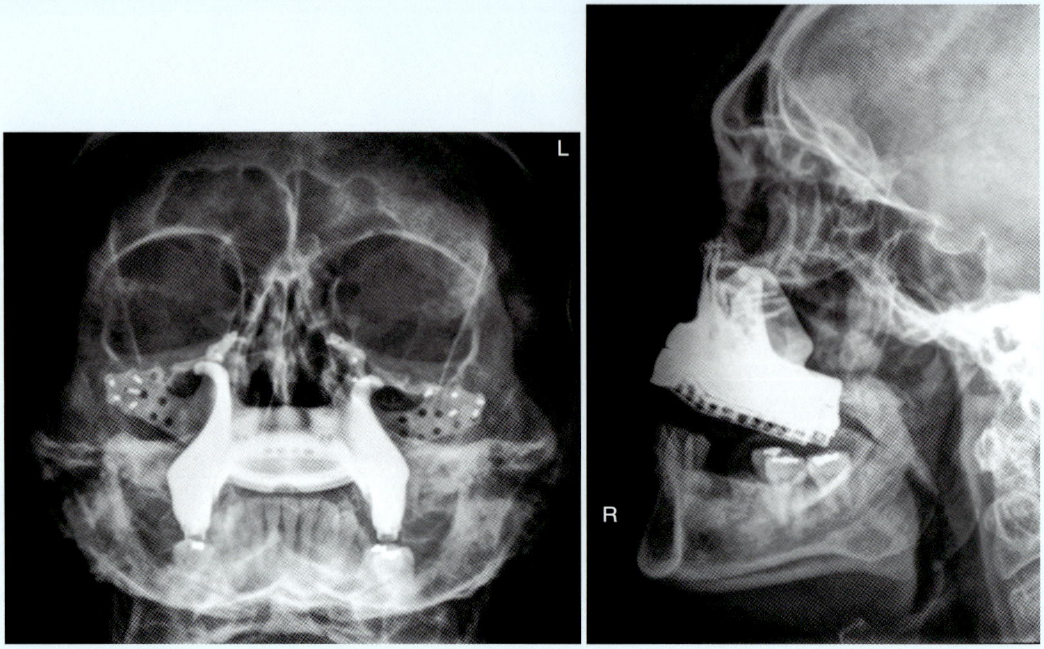

FIGURE 7-103. Despite detailed consideration of the positioning of the occlusal plane, its placement is incorrect, and extensive occlusal grinding was required at the time of overdenture placement. The use of a mandibular biomodel as a functional articulator is crucial to prevent this potential problem.

RECONSTRUCTION OF THE MANDIBULAR DENTITION

The options for reconstruction of two bounded saddles in the mandibular dentition included:

1. Partial denture;
2. Dental bridge;
3. Endosseous dental implants and dental crowns;
4. MDIs and dental crowns;
5. MDIs and overdenture with connecting lingual plate or lingual bar;
6. MDIs with two small removal bridges and MiniDentures (Peckitt)[15] (Figures 7-104 to 7-107).

CASE DISCUSSION 5 Customized Hybrid Implant Systems—cont'd

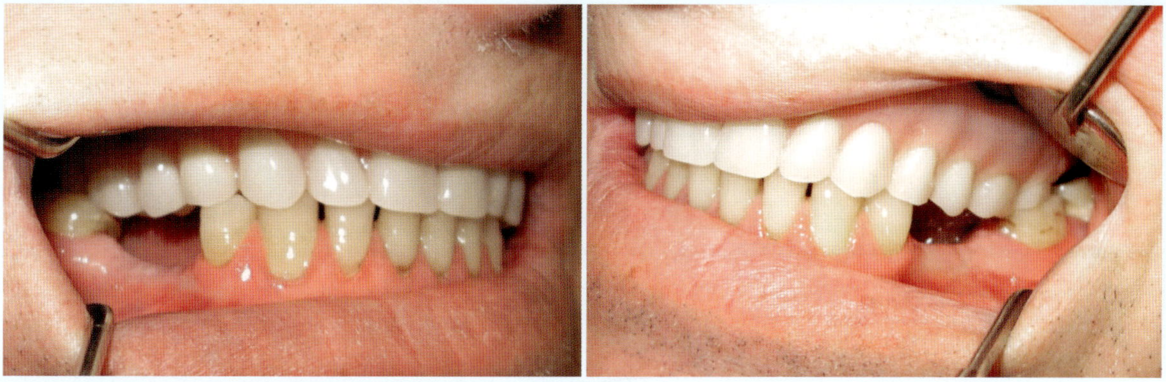

FIGURE 7-104. Oral rehabilitation with MDI system.
In this case, the MDI options included:
- Lower overdenture with lingual bar or lingual plate;
- Two removable bridges (MiniDentures);*
- MDI-retained fixed crown and bridge work.

(*Option chosen for reasons of cost, comfort, absence of lingual bar, minimal soft tissue coverage).

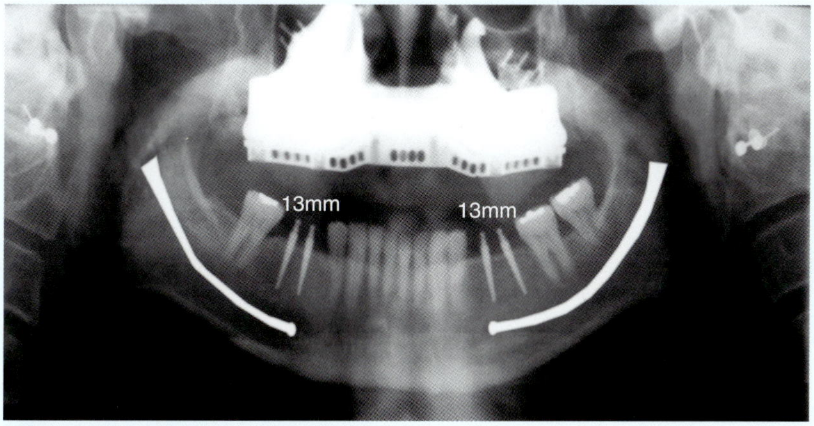

FIGURE 7-105. Four 13-mm MDI Max have been placed in the body of the mandible for the replacement of 19, 20, 29 and 30 with panoramic planning and nerve identification.

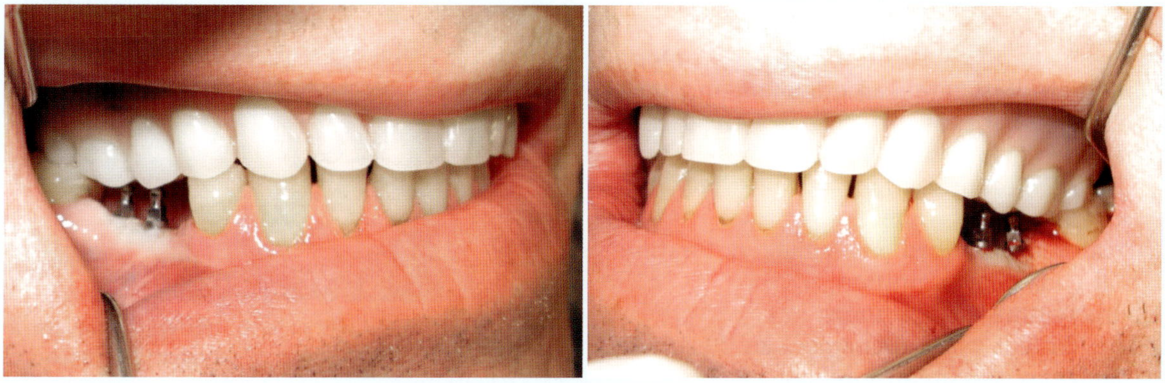

FIGURE 7-106. MDI placement (surgery).

CASE DISCUSSION 5 Customized Hybrid Implant Systems—cont'd

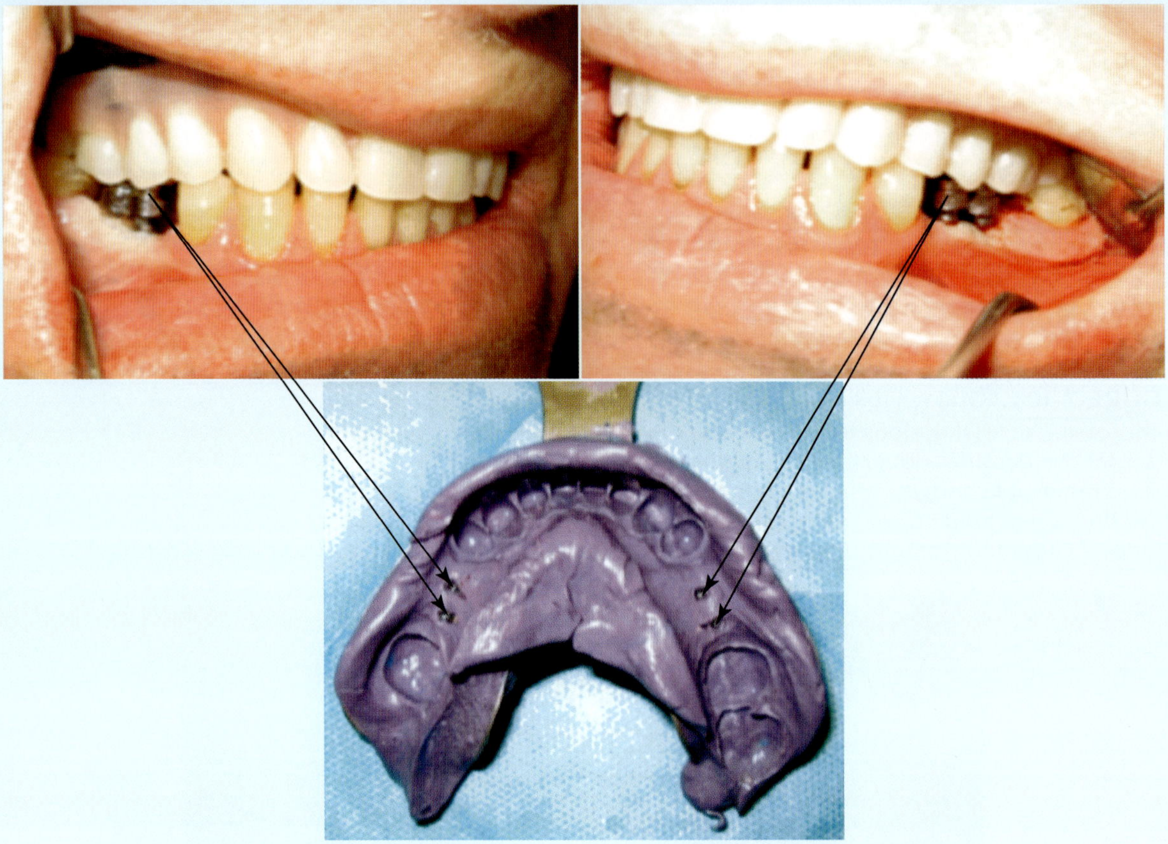

FIGURE 7-107. Housings are placed and a rubber base impression is taken without shims.

Four 13-mm Sendax MDI Max were placed as a secondary procedure at the patient's request in areas 19, 20, 29 and 30 (see Figures 7-105 to 7-108) The reconstruction was stable at 6 months (Figures 7-108 to 7-115).

DISCUSSION

The combination of EAS and MDI technology produced an outstanding and dramatic outcome for this patient at approximately 50% the cost of advanced free flap transfer. It is to be noted that:

1. Midface Reconstruction was possible as a single stage procedure;
2. Treatment included immediate restoration of the maxillary dentition;
3. Surgery time was 1.5 hours;
4. The patient was discharged at 20 hours (dame-day outpatient surgery);

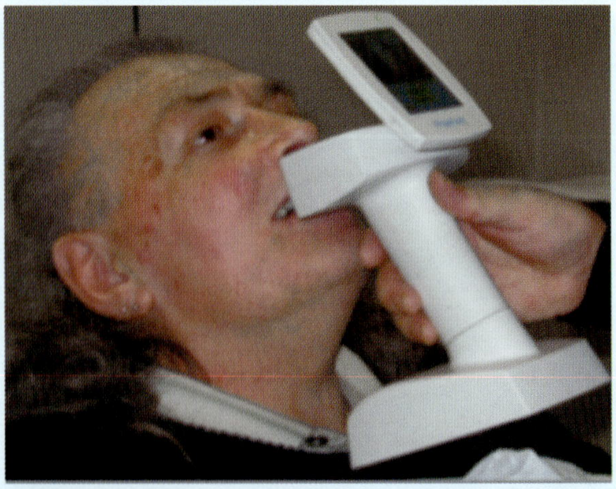

FIGURE 7-108. DeguDent Shadepilot was used to take the shade guide for the MiniDenture. (Courtesy Liz Woodward, Densply Ltd, New Zealand.)

CASE DISCUSSION 5 Customized Hybrid Implant Systems—cont'd

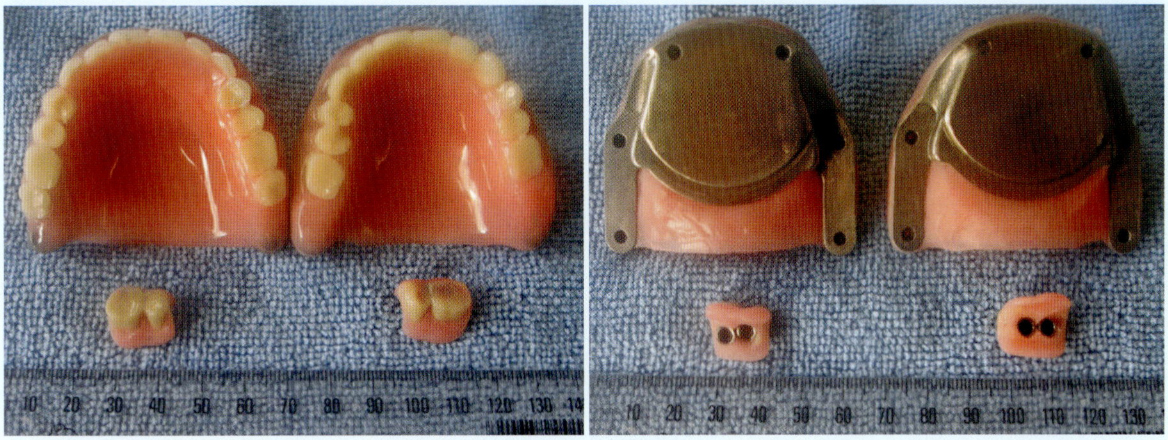

FIGURE 7-109. A spare upper overdenture has been constructed with a pair of MiniDentures. (Courtesy Lesley Williams, Broadway Dental Laboratory, Palmerston North, Manawatu-Wanganui, New Zealand.)

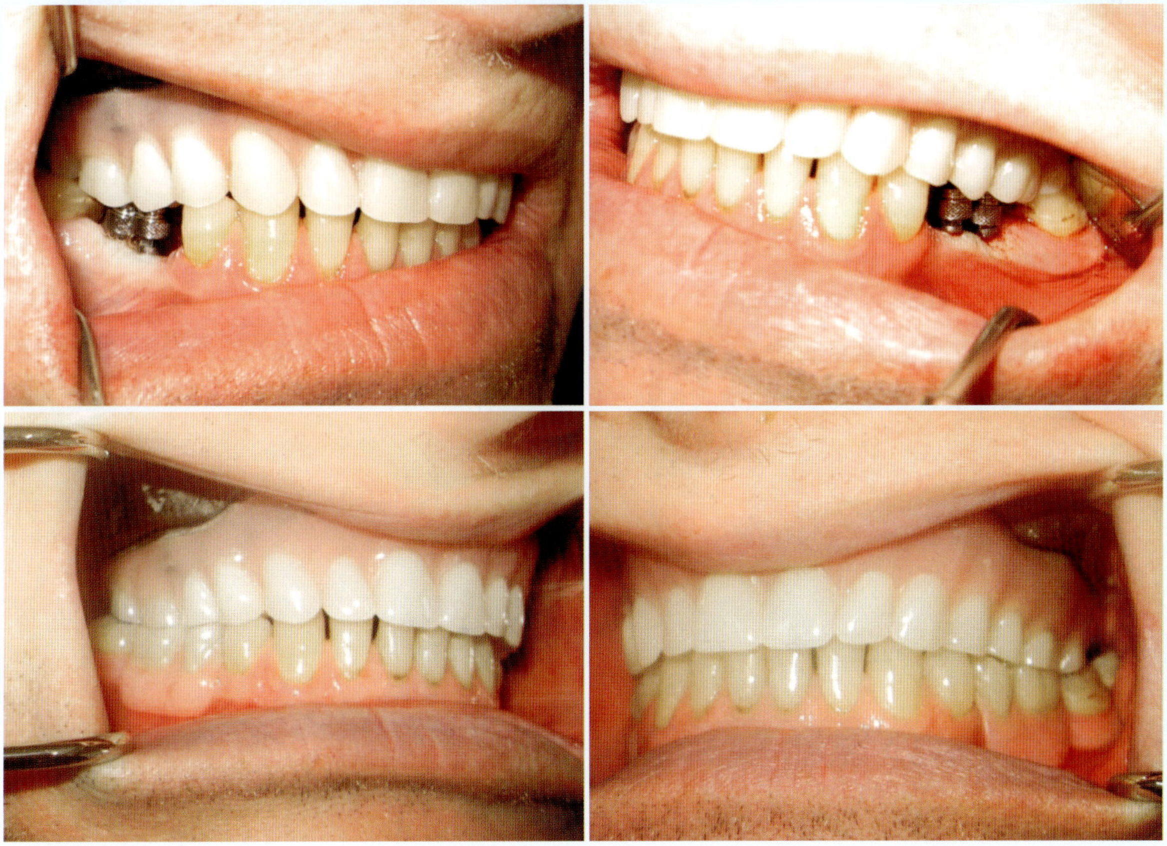

FIGURE 7-110. Accommodation of the MiniDentures required adjustment of the upper occlusion.

CASE DISCUSSION 5 Customized Hybrid Implant Systems—cont'd

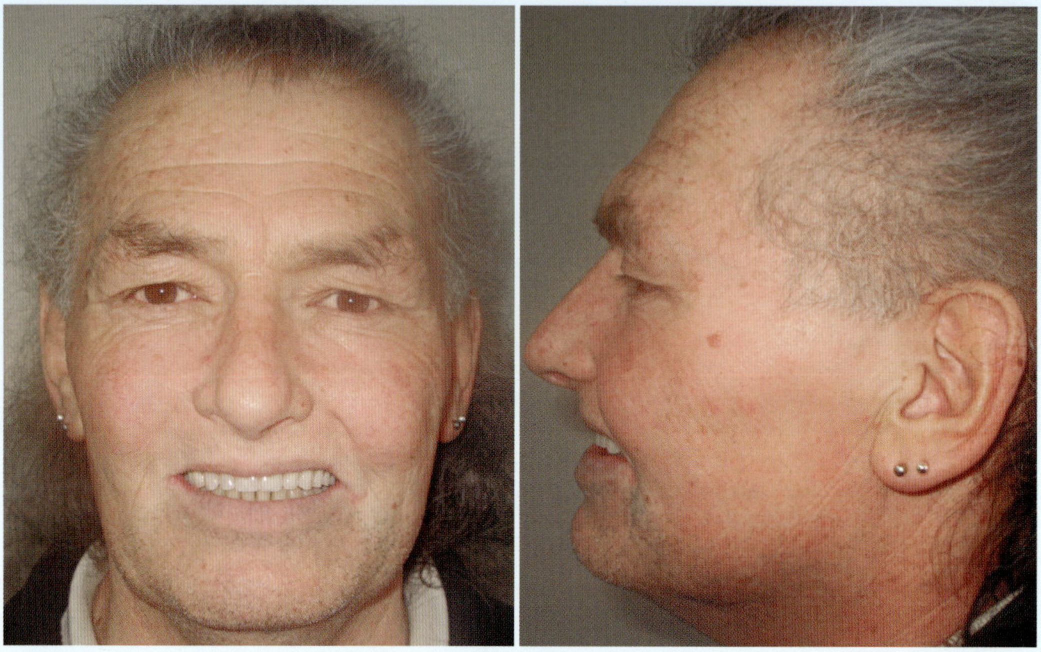

FIGURE 7-111. Normal anatomy has been precisely replicated without major surgery and without any facial scarring by using an adaptation of the Sendax MDI overdenture O-ring system in the maxilla and the Sendax MDI system in the mandible. This treatment has produced a life changing outcome for this patient with restitution of a normal quality of life.

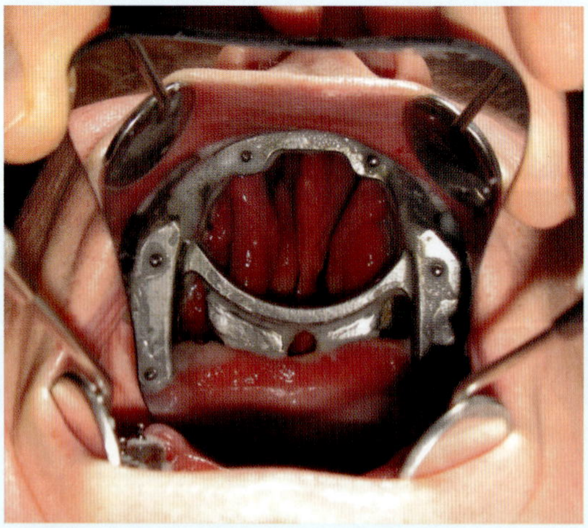

FIGURE 7-112. The nasal escape in the region of the post dam has been eliminated with a resin obturator extension on the palate.

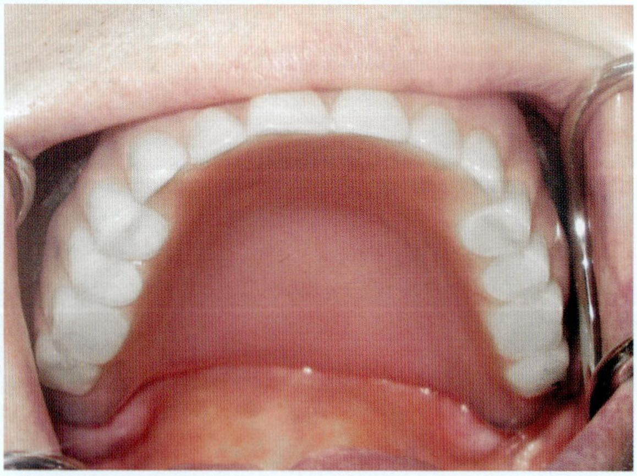

FIGURE 7-113. The nasal escape in the region of the post dam has been eliminated with a resin obturator extension on the palate.

CASE DISCUSSION 5 Customized Hybrid Implant Systems—cont'd

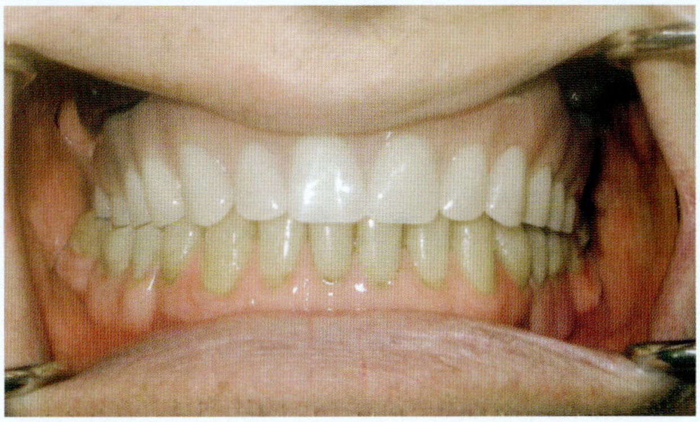

FIGURE 7-114. A good functional occlusion has been obtained with minimum surgical trauma at approximately 50% the cost of complex composite free flap surgery.

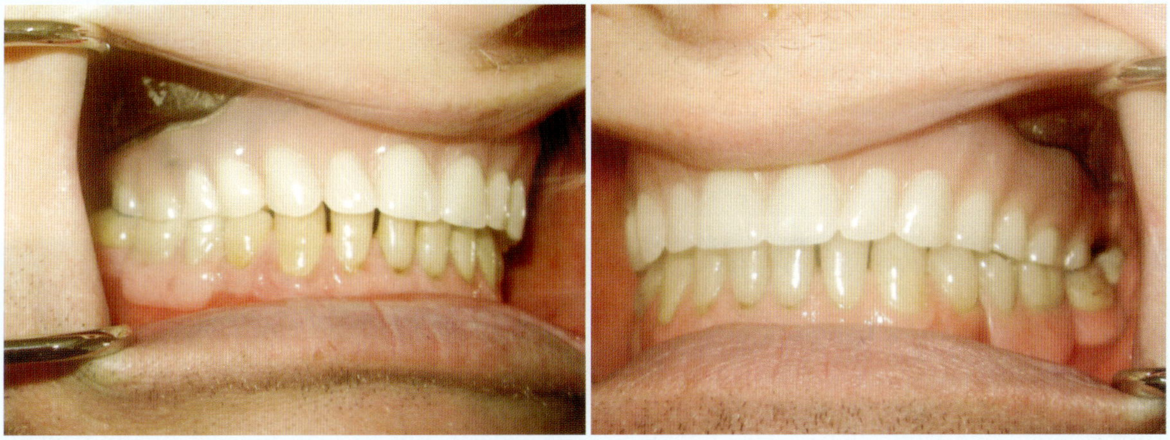

FIGURE 7-115. Note the improvement is shade estimation in the MDI-retained MiniDenture with DeguDent Shadepilot. This system is advocated to reduce the incidence of operator error and is a good example of EAS in practice.

5. Concomitant reconstruction of the mandible was delayed at the patient's request until the midface outcome was known;
6. Facial and dental esthetics were both excellent;
7. Retention of the overdenture was provided by six abutments and the MDI O-ring system; retention is excellent and overdenture removal required a special instrument;
8. Phonation speech and swallowing are normal;
9. This treatment modality restored the quality of life for this patient with minimal surgical trauma;
10. With current long-term stability demonstrated in the United Kingdom at 16 years, EAS is a consideration for the primary treatment option for these cases. Further research is required on larger numbers of patients to increase the evidence base for this innovative solution.

RADIOTHERAPY ISSUES

The potential modification of the radiation dose received at the bone-titanium (plate and screws) interface and bone-soft tissue interface has been investigated for the 2.4-mm reconstruction plate.[8]

CASE DISCUSSION 5 Customized Hybrid Implant Systems—cont'd

Using an adult head and neck (ex vivo model), a medical grade 6 hole plate (2.4 mm) was fixed in the midline of the mandible. The mandible was then irradiated using 6-MV photon beams. Thermoluminescent dosimeters were used to measure the radiation doses anterior and posterior to the mandible. The experiment was then repeated without the plate and screws.

The differences between the average doses to the mandible with plate and screws versus without plate and screws was +2.1% at the buccal aspect of the mandible and +3.0% at the lingual aspect; *P* values were 0.741 and 0.323, respectively. The results are not statistically significant.

The authors concluded that there was no significant influence on titanium alloy plate and screws on the radiation doses received by tissues anterior or posterior to the mandible. This evidence supports the contention that the concomitant placement of MDI at the time of mandibular resection is appropriate:

- Trismus is not usually an issue at the time of resection but may be an issue in the secondary placement of implants. Trismus after jaw resection is not uncommon and may complicate the placement of endosseous dental implants, especially MDIs, which by the virtue of their length can be difficult to place, especially in the posterior mandible and maxilla.
- Radiotherapy dose and shielding of radiation fields does not appear to be an issue with customized implants (1 mm thickness) nor with MDI components.
- The employment of customized titanium hybrid systems with removable sections facilitates direct inspection of the radiation field and the use of these systems with adjuvant radiotherapy.

CASE DISCUSSION 6 Panfacial Resection and Reconstruction

The combination approach of EAS planning, biomodel analysis, and biomodel surgery combined with the design and fabrication of MDI-retained prostheses greatly simplifies the case management of patients presenting with huge facial tumors.

A 42-year-old Fijian man attended with a huge rapidly growing tumor of the midface. Biopsy confirmed a diagnosis of fibrosarcoma. CT scans used in the staging of the tumor were reformatted into STL file format for biomodel manufacture. Light sensitive Stericol resin and color stereolithography permitted biomodel tumor mapping and biomodel surgery to show the feasibility of tumor resection (Figures 7-116 to 7-119).

TREATMENT PLAN

A fine-needle aspirate of the jugulodigastric node revealed no evidence of metastatic tumor. Although biomodel surgery confirmed the feasibility of tumor resection, a massive resection of the maxilla and mandible was required to deliver the tumor. Treatment was performed with Dr. Mark Izzard's head and neck surgical team in Auckland, New Zealand.

The treatment plan was essentially palliative rather than curative and designed to maintain a good aesthetic quality of life with minimum surgical trauma:

1. Hemimaxillectomy distal through the socket of 11 with resection of the right pterygoid plates at the base of skull with the right side of the soft palate; preservation of the orbit and the orbital floor;
2. Clearance of the infratemporal fossa with the option of a zygomatic arch osteotomy to facilitate superior access to the upper tumor margins;
3. Access to the tumor required a hemimandibulectomy with resection of the right condyle;
4. The external skin of the cheek and middle and lower branches of the facial nerve were to be sacrificed.

CASE DISCUSSION 6 Panfacial Resection and Reconstruction—cont'd

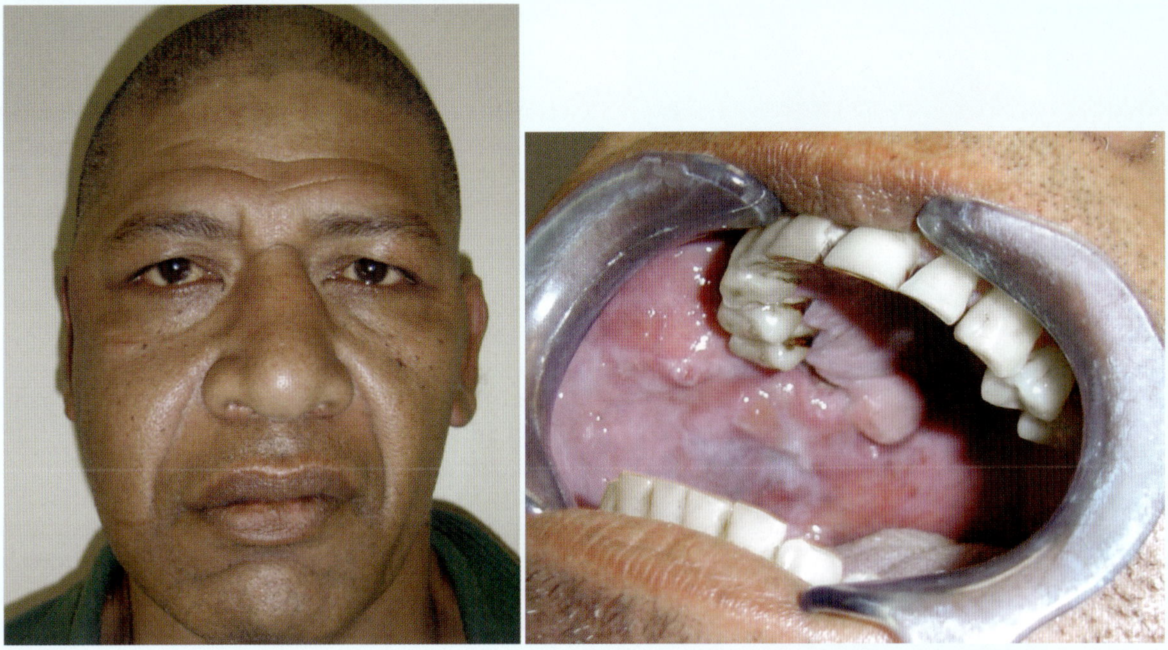

FIGURE 7-116. A huge sarcoma is invading the cheek, maxillary sinus, palate, infratemporal fossa, and abutting onto the base of skull.

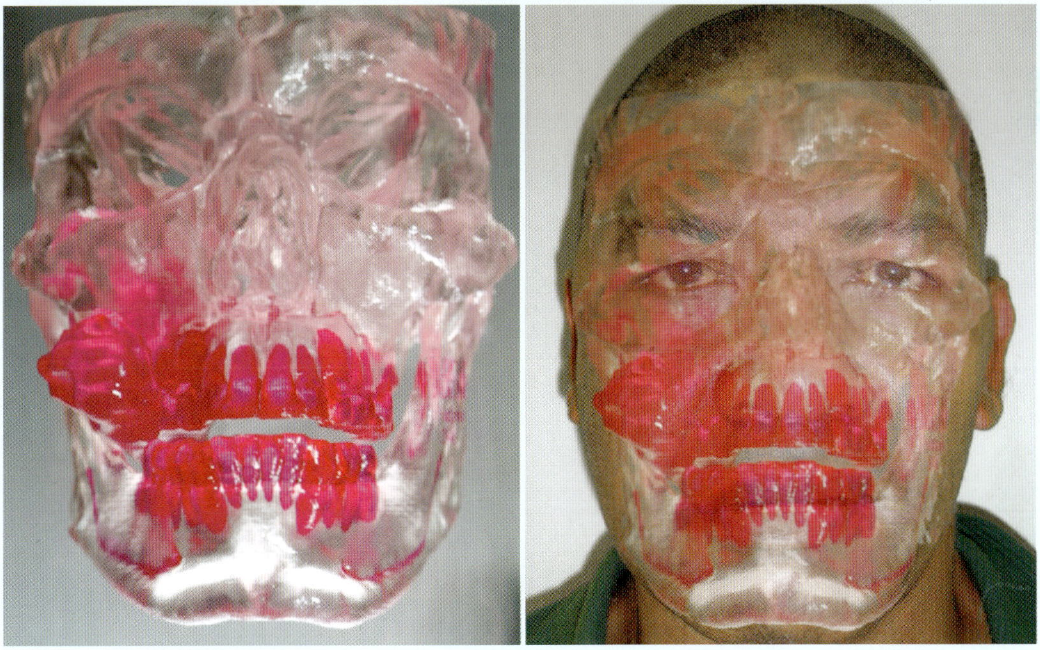

FIGURE 7-117. Tumor mapping is possible with colorable resins.

CASE DISCUSSION 6 Panfacial Resection and Reconstruction—cont'd

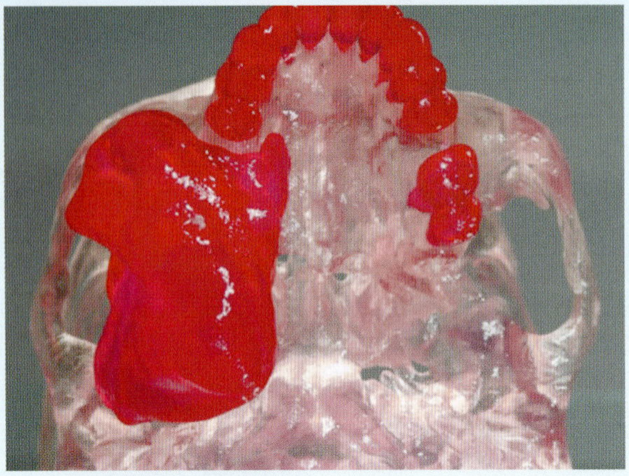

FIGURE 7-118. Submentovertex view of the cranial base before model surgery.

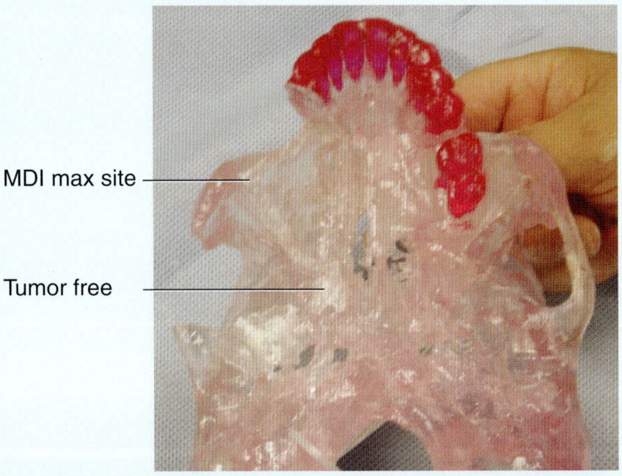

FIGURE 7-119. Model surgery permits a tumor resection plan.

PANFACIAL RECONSTRUCTION

The logistics of the reconstruction were formidable. Mandibular and temporomandibular joint reconstruction was to be achieved with a free fibula flap and reconstruction plate and concomitant placement of 13-mm MDIs Max in the fibula. The mandibular condyle would be reconstructed by cutting the reconstruction plate short of the glenoid fossa and fixing it in place with suspensory nylon sutures from the periosteum and soft tissues around the glenoid fossa.

Plans to reconstruct the cheek with a radial forearm flap were not possible because of radial artery anatomy, and the option of a lateral thigh flap was method finally chosen. Reconstruction of the right maxilla could have been undertaken with a free flap but this would have added to the surgical trauma and increased the likelihood of significant postoperative facial deformity. The real possibility of local recurrence invading the free flap reconstruction would also affect the quality of palliation.

The option of a maxillary obturator was problematic because available retention for such a tissue borne device was inadequate and bone was insufficient for conventional endosseous dental implant stabilization.

The solution was to design a maxillary obturator which would be MDI-retained, using a combination of the Sendax MDI system and a subperiosteal MDI option (ComputerGen Implants Ltd, Worldwide Patents Pending) (Figures 7-120 to 7-125).

Surgery was completed in 10 hours (Figures 7-126 to 7-145).

CASE DISCUSSION 6 Panfacial Resection and Reconstruction—cont'd

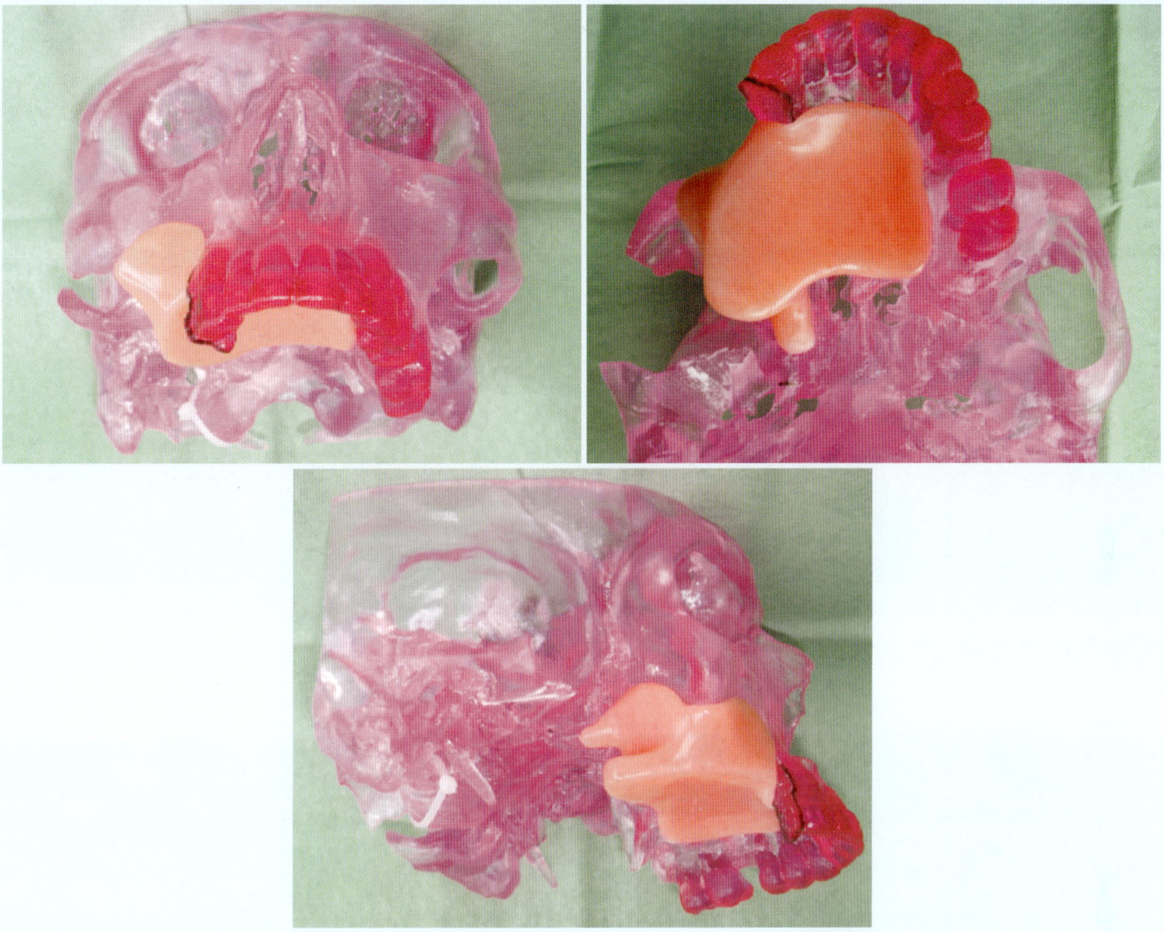

FIGURE 7-120. Reconstruction of the mandible will require a free fibula flap with concomitant placement of MDIs for overdenture attachment.

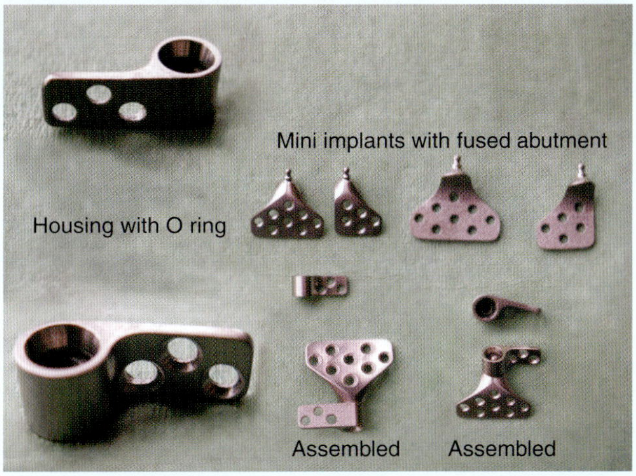

FIGURE 7-121. A subperiosteal implant system was designed for use in conjunction with Sendax MDIs for obturator fixation.

CASE DISCUSSION 6 Panfacial Resection and Reconstruction—cont'd

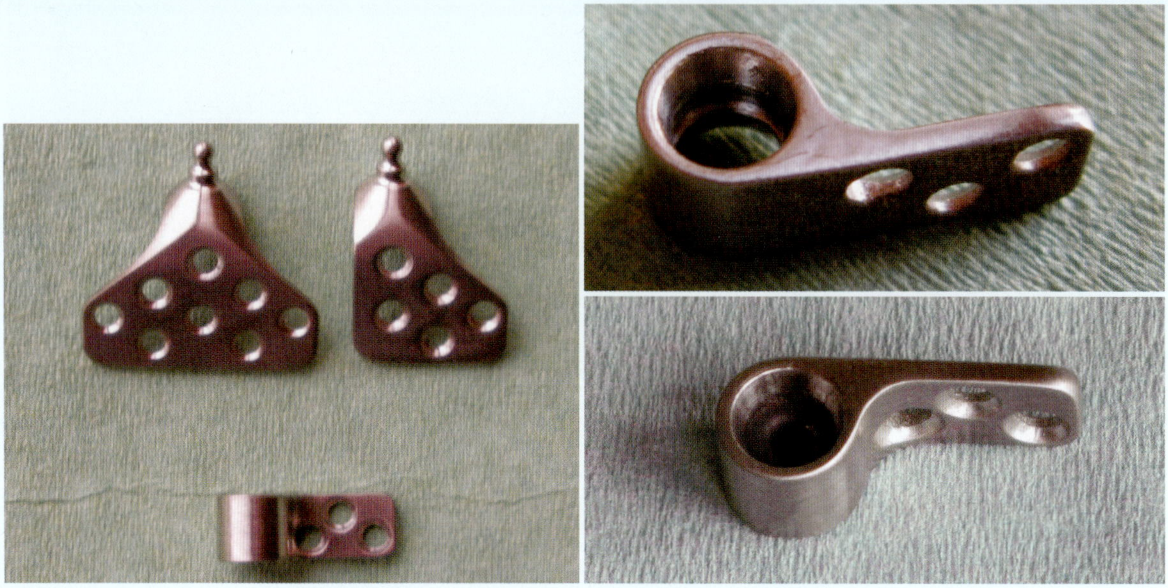

FIGURE 7-122. Note the bidirectional housing with and without the MDI O ring. This gives greater versatility to endosteal osteosynthesis. The housing is fixed to the facial skeleton with 1.5-mm or 2.0-mm screws.

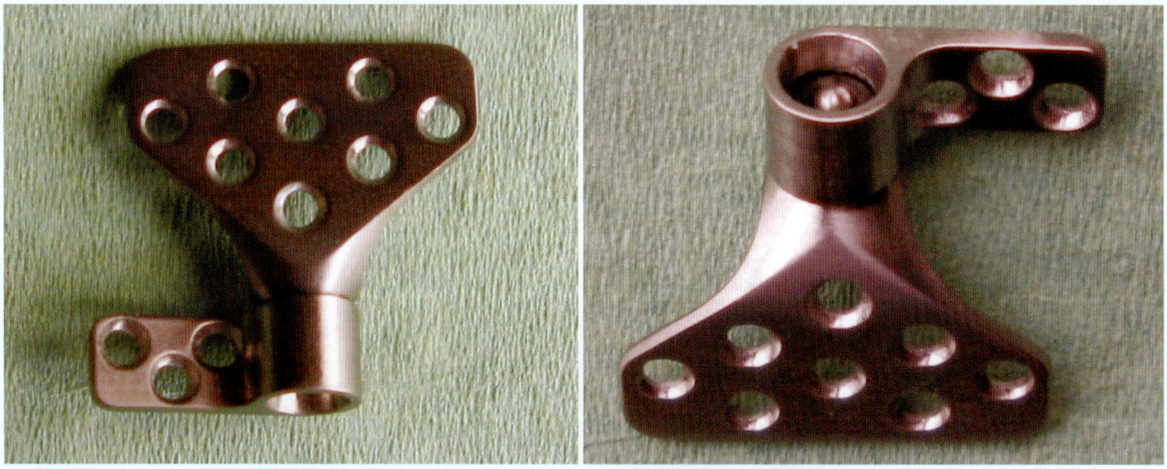

FIGURE 7-123. Assembled system, bidirectional abutments.

CASE DISCUSSION 6 Panfacial Resection and Reconstruction—cont'd

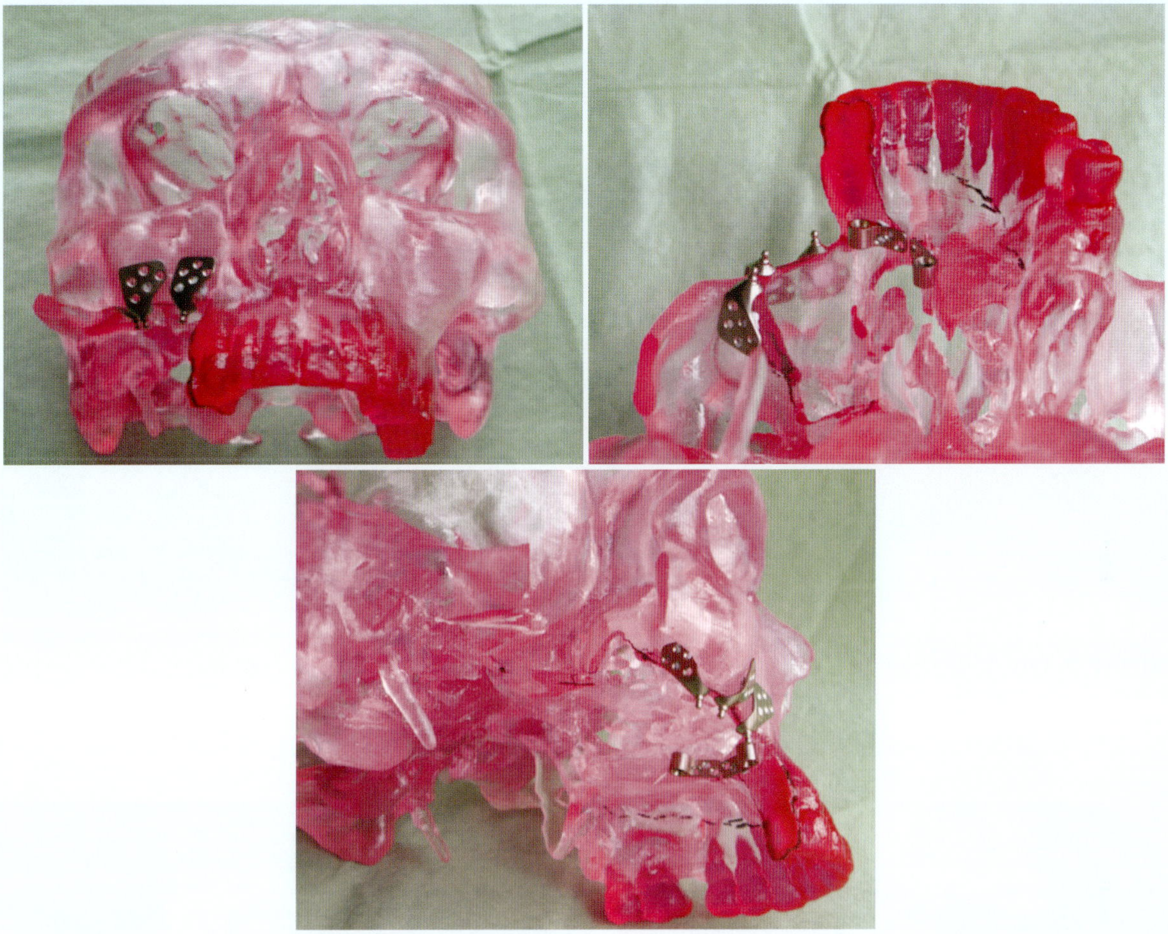

FIGURE 7-124. The system components of a SLA model. The bidirectional housings are fixed to the medial osteotomy cuts and medial aspect of the palatal shelf.

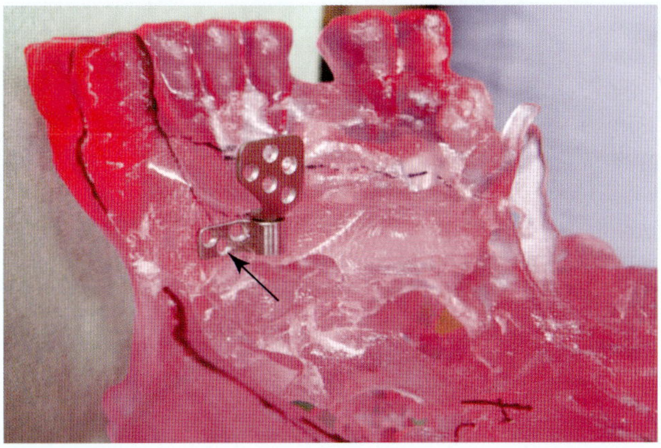

FIGURE 7-125. The assembled system of subperiosteal abutment and bidirectional housing, which in this case is fixed to the anterior osteotomy cut. The abutment is located in the denture base, and the system permits the use of a straight abutment.

CASE DISCUSSION 6 Panfacial Resection and Reconstruction—cont'd

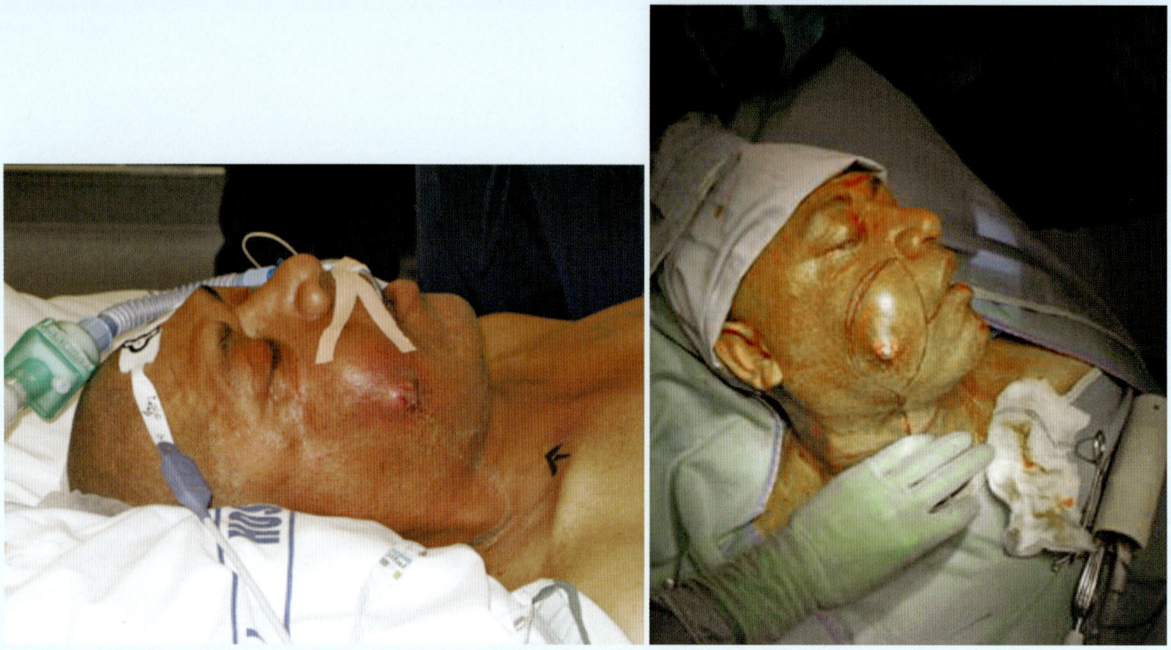

FIGURE 7-126. Right panfacial resection, maxillary obturator, free fibula flap—mandible, lateral thigh flap—cheek. (Courtesy Mark Izzard FRACS, ORL/Head and Neck/Facial Plastic Surgeon, Auckland, Australia.)

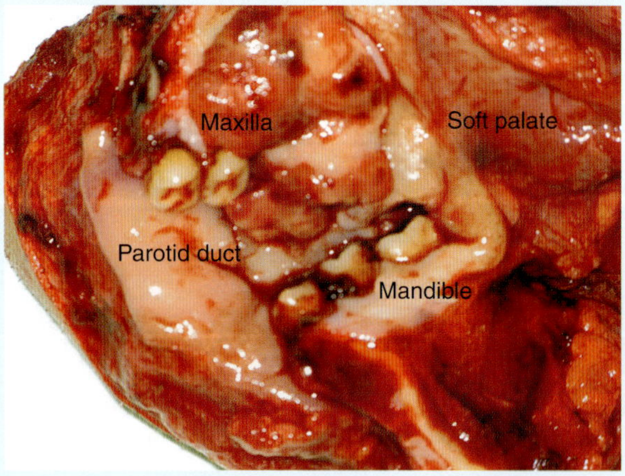

FIGURE 7-127. Functional neck dissection. 33 nodes all clear, invasion of the external jugular vein, clear margins.

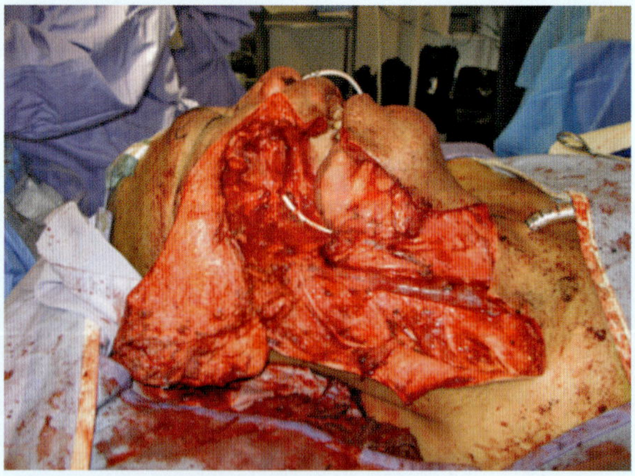

FIGURE 7-128. A hemimaxillectomy and hemimandibulectomy (including the condyle) has been completed. A functional neck dissection has been completed.

CASE DISCUSSION 6 Panfacial Resection and Reconstruction—cont'd

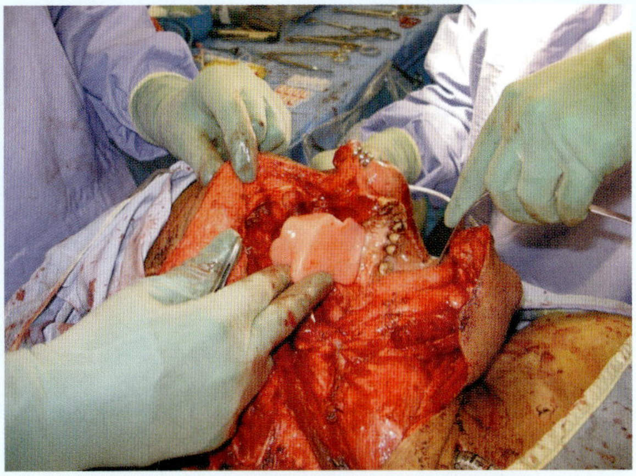

FIGURE 7-129. Try-in obturator.

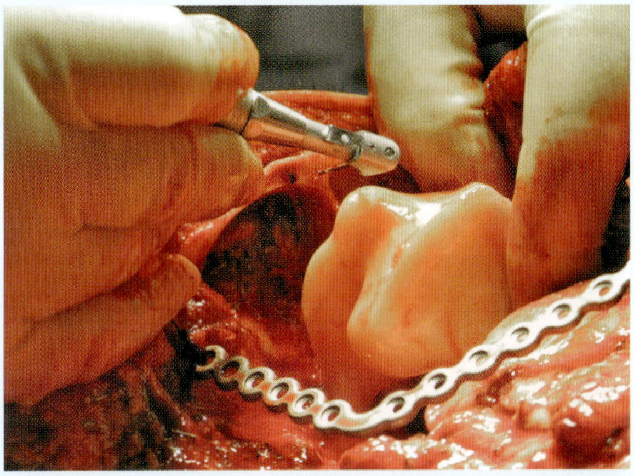

FIGURE 7-130. The maxilla in this case has good width for placement of a single 10-mm MDI Max in the anterior wall of the maxillary sinus at its junction with a bony septum. The pilot hole was drilled with a 1.1-mm drill to a depth of 10 mm to avoid implant fracture. Bone density Misch D1.

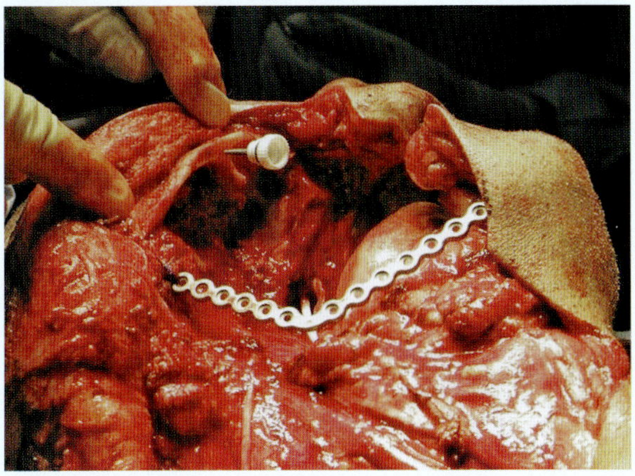

FIGURE 7-131. Placement of MDI Max (10 mm) with finger driver.

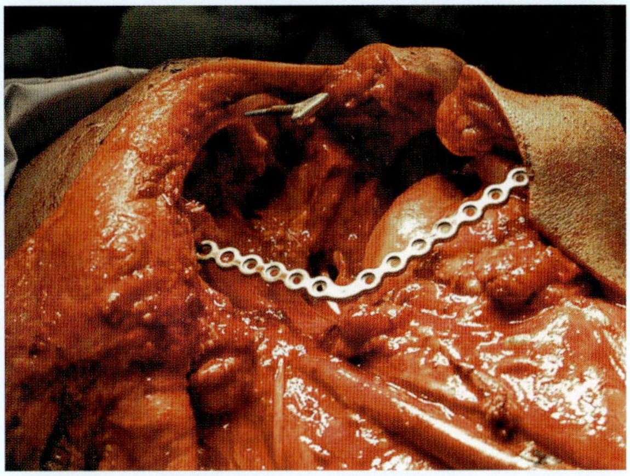

FIGURE 7-132. Bone density D1 prevented placement of the MDI down to the collar.

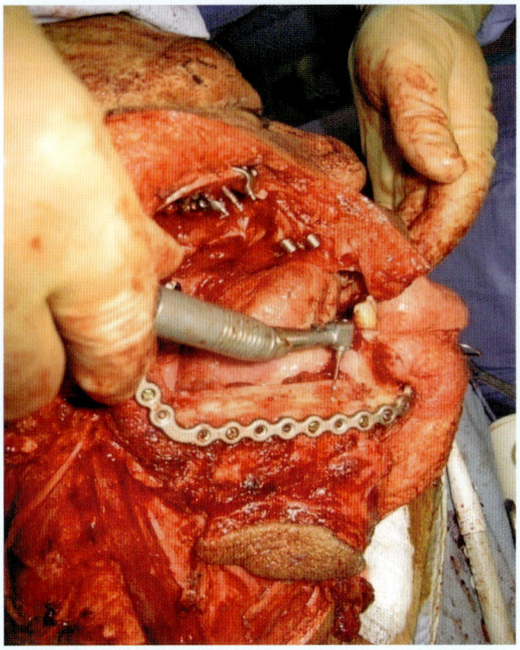

FIGURE 7-133. The problem of seating MDIs correctly with a 1.1-mm pilot drill was also found in the mandible. The fibula was also graded as D1 bone and a 1.8-mm drill was required to facilitate placement of the 10-mm MDI Max in the fibula.

CASE DISCUSSION 6 Panfacial Resection and Reconstruction—cont'd

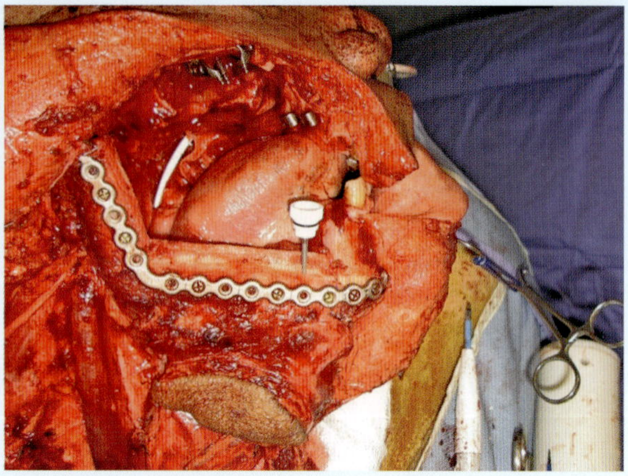

FIGURE 7-134. Initial placement of 13-mm MDI Max (free fibula flap) with finger driver.

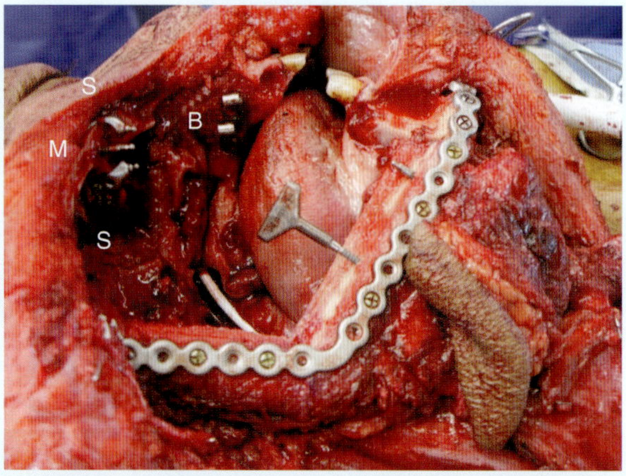

FIGURE 7-135. Two 13-mm MDI Max have been placed in a free fibula flap. The condyle has been resected and a 2.4-mm reconstruction plate has been cut short to produce an arthroplasty gap. With the teeth in occlusion, the reconstruction plate is secured to the periosteum and adjacent remnant of lateral pterygoid around the glenoid fossa with suspensory sutures to produce a functioning pseudo temporomandibular joint. A conventional MDI (*M*) is accompanied by two subperiosteal MDIs (*S*). Two bidirectional housings (*B*) are located on the anterior and medial osteotomy cuts near the pyriform fossa of the nasal aperture.

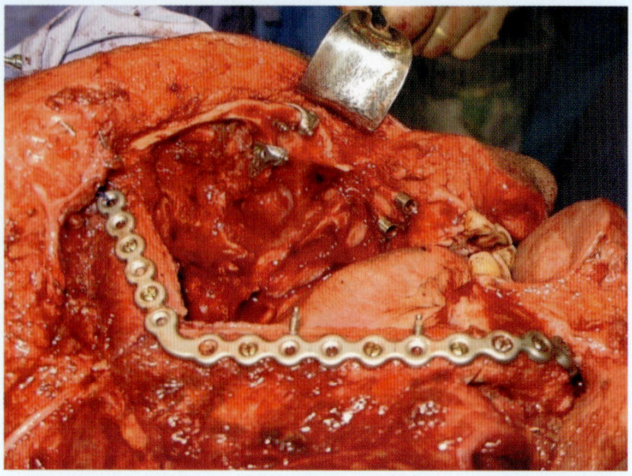

FIGURE 7-136. Mini endosteal and flanking subperiosteal implants are located in the anterior maxilla. Bidirectional housings are located on the medial maxillary osteotomy cut distal to 11. Note the parallel placement of the implants and housings. Two MDIs are located in the mandible. The suspensory suture for temporomandibular joint reconstruction is seen.

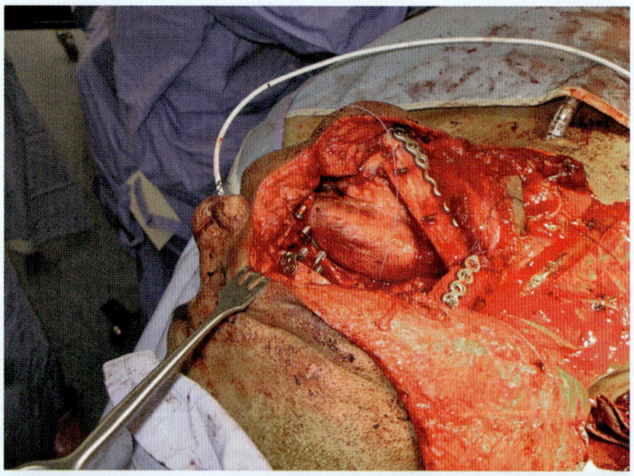

FIGURE 7-137. Shims have been placed. Note that the MDIs can only be placed in the dense bone of the fibula with a larger 1.8mm pilot hole.

CASE DISCUSSION 6 Panfacial Resection and Reconstruction—cont'd

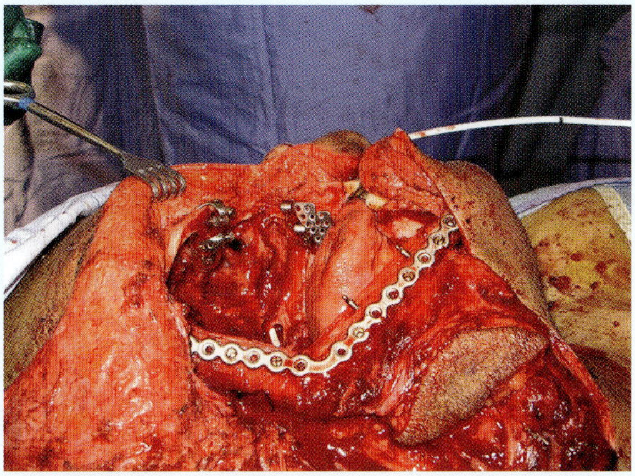

FIGURE 7-138. Placement of MDI housings over MDI and subperiosteal implants. Placement of subperiosteal implant abutments into bidirectional housings. MDI Max Implants could also have been used for location in the denture base.

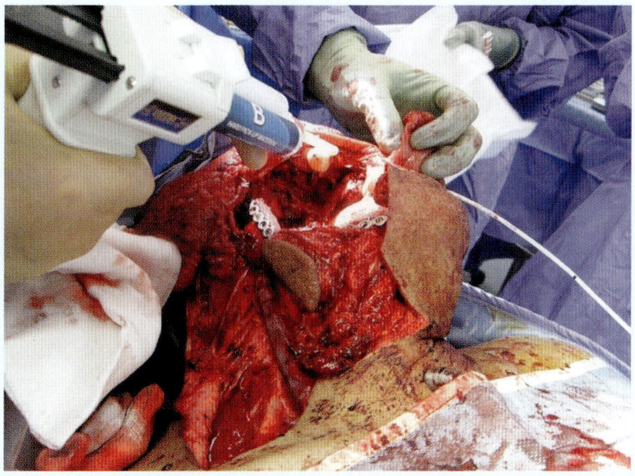

FIGURE 7-139. Undercuts have been blanked out with bone wax and a locating impression is taken with hard pickup resin.

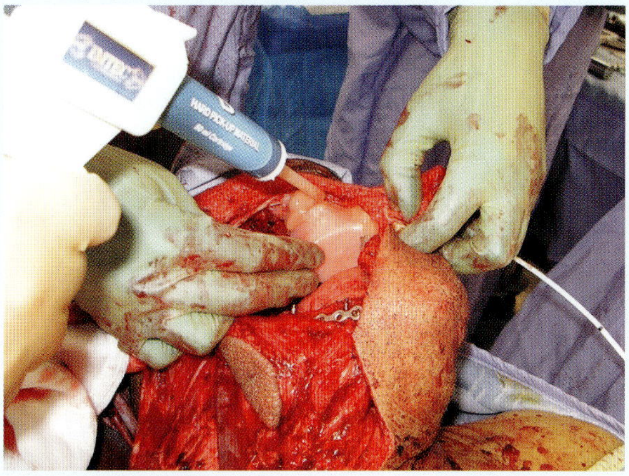

FIGURE 7-140. The obturator is rebased with hard pickup resin.

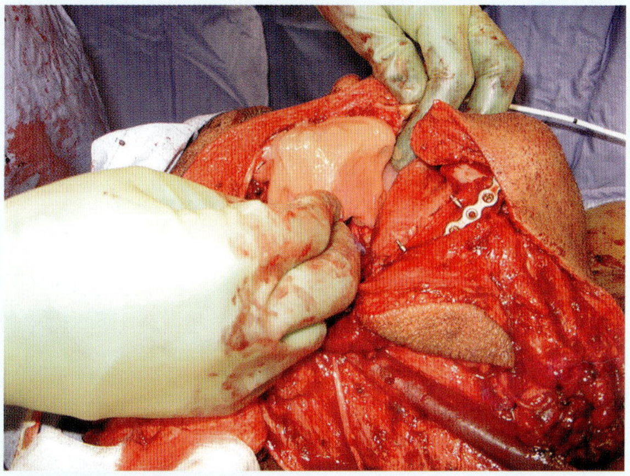

FIGURE 7-141. The resin is allowed to set and the obturator removed.

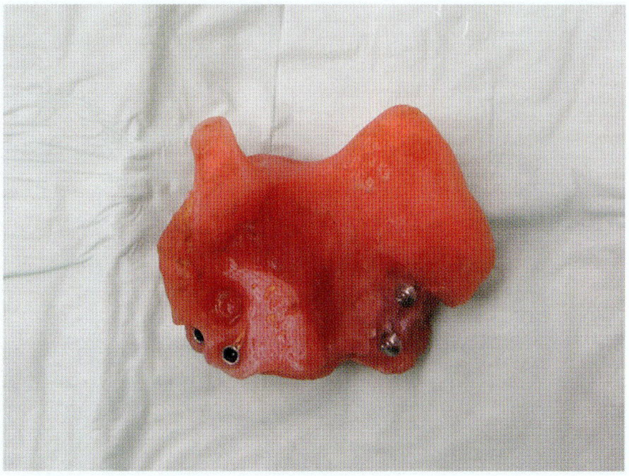

FIGURE 7-142. The housing related to the most posterior (subperiosteal implant) was removed to alleviate seating difficulties in the orbital rim.

CASE DISCUSSION 6 Panfacial Resection and Reconstruction—cont'd

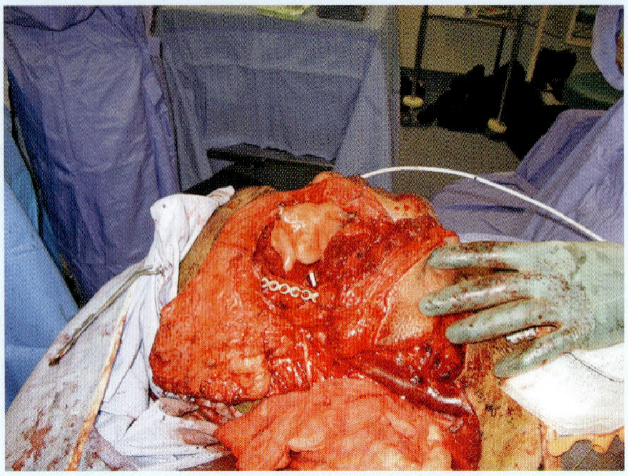

FIGURE 7-143. Excellent stability and retention was of the obturator was achieved with the MDI systems.

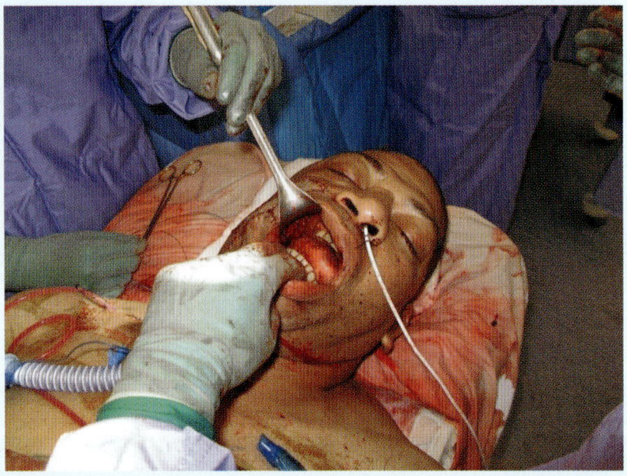

FIGURE 7-144. The lateral thigh flap has effectively reconstructed the buccal mucosa.

OUTCOME

The combination of EAS planning, biomodel mapping with color stereolithography, and model surgery confirmed the feasibility of the surgery in this difficult case. The surgery was greatly simplified, and this affected the cost of palliative treatment. The esthetic outcome was judged to be excellent (Figures 7-146 and 7-147).

DISCUSSION

The implants were designed to provide a solid base for the obturator on the affected side, which would prevent rocking, and to provide adequate retention for the obturator.

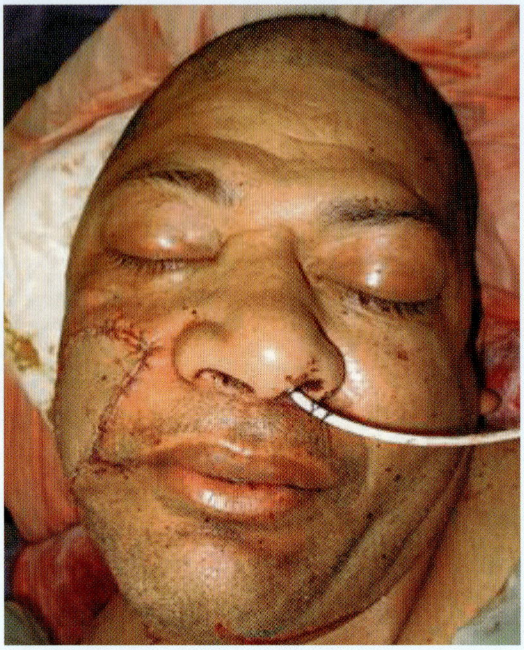

FIGURE 7-145. Good esthetic outcome. Almost normal cheek contour.

The main difficulty with this case was related to the location of the mini abutments in the orbital rim and the contracture of the reconstructed cheek around the osteotomy cut. This contracture made removal and replacement of the obturator difficult because soft tissue began to encroach on the abutments.

A potential solution to address for this problem is to cantilever linked obturator attachments from the MDIs more inferiorly into the maxillary sinus, away from the soft tissues. This implies the development of a family of possible screwless abutment systems, which would facilitate the restorative dentistry components of this system.

ADVANTAGES OF IMPLANT-RETAINED OBTURATORS

The advantages of a removable implant-retained obturator systems over free flap transfer in the maxilla are listed as follows:

1. Low cost;
2. Reduction in surgical trauma;
3. No donor site surgery required;
4. Reduction in the use of hospital resources;
5. Reliability of osseointegration;
6. Promotes optimum esthetics;
7. Facilitates simple oral rehabilitation solutions;

CASE DISCUSSION 6 Panfacial Resection and Reconstruction—cont'd

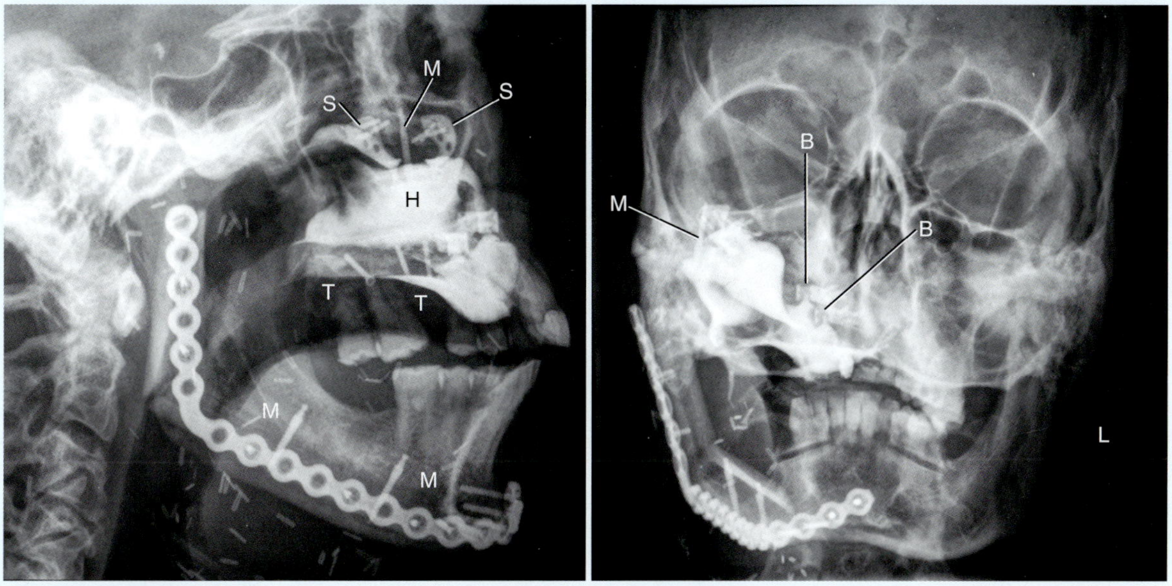

FIGURE 7-146. The MDI abutment is located in the housing located in the overdenture base. The abutments located in the overdenture base are located in the bidirectional housings (*B*).
M: MDI Max
S: Subperiosteal MDI
H: MDI housing
B: Bidirectional housing
T: Transpalatal screw

8. Facilitates inspection and biopsy of the cranial base;
9. Facilitates possible salvage procedures;
10. The obturator cannot be invaded by recurrent tumor;
11. Conversion to a semifixed or fixed customized cantilevered maxillary implant system is feasible after the patient has been declared tumor free; advanced (and more costly) reconstructive treatment can be reserved for patients who are more likely to survive the tumor;
12. Optimum possible palliation in conjunction with an EAS plan should be achievable for the tumor stage at presentation.

COMPLICATIONS OF IMPLANT-RETAINED OBTURATORS

Trismus may cause problems with insertion and removal of the obturator. This is particularly relevant with postoperative radiotherapy.

Implants may be lost after radiotherapy. Hyperbaric oxygen protocols may be indicated.

Soft tissue retraction or encroachment over abutments may be overcome with design modifications.

CASE DISCUSSION 6 Panfacial Resection and Reconstruction—cont'd

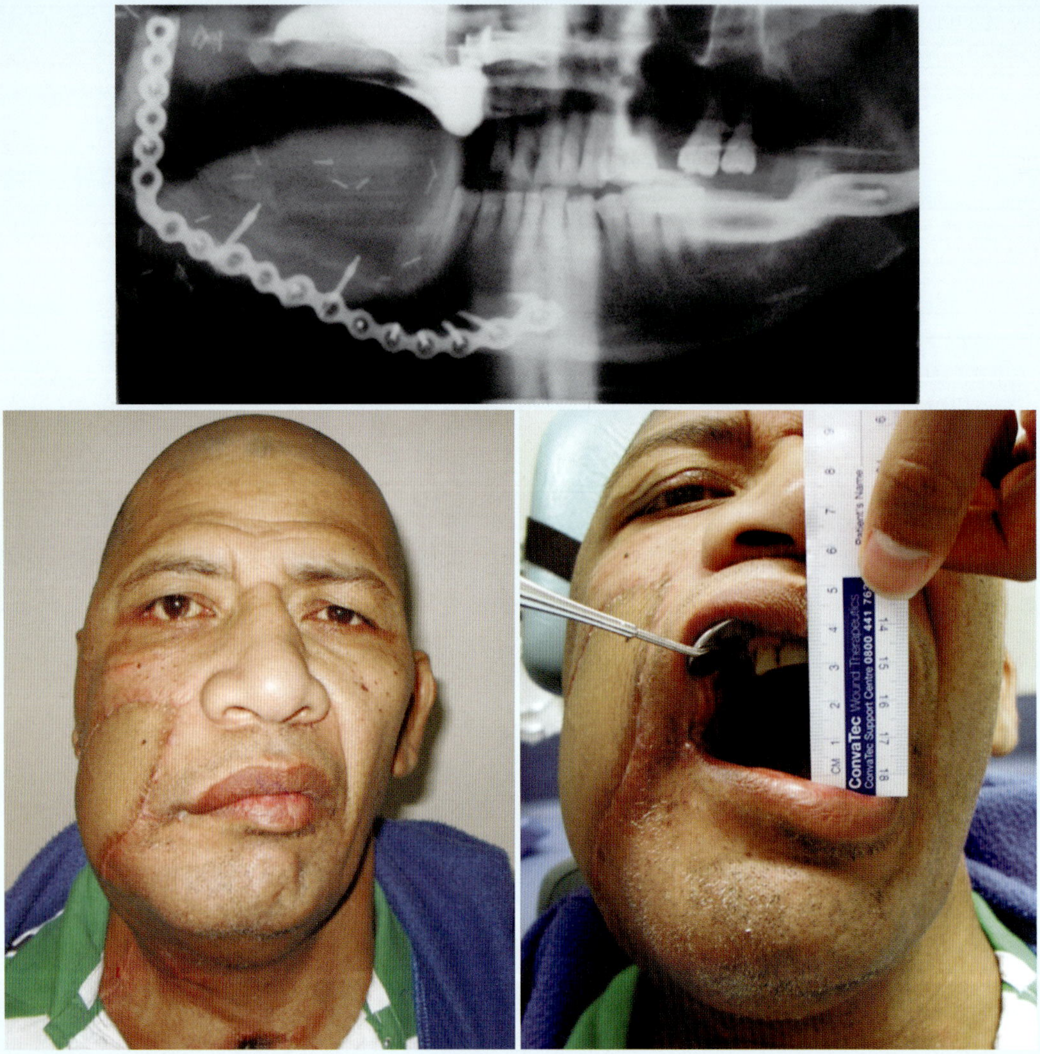

Opening 30mm

FIGURE 7-147. Note the good facial contour of cheek and mandibular angle. There is excellent chin positioning and excellent function of the temporomandibular joints. The obturator was removed on several occasions for further biopsy of the cranial base, especially in the region of the resected pterygoid plate. All biopsies were negative for tumor. At 1 month the obturator became loose and required replacement under general anesthesia. The tissue surrounding the osteotomized maxilla in the infraorbital area was undergoing contracture making it difficult to locate the housings onto the implants. The superior aspect of the lateral thigh flap was freed with a transcutaneous incision down onto the orbital rim and the obturator replaced. The retention was reinforced with two left-sided (2 mm) transpalatal screws.

The patient completed a course of radiotherapy and 3 months after treatment developed a large recurrence in the infratemporal fossa, which invaded the base of skull. No further surgery nor radiotherapy was possible. The perceived aggressiveness of this tumor and subsequent recurrence justifies the decision not to place an additional free flap into the maxillary defect, which would have become invaded by recurrent tumor.

Cost of MDI system $7,805 (New Zealand) $4,550 (United States)

Conclusion

The introduction of EAS and its association with MDI and in particular the Sendax MDI system has produced a paradigm shift in:

- Presurgical planning with enhanced accuracy;
- Reduced surgical trauma;
- Rehabilitation of complex maxillofacial cases;
- Enhanced outcome;
- Lower cost per intervention.

Acknowledgements

Engineering Team

Massey University Centre of Engineering Assisted Surgery

Gurvinder S. Virk, Prof. of Robotics, Wellington, New Zealand
Dr. Liqiong Tang, Palmerston North, New Zealand
ComputerGen Implants Ltd, New Zealand
A/Prof. Ninian Peckitt
Axia 3D Design Group Ltd, New Zealand
Andrew Kersley
Arcam AB Sweden
Magnus René, President
Camplex Ltd, New Zealand
Chris Whittington
Medical Modeling Inc, United States
Andy Christensen
Delcam Ltd, United Kingdom
Jason Hogan
IMTEC Inc, United States
John Davies European Representative
Broadway Dental Laboratory, New Zealand
Ashley Hughes
Lesley Williams
Dental Art Dental Laboratory, New Zealand
Barry Williams
Enztec Ltd,* New Zealand
Paul Morrison*

Clinicians

A/Prof. Ninian Peckitt, OMFS, Palmerston ,North New Zealand
Dr. Mark Izzard, ORL/Head and Neck, Auckland, New Zealand
Dr. John Chaplin, ORL/Head and Neck, Auckland, New Zealand
Dr. Nick McIvor, ORL/Head and Neck, Auckland, New Zealand
Dr. Irene Kennedy, Prosthetic Dentistry, Auckland, New Zealand
Dr. Richard Hart, Oculoplastic, Auckland, New Zealand
Dr. Bruce Murdoch, OMFS, Palmerston North, New Zealand
Dr. Phillip Marshall, Hospital Dentistry, MidCentral DHB, New Zealand
Dr. N. Manoharan, ORL, MidCentral DHB, New Zealand
Dr. P.J. Famanui, ORL, Wanganui DHB, New Zealand
Dr. Nick Nidev, Radiation Oncologist, MidCentral DHB, New Zealand
Dr. Norman Andrews, Dental Surgeon, Clay Cross, United Kingdom
Dr. Aneu Sood, Dental Surgeon, Nottingham, United Kingdom
Dr. Victor Sendax, MDI Sendax Concept, New York City, United States

Institutions

Medsafe, New Zealand http://www.medsafe.govt.nz
MidCentral District Health Board, New Zealand
Stuart Johansen, Surgical Business Manager
Department of Dental Surgery, MidCentral DHB
Dr. Phillip Marshall, Director, Dental Surgery
Department of Radiology
Dr. John Goulden, Clinical Director
Jackie Cook, Senior Radiographer, CT scans
Department of Medical Photography
Gary Hutchinson
Auckland District Health Board, New Zealand
Wanganui District Health Board, New Zealand
Southern Cross Hospitals, New Zealand
Andrew Lesperance, Hospital Manager, Palmerston North, New Zealand
Gillies Clinic, Auckland, New Zealand
Accident Compensation Corporation, New Zealand
AIG Life Health Insurance, New Zealand
University of De Montfort Leicester, United Kingdom
Prof David Wimpenny
AMRC with Boeing, University of Sheffield, United Kingdom
Adrian Allen, Commercial Director

Media

RSVP Productions Ltd, New Zealand

*Enztec Ltd withdrew from the Engineering Assisted Surgery Programme in 2008.

Robyn Scott-Vincent, Television Documentary Producer who has produced numerous documentary reports with great sensitivity.

The Patients

The consent and cooperation of all patients in the presentation of their cases is gratefully acknowledged.

References

1. American Cancer Society. http://www.cancer.org
2. American Cancer Society Cancer Facts and Figures: 2005, http://www.cancer.org/downloads/STT/CAFF2005f4PWSecured.pdf.
3. American Joint Committee on Cancer: Manual for Staging of Cancer Third Ed. In Beahrs OH, Henson DE, Hutter RVP, Myers MH, editors: *Purposes and Principles of Staging: Chapter 1 pp 3-10*, 1988, Lippincott Company Philadelphia.
4. British Dental Association http://www.bda-dentistry.org.uk
5. Better Care for the Severely Injured: British Orthopaedic Association / Royal College of Surgeons of England Joint Publication, 2000, http://www.rcseng.ac.uk/publications/docs/severely_injured.html.
6. Cancer Registration Statistics 1979-1989 Series MB1 nos 11–22, OPCS
7. Cancer Research Uk United Kingdom Oral Cancer Mortality Statistics http://info.cancerresearchuk.org/cancerstats/types/oral/mortality/?a=5441
8. de Mello-Filho FV, Auader M, Cano E, Carrau RL, Myers EN, Miles E: Effect of mandibular titanium reconstructive plates on radiation dose, *American Journal of Otolaryngology* 24(4):231–235, 2003.
9. The Golden Ratio http://en.wikipedia.org/wiki/Golden_ratio
10. Levin Eddy, The Golden Ratio http://www.goldenmeangauge.co.uk/fibonacci.htm
11. Lovel T: Palliative Care and Head and Neck Cancer – Editorial, *British Journal of Oral & Maxillofacial Surgery* 38:253–254, 2000.
12. Marx RE, Carlson ER, Eichstaedt RM, Schimmele SR, Strauss JE, Georgeff KR: Platelet-rich plasma: Growth factor enhancement for bone grafts, *Oral Surg Oral Med Oral Pathol Oral Radiol Endod* 85(6):638–646, 1998.
13. Mortality Statistics: Cause 1979-1989 England and Wales OPCS
14. Oral Cancer Fact Sheet 1993 14.1, Cancer Research Campaign, 6-10 Cambridge.
15. Peckitt N.S. http://www.maxfac.com
16. Peckitt NS: *Tissue Engineering Maxillary Atrophy Dentistry Scotland Clinical* 3(3):22–29, 2007.
17. The Edentulous State: a need for change: Ninian Peckitt CPD in Practice: Implant Dentistry Ref CPD-13 pp 36–39
18. Clinical Evidence: Mini dental implants: a versatile system Ninian Peckitt, *Private Dentistry* 16–24, 2006.
19. The edentulous state: the need for change part one, *Ninian Peckitt Dentistry* 28, 2006.
20. The edentulous state: the need for change part two, *Ninian Peckitt Dentistry* 27, 2006.
21. The edentulous state: the need for change part three, *Ninian Peckitt Dentistry* 15, 2006.
22. Stereoscopic Lithography and the manufacture of customized titanium implants in orofacial reconstruction. Peckitt N.S, *British Journal of Oral and Maxillofacial Surgery* 37:353–369, 1999.
23. Rapid Product Manufacture http://www.arcam.com
24. Screening for Oral Cancer 1994 Department of Dental Sciences, Royal College of Surgeons of England.
25. Spiro RH, Alphonso AE, Farr HW, Strong EW: Cervical node metastasis from epidermoid carcinoma of the oral cavity and oropharynx. A critical assessment of staging, *American Journal of Surgery* 128:562–567, 1974.
26. Adult Dental Survey, Oral Health in the United Kingdom: Social Survey Division of the Office for National Statistics in collaboration with the Dental Schools of Birmingham, Dundee, Newcastle and Wales, and the Central Survey Unit of the Northern Ireland Statistics and Research Agency. In Walker Alison, Ian Cooper, editors: London, 1988, The Stationery Office.

Chapter 8

The Maxillofacial Prosthodontist's Role in Postcancer Rehabilitation Using Mini Dental Implants

GEORGE C. BOHLE III GREGORY C. BOHLE

Outline

Patients who have been diagnosed with cancer or had traumatic injuries are often unwilling or unable for a variety of reasons to undergo oral or maxillofacial rehabilitation with dental implants. Although some of the reasons are also relevant to patients without trauma or cancers, the additional factors of a cancer diagnosis or traumatic injury must be taken into consideration when formulating treatment plans. Patients will use age as a reason not to consider implant therapy and, although this is a valid argument in their mind, they are unaware of the minimal procedure needed for mini dental implant (MDI) placement and the immense improvement the implants will make in the comfort and function of their prostheses. Financial concerns are given as reasons for patients to reject implant therapy. For patients suffering from traumatic injuries or who have undergone ablative cancer surgery to the oral cavity, implant rehabilitation in most instances is now a medical service. Proper Current Procedural Terminology (CPT) codes rather than Current Dental Terminology (CDT) codes aid in providing the correct coverage patients need for their rehabilitation treatments. Although each insurance provider has specific regulations, a letter explaining the medical necessity of the implants is often required for reimbursement. The prognosis of the patient should be taken into consideration because those who have undergone multiple procedures or are terminally ill may not wish to undergo any seemingly unnecessary treatment. The use of MDIs could be indicated for these patients because the surgical placement is usually less invasive than for conventional implants, which makes recovery easier. Finally, the patient's general psychological outlook must be considered to ensure that the final prosthesis will meet realistic expectations of both patient and practitioner.

Treatment of patients with head and neck cancer, trauma, or developmental defects requires a multidisciplinary team approach. Depending on the trauma or disease and treatment to be rendered, this team may include a surgeon(s), prosthodontist, radiation oncologist, medical oncologist, speech and language pathologist, physical therapist, psychiatrist, nursing, and social worker. Before starting any treatment—whether a single or multiple modality of surgery, radiation, or chemotherapy—a prosthodontist trained in maxillofacial prosthetics should be consulted because each of the above will have varying degrees of impact on function and future treatment that can be rendered. Anatomical variations and changes in functional jaw movement from cancer or trauma surgery, alterations in healing capacity, and oral homeostasis after radiation therapy, and changes in the immune status, healing, and physiologic balance from chemotherapy will be accounted for by the prosthodontist in determining necessary treatment before, during, and after therapy. Prosthodontic rehabilitation of the oral cavity, specifically the use of dental implants for this patient population, has been a controversial subject. The paradigm is changing, and the use of MDIs is aiding this shift in care.

Treatment of Patients Receiving Radiation and/or Chemotherapy

Patients who have been referred for disease management through nonsurgical means with either radiation or chemotherapy alone or combined should be seen before initiating their cancer care. A thorough examination with appropriate dental radiographs should be completed, looking specifically for teeth with a poor or hopeless prognosis. Teeth that are not able to be restored and that are in the field of radiation should be extracted as far in advance of commencement of the treatment as possible to allow for healing.[11] Ideally 21 days before treatment is desirable but depending on the aggressiveness of the disease this is not always possible. The remaining teeth should be in good periodontal health and either be caries free or have sound conservative restorations. The patient should be instructed on to proper homecare regimens: brushing after every meal, flossing, daily use of a fluoride supplement such as 1.1% sodium fluoride (PreviDent 5000 Plus, Colgate Oral Pharmaceuticals, New York, New York), and seeking routine professional dental care every 3 to 4 months with a local general practitioner and hygienist for the remainder of their life.[9]

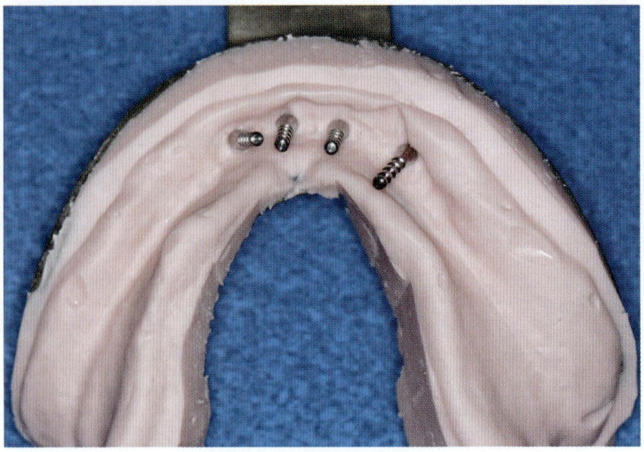

FIGURE 8-1. Primary irreversible hydrocolloid impression with MDI laboratory analogs in place.

If the patient currently has MDIs or conventional implants in the field of radiation a protective mouth guard can be fabricated to lessen the effects of backscatter that cause an increase in mucositis to the adjacent soft tissues or tongue.[3] The mouth guard is fabricated by making an impression with irreversible hydrocolloid, placing laboratory analogs in the impression, pouring a cast from improved stone, and using a vacuum formed material such as 0.15-inch thickness resilient material (Mouthguard Regular Clear .150, Henry Schein Inc., Melville, NY) similar to an athletic mouth guard or a combination material for a soft lined rigid protector (Proform Dual Laminates, Keystone Industries, Cherry Hill, NJ) (Figures 8-1 to 8-3). This will provide spacing between the metallic restorations and the adjacent soft tissue. It is important to note that the patient must have the mouth guard(s) in place during the simulation appointment while the positioning mask appliance is being fabricated by the radiation oncology team. Several studies have confirmed that backscatter in the bone and around the soft tissues of irradiated implants occurs; however, the negligible amount does not necessitate trephine removal of the implant.[23,2]

During radiation and/or chemotherapy, elective procedures should be avoided for both patient safety and comfort. The ensuing mucositis places the patient at increased risk for infection and delayed healing, and the oral cavity is generally too uncomfortable to tolerate surgical procedures. If MDI placement is deemed necessary at this time, active chemotherapy is not an absolute contraindication.[14,22] Current laboratory blood counts should

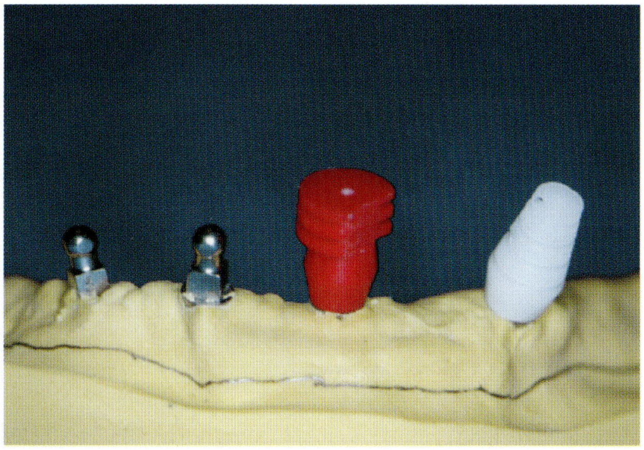

FIGURE 8-2. Close-up view of the four analogs illustrating no additional retention or the use of either 2.9-mm impression coping (*red*) or 2.9-mm immediate temporization cap (*white*).

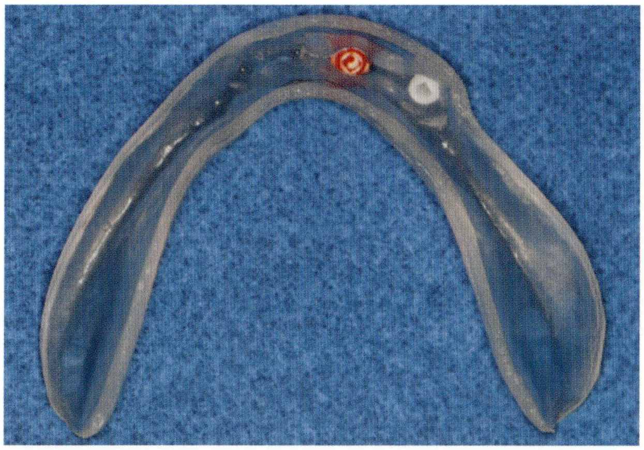

FIGURE 8-3. Completed mouth guard using a dual laminate material, providing a soft lining, that engages the O ball design or retains either the 2.9-mm impression coping (*red*) or 2.9-mm immediate temporization cap (*white*).

be obtained, paying particular attention to overall platelet count, clotting time (international normalized ratio [INR]), and immune status (specifically the absolute neutrophil count [ANC]). Because most MDIs are placed with a flapless surgical approach previously described and bleeding is minimal, a recommended platelet count of > 50,000, an INR ≤ 2.5, and an ANC >1.0 could be considered safe. The use of systemic or local antibiotics both prophylactically or adjunctly is empirical and can be used at the practitioner's discretion (Esposito et al. 2008).[8,18]

After radiation and/or chemotherapy, a patient can be considered for MDI treatment for removable or fixed prosthodontics. Regarding chemotherapy, the patient should meet the criteria described above for blood counts that will allow healing properties to return to near normal even if they are on several maintenance drug therapies.[15] Research and debate regarding dental implant treatment and patients using oral or intravenous (IV) bisphosphonates exists. Grant et al.[10] published a review of 115 patients who were taking oral bisphosphonates and showed no deleterious effect on osseointegration or the complication of osteonecrosis of the jaw. Patients who have used or currently use IV bisphosphonates should not be considered implant candidates until further research is completed and the risks for osteonecrosis of the jaw are fully understood by patients and practitioners.[21,13] The authors have successfully placed a very limited number of MDIs in oncology patients using both forms of bisphosphonate drugs, but long-term follow-up is not available, and therefore this is not recommended.

For placing MDIs in irradiated patients, several factors must be considered. The type, dose, and field of radiation play a significant role in this decision. The dose of 5500 cGy is often quoted as the cut off, presenting a relative low risk for development of osteoradionecrosis (ORN). Patients, however, must be educated about this risk, possible alteration of osseointegration, and documentation of this possibility should be made in the informed consent.[17] The use of hyperbaric oxygen is controversial and debate continues today and is not advocated because current literature fails to prove its efficacy in preventing or treating ORN (Esposito et al. 2008).[7,20] The flapless placement technique should lessen the risk for developing ORN because the periosteum is not manipulated to the extent as in an open procedure. Another controversial subject is the timing of implant surgery after radiation therapy. Proposed theories of bone healing alterations after radiation therapy are: decreased healing capacity is immediate and lifelong or decreased healing capacity does not occur in the first 6 months post radiation then worsens in the remaining lifespan.[16] Despite the healing mechanism alterations, studies fail to show a clinically significant difference in osseointegration rates.[19,6] A review of the clinical practice concurs with these published findings. When possible, implants are placed at the time of surgery, but previous radiation therapy is not an absolute contraindication. Antibiotic use is empirical, and we will routinely prescribe 0.12% chlorhexidine gluconate (PerioGard,

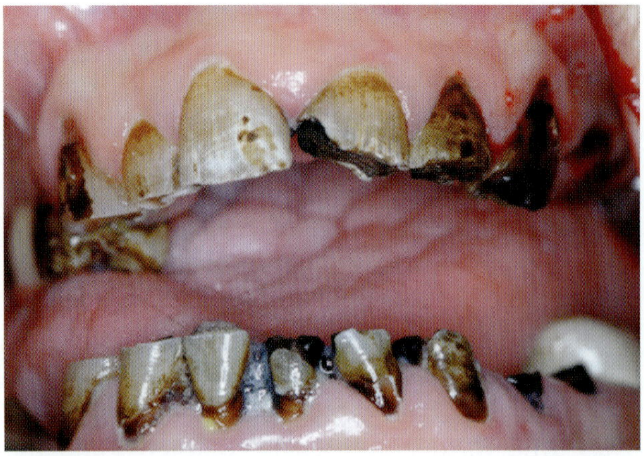

FIGURE 8-4. Generalized severe caries secondary to xerostomia from radiation therapy for unknown primary. Note the ropey saliva present on the anterior mandibular teeth.

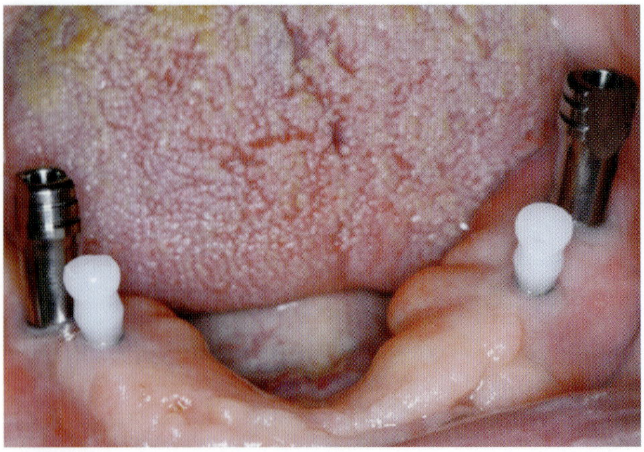

FIGURE 8-5. MDIs and Endure (IMTEC Inc., Ardmore, OK) implants with impression copings before final impression. The implants were placed at the time of extraction using the MDIs for immediate stabilization while the conventional implants integrated.

Colgate Oral Pharmaceuticals, New York, New York) to be used twice daily for 7 to 14 days after implant placement.

The next consideration in treatment planning implants in the irradiated patient is anatomical site. The maxillary arch has greater blood flow than the mandible. Therefore, MDIs placed in the maxilla may have a lower risk for developing ORN than those placed in the mandible. Patients who have had radiation and/or chemotherapy can be candidates for implants with proper planning and patient education. Consultation with the radiation oncologist, radiation physicist, and medical oncologist when planning MDIs for irradiated patients will provide definitive answers to the total dose, delivery method, anatomical site, and overall healing capacity of the patient, allowing for predictable and safe implant placement (Figures 8-4 to 8-7).

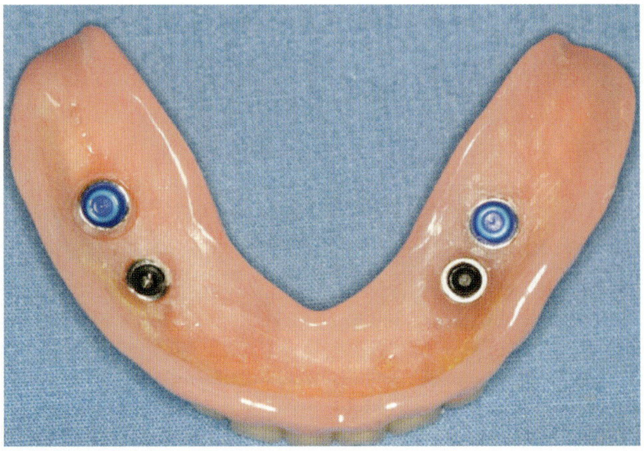

FIGURE 8-6. Completed denture using both O ring and locator attachments.

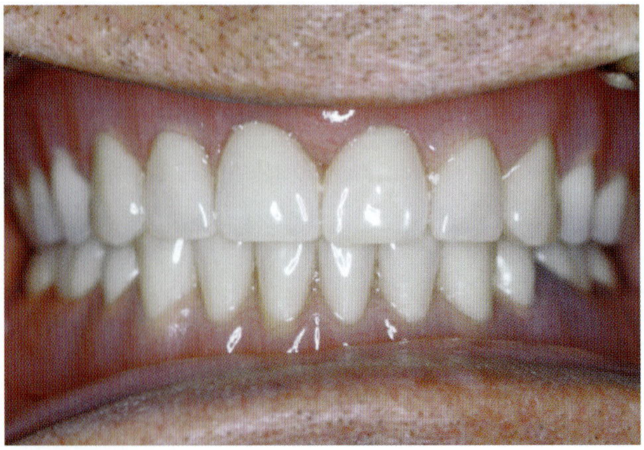

FIGURE 8-7. Completed maxillary and mandibular dentures.

Treatment of Patients Before and After Surgical Resection

Hard Palate Defects

Patients that are referred before surgical resection of lesions involving only the hard palate and adjacent structures will be examined as previously described. If the patient is fully dentate then a discussion of surgical, interim, and definitive obturator prostheses procedures, expected results, and sequelae would take place. An irreversible hydrocolloid impression of the maxillary and mandibular arches is made, and a facebow recording is completed. The casts are poured in stone as a permanent record for future reference. A second impression of the maxillary arch or a duplicate of the stone cast is used to fabricate the surgical obturator. The proposed surgical resection is outlined, the tumor if visible is removed and any teeth that may be in the resection, and an acrylic resin surgical obturator is fabricated.[12] This obturator is delivered in the operating room at the time of tumor resection and is held in place with orthodontic ligature wires around the remaining teeth. In approximately 10 days, the surgical obturator is removed and the interim obturator is delivered. The interim obturator is fabricated on the mounted cast that was used to fabricate the surgical obturator. If any additional teeth were removed during the surgery, they can be removed from the cast before the interim being made. Wrought wire (18 gauge) and ball clasps are contoured to the remaining teeth on the cast, denture teeth are set to the mounting, and the interim prosthesis is waxed and processed in heat polymerized acrylic resin. After removal of the surgical obturator and all remaining surgical packing, the interim obturator is fitted to place and adjusted for comfort and occlusal stability. A resilient material such as tissue conditioner (COE Comfort, GC America, Alsip, IL) is used to fabricate the obturator portion of the prosthesis. After a minimum of 3 months, longer if postoperative radiation therapy is necessary, the definitive obturator may be fabricated. The definitive obturator differs from the interim in that the healing around the defect has stabilized and a cast framework is made rather than an interim entirely from acrylic resin. The process for fabricating the cast framework closely follows procedures used for a removable partial denture framework. A diagnostic cast is surveyed for optimal placement of rest seats, placement of major/minor connectors, and development of the obturator portion of the prosthesis. The tooth preparations are completed, a master cast is made, and the laboratory fabricates the framework. After verification of the fit of the framework, a corrected cast procedure is completed to record the defect area. The trial prosthesis in wax is verified, processed, and delivered.

Patients who are partially or completely edentulous are faced with a greater prosthetic rehabilitation challenge due to the varying degree of stability from the lack of teeth. When evaluating these patients before the maxillectomy, discussion involving implants must be included. Although the patient may choose not to have implants placed at the time of resection, most will choose to have this done while they are under anesthesia. Additionally, educating the patient about the probable need for postoperative radiation therapy placement will allow for 6 to 8 weeks of integration and make the transition from the surgical to interim obturator easier. The procedures involved in preparing partially or completely edentulous patients closely mimic the steps describe above for dentate patients. One difference is that when fabricating the surgical obturator either a trough can be created or holes can be placed before or at the time of surgery to fit around the implants. The number of implants will vary with the anatomical volume remaining after the resection; however, all available bone should be used. The 1.2-mm osteotomy drill is used to pierce the soft tissue and just puncture the maxillary bone. The 2.4-mm MDI MAX is then allowed to self-advance through the bone using the finger, winged, and ratchet drivers until properly seated.[4] If a flap is reflected, closure with sutures will complete the placement and the surgical obturator will be delivered (Figures 8-8 to 8-11). The surgical obturator is then fixed by wiring around the remaining teeth, suturing the obturator to place, using orthopedic fixation screws into the remaining palate, or transalveolar wiring. Transalveolar wiring can be accomplished using a surgical awl, sternum wiring kit, or 1-mm drill and passing the wire from buccal to lingual. After all the wires (usually 3 to 4) have been passed through, the surgical obturator can be "threaded" with the wires and seated to place. The wires are then twisted clockwise until tight and the excess cut leaving a 6-mm tail that is shaped like a rosette.

After 5 to 14 days of initial healing and at the surgeon's discretion, the surgical packing and obturator is removed and the defect cleaned. The implants are evaluated for mobility and a panoramic radiograph is taken. The interim obturator is modified to seat fully over the implants and the extensions are adjusted for comfort. Using a resilient material of choice, the obturator portion is fabricated. At this point, either the metal housings containing the O rings can be incorporated into the obturator or the tissue conditioner can be used until the tissues are less sensitive (Figures 8-12 to 8-15). The patient's occlusion is adjusted as necessary but will be con-

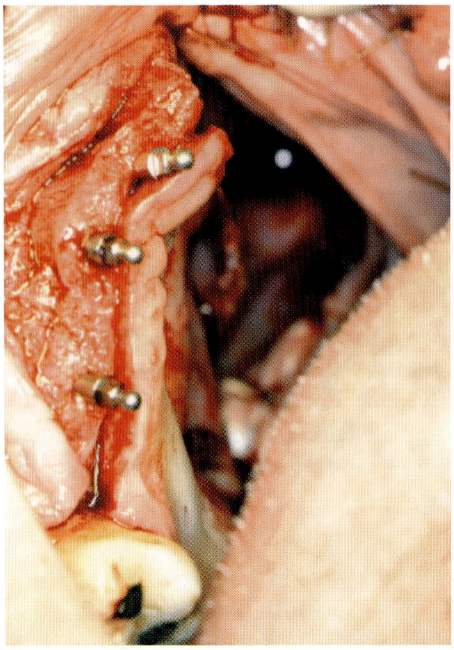

FIGURE 8-8. MDIs placed by reflecting a flap done at the time of the left maxillectomy while waiting for the results of the frozen sections of the margins.

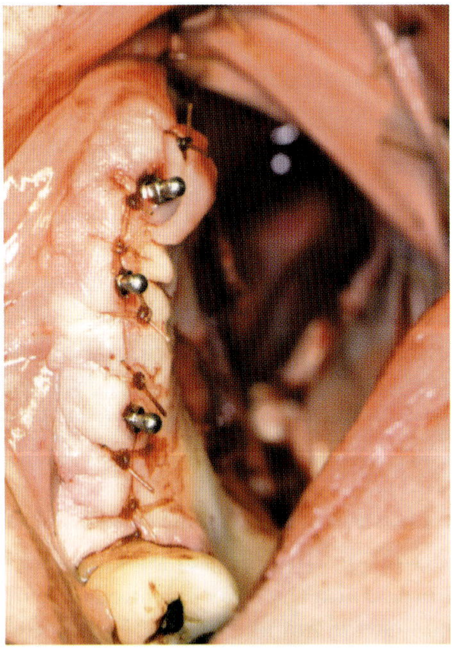

FIGURE 8-9. The flap is sutured closed using 3-0 chromic sutures before packing placement.

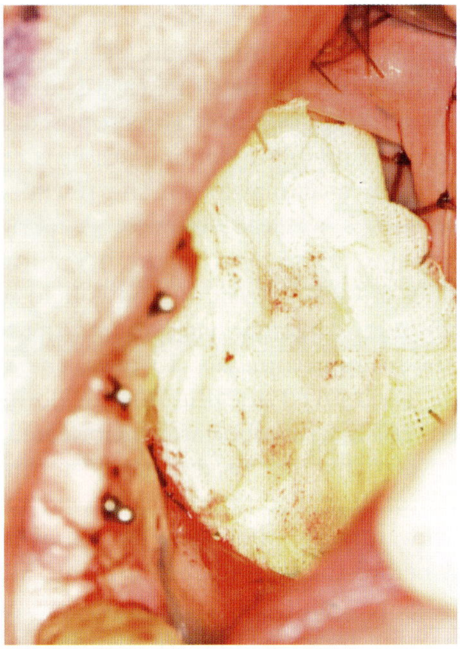

FIGURE 8-10. Xeroform gauze (*yellow*) is packed into the defect, providing pressure to the skin graft on the buccal mucosa and primary obturation of the defect.

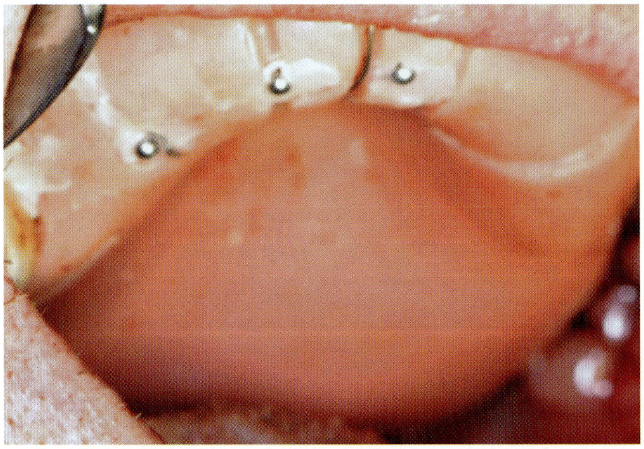

FIGURE 8-11. Holes are drilled into the surgical obturator to fit around the MDIs. The obturator is then wired to place and will remain for approximately 1 week.

tinuously monitored during the next few weeks as healing continues. The occlusion at this point is usually guarded from edema and pain of the surgical site, temporomandibular mandibular joint, and muscles of mastication. Patients and caregivers are shown how to insert, remove, and care for the prosthesis. Gentle rinsing of the resilient liner will protect against damage, and the obturator should be removed while sleeping and placed in a container of clean water, allowing the remaining supportive structures recovery time. Fabrication of the definitive obturator with MDIs in place should not begin for a minimum of 3 months after surgery to allow for complete healing. If postoperative radiation therapy is performed, the interim obturator should be worn throughout the therapy and an additional

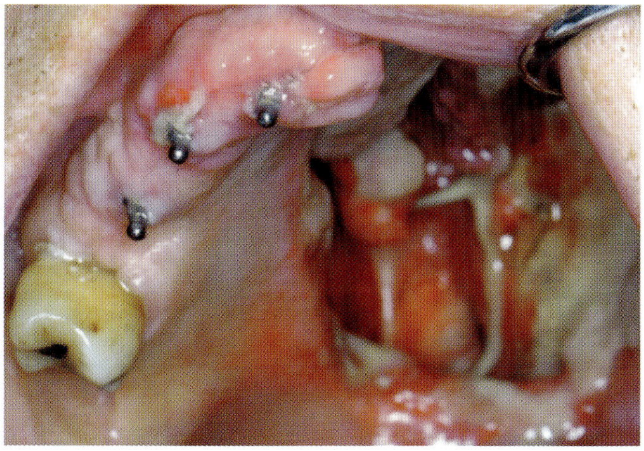

FIGURE 8-12. Initial appearance of maxillary arch after surgical obturator and packing removal.

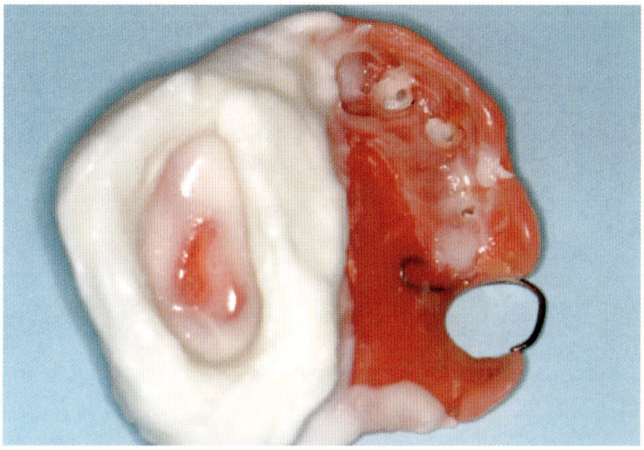

FIGURE 8-13. The interim obturator is relieved for complete seating and the obturator portion is formed with tissue conditioner.

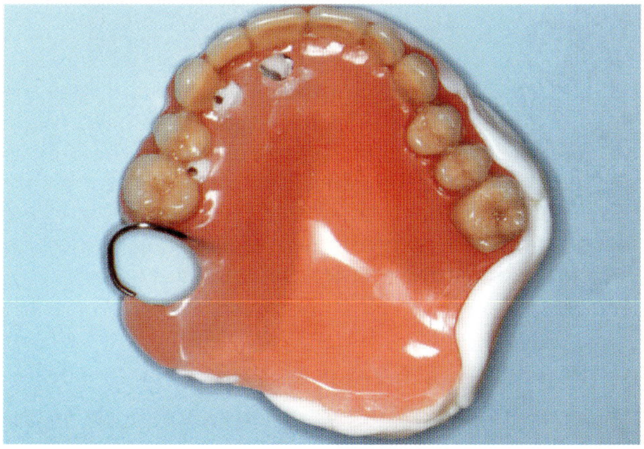

FIGURE 8-14. During the initial stages of the interim obturator delivery, the tissue conditioner can be used for engagement of the O balls or metal housings can be incorporated at this time.

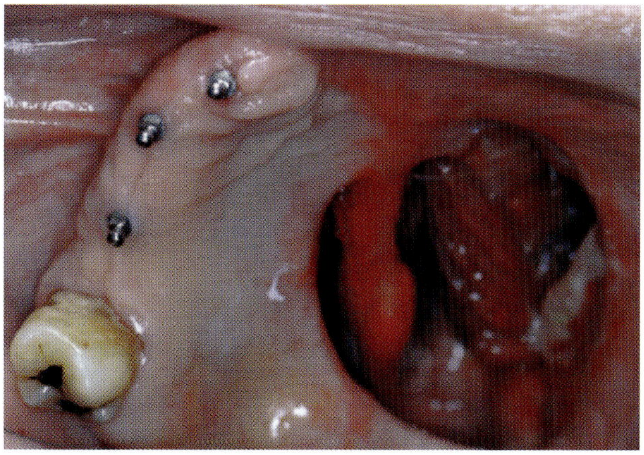

FIGURE 8-15. One month postoperative photo of the maxillectomy defect.

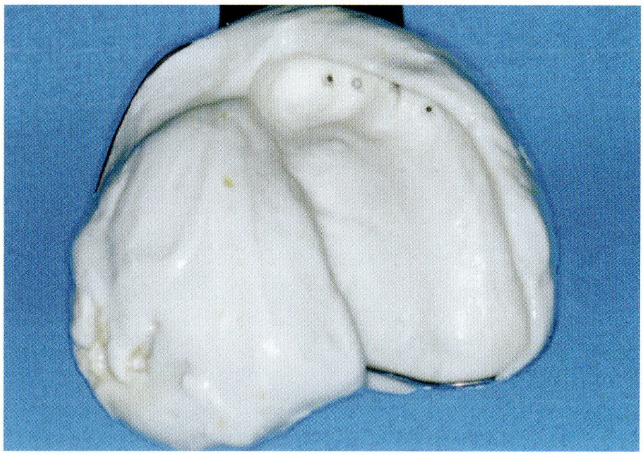

FIGURE 8-16. Primary irreversible hydrocolloid impression of the four MDIs in place for definitive obturator fabrication.

healing time of 3 to 6 months given at the cessation of the radiation therapy. For partially edentulous patients, the MDIs will augment the retention of the obturator. Conventional clasp design remains the principle means of retention and resistance with the O rings adds to this. At the time of the framework try-in, the metal housings containing the O rings can be attached to the framework with autopolymerizing acrylic resin. The occlusal record can then be completed, the wax up verified, and the prosthesis processed as normal. In completely edentulous patients, the primary impressions of the implants is marked with indelible ink or laboratory analogs can be placed before pouring the casts (Figures 8-16 and 8-17). The ink transfers to the custom tray so a window can be produced or, if implant analogs were used, relief can be provided, allowing complete seating of the tray (Figures 8-18

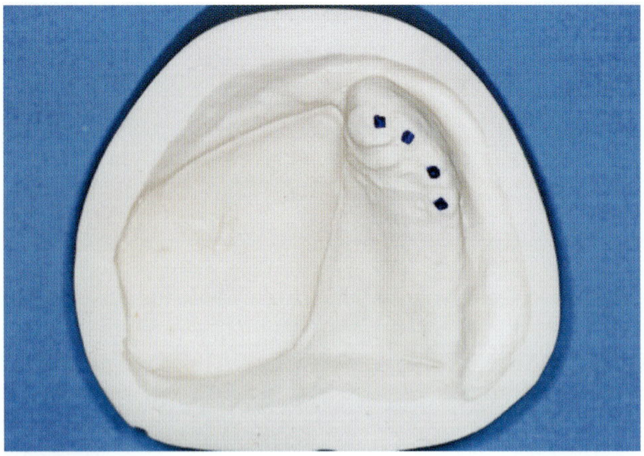

FIGURE 8-17. Primary plaster cast demonstrating the blue ink transfer of the MDI location from the primary impression.

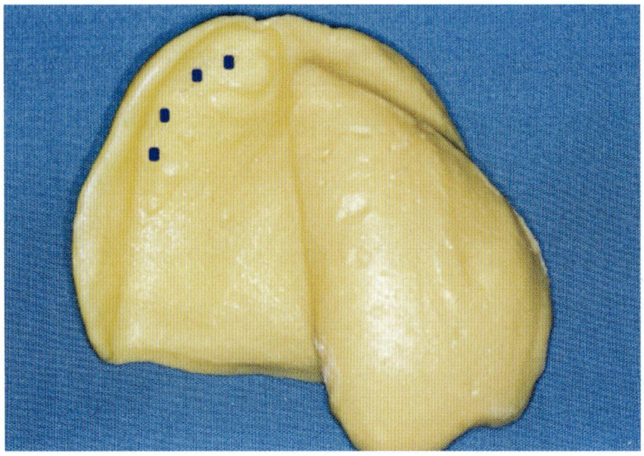

FIGURE 8-18. Minimal blockout of undercuts allows for the fabrication of the custom tray into the defect, and the blue ink transfer provides visualization of the MDI sites.

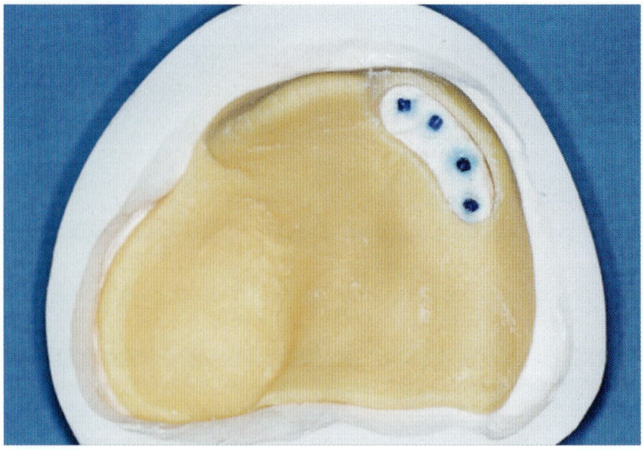

FIGURE 8-19. The completed custom tray with a window around the implants to ensure complete seating and direct intraoral incorporation of the metal housings to the tray.

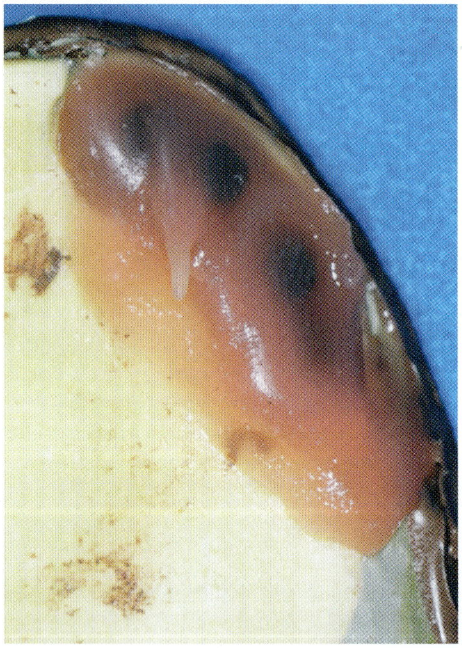

FIGURE 8-20. Metal housings incorporated into the custom tray after the final impression has been made with Secure (IMTEC, Inc.), ensuring that the tray is fully seated. If the housings are incorporated before the impression being made, it is possible to have material interfere with complete seating and renders an inaccurate implant-to-patient relationship.

to 8-19). The tray is tried in the patient's mouth and adjusted as needed for complete seating and comfort. The impression of the arch and defect is completed with the material of choice, and metal housings are incorporated into the tray using autopolymerizing acrylic resin (Secure, IMTEC inc., Ardmore, OK) (Figures 8-20 and 8-21). Laboratory analogs are incorporated into the stone cast and a base plate with the metal housings, and O rings will be placed in the base plate for more accurate records. The occlusal records and teeth verification is completed and the obturator processed in a normal fashion.

Patients must be made aware before and reminded after delivery that the implants will not reduce all movement. The obturator will move under function but will not become dislodged without manual manipulation. All movement cannot be eliminated because the obturator requires the standard denture-bearing areas for support, and these areas were reduced due to the surgery. The implants are meant to assist in stability and provide better efficacy;

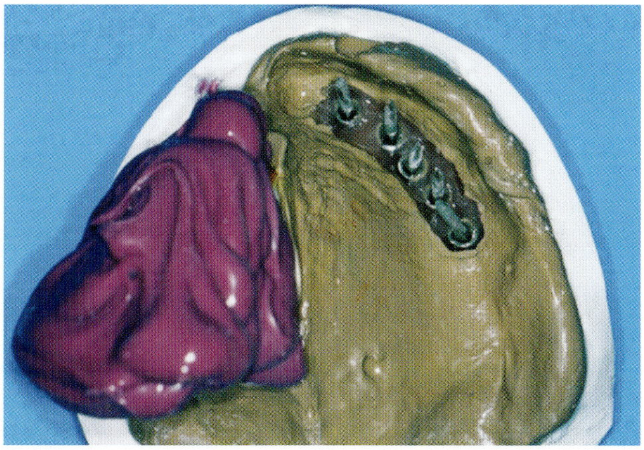

FIGURE 8-21. Multiple materials can be used for the final impression. MDI laboratory analogs are placed in the incorporated housings, the final impression is boxed, and the cast is poured.

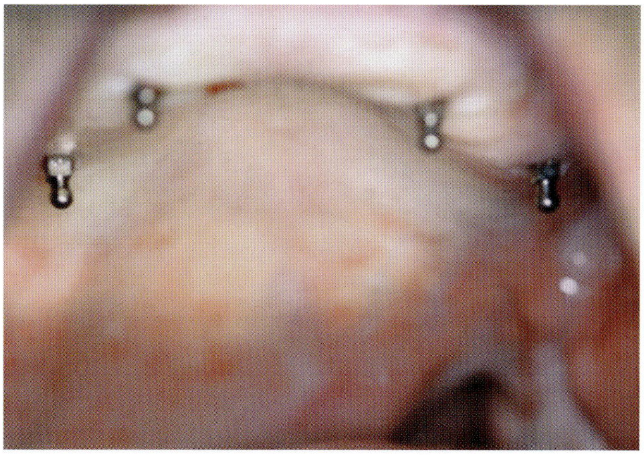

FIGURE 8-22. MDIs placed to aid in stabilizing an edentulous soft palate obturator after surgical resection to the left soft palate and tonsil.

the obturator will not become dislodged under regular function of speaking, swallowing, and chewing.

Soft Palate Defects

Patients with soft palate issues can be classified under the umbrella term velopharyngeal inadequacy. This inadequacy is characterized by one of three categories: (1) velopharyngeal insufficiency, meaning that an anatomical defect of the soft palate prevents formation of the sphincter; (2) velopharyngeal incompetence, meaning that an intact soft palate does not function adequately to form the sphincter mechanism; or (3) a combination of the two, meaning that an anatomical defect exists and the remaining soft palate function is compromised. These issues can arise from trauma, surgery, radiation therapy, or developmental defect at birth. Treatments of these issues involve either surgical reconstruction and/or a variety of maxillofacial prosthetic appliances.

Patients with velopharyngeal insufficiency will require obturators to restore the area of the defect to allow competency in swallowing and speaking. If patients are seen before surgery, the steps for fabricating the surgical obturator are similar to those outlined above for the hard palate obturator. If a patient is fully dentate, an impression is made, and the cast is altered to the anticipated surgical outlines. The surgical obturator is then delivered and, again, after 5 to 10 days of healing and at the surgeon's discretion, the surgical obturator is removed and an interim soft palate obturator is delivered. The interim prosthesis is similar to the interim hard palate obturator except that the extension into the oropharynx separating the nasopharynx is fabricated using resilient lining material as described above with the patient moving the head to the right and left touching the chin to the chest and moving it back as well as swallowing small sips of water and speaking to help form the resilient material in a functional impression. The excess material is removed, and the patient will practice insertion and removal. Care for the interim obturator is similar to the interim hard palate obturator. If radiation is not necessary, the definitive obturator can be fabricated on a cast framework, which can be started at 3 to 4 months of healing. This type of prosthesis in a fully dentate patient is retentive and provides the patient with effective speech and swallowing.

Partially and completely edentulous patients pose similar challenges as patients with hard palate obturators. If these patients are seen before surgery, discussion of the use of implants is necessary. Following the fabrication process for a surgical obturator described above, the MDIs can be placed at the time of the surgery in the remaining hard palate to provide stability for the soft palate obturator in the interim and definitive phases (Figures 8-22 to 8-24). From the initial cast, rest preps for the remaining teeth in a partially edentulous patient can be planned. The custom tray is fabricated and a secondary impression is made. A framework is fabricated and upon verification a corrected cast impression of the soft palate defect is completed. This corrected cast impression can be done in a variety of different materials; we

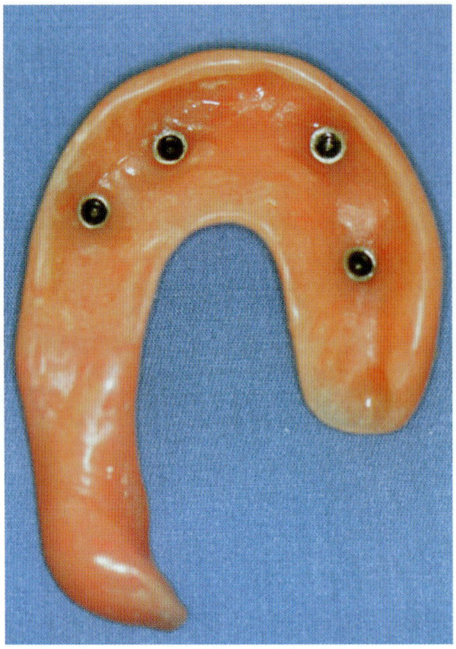

FIGURE 8-23. Soft palate obturator with four O rings for retention, allowing more open palatal contours.

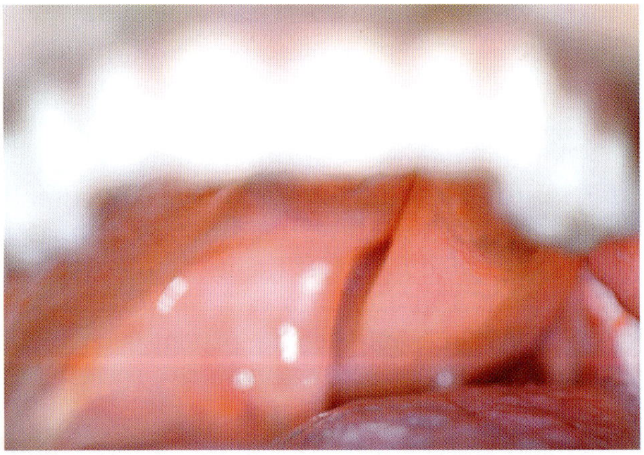

FIGURE 8-24. Soft palate obturator in place, allowing for intelligible speech and competent swallowing.

prefer modeling compound so the periphery can be reduced by 2 to 3 mm, and a tissue conditioning material is applied. The patient will then functionally generate the impression of the defect. The lateral extensions of the prosthesis must be monitored to ensure that no overextension occurs that will lead to sore areas where the palate will drape. After the secondary impression has been made, a framework is made to extend the meshwork into the defect. The laboratory prescription must inform the technician to allow for approximately double the normal block out so that there is adequate room

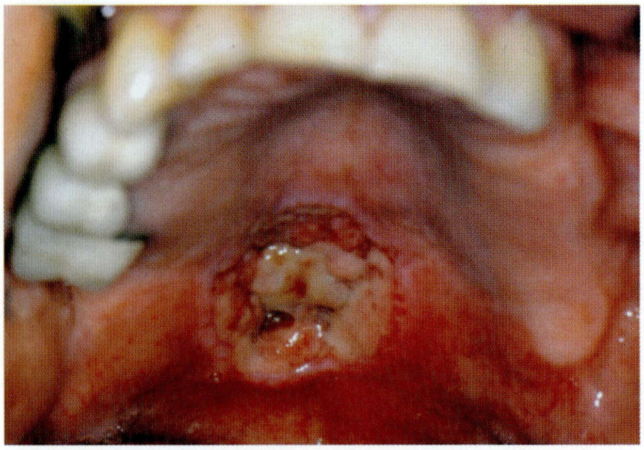

FIGURE 8-25. Adenoid cystic carcinoma of the junction of the hard and soft palate.

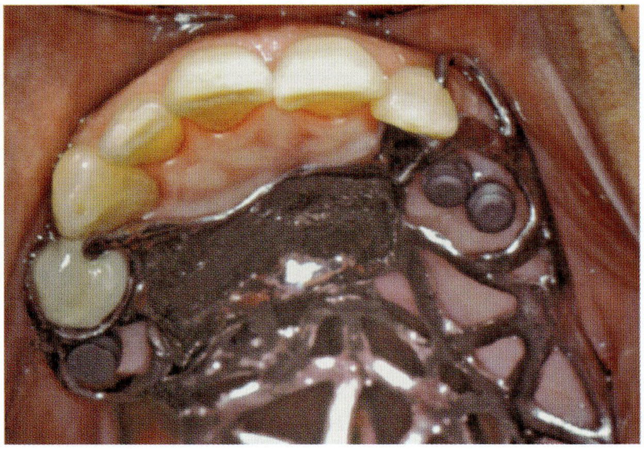

FIGURE 8-26. Metal framework in place, demonstrating conventional clasping and three MDIs to augment retention. The metal housings will be attached to the framework with autopolymerizing acrylic resin.

for adjustment before encroaching upon the metal framework.

For edentulous patients, processed-based plates are recommended so that jaw record relations and wax teeth trial denture verifications are more accurate. In partially edentulous patients, after verification of the framework, the metal housings with the O rings are best picked up directly in the mouth using autopolymerizing acrylic resin. This can then be used to verify the position of the implants in the master cast (Figures 8-25 to 8-28). For completely edentulous patients, the metal housings containing the O rings can be picked up in the processed-based plate, and the prosthesis can be processed in a routine manner. Without implants to aid with stabilization and retention, upon function the posterior pharyngeal wall will dislodge the prosthesis

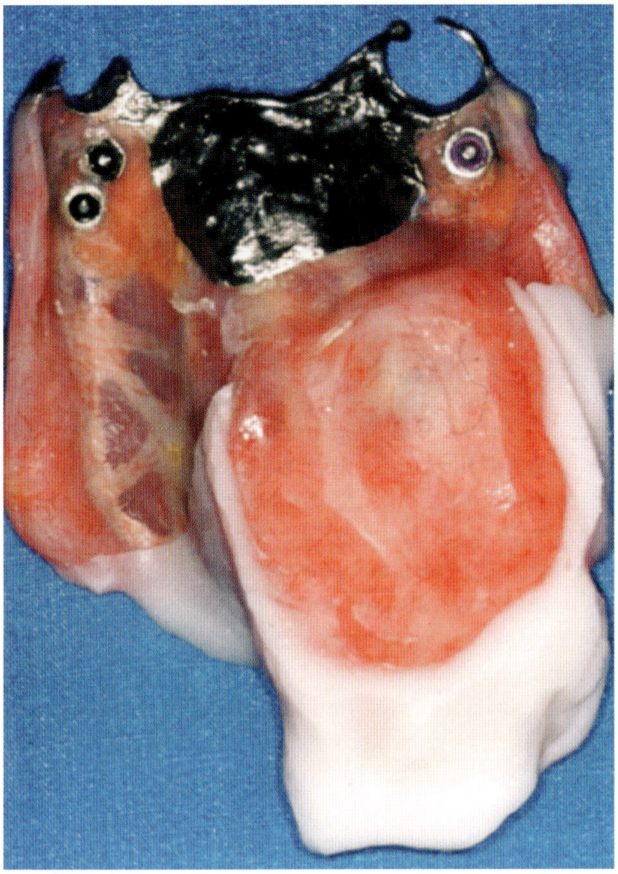

FIGURE 8-27. A base plate is attached, and at a subsequent visit, final registration of the defect can be obtained.

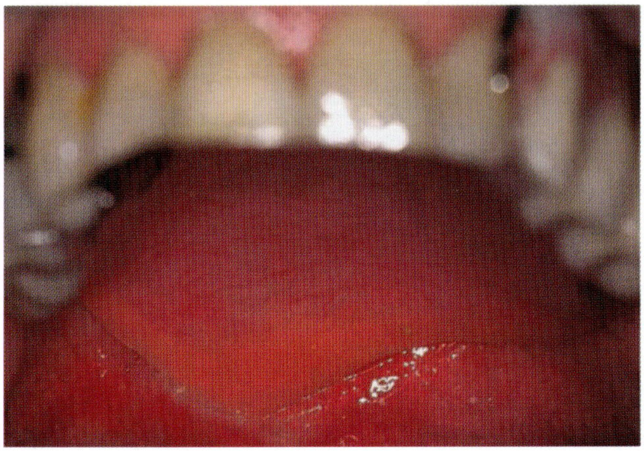

FIGURE 8-28. Soft palate obturator in place after functional molding.

anteriorly and the lateral pharyngeal walls will push the prosthesis medially, overcoming any type of dental adhesive. This dislodgement of the prosthesis allows for leakage of foods and liquids and hypernasality in speech.

For patients presenting with velopharyngeal incompetence, a palatal lift prosthesis will aid in speech and swallowing. Completely dentate patients will have less trouble with retention of the prosthesis because the teeth will provide adequate retention for the framework and support in lifting the soft palate. Partially or completely edentulous patients are at a severe disadvantage for retention and stability of this type of prosthesis because attempting to lift and maintain the soft palate in an elevated position places great stress on the prosthesis. A discussion of the placement of implants to aid in mechanical retention and to provide stability and overcome the downward force of the elevated soft palate will greatly improve the function of the prosthesis. Fabrication of this type of prosthesis begins with a primary impression of the maxillary arch and soft palate in entirety. If the patient has a gag reflex, this must be compensated for by using either topical or local anesthetics to obtain an accurate impression for the prosthesis. If the gag reflex prevents making the impression, a patient can attempt to desensitize the reflex by practicing with a spoon in the roof of the mouth or by using over-the-counter medicaments such as sprays or throat lozenges. After the gag reflex has been desensitized, the prosthesis can be attempted. Often for the initial impression, the custom tray is fabricated and tried in the mouth. Modeling compound is then put into the tray to elevate the soft palate to the level of the hard palate so that when the practitioner looks into the mouth, the posterior wall of the oropharynx should be easily visible. For completely edentulous patients, implants are relied upon as the sole means of retention.

If patients have a combination of velopharyngeal incompetence and insufficiency, combinations of the above prostheses and, if the tongue is involved in the surgery, possibly palatal augmentation prostheses are used. Dentate patients do reasonably well in terms of retention and stability of these types of combination prostheses, but partially and completely edentulous patients have a more trying time. The steps for fabricating such prostheses are described above, with the exception of how an augmentation segment, if necessary, is added to the prosthesis. The above steps for the prosthetic appliance are followed, then a resilient lining material is placed into the palate vault, and the patient is asked to speak, swallow, and to move the remaining tongue to functionally form the new palatal contours. These new palatal contours aid in clarification of speech and, in the transit phase, maneuvering a bolus of food to the oral pharynx for swallowing. Regardless of the type of prosthesis necessary in dealing with soft palate rehabilitation, it is beneficial to collaborate with a speech and language pathologist who may aid not in only helping to form the prosthesis for clarification of speech but can also provide exercises for patients to improve swallowing.

It is important to educate the patient that these prosthetic devices are a static piece of acrylic resin attempting to replace a functional muscle used for all speech sounds and every type of swallowing. A static prosthesis is not going to compensate for every muscle action, leakage can occur occasionally; and a difference in the voice may be noticeable. These differences have been studied extensively in the literature and found that, based on intelligibility scores, a patient can be adequately rehabilitated.[5] Secondly, the patient must be educated in that if the tongue, oropharynx, hypopharynx, and/or esophagus have been affected, either due to neurological, surgical, or radiation alterations, the prosthesis will not aid in any of the swallowing phase other than separating the nasopharynx from the oropharynx. Patients will often be concerned if they continue to have difficulty in swallowing and must be made aware that the musculature that moves the bolus of the food from the oropharynx to the hypopharynx esophageal junction is not affected by this type of prosthesis, regardless of being dentate or having implant stability. Implants in these patients, however, make a huge difference in the efficacy of the prosthesis and should be considered for all patients missing multiple teeth or who are completely edentulous to improve their quality of life.

Mandibular Defects

Cancers of the mandible, mandibular gingiva, floor of the mouth, retromolar trigone, tonsil, base of tongue, or oral tongue can result in two classifications of surgery. A marginal mandibulectomy is when a piece of the mandible has been removed yet the continuity of the mandible has not been disturbed. The inferior cortex of the mandible remains intact and the affected area with tumor has been removed. Dentate and partially dentate patients fare well with a resection appliance because the remaining teeth will provide the retention and stability necessary for this removable appliance. Completely edentulous patients with a marginal mandibulectomy may be able to compensate with a well constructed resection appliance; however, the alteration in anatomy and scarring of the floor of mouth, buccal mucosa, and/or labial mucosa, depending on the surgical site, will have a direct effect on the retention and stability of this prosthesis. MDIs should be considered to help stabilize the resection appliance to improve function and comfort. Most of these patients will undergo radiation therapy, and placement of these implants in an irradiated patient has been discussed earlier. MDIs can routinely be placed without reflecting a flap; therefore, these patients should be considered for a minimum of two implants to aid in stabilization of the resection appliance. The second classification involves the patients who undergo a segmental mandibular resection. This classification of patients can be further subdivided into segmental mandibulectomy with and without reconstruction.

Patients who have had a segmental mandibulectomy with a vascularized flap reconstruction using the fibula free flap are candidates for MDIs. Often after ablation of the tumor and reconstruction with the fibula free flap, patients will be subjected to radiation therapy and will present with obliterated buccal and lingual vestibules. Due to the risk for osteoradionecrosis, most surgeons will opt for the least invasive prosthetic rehabilitation possible, which would be a removable resection appliance. These resection appliances, however, are difficult for even the dentate patient due to the lever action and altered soft tissue anatomy. Often the fibula flaps are placed laterally to provide good facial contours, but the remaining arch form is lingual to the fibula. This alteration in anatomical structure does not provide for optimum functional capacity of the prosthesis because the clasping situation does not provide maximum comfort and efficiency in function. One alternative to conventional dental implants should the surgeon not wish to violate the previously irradiated site or the plastic and reconstructive surgeons be willing to remove the mini plate hardware that is often in the area where the implant should be placed, the MDI can be planned as it is. With the growing use of cone-beam computer tomography, implant planning software, and surgical guides, flapless implant placement between the orthopedic stabilization screws can be accomplished (Figures 8-29 to 8-31). One of the drawbacks

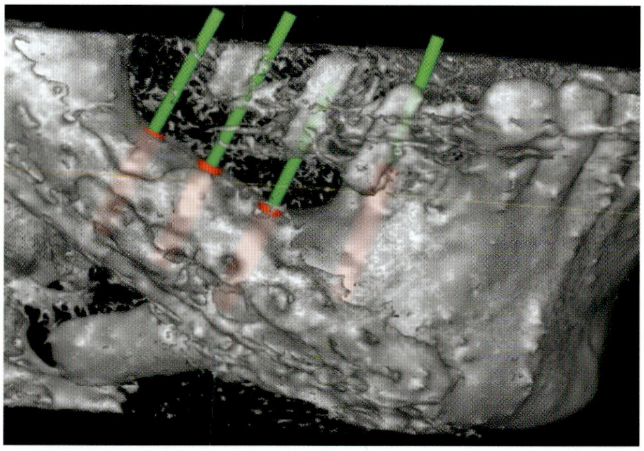

FIGURE 8-29. Three-dimensional rendering (ILUMA cone beam CT scan, IMTEC, Inc.) of an adolescent patient who underwent a fibula free flap reconstruction now in need of dental implants. MDIs are being used as long-term provisionals that can be removed and replaced with conventional implants when he reaches adulthood.

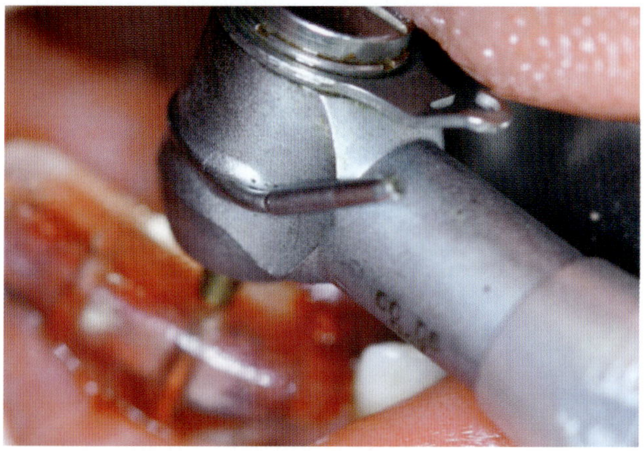

FIGURE 8-30. CAD/CAM fabricated implant surgical guide (Medical Modeling, Inc., Golden, CO) for implant surgery.

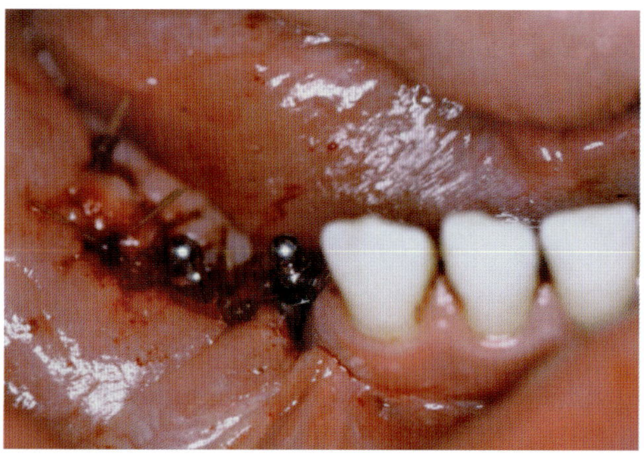

FIGURE 8-31. Three MDIs in place in the reconstructed fibula.

of using the MDI can be the tissue thickness over the fibula. This can be overcome by asking the plastic and reconstructive surgeon to thin the flap, or, if this is not possible, placement of the implant will require fabrication of a custom abutment. In the case of a fixed prosthesis, custom abutments are verified, jaw record relations completed, and cementation of the prosthesis is performed. Temporary cement is all that is necessary because the abutments will create accurate parallelism to provide the resistance form, obviating the need for a luting agent. In the case of a removable prosthesis that is stabilized by the implants, direct attachment of O rings into the prosthesis can be accomplished using the steps outlined above for obturator prosthesis. In the case of patients with a marginal mandibulectomy whose anatomical landmarks have been changed, MDIs can be of value in providing an increase in stabilization of the removable resection appliance and thus increasing the comfort of the prosthesis. Should there be recurrent disease or need for further surgery, the implants can be trephined out or removed en bloc with little difficulty.

Mandibulotomy Approach

One other surgery involving the mandible that does not result in the loss of continuity of the mandibular arch but can result in the loss of a tooth or teeth is the mandibulotomy approach. This surgical approach is used mainly for tumors of the base of tongue and tonsil and requires an osteotomy to be made through the interdental space between two teeth. Typically these teeth are the canine and first bicuspid, but some surgeons may choose to make the cut between the central incisors or a central and lateral incisor. If the osteotomy is made without extracting a tooth, after the mandibulotomy a tooth or teeth can be lost due to being devitalized from the osteotomy (Figures 8-32 and 8-33). If one tooth is lost, sometimes the space is not adequate for a conventional implant. The choices to prosthetically rehabilitate the edentulous space become a resin bonded fixed partial denture (Maryland bridge), a fixed partial denture, removable partial denture, or an MDI. The MDI allows for restoration of this space without performing any preparations to the virgin teeth adjacent to the edentulous space. A diagnostic panoramic radiograph is taken and when the mandibulotomy surgical site appears well healed, the MDI can be placed following standard

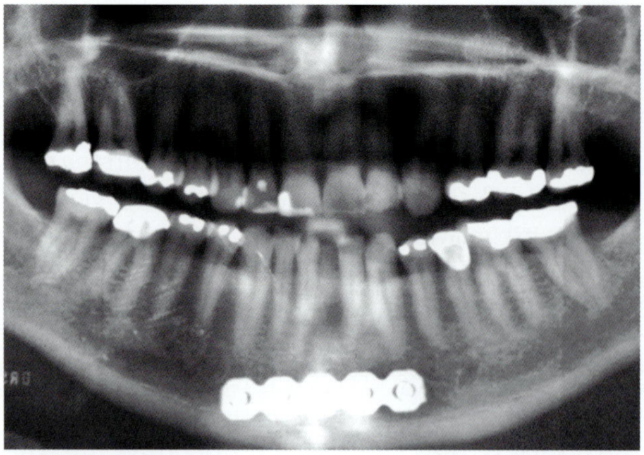

FIGURE 8-32. Panoramic radiograph showing a well-healed mandibulotomy approach with missing left central incisor.

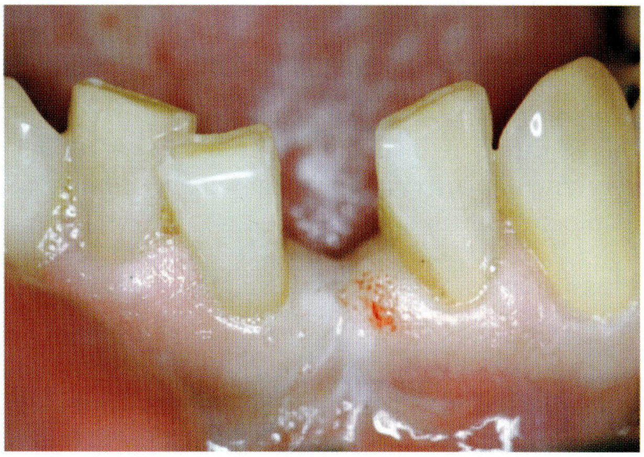

FIGURE 8-33. Missing mandibular left central incisor after a mandibulotomy approach for a base of tongue cancer.

surgical protocol. After placement of the implant, an impression is made, preferably with vinyl-polysiloxane, and an immediate provisional prosthesis can be placed. The impression is taken to the laboratory and an appropriate laboratory analog is placed. Improved stone is poured and a master cast is used to fabricate the prosthesis (Figure 8-34). After the porcelain is fused to the metal crown, the provisional prosthesis is removed, the implant is evaluated for any mobility, and, if any mobility is present, the implant is considered a failure. If there is no mobility, the crown is tried to place, adjusted, and cemented with the practitioner's choice of luting agent (Figures 8-35 to 8-37). The luting agent can be temporary cement or any of the various permanent luting agents. The MDI is a great treatment option for these narrow spaces, preserving actual

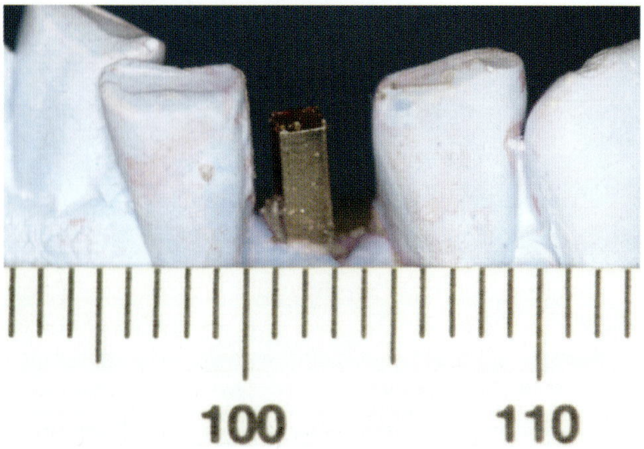

FIGURE 8-34. Standard wall MDI laboratory analog showing the limited edentulous space available.

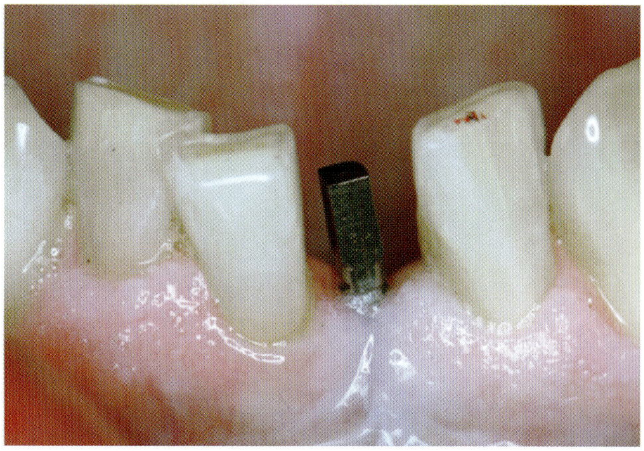

FIGURE 8-35. MDI at the time of surgery before placement of the provisional crown.

tooth and providing an immediate prosthetic rehabilitation to the surgical area.

Maxillofacial prosthetics:

The MDIs can also be considered to stabilize extra oral prosthetics. Although a very limited number of patients have been selected and actually utilized this treatment plan, further research is necessary for a long-term follow-up and true scientific proof of use. The first of two patients to use the implants was a 17-year-old female with hemi-facial microsomia with no formation of an inner ear complex on the left side. Utilizing a CT scan and implant planning software three MDIs were placed in the temporal bone to aid in retention of her auricular prosthesis. The implants can be altered in length using a sterilized carborundum disc with copious irrigation to remove debris. However, the major drawback to using the MDI is that altering the retentive appliance is difficult. The patient is treatment planned for o-ring retention were

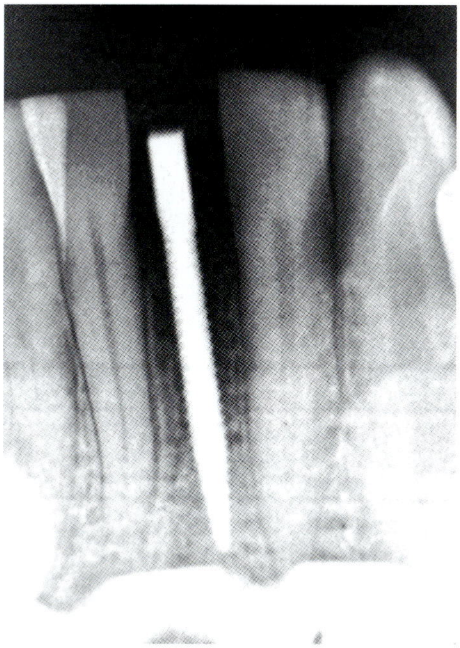

FIGURE 8-36. Periapical radiograph showing the position of the 1.8-mm MDI in relation to the adjacent teeth.

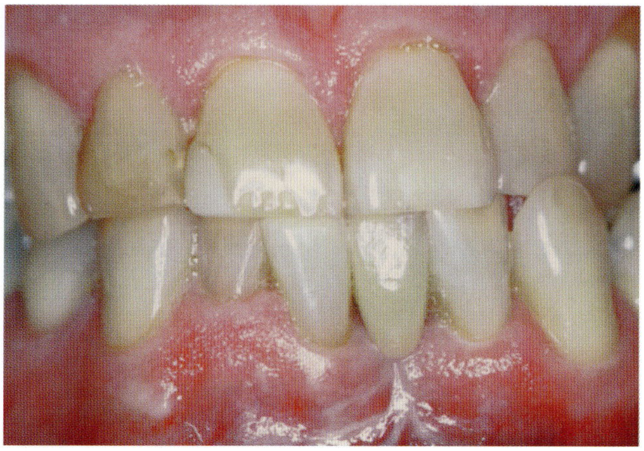

FIGURE 8-37. Completed porcelain fused to metal crown replacing the missing mandibular left central incisor.

as if a conventional craniofacial implant is use a multitude of bars, magnets, clips are at the practitioner's disposal. The second patient that was attempted with success was 62-year-old female status post a maxillectomy, radiation therapy, and partial rhinectomy with a failed attempt at reconstruction. The patient was fitted with an adhesive retained nasal prosthesis, however, desired mechanical retention as well. Two MDIs were placed utilizing a CT scan and implant planning software to aid in retention of her nasal prosthesis (Figs. 8-38 to 8-41).

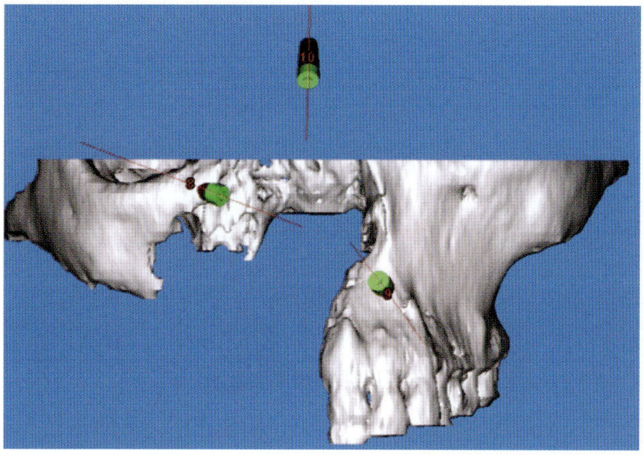

FIGURE 8-38. Implant plan for MDIs to retain the patient's nasal prosthesis.

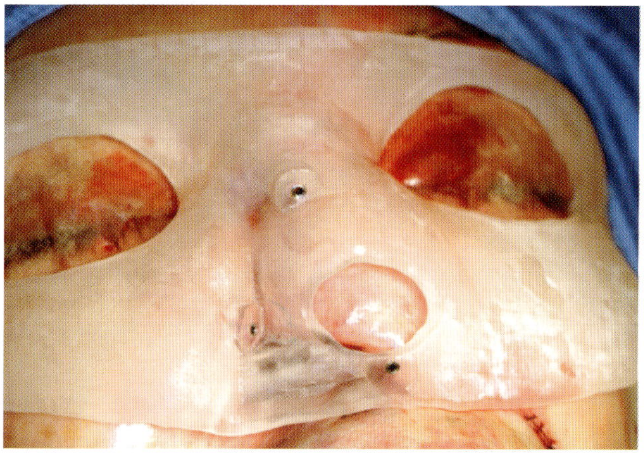

FIGURE 8-39. MDI surgical guide in place for placement of the implants.

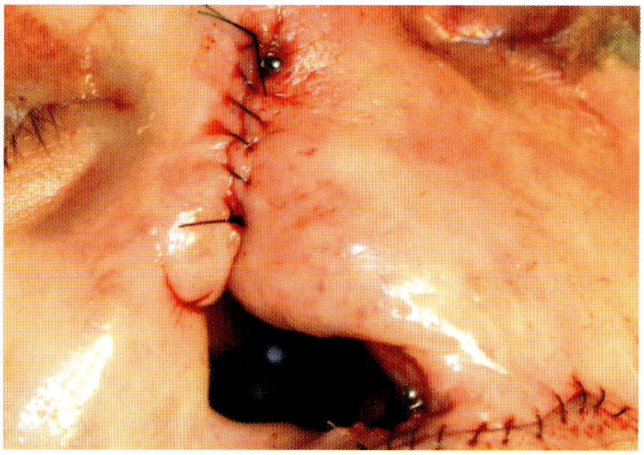

FIGURE 8-40. Two MDIs placed at the same time the plastic and reconstructive team revised the patient's scars.

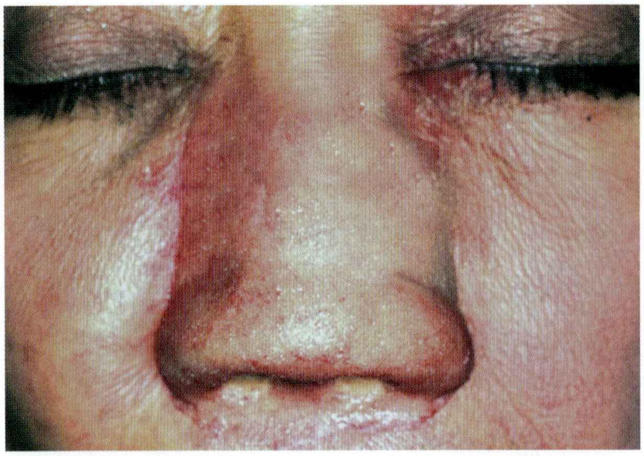

FIGURE 8-41. Final prosthesis in place using O rings for primary retention and minimal liquid adhesive to secure the edges of the prosthesis.

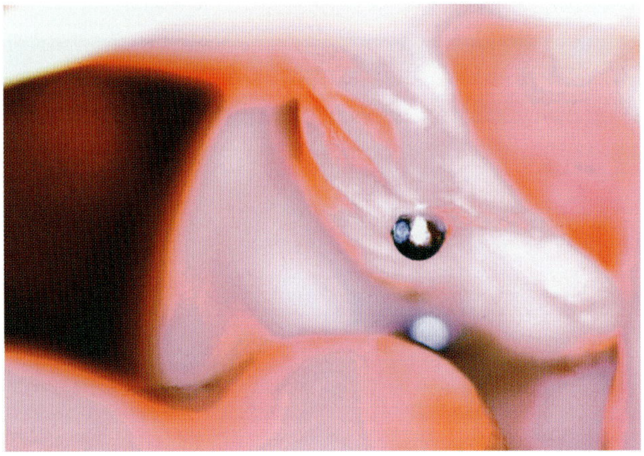

FIGURE 8-42. Two MDIs in the left maxillary segment of an infant with cleft palate.

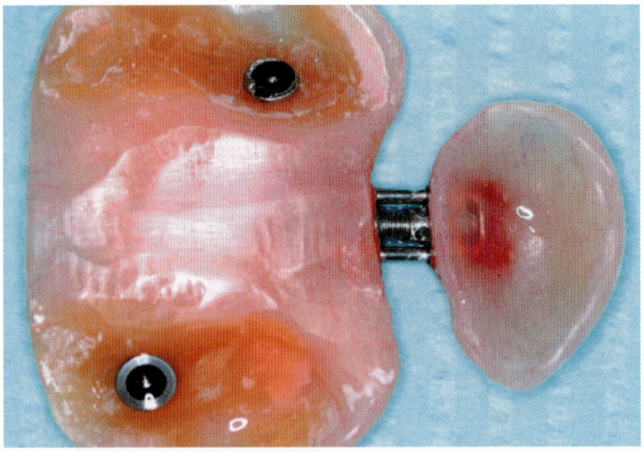

FIGURE 8-43. O rings incorporated into cleft palate appliance with jack-screw.

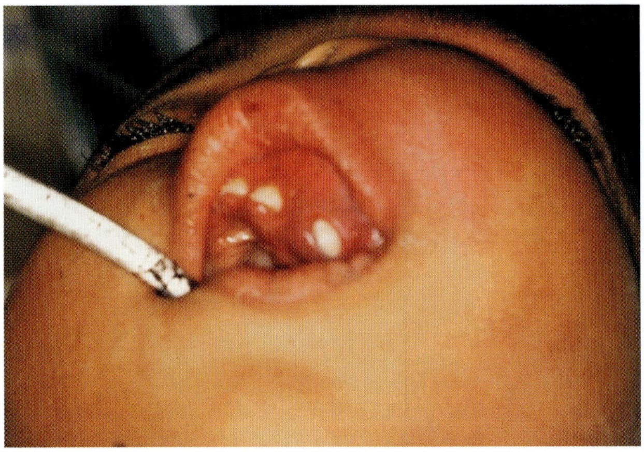

FIGURE 8-44. Infant with osteofibroma of the left maxillary sinus.

One other maxillofacial prosthetic application of MDIs explored was in the pediatric cleft palate and oncology patient population. Two male infants ranging in ages of 22 months and 26 months had MDIs placed in the bilateral cleft segments in the hopes of retaining a nasoalveolar molding appliance (Figures 8-42 and 8-43); 10-mm length implants were adjusted to be 5 to 6 mm long and were placed in the infantile maxillary bone. The surgical placement of the implants went without complication; however, the infantile bone density is so soft that the implants were lost within 10 days. The implant sites failed within 5 to 7 days without other complication— but the patients were subjected to a procedure that was not successful. A third infant was selected for implant placement; a 28-month-old boy had an osteofibroma of the left maxillary sinus. The tumor was ablated, and three MDIs were placed in the remaining maxilla. The prosthesis was immediately stabilized by these implants, which were successful until the age of 38 months (Figures 8-44 and 8-45). The implant sites healed without complication. Therefore MDIs for maxillofacial prosthetics both intra- and extraoral can be used with a relative degree of success, but not in the infantile cleft palate population. The extraoral application of the implants in the two patients described was successful, but consideration to conventional craniofacial implants should be given due to the increased diameter lending to greater surface area and the ability to alter the attachment apparatus. These implants, however, can be considered for the patients who have no other means of attachment or cannot afford the other procedure as described.

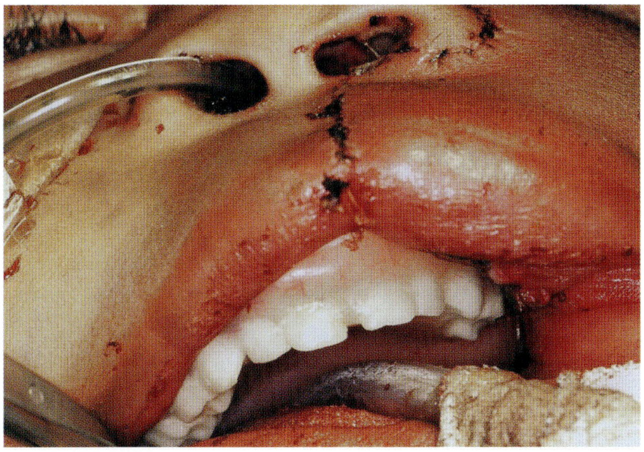

FIGURE 8-45. Surgical obturator delivered after maxillectomy and MDI placement.

References

1. Alsaadi G, Quirynen M, Komárek A, et al: Impact of lack and systemic factors on the incidence of late oral implant loss, *Clin Oral Impl Res* 19:670–676, 2008.
2. Beyzadeoglu M, Dirican B, Oysul K, et al: Evaluation of scatter dose of dental titanium implants exposed to photon beams of different energies and irradiation angles in head and neck radiotherapy, *Dentomaxillofac Radiol* 35:14–17, 2006.
3. Binger T, Seifert H, Blass G, et al: Dose inhomogeneities on surfaces of different dental implants during irradiation with high-energy photons, *Dentomaxillofac Radiol* 37(3):149–153, 2008.
4. Bohle GC, Mitcherling WW, Mitcherling JJ, et al: Immediate Obturator Stabilization Using Mini Dental Implants, *J Prosthodont* 17(6):482–486, 2008.
5. Bohle GC 3rd, Rieger J, Huryn J, et al: Efficacy of speech aid prostheses for acquired defects of the soft palate and velopharyngeal inadequacy- clinical assessments and cephalometric analysis: a Memorial Sloan-Kettering Study, *Head Neck* 27(3):195–207, 2005.
6. Colella G, Cannavale R, Pentenero M, et al: Oral implants in radiated patients: a systematic review, *Int J Oral Maxillofac Implants* 22(4):616–622, 2007.
7. Esposito M, Grusovin MG, Patel S, et al: Interventions for replacing missing teeth: hyperbaric oxygen therapy for irradiated patients who require dental implants, *Cochrane Database Syst Rev* 23(1):CD003603, 2008.
8. Esposito M, Grusovin MG, Talati M, et al: Interventions for replacing missing teeth: antibiotics at dental implant placement to prevent complications, *Cochrane Database Syst Rev* 16(3):CD004152, 2008.
9. Fischer DJ, Epstein JB: Management of patients who have undergone head and neck cancer therapy, *Dent Clin North Am* 52(1):39–60, 2008.
10. Grant BT, Amendeo C, Freeman K, et al: Outcomes of placing dental implants in patients taking oral bisphosphonates: a review of 115 cases, *J Oral Maxillofac Surg* 66(2):223–230, 2008.
11. Hancock PJ, Epstein JB, Sdler GR: Oral and dental management related to radiation therapy for head and neck cancer, *J Can Dent Assoc* 69(9):585–590, 2003.
12. Huryn JM, Piro JD: The maxillary immediate surgical obturator prosthesis, *J Prosthet Dent* 61(3):343–347, 1989.
13. Hwang D, Wan HL: Medical Contraindications to Implant Therapy: Part I: Absolute Contraindications, *Implant Dent* 15(4):353–358, 2006.
14. Karr RA, Kramer DC, Toth BB: Dental implants and chemotherapy complications, *J Prosthet Dent* 67(5):683–687, 1992.
15. Kovács AF: Influence of chemotherapy on endosteal implant survival and success in oral cancer patients, *Int J Oral Maxillofac Surg* 30(2):144–147, 2001.
16. Marx RE, Johnson RP: Studies in the radiobiology of osteoradionecrosis and their clinical significance, *Oral Surg Oral Med Oral Pathol* 64(4):379–390, 1987.
17. Oh WS, Roumanas E, Beumer J III: Maxillofacial Restoration after Head and Neck Tumor Therapy, *Compendium* 28(2):70–77, 2007.
18. Resnik RR, Misch C: Prophylactic Antibiotic Regimens in Oral Implantology: Rationale and Protocol, *Implant Dent* 17:142–150, 2008.
19. Schepers RH, Slagter AP, Kaanders JH, et al: Effect of postoperative radiotherapy on the functional result of implants placed during ablative surgery for oral cancer, *Int J Oral Maxillofac Surg* 35(9):803–808, 2006.
20. Schoen PJ, Raghoebar GM, Bouma, et al: Rehabilitation of oral function in head and neck cancer patients after radiotherapy with implant-retained dentures: effects of hyperbaric oxygen therapy, *Oral Oncol* 43(4):379–388, 2007.
21. Scully C, Madrid C, Bagan J: Dental endosseous implants in patients on bisphosphonate therapy, *Implant Dent* 15(3):212–218, 2006.
22. Steiner M, Windchy A, Gould AR, et al: Effects of chemotherapy in patients with dental implants, *J Oral Implantol* 21(2):142–147, 1995.
23. Wang R, Pillai K, Jones PK: Dosimetric measurement of scattered radiation from dental implants in simulated head and neck radiotherapy, *Int J Oral Maxillofac Implants* 13(2):197–203, 1998.

Chapter 9

The Orthodontist's Role in MDI Therapeutics

ORTHO Transitional Anchorage Devices (TADs) and Related Applications

FRANS CURRIER   ONUR KADIOGLU

Outline

Introductory Background by Dr. Victor Sendax

Early on in the development of the mini dental implant (MDI) concepts, it became increasingly evident that applying a modified Sendax insertion protocol to the problems of achieving orthodontic anchorage was originally a niche procedure that now offered significant benefits in a setting that was ripe for innovation.

The key advantage gained by inserting these ultra-streamlined transitional anchorage devices into mature bone with virtually no invasive bony drilling was the achievement of immediate functional resistance to opposing force, essential for any measurable orthodontic movement, and often without exclusive reliance on traditional intraoral or extraoral orthodontic appliances. An added potential benefit thus came to the fore when considering that these mini implant devices typically can also play a more long-term definitive role in selected cases, in which lost dentition required fixed prosthodontic replacement, along with reliably stable retention for removable systems.

As a prime center for orthodontic research, University of Oklahoma has contributed the following section as a review of its research and clinical perspectives on temporary anchorage devices (TADs) for the orthodontic domain:

Dr. Frans Currier, Member of Founding Faculty and Professor of Graduate Orthodontics, University of Oklahoma, summarizes his extensive experiences with MDI orthodontic applications. Dr. Onur Kadidoglu, Assistant Professor of Orthodontics at University of Oklahoma, has been instrumental, in association with Dr. Currier, in advancing the specialized research and development supporting the use of TADs.

Introduction to Anchorage and Biomechanics

The use of anchorage is important in orthodontic biomechanics. Root lengths, shapes, and surface areas help differentiate teeth that resist tooth movement.[67] Reciprocal effects influence the teeth that do not have direct forces applied, and collateral effects are secondary involving the teeth to which the force is applied.

Areas of anchorage have been classically designated by area—extraoral versus intraoral. This labeling is done both for the force system itself and anchorage considerations.

Extraoral anchorage is the oldest anchorage system in contemporary orthodontics and includes both facebow and J-hook headgears in Class II correction or anterior retraction compared with the facemask, which is used in maxillary protraction for cases of Class III maxillary deficiency problems. The application of headgears is usually labeled as occipital anchorage whether it involves high, straight, or low pull. The neck strap is related to the low pull headgear, which can be identified as the Kloehn type that was introduced in the 1940s.[36]

The intraoral application of anchorage can be divided by arch and teeth. Palatal anchorage has been used for more than 150 years for the maxillary dentition; the mandible is newer, was originally called Baker anchorage when it was introduced in the 1890s, and is weaker in the mandible due to its form and flexibility. Dental anchorage is best used cross-arch rather than by quadrant. Individual tooth anchorage is weak.

Anchorage units are basically dictated by surface area and the type of adjacent bone, maxilla versus mandible. The usual cross-arch systems in the mandible include the lingual arch or lip bumper and in the maxilla the Nance holding arch, transpalatal bar or arch, or the vertical holding arch.

The word *anchorage* is used differently than as used in engineering. One can define it as resistance to unwanted tooth movement. Using Newton's Third Law, which states that for every action there is an equal and opposite reaction, anchorage can be defined as resistance to the orthodontic reactive forces, which are those reacting to ones created from the appliances on the teeth that the orthodontists wish to move. These inevitable reactive forces do have the ability to move teeth just like the applied forces. Therefore, in planning orthodontic biomechanics, it would be inadequate to only concentrate on the movement of the teeth that are desired to be moved. Successful and efficient biomechanics can be achieved by knowing how to deal with the unwanted reactive forces or at least by being able to minimize them.

There is no doubt that temporary anchorage devices (TADs) can revolutionize the treatment mechanics in orthodontics. Complicated movements such as molar intrusion, arch intrusion, and retraction of anterior teeth or protraction of posterior teeth without reciprocal movement of the reactive units have previously been managed through various types of modified force systems, such as the manipulation of moment arms, pitting anchorage units with greater resistance against the tooth or teeth to be moved.[31] An important biomechanical aspect in the use of TADs is related to the direct application. Forces are different than moments. A moment is the tendency of a force to rotate an object about a point. Therefore, in orthodontics, forces are linear but moments circular. Couples are force systems separated by a distance and have equal and opposite vectors (i.e., edgewise brackets). Both couples and moments created in conventional retraction and protraction mechanics are not present when direct anchorage methods are used with the TADs. The TADs will not create any counteracting moments to cancel those in the active unit, which the anchorage teeth (reactive units) would create with conventional biomechanics. Because of this, when planning anchorage with TADs, clinicians should evaluate the mechanical setup carefully to understand the lack of reciprocal effects on the teeth. Basic biomechanical considerations still apply. Application of a force vector that does not pass through the center of resistance (biologic entity at furcation of multirooted teeth or one third the distance from the cementoenamel junction to the root apex in single-rooted teeth) still results in rotational movements. Centers of rotations, however, are defined by the moments about them and their resistance. Again, for every action there is an equal and opposite reaction. What changed with TADs was where the equal and opposite reactive forces occurred.[31] The reactive forces with TADs are dissipated in the skeleton. Knowing this not only changes the mechanics but, in fact, directs the clinician to greater attention in the biomechanical planning of the particular case.

Using various lever arms, one can control the point of force application and achieve desired intrusive or extrusive effects during retraction according to the patients' needs.[52,55]

In a series of articles by Cornelis et al.[8] and De Clerck et al.,[12,13] the biomechanical considerations in extraction versus nonextraction cases and intrusion mechanics were discussed. Although these authors focused on using mini plates, the same principles can apply to the mini screw TADs. They noted that regardless of the appliance used, the undesirable frictional forces may actually help correct the overjet in the early stages of treatment, thus reducing overall treatment time. In conventional sliding mechanics without TADs, permanent canines are distalized with elastics between the permanent canines and molars. The compensating moments are generated and cancel each other out, thus resulting in canine distalization with minimal overjet correction. However, if the TADs are used as the direct form of anchorage and if there is no contact between the maxillary and mandibular permanent incisors, the resulting force from the archwire will retract the four maxillary permanent incisors distally, thus reducing the overjet and the total treatment time. The authors also discuss the faciolingual aspect of the posterior teeth. The rotational moment of the reactive unit is again not present with TADs. The only moment is on the permanent canine, and it is not being neutralized. Therefore the arch wire will keep tilting, causing a crossbite on the distalization side of the canine. To prevent this, a transpalatal bar is recommended. These devices may also be used when intruding the posterior teeth in the maxillary arch, similar to a fixed lingual arch in providing control for intrusion of the mandibular posterior teeth. Some clinicians suggest the use of palatal TADs for better control on the maxillary permanent molars during intrusion.

Immediate loading of the TADs has been under investigation for more than a decade. Current literature is inconclusive whether the clinicians should immediately load the TADs. However, immediate loading seems to be acceptable with reduced forces.[45,46,9] These light loads are between 25 and 50 grams.

Owens et al.[48] evaluated the stability of TADs in relation to the timing, amount, and location of force application. They tested 56 TADs on skeletally mature male beagle dogs. The maxillary TADs were divided into two groups of immediate loading and delayed loading. In the mandible all the TADs were immediately loaded. The experimental TADs had a corresponding unloaded control. They presented an overall success rate of 93% with no significant effects of timing, amount, or location of force applied. No correlations were reported between the timing of force application and the success rate.

Temporary Anchorage Devices

The application of skeletal anchorage devices in orthodontics currently has come from the extensive use of skeletal implants used in restorative dentistry. These osseointegrated devices have directed dentistry in new directions from surgical management through the restoration of the implants. These changes include input from general dentistry, oral surgery, and periodontics. The application in orthodontics has included osseointegrated bars and screws as well as onplants.[60-63,3] The trend is toward screws that are not osseointegrated for bony anchorage that make tooth anchorage more strong, either in an indirect or direct manner.

Many articles have been published describing this novel method of attaining seemingly absolute anchorage, especially after Kanomi's 1997 article,[30] which gave rise to the modern TADs that are being used today.

The traditional implants as skeletal anchorage have not reached wide-spread use in orthodontics for several reasons. The traditional implants used in dentistry, such as the Brånemark system, have limitations that make their use in orthodontics problematic. These implants are often too large to be placed in convenient places, remain costly, and require a fairly invasive surgical procedure, followed by extended healing time.[6] These limitations have spurred a number of innovative implant designs and sizes in recent years.

The advent of mini- or microimplants now provides the orthodontic profession with a viable option for skeletal anchorage. A recent term used to describe these implants for skeletal anchorage is *temporary anchorage device* (TAD). Considering the traditional implants in dentistry that are designed and manufactured for long lasting prosthetic replacements or for stabilization of removable prostheses, the term is fitting for the implants use in orthodontics. The word *temporary* indicates the removal of the TADs after the desired orthodontic movement is completed.

Some researchers prefer *temporary skeletal anchorage device* (TSAD). TSAD may be a more descriptive term for these mini screws. However, due its wide acceptance, the term TADs will be used here.

Numerous reports have been published about the success of TADs in supplying anchorage for orthodontic tooth movements. They are becoming more and more widely used in clinical orthodontics.

Much has improved since the introduction of TADs in 1945 by Gainsforth and Higley[15] from the University of Iowa. They were the first investigators who thought it was time to investigate alternative anchorage resources in orthodontics and tried using the basal bone with an animal model. They were inspired by a series of surgical techniques described in Shaar and Kreuz's 1943[63] text *Manual of Fractures*. Vitallium, being the most biocompatible and inert alloy at the time, was the choice of material for the screw hooks. Their screws were 13 mm in length with a diameter of 3.4 mm. They were placed in the ramus immediately distal to the last molar. Maxillary canines were banded in each of the six dogs, and four of the dogs had an orthodontic appliance using an elastic that stretched from the implant to a jig in the maxillary arch and then to the maxillary canine for orthodontic traction. The remaining two dogs served as controls with no traction forces applied on their teeth. Placement of the implants occurred under general anesthesia using sterile techniques. The implants were immediately loaded after placement with an elastic force of 140 to 200 g. Although the hope for basal bone anchorage existed, their results were not supportive of the idea. None of the screws stayed more than 31 days, but the teeth moved a few millimeters with minimal anchorage loss, which was not enough to inspire the profession.

After Gainsforth and Highley's unsuccessful attempt, further research into skeletal anchorage in orthodontics was limited for some time. More than 20 years later, Linkow of New York published the next article on the subject of implants and their usage as skeletal anchorage units in orthodontics in 1969.[41] His article described the use of an endosseous blade implant in orthodontics. These implants had been successfully used in dentistry for several years before his report, but the orthodontic community was relatively skeptical of the ideas brought forth by Linkow. One year later, Linkow[40] published a follow-up article in 1970 that established his position in the development of implants in orthodontics. He noted that most of the emphasis in implantology to that time was placed on perfecting implant design and techniques. He added that several years of proven success made it possible to broaden the range of implant applications, and he advocated implant use as an adjunct to conventional orthodontic therapy. In this article he listed problems that could benefit from the use of endosseous implants. The six cases that Linkow selected were patients with missing teeth or with teeth that were lost in the course of orthodontic treatment. The implant functioned to replace these missing teeth, either to maintain space or as anchorage on which the force systems were applied directly to the restored implant. He argued that implants could be used to prevent drifting of teeth and act as an anchorage point. Linkow asserted that implants could eliminate the need for extraoral anchorage devices.

The transition into a more contemporary look for the implants took another 13 years. Creekmore and Eklund[10] presented a case report of a 25-year-old woman. This was the first temporary anchorage device placed specifically to aid orthodontic mechanics and had a screw type design. The investigators placed a Vitallium bone screw just below the anterior nasal spine and used a light elastic thread to it, on which they attempted to intrude the maxillary incisors to correct her deep bite. They were able to intrude and torque the maxillary central incisors with the help of the screw. The Vitallium screw remained stationary for a year until the mechanics were completed. They posed the question "Might skeletal anchorage be applied to orthodontic tooth movement and orthopedic jaw movement?" In the same year, the stability of the Vitallium screws was confirmed on a histologic animal model by Gray et al.[19]

The advances in biomaterials introduced titanium to dentistry. After the report[1] of the American Dental Association (ADA) Council on Scientific Affairs in 1996, the use of endosseous implants increased. The ADA accepted the use of both pure titanium and titanium alloy implants. Although the clinical data for long-term success of the endosseous implants is still lacking, titanium has been used for more than 25 years and used for both endosseous and subperiosteal implants in many different forms such as rods, posts, blades, and finally mini screws. The process of living tissues becoming structurally and functionally connected with the oxide surface of the body of the implant is called *osseointegration.* This process is necessary for the prosthodontic use of implants. However, it is not a requirement for a successful application of an orthodontic mini screw. Although a recent report[34] promotes the need for partial osseointegration for orthodontic mini screws, it may complicate their removal as temporary anchorage devices and may not be widely accepted under the presence of numerous successful clinical studies.

In the late 1990s, the contemporary designs made with pure titanium and titanium alloys were introduced, and clinical trials were initiated. In 1995 Block and Hoffman[3] introduced the "onplant" and evaluated possible palatal applications. They used a design that measured 10 mm in diameter and 2 mm in height. The implant itself was a disk with one side textured in addition to a hydroxyapatite coating. On the opposite side, it had an internal thread for attachments. The onplant resided on the surface of the palatal bone, and after osseointegration, it could withstand enough force to be used for orthodontic anchorage. The onplant was tested in both animal and human models and proved safe and effective for intraoral anchorage. However, its use resulted in limited acceptance due to a large surgical flap on the palate for both placement and removal.

The palatal trend has been similar to facial applications whereby the initial versions were endosseous and later were being replaced by mini screw type, nonosseointegration TADs. Wehrbein et al.[69] introduced an anchorage setup through a transpalatal bar for en masse retraction of maxillary anterior teeth. It was done without the use of compliance-dependent appliances such as headgear or elastics. They reported a mean anchorage loss of 0.7 mm on the right side and 1.1 mm on the left side.

Numerous studies have been published investigating the possibilities of using palatal TADs either by assisting holding arches or by assisting intraoral distalization appliances in an indirect manner. In 1997, Kanomi[30] reported using miniscrew for anchorage in an intrusion case. His work initiated the concept of modern TADs. In 1998, zygoma ligatures were proposed as an option for maxillary anchorage.[47] In 1999 Umemori et al.[68] discussed skeletal anchorage systems and titanium miniplates for correction of open bites.

In the last decade, efforts have been made in Asia and Europe to achieve skeletal anchorage with the use of small titanium screws, palatal implants, and miniplates with screws. The lack of Food and Drug Administration clearance discouraged pursuit of this research topic in the United States. Mini screws were found to be minimally invasive, had few anatomical limitations, could be used in the palate and with adolescents, were less expensive than osseointegrated dental implants, and could be immediately loaded because osseointegration was not a prerequisite. The FDA approval of titanium screws for anchorage in orthodontics first came in effect in 2003. Since then, the number of the screw systems has increased by the introduction of new systems in the United States market. Today there are about 15 mini screw systems available for use in the United States.

Biological Considerations

A number of studies in the dental literature look at osseointegration and bone remodeling around the endosseous implants. Huja et al.[23-25] studied bone adaptation and response to TADs.

In their studies, they looked at the effect of micro cracks in the bone caused by the insertion of the TADs. Their results indicated that regional bone turnover was elevated. The increased rates noted were 100% to 200% recorded during the healing period of 6 to 12 months. This was in contrast to normal cortical bone turnover rate, which was 2% to 20% per year.[24] The authors called this phenomenon a localized bone adaptation response.

Indications and Applications

The application of TADs in orthodontics has its use in the young permanent dentition, the adolescent dentition (all 28 permanent teeth erupted), or the adult dentition. Its use for patients younger than 12 years old is limited, so interception of malocclusion in the primary and transitional dentitions with TAD anchorage can be substituted with either other intraoral devices or extraoral anchorage. Sex and race are not associated with limitations in the use of TADs.

The three planes of space model are used in contemporary orthodontics. The transverse plane of the face and the arches matures the earliest. Therefore correction of posterior crossbites or narrow dental arches needs to be done early, preferably younger than the age of 12 years. These transverse skeletal problems are resistant to surgical intervention in late adolescence or in the young adult. The TADs have limited application in this plane of space.

Angle's classification is a dental classification of the arches based upon the position of the maxillary permanent first molars. It is a system that emphasizes the sagittal plane. Most anomalies of the dentition are related to Class I malocclusions. If extraction of premolars is needed in these cases, TADs might be helpful. The application for nonextraction therapy of these cases is limited.

Class III malocclusions are not common, and many are centered around a maxillary deficiency that necessitates maxillary expansion and protraction early. These are nonextraction orthodontic cases in the maxilla unless it is surgical case of maxillary advancement after growth is complete. The use of the osseointegrated plate with protraction facemask could be considered here. However, the use of TADs is limited.

Class II malocclusions have a spectrum of presentations. These can be skeletal or dental in origin. The Class II, division 2 malocclusion is much rarer than the Class II, division 1 malocclusion. The II-2 pattern usually presents more as a Class I skeletal deep bite problem with vertical maxillary central incisors. These nonextraction cases need to be treated during growth. Extraction of first premolars in the maxilla usually does not allow favorable esthetic results. The application of TADs could be used for mandibular anchorage to prevent the lower arch from coming too far forward. However, the use of TADs in the lower arch is similar to the fixed lingual arch in that it reduces normal vertical increases with the posterior tooth eruption and, therefore, can adversely affect the anterior overbite. These patients usually have low smile expressions and deep bites that prevent the use of TADs in the maxillary anterior to open the bite.

The Class II, division 1 malocclusion presents either extraction or nonextraction protocols for the premolars. If extractions are indicated in the maxilla, TADs can assist in anterior retraction. If extractions are indicated in the mandible, TADs can assist in either anterior retraction or posterior protraction. Many end-to-end malocclusions can be treated with maxillary molar rotations and nonextraction therapy with maximum mandibular anchorage.

Three masters' theses on TADs have been completed at the University of Oklahoma. The first investigated the anchorage possibility of TADs in extraction cases for the maxilla and the other in the mandible. The third one investigated the anchorage use of TADs in nonextraction Class II treatment protocol with fixed functional appliances. All three studies were approved and periodically reviewed by the Institutional Review Board of the University of Oklahoma Health Sciences Center. The TAD system used for all three studies was the Ortho Implant (IMTEC, Ardmore, OK). The initial version of this system was an established FDA-approved mini implant system (Sendax MDI) that had been modified for an off-label, novel use in orthodontic patients as anchorage. Currently it is marketed as Ortho Implants specifically for orthodontic use.

The first study[20,21,22] investigated the retraction of maxillary permanent canines.

The study[22] comprised 16 subjects who had maxillary first premolars extracted. TADs were placed between the roots of the maxillary permanent first molars and the second premolars by one oral surgeon. All retraction was accomplished on 0.017 × 0.025-in stainless steel archwires in 0.022-in slots by using nickel-titanium springs stretched from the implant head to the brackets on the permanent canines. Because this was the first study completed in the department, investigators tested different placement protocols. In the first protocol, the investigators used a noninvasive protocol. However, it resulted in the loss of 51% of the implants (19 of 39); the second protocol required a small flap surgery and resulted in 100% stability (10 of 10). The

TABLE 9-1

Calculated Monthly Canine Retraction Rates

Total Time (d)	Left Side Total Distance (mm)	Calculated Mean Rate (mm/mo)	Patient	Total Time (d)	Right Side Total Distance (mm)	Calculated Mean Rate (mm/mo)
64	4.1	1.9	1	64	4.2	2
107	6.3	1.8	2	72	5.6	2.4
28	1.6	1.8	3	28	2.1	2.2
113	**5.75**	**1.5**	4	**113**	**5.72**	**1.5**
83	**4.3**	**1.5**	5	**83**	**2.5**	**0.9**
152	**6.4**	**1.3**	6	**152**	**5.4**	**1.1**
114	4.6	1.2	7	**114**	**6.8**	**1.8**
91	3.5	1.2	8	91	2	0.7
98	3.75	1.15	9	**98**	**1.42**	**0.4**
152	**4.3**	**0.9**	10	**152**	**6.7**	**1.2**
126	3.8	0.9	11	91	3.6	1.2
91	**2.66**	**0.9**	12	**91**	**2.51**	**0.9**
98	2.25	0.7	13	98	1.89	0.5
126	2.5	0.6	14	126	4.4	1.1

Bold numbers indicate the second protocol was used.
Data from Herman RJ, Currier GF, Miyake A: Mini-implant anchorage for maxillary canine retraction: a pilot study. *Am J Orthod Dentofac Orthop* 130:228, 2006.

calculated monthly canine retraction rates varied widely from 1.5 to 6.1 mm per month (Table 9-1). The researchers also noted excessive crown tipping into the extraction spaces in four of the 28 retracted canines, and this was related to the method of ligation of the canine to the archwire. They were able to preserve anchorage and concluded successful results in canine retraction.

The second study[60] evaluated en masse retraction of the mandibular incisors and retraction of mandibular permanent canines in selected cases. The sample contained 10 patients who had mandibular first premolars extracted for orthodontic treatment. TADs were placed laterally in the mandibular alveolar ridge between the roots of the permanent first and second molars by one oral surgeon. TADs were ligated to the bracket of the mandibular permanent first molars, providing indirect anchorage for retraction of the mandibular anterior teeth. All patients were treated with the 0.022-in slot Damon 2 appliance (Ormco, Glendora, CA). En masse retraction of the mandibular anterior teeth (n = 7) was accomplished on 0.019 × 0.025-in stainless steel archwires, and in certain cases canine retraction (n = 3) was accomplished on 0.018-in HiTi stainless steel archwires using nickel-titanium springs stretched from the mandibular permanent first molar brackets to anterior hooks soldered to the archwire or to the hooks on the canine bracket during en masse or canine retraction, respectively. Monthly rate of retraction was calculated for each mandibular canine. In the en masse retraction group of seven, total mean retraction for the canines was 0.61 mm per month with an arch length change of 0.56 mm per month. The canine retraction group of three demonstrated a total mean retraction rate of 1.75 mm per month for the canines. Overall, the reported retraction rates seemed appropriate compared with the findings of similar studies. Stability of the implants was reported to be very good, and results indicated minimal anchorage loss and good vertical control of the mandibular posterior dentition.

Similar findings from both studies were as follows: the soft tissue reactions were excellent; patient acceptance and tolerances were reported to be very high; and the Ortho Implant proved to be an effective TAD in the posterior maxilla or mandible to assist in retracting maxillary or mandibular anterior teeth (Table 9-2). After serving as anchorage devices, the implants were easily removed without any complications in both studies.

The third study investigated the skeletal, dental and soft tissue changes with Forsus fatigue resistance appliance with and without TADs.[27] Forsus appliances are fixed functional appliances used to correct Class II malocclusions. As they assist in correcting the Class II malocclusion, they tend to move the mandibular teeth forward, particularly the anterior ones, resulting in anchorage loss. The TADs were used to prevent this side effect from these fixed functional appliances. The stability, soft tissue health, and patient acceptance of TADs were also evaluated similar to the previously completed studies. A total of 20 patients in the permanent dentition, between 11 to 17 years of age, with Class II or end-on-end molar relationships and with an indication for nonextraction orthodontic treatment were randomly selected to participate. MBT prescription low profile Victory Series 0.022 × 0.028-in fixed orthodontic appliances were selected for bonding all the teeth, except for the maxillary permanent first molars, which were banded for application of the fixed functional appliances.

After leveling and aligning stages and the space closures, the Forsus appliances with or without TADs were delivered for correction of the Class II malocclusion. Cone Beam CT (CBCT) images were used for accuracy in locating the insertion site. Axial, coronal, and sagittal slices were used to determine the safest location between the roots of the mandibular second premolars and the permanent first molars. The level of insertion was measured from the orthodontic wire toward the apices of these teeth using the Dolphin 3D, Dolphin Imaging Version 10.1 (Dolphin Imaging, Chatsworth, CA) (Figure 9-1). Measurements were done using the software and then transferred to the patient using periodontal probes.

Group I included 11 patients, seven boys and four girls, with an average age of 12 years 3 months, and Group II included nine patients, seven boys and two girls with an average age of 12 years 9 months. Class II correction was continued until an edge-to-edge incisor relationship was achieved. The Forsus appliances were removed, and patients were instructed to wear Class II elastics half-time for the final settling of the occlusion. All TADs in this study were placed by one resident under the supervision of one orthodontic faculty. The preliminary results showed that the overbite was corrected as a result of proclination and intrusion of the mandibular permanent incisors and extrusion of the mandibular permanent first molars as well as growth of the mandible. Overjet and the Class II relation were corrected by proclination of the mandibular incisors and forward movement of the mandibular dentition as well as distal movement and tipping of the maxillary permanent molars.

In the group that received TADs, the anchorage loss was minimized in the mandibular dentition. The forward movement of the mandibular teeth was considerably less in the TAD group compared with the control group. The investigation also showed that the maxillary growth was better in the TAD group. TADs provided better vertical and

TABLE 9-2

Preliminary Summary of the Combined Data From Three Studies on Soft Tissue Health, Stability of TADs, and Patient Acceptance

		Soft Tissue Health			Stability of TADs			Patient Acceptance			
	# of TADs	A	B	C	A	B	C	A	B	C	# of Patients
Study 1	N = 39	19	10	10	19	–	20	10	5	1	N = 16
Study 2	N = 22	10	10	2	17	3	2	6	4	0	N = 10
Study 3	N = 18	3	15	0	14	2	2	7	2	0	N = 9
Totals	79	25	35	12	50	5	24	23	11	1	35
		A: Healthy. B: Erythematous. C: Purulent or necrotic.			A: No instability. B: Slight instability (< 1 mm). C: Mobile (≥ 1) or loss.			A: No discomfort. B: Slight discomfort. C: Moderate to severe discomfort.			

TADs, Transitional Anchorage Devices.

anteroposterior control for the maxillary posterior teeth that assisted in the correction the Class II malocclusion (Figure 9-2).

Nonextraction treatment of Class II malocclusions require more compliance from the patients and, therefore, could be more difficult. Park et al.[56] published a study on the group with distal movement of teeth using TADs. The sample included 13 patients with a mean age of 17.9 ± 5.7 years, and the authors used dental casts and cephalograms for

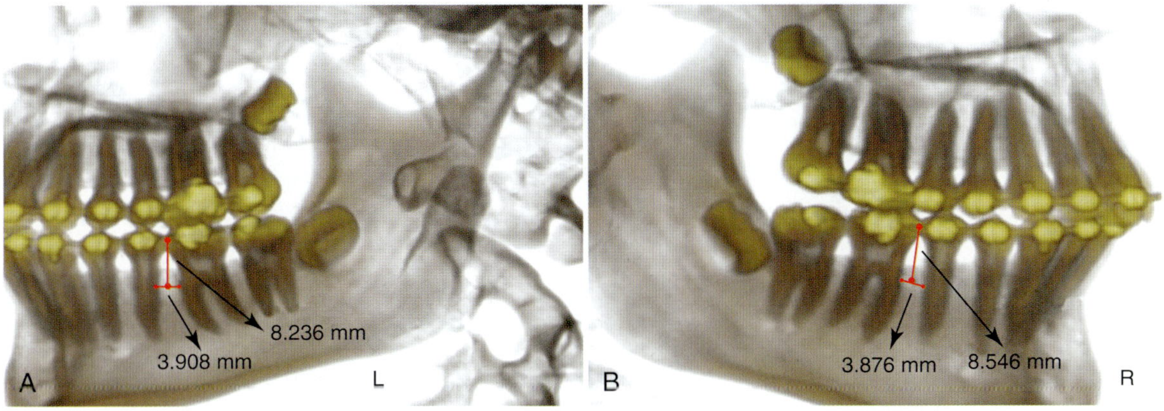

FIGURE 9-1. A, Right CBCT image before placement of TADs. **B,** Left CBCT image before placement of TADs.

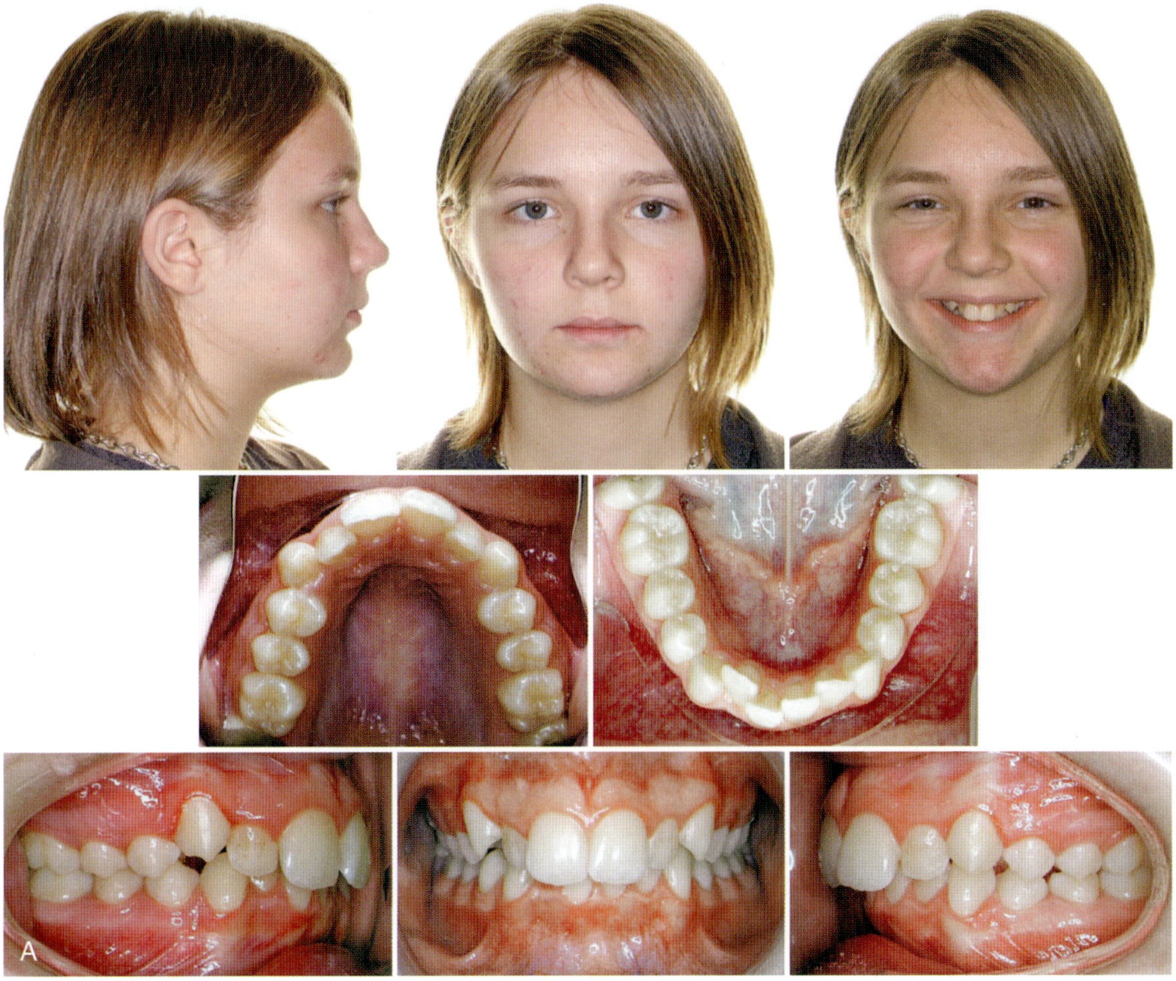

FIGURE 9-2. A, Records of a case from Group 1. Initial photos before treatment. Chronologic age: 13-4.

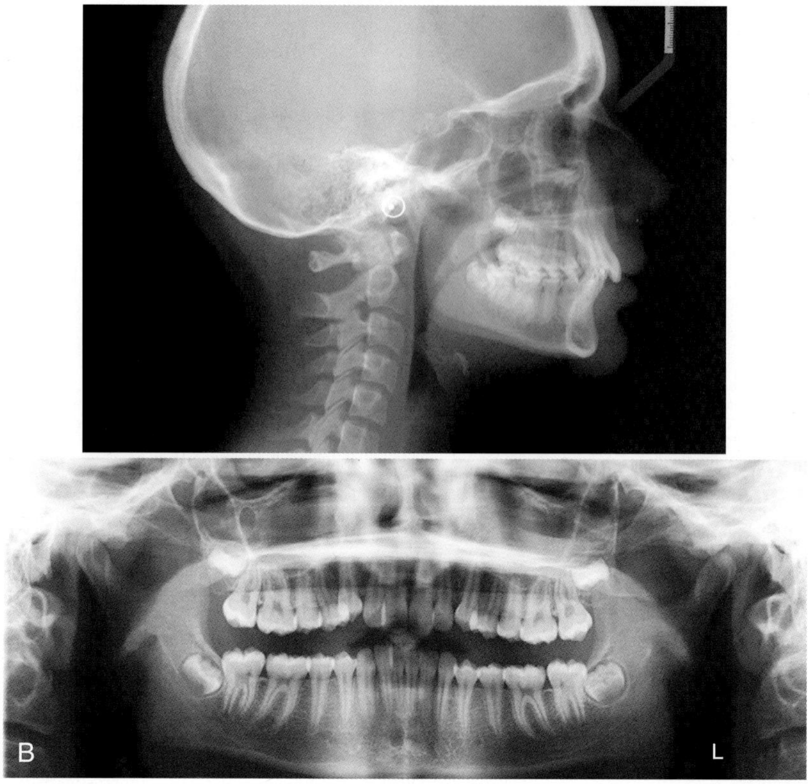

FIGURE 9-2—cont'd B, Initial lateral cephalometric and panoramic radiographs before treatment. Chronologic age 13-4.

evaluations. All patients were treated with a nonextraction orthodontic protocol, except for one patient who had been treated with maxillary first premolar extraction and distalization of the maxillary anterior teeth. A total of 11 patients had mandibular microscrew implants to distalize the entire mandibular dentition; four patients had maxillary microscrew implants, and two of these four patients had mandibular implants as well. They reported statistically significant differences between pre- and postrecordings, indicating that the teeth were effectively distalized. In addition, they did not observe any reciprocal side effects on the maxillary anterior teeth as one might normally expect when using molar distalizing appliances. Although statistically insignificant, simultaneous distalization of all the maxillary teeth could be noted as a worthwhile finding from the study. The authors also reported that all maxillary teeth showed intrusion during distalization. Mild distalization of the mandibular teeth was also noted. They showed a 90% success rate and concluded that TADs could provide significant anchorage for distalization mechanics, thus preventing back-and-forth movements and round tripping.

When distalizing the entire maxillary dentition with TADs, some researchers have advocated using mini plates instead of mini screws. Cornelis et al.[9] have been working with mini plates since the early 2000s, and they recently published a clinical study on 17 nongrowing patients who underwent en masse distalization of the maxillary arch for treatment of the Class II malocclusion using mini plates placed in the infrazygomatic crest. They loaded the mini plates 3 weeks after surgery with a 150-g force to distalize the molars. They were able to achieve an overtreated Class I relationship in all patients in 7 ± 2months. The authors concluded that maxillary molar distalization with mini plates was a predictable treatment modality for patients with Class II molar relationship.

There are six areas of orthodontics— preventive, interceptive, adjunctive, corrective, functional orthopedic, and orthognathic surgery. The use of TADs can be selectively used in corrective for various malocclusions as discussed but also in adjunctive orthodontic therapy. These adult adjunctive cases need selected tooth movement mostly for better fixed prosthodontics and for some removable

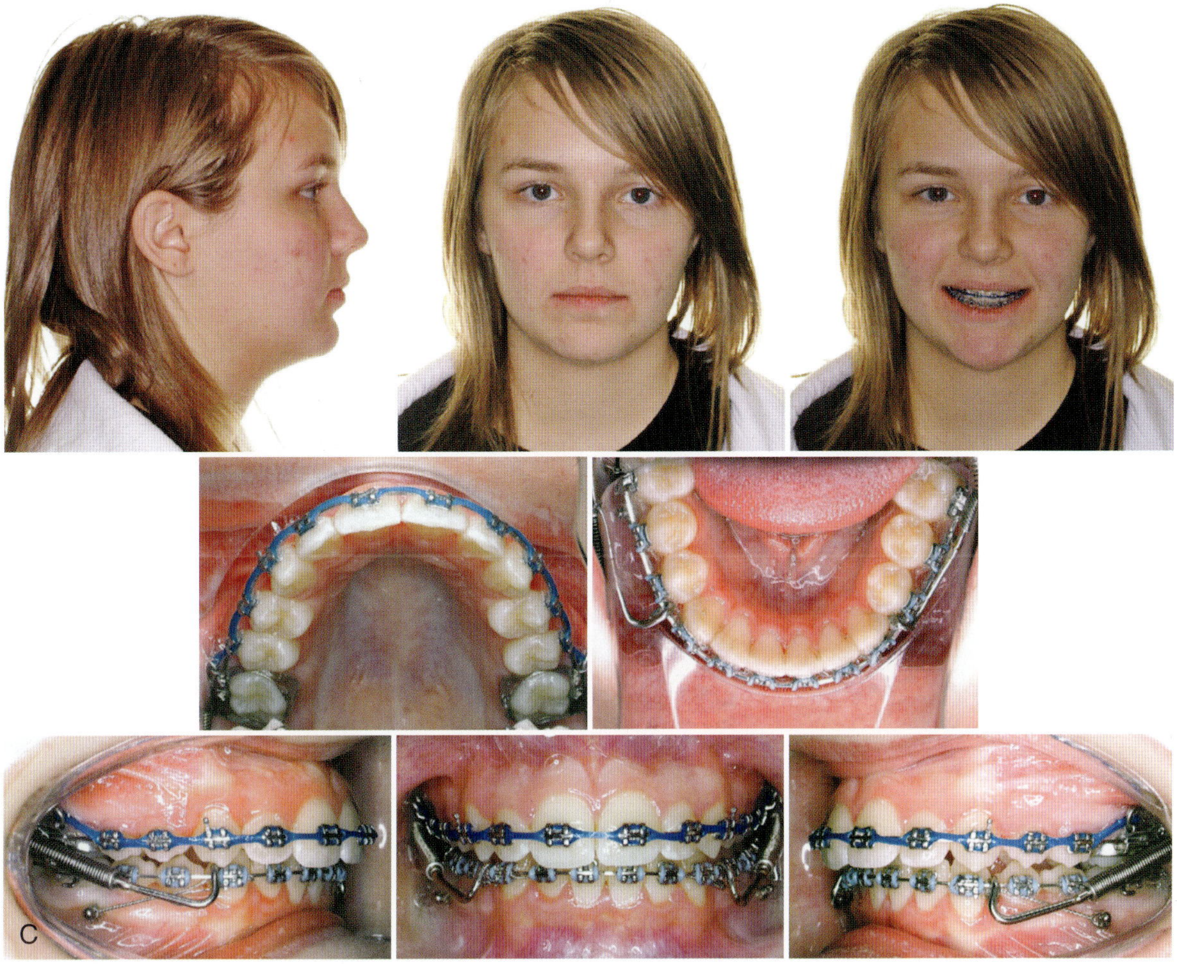

FIGURE 9-2—cont'd C, Progress photos after leveling and aligning with delivery of the Forsus device and TADs. Chronologic age 14-2.

prosthodontics. These TADs in the middle of an edentulous ridge with a surrounding composite/band allows reevaluation of the needs for more complicated cross-arch anchorage. Fixed functional appliances could also benefit from mandibular TAD anchorage.

The classification of the face assists in the analysis of those cases where TADs might be helpful. The vertical face is divided into anterior and posterior with the posterior identified inferior to the ears. These two areas do not correlate well. In preschoolers, they are both short. However, as one grows and matures, the relationship is usually inverse, with the anterior long/posterior short or the anterior short/posterior long. These are the extremes. Usually the posterior develops more due to the sigmoid curve of growth and the skeletal muscular system enlargement in adolescence.

Because everyone starts with short face syndrome, the orientation is toward nonextraction therapy. Patients with short face syndrome usually have short anterior faces, longer vertical noses, and very short faces inferior to the nose. These are nonextraction cases. TADs might be helpful only in preventing the lower arch from coming too far forward.

Patients with long faces can be identified early because they look mature for age. Not only is there a longer anterior face, but also the area inferior to the nose is much longer than normal. Many times these cases have short posterior vertical faces, which allow for the mesial components of force that naturally occur for the permanent molars to move anteriorly more rapidly. The use of TADs for either arch can be helpful. The use of TADs to prevent a vertical expression of the changes in

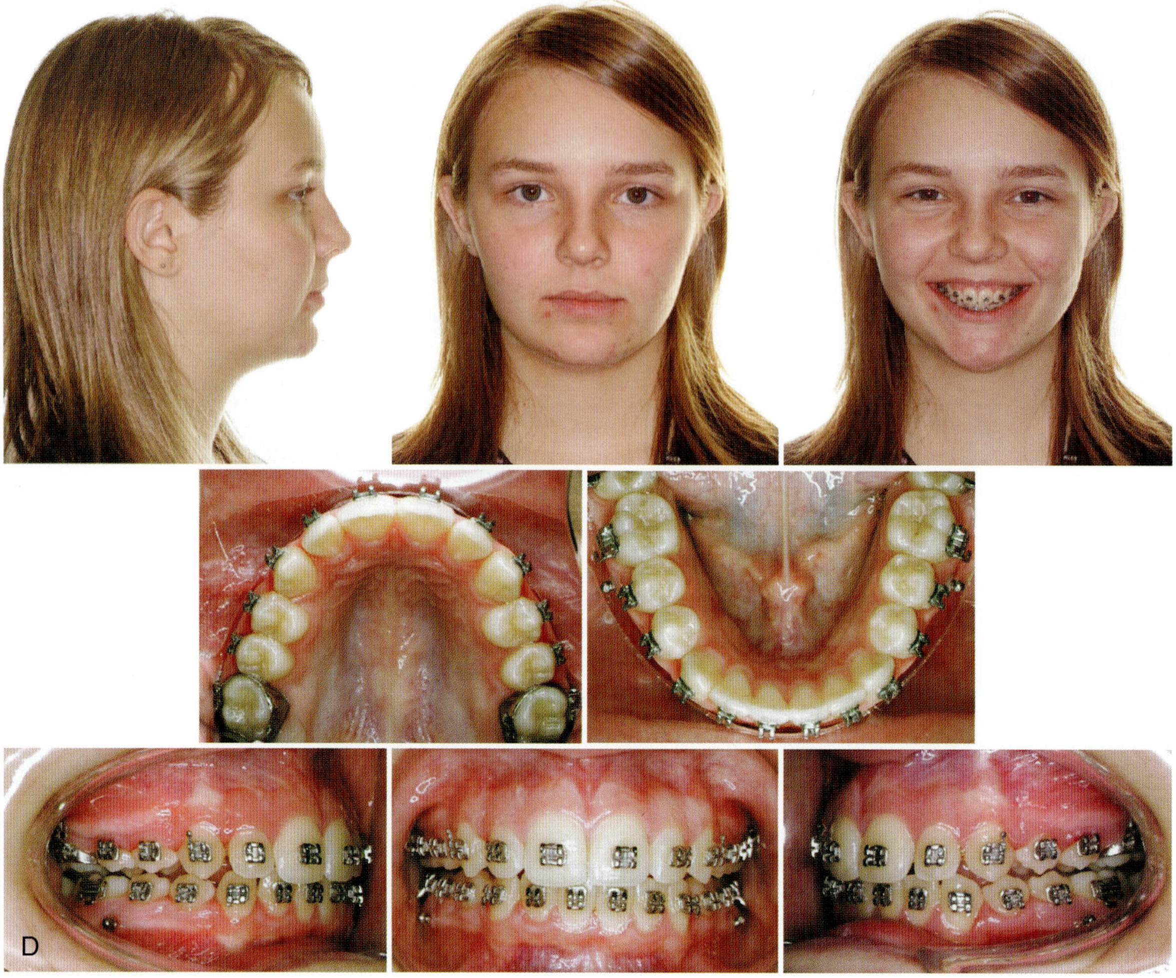

FIGURE 9-2—cont'd D, Progress photos after Class II correction. Chronologic age 14-7.

the occlusion can be also be very helpful. Patients with long faces have a thicker sagittal expression of the soft tissues compared with patients with short faces.

The relationship of the posterior face to the anterior is important and independent of the anterior face. The higher the mandibular plane to the occiput (skull), the greater the chance of posterior space loss. These are considered high angle cases, and the use of TADs could certainly be beneficial. The low angle cases, ones in which the mandibular planes do not intersect into the skull, will not need TADs as much because the posterior teeth do not naturally drift mesially as easily.

Location

Where to place TADs has been of great interest for investigators. Various studies have been published on this issue, and different auxiliaries have been recommended. Selection of the location and placing the TAD is a technique sensitive procedure, and there is no doubt that it has a learning curve.

Having a protocol designed specifically for the needs of the clinic or practice where TADs will be used is highly recommended. There are many samples provided by the various companies. However, the various items listed may not suit the needs of the practitioner's office.

Current literature suggests that the success rates are 90%, and this is what we see at our graduate orthodontic clinic. Most current data suggest that sex, chronologic age, and even the load do not seem to have a marked effect on success, but the location and the type of the tissue around the TAD do have an effect.[5,7] Hard and soft tissue thicknesses and the amount of attached mucosa play a role in the success of TADs.

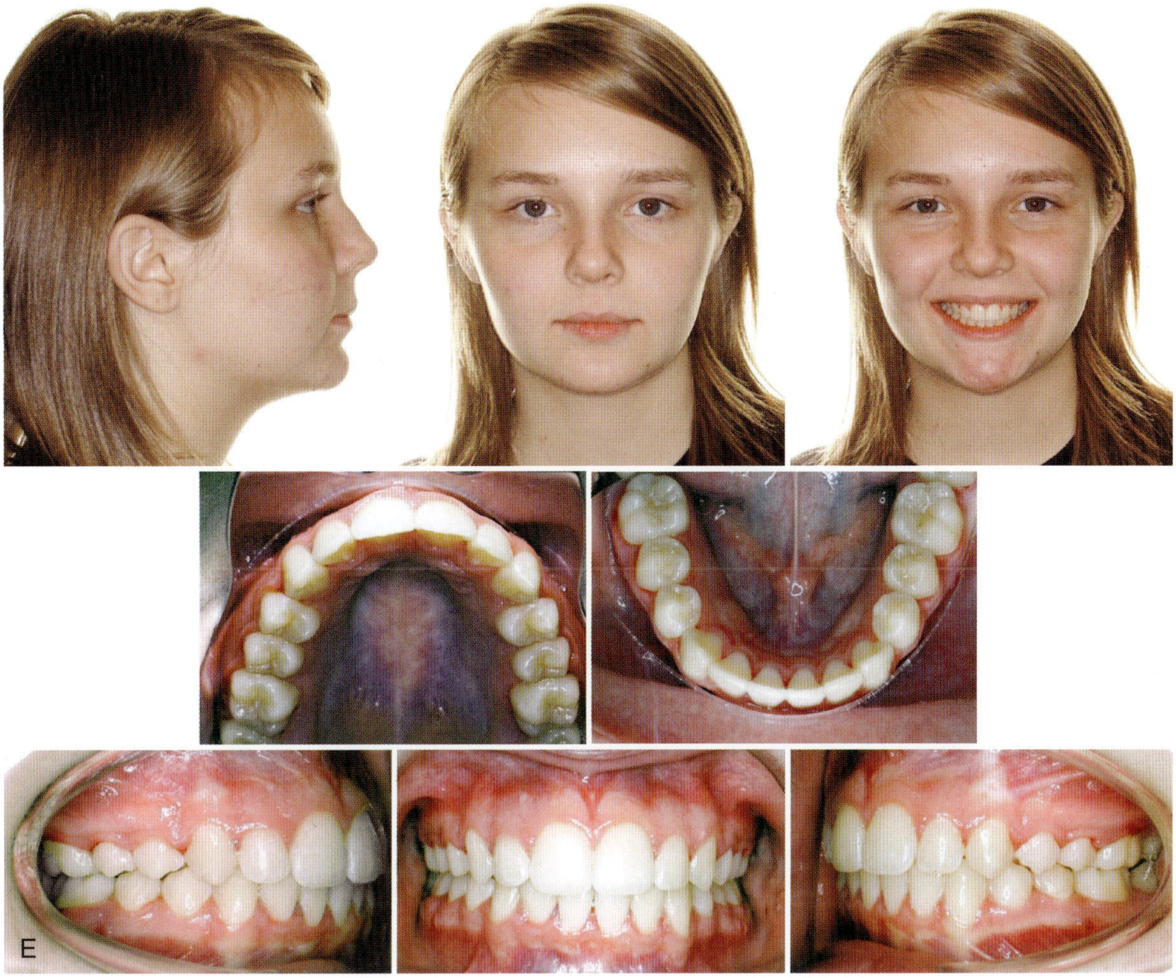

FIGURE 9-2—cont'd E, End of active treatment photos. Chronologic age 14-10.

The design of the TAD system and its threaded functional unit may also indirectly affect the location. Particularly, in selecting the right length of TADs for systems like the IMTEC Ortho Implant, it may even play a more important role than the thickness of the cortical bone.[6] The use of longer TADs is recommended if the soft tissue thicknesses are greater than 1.5 mm. The Ortho Implant has 4 mm of tapering body and 2 mm full thickness cylindrical threaded body, which is 1.8-mm in diameter. For better anchorage, the cylinder of full thickness diameter should reside in the cortex. Therefore, if the soft tissue thickness is more than 1.5 mm, the neck of the Ortho Implant would be too close to the soft tissues and possibly could become submerged, which would require the use of a longer TAD.

Locations like the posterior mandible and those that are surrounded by the unattached mucosa are more prone to failure and infection. Conversely, TADs placed in the posterior maxilla and in the keratinized mucosa seem to have higher survival rates. One guideline to keep in mind is that, in general, men will present with greater soft tissue thicknesses than women.

Beside the soft tissues, the thicknesses of the cortical plates that house the threads of TADs play an important role by providing anchorage and stability by housing the anchoring threaded portions of TADs. Therefore, to achieve adequate anchorage, it is necessary to know the thicknesses and the densities of the cortical bone in various parts of the jaws and the soft tissue characteristics of the area where one would like to place the TAD. Experience with dental implants has shown that the denser the bone the higher the success of the implant.[26]

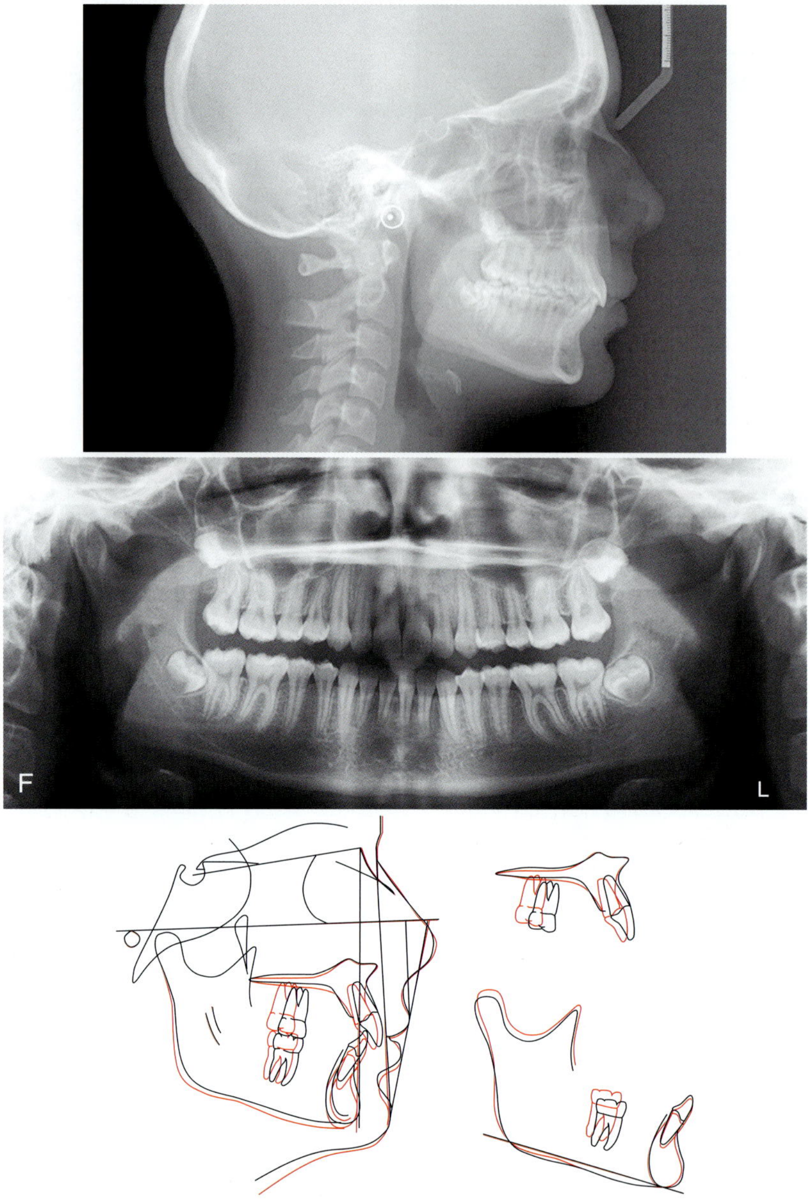

FIGURE 9-2—cont'd F, End of active treatment lateral cephalometric and panoramic radiograph. Chronologic age 14-10. G, Superimpositions of completed active treatment on the original tracing in an 18-month period.

Maxilla

Facial

The most widely used location is the facial interradicular space in the posterior maxilla. Most orthodontic mechanics is on the facial, which makes it easier and widely accepted for clinicians to use the buccal alveolar ridges for the placement of TADs. The posterior maxilla also has a dense cortical plate. Kim et al.[32] noted that the buccal soft tissues were thickest closest to and farthest from the cementoenamel junction and thinnest in the middle.

Another good location for TADs in the posterior maxilla is the infrazygomatic crest. The crest is considered an ideal location for mini plate applications. However, it is becoming more popular for TADs as well. Liou et al.[43] presented a study in which they looked at thickness of this location and the best angle for TAD placement to prevent contact with the roots of the permanent first molars. Using CBCT images, they were able to measure the thickness of the infrazygomatic crest and the insertion angle of the TAD at five degree increments from 40° to 75° to the maxillary occlusal plane. The authors recommended that the ideal location is at 14 to 16 mm above the maxillary occlusal plane and at an angle between 55° to 70° from the maxillary occlusal plane.

The least amount of bone thickness in the maxilla is reported to be in the tuberosity area.[51]

Placement protocols on the anterior facial provides vertical control for the anterior teeth for both direct and indirect applications. Radiographic examination is required for the best location within the interradicular spaces mesial to the permanent maxillary canines. For vertical control when the rigid orthodontic wires are in place, an indirect use of a single TAD placed between the roots of the permanent maxillary central incisors seems to provide adequate anchorage. For direct applications, two TADs between the roots of the permanent maxillary lateral incisors and canines is a better option because two TADs can provide a more symmetrical pull for the anterior dentition. One of the limitations of the anterior segment is the slope of the alveolar bone. In order to prevent any tissue impingements, long head designs are preferred. However, care must be taken to avoid irritating the labial mucosa. This area is covered with a thick soft tissue.[4]

Poggio et al.[58] published a landmark study in which they tried to provide an anatomical map to assist clinicians in safe placement of TADs between dental roots. They used CBCT volumetric images of 25 maxillary and 25 mandibular interradicular spaces. They measured the mesiodistal widths of the interradicular spaces at 2, 5, 8, and 11 mm from the alveolar crest. They reported that the midarch areas between the permanent canines and the first premolars and first premolars and second premolars had adequate spaces at 5-, 8-, and 11-mm levels, which could serve as suitable locations; 3 mm of mesiodistal width was defined as adequate so that an average TAD with 1.5 mm of thickness could be placed and still would have a distance of half a millimeter to the periodontal ligament of the teeth.

Park et al.[55] presented an investigation in which they tried to quantitatively evaluate the density of the alveolar and basal bones of the maxilla and the mandible. They noted the highest bone density levels in the buccal maxilla were in the permanent canine and premolar areas.

With numerous case reports on retraction of anterior teeth, the literature still lacks long-term clinical studies. One of the earlier case reports[50] described a patient treated with TADs. The patient previously had maxillary first premolars extracted, and, with TADs, Park[50] was able to retract the maxillary anterior teeth bodily using sliding mechanics and intrude them 4 mm with 1.5 mm of distal movement of the posterior teeth. TADs remained stable for the duration of treatment. Instead of losing anchorage, a gain was seen.

In another article published in 1999, Park and Kim[51] evaluated the efficacy of skeletal cortical anchorage using TADs. They examined 14 patients with a total of 28 TADs placed in the maxillary and mandibular alveolar bones. These authors reported five implant failures, which were attributed to excessive force during orthodontic mechanics. Their results revealed 1 to 2 mm of posterior movement of the posterior teeth, and they concluded that TADs might be an excellent method of anchorage control in orthodontics for cases that require maximum anchorage.

In a later case report, Park et al.[53] described the mechanics of bodily tooth movement. By using forces with vectors passing near the center of resistance of the maxillary anterior teeth, they were able to achieve bodily intrusion and retraction of the maxillary anterior teeth.

Park et al.[52,55] published two more articles in two different journals. The authors estimated the center of resistance of the six anterior teeth to be halfway between the center of resistance of the four maxillary permanent incisors and canines. They favored using upward and backward forces passing near the center of resistance, which resulted in bodily intrusion and retraction of the maxillary teeth. They noted that the occlusogingival position of TAD would determine the force direction, and thus the retraction of the anterior teeth could easily be controlled, depending upon the needs of each case. Another method of changing the direction of force as described by the authors was the vertical position of the anterior hooks. They noted that with the use of short anterior hooks the vertical component of the force would increase and the horizontal component of the force would decrease, and vice versa. Although variability was large, the authors also provided some measurements for the placement of the hooks. They noted for that bodily retraction of the anterior teeth with a slight intrusion, the proper position of the maxillary TADs would be 8 to 10 mm apical to the bracket slot with the anterior hooks 5 to 6 mm gingival to the bracket slot.

Thiruvenkatachari et al.[66] compared the amount of anchorage loss with TADs and conventional molar anchorage during canine retraction. Subjects in this study included 10 orthodontic patients (seven women and three men) with a mean age of 19.6 years and a range of 18 to 25 years. The treatment plans included extraction of all first premolars. After the cephalometric evaluation, the researchers noted the amount of molar anchorage loss an average of 1.6 mm in the maxilla and 1.7 mm in the mandible on the molar anchorage side. No anchorage loss was recorded on the TAD side. They concluded that the TADs could function as direct and efficient anchors for canine retraction when maximum anchorage was desired.

Garfinkle et al.[17] clinically evaluated the TAD anchorage in premolar extraction cases and success rates, loading, and patient acceptance. Their study involved 13 patients, eight female and five male patients with an average age 14 years 10 months, who were treated with 82 TADs measuring 1.6 mm in diameter and 6 mm in length that were placed in the buccal alveolar bone one unloaded and one loaded/quadrant. They randomly selected the right or left side of each arch for immediate loading up to 250 g of direct force and loaded the contralateral side 3 to 5 weeks later. Their results indicated an overall TAD success rate of 71%. No statistically significant differences were found between the success rates of immediately loaded TADs and those that were loaded later. However, the combined success rates for loaded TADs (80.5%) were significantly higher than that of unloaded TADs (61.0%). They noted that the patients' motivation for treatment with TADs was primarily to avoid the wearing of headgear.

For vertical control, maxillary posterior and anterior facial locations are commonly preferred by clinicians. The transverse dimension of maxillary and mandibular arches should be carefully evaluated to deliver the most optimal biomechanics. In a case report by Park et al.,[54] a 16-year-old girl with an anterior open bite was treated with nonextraction therapy that included intrusion of the maxillary and mandibular posterior teeth with TADs, which were placed in the alveolar bone near the posterior teeth. To prevent adverse side effects of buccoversion or linguoversion of the posterior teeth during intrusion, the authors used a transpalatal bar in the maxillary arch and a fixed lingual arch in the mandible, which are becoming more common while using TADs for intrusive mechanics. The authors were able to correct the 3-mm anterior open bite in 11 months by intrusion of both maxillary and mandibular posterior teeth, thus creating a favorable autorotation of the mandible. They noted that the posterior intrusion showed some relapse in the early stage of retention at 8 months. After that, no obvious relapse was seen in the vertical position of the molars and the mandibular plane angle. They recommended following such cases carefully for the potential of relapse. This is a very important concept, but the literature still lacks long-term data on intrusion mechanics with TADs.

Yao et al.[71] had a larger sample of patients and looked at intrusion of over-erupted permanent molars with TADs. Their sample included 22 patients with a mean of 27.6 years. Although they used two different modalities, mini plates or TADs, the forces applied were between 150 and 200 g, which effectively intruded the over-extruded molars.

Paik et al.[49] presented a case report in 2003 outlining treatment of vertical maxillary excess in an adult patient using TADs. In this case, the group utilized 1.6-mm diameter implants with a length of 8 mm between the maxillary and mandibular permanent first and second molars. The implants were then used as skeletal anchorage to allow maxillary anterior intrusion with resulting mandibular autorotation. The results of this case lead them to believe vertical correction that could once only be treated with surgery might be possible with orthodontic treatment and the added use of implants. Further research on larger samples and long-term evaluations is needed in vertical control.

Palatal

As described earlier, the palate has been considered a suitable location for TAD placement. It is in fact an advantageous area with no anatomical structures in most areas, such as nerves, blood vessels, or roots that can impede the placement of TADs. It allows for direct applications such as holding the premolars for protraction of permanent molars or as a Nance holding appliance to hold the molars for retraction of the anterior permanent teeth and indirect applications such as posterior molar intrusion. The attached soft tissues provide a healthy environment for TADs. However, thicknesses must be considered. The midpalatal suture has thick dense bone. The interdigitation of the bone lasts until late teen years. Therefore caution should be taken for growing adolescents due to the high rates of bone turnover that may interfere with the adaptability of the screw within the bone. For these patients, it is recommended to place the TAD just lateral to the midpalatal suture. However, if the plan is to deviate more than 1 mm away from the suture, placing it further posterior or using a shorter TAD is not recommended.

Palatal tori may also be used. However, for all palatal applications as well as tori, bone density should be carefully studied. Screw thicknesses less than 2 mm are not recommended due to higher torque values that may be generated during placement, which could lead to breakage of the screws. This may be eliminated by the use of pilot drills for these areas. For interradicular applications, lesser diameters can be used.

Common locations are the midpalatal suture distal to the incisive foramen and on the palatal interradicular spaces of the premolars and molars, which, in general, are lined with wide and thick cortical plates bordered by the palatal roots of the permanent maxillary molars. As a guideline, the midpalatal area within 1 mm of the midsagittal suture has the thickest bone available in the whole palate. From there, the thickness tends to decrease laterally and posteriorly.[29]

These median and paramedian areas can be the site of choice for TAD placement. More specifically, Gracco et al.[18] reported that the most optimal areas were either with one at 6 mm from the median suture and 4 and 8 mm from the incisive foramen or at 3 mm from the suture and 16 and 24 mm from the foramen. Researchers recommend careful length selection to avoid penetration into the nasal cavity but to allow full thickness of the cortical plate to be used in the anchorage. Longer TADs can be used for the anterior parts, whereas shorter ones are recommended for the midpalatal and posterior parts.

The functional lengths of TADs should be taken into account with the thickness of the mucosa because the thickest soft-tissue measurements are at 4 mm posterior to the incisive papilla and from there the depth remains the same. Kim et al.[32] noted that the palatal soft tissues were found to have a thickness that increased gradually from the cementoenamel junction toward the apical region and the midline.

Taking CBCT images may be advantageous because Kang et al.[29] in studying the bone thicknesses in the palate noted large individual differences. Although not usually obtained, CBCT images provide the best data for the availability of cortical bone and guide the clinicians in preventing contacts with anatomical structures.

Mandible

In general, the cortical bone density in the mandible is greater than the maxilla. An increasing and decreasing pattern of density in the maxilla is seen when looking from anterior toward the posterior. The mandible, however, shows only an increasing pattern that progressively increases from the incisors to the retromolar area.[56]

Lingual TAD application in the mandible is limited due to the possibility of discomfort to the patient and a high failure risk due to the presence of a very active muscle mass, the tongue.

The greatest amount of mesiodistal dimension in the mandible is between first and second premolars, and the least amount of bone is between the first premolar and the permanent canine.

Initial investigations reported high failure rates for the buccal mandible. Some have alluded that this is due to the dense nature of the bone and the heat generated during the use of the pilot drills to place TADs into this dense structure. Failure rates in the mandible do seem to decrease and are becoming close to those of the maxilla due to the increased usage of self-drilling TADs.

Posterior Facial

This location provides good direct and indirect anchorage for retraction of the mandibular incisors as well as controlling the unwanted movements of the entire mandibular dentition or posterior dentition when used in conjunction with conventional orthodontic mechanics. For two of the clinical studies completed in our department, the posterior mandible was the location of choice. We had a 90% success rate. Mild inflammation was present throughout the treatment. However, failure occurred only in 10% of TADs. According to Poggio et al.,[59] the mesiodistal widths of the interradicular space are more favorable between the mandibular permanent first and second molars at almost every level, starting 2 mm below the alveolar crest. The second best location in this region is between the mandibular permanent first molar and the second premolar. However, available space can be found 8 mm below the alveolar crest for this location, which may not be favorable due to the presence of unattached gingiva.

Dense cortical plate is present in the retromolar area, ramus, and the external oblique ridge, and it could be beneficial for direct applications on patients with Class III malocclusions for retraction of the mandibular dentition. The soft tissues are thickest in this area and are not attached, which can create an unfavorable environment for TADs.[4] The possibility of full tissue coverage is high.

Anterior Facial

The anterior facial mandibular region has the least dense bone. As long as the interradicular spaces allow, this region may provide direct anchorage for intrusion of the mandibular incisors. Due to the limited attached gingiva, inflammation may lead to totally covered TADs, and this is not uncommon.

Root proximity is another factor that may result in failure of TADs. To investigate this, Kuroda et al.[39] did a study with dental radiographs and CT images to examine 216 titanium TADs in 110 patients. They defined success as having a force applied on the TAD for 1 year, or until completion of orthodontic treatment, without complications. Their results indicated a high success rate of 80%. The authors were able to show a significant correlation between success rates and root proximity of the TADs. They noted that the closer TADs were to the roots the lower the success.

Researchers also investigated the use of TADs for bone-borne applications. One of the earlier animal studies by Smalley et al.[65] evaluated titanium implants for maxillofacial protraction in monkeys. They used an extraoral traction appliance that was attached to implants located in the maxillary, zygomatic, frontal, and occipital bones of the monkeys. They found the implants remained stable with a force of 600 g for 12 weeks in two groups and 18 weeks in two additional groups.

Although mini plates were preferred for skeletal applications, such as bone-to-bone or from bone to an extraoral device, it is worthwhile to mention some work with these mini plates has presented striking results. Hugo De Clerck[11] presented promising results on young cases with Class III malocclusions. They were placing four mini plates, two in the maxillary buttress and two in the mandibular anterior, and running Class III elastics to address the skeletal discrepancies early. Similar to this approach, in a preliminary study by Kircelli et al.,[35] two mini plates were placed under and on either side of the anterior nasal spine, and elastics were used to a reverse pull headgear in growing cases with Class III malocclusions. They were able to achieve dramatic changes with this approach.

Placement

Who Places TADs?

The use of a TAD can have a profound effect in the biomechanics in a particular case. In some ways, it can be a substitute for an intraoral anchorage device like a Nance holding arch or lingual arch. However, because of root proximity, the timing in placement of the TAD can be done after root divergence so that the TAD has a more favorable placement. Because the one doing the tooth movement plans the direction and types of the tooth movement, the orthodontist can be the best individual to place TADs. The use of more profound topical anesthesia has helped orthodontists place TADs facially. Practitioners who may not be used to this newer method of anchorage might be more comfortable in having another colleague place them. This could be done not only due to lack of familiarity with TADs but also the way a practice is setup to treat patients. Otherwise, the family dentist, the periodontist, or the oral surgeon may place them. There are cost considerations with this referral.

Sizes and Designs

There are various TAD systems on the market that can be purchased. Sizes and designs vary. A system may offer thicknesses ranging from 1 to 2 mm. These should be used in evaluating the need for the anchorage and in the locations of TADs. Recent research favors TADs that are greater than 1.5 mm. The greater the thickness the higher the potential for damaging anatomical structures. Therefore site evaluation is critical in selecting the right thickness. Conically shaped functional designs are favored due to easy removal of the TADs. Conical designs have a better chance to provide primary stability. Generally after insertion a TAD should be solid and have no signs of mobility. If primary stability is not achieved, a clinician should realize that the TAD will probably fail.

Length of a TAD is another critical factor. Few in the initial applications recommended the use of bicortical anchorage, meaning that the tip of the TAD would reach the contralateral cortical plate and provide better anchorage and stability. This would require the use of much longer TADs, but their application is now limited. Shorter lengths are preferred by most the clinicians. Generally, these vary from 6 to 12 mm.

The head of a TAD is part of the screw that stays above the surface of the mucosa and allows for different active and passive members, such as power chains, coil springs, or ligature ties to be used. Different head designs are available. Most systems offer bracket designs because this type seems to be more user friendly for clinicians. Button heads, hook heads, or ball heads are also available. Regardless of the design, most of the heads will have a hole to allow for threading different auxiliaries when needed.

Locations Guides

Panoramic radiographs provide information on the available bone and the anatomical structures. A panoramic film is obtained before planning of a TAD. However, panoramic radiographs have a tendency to overestimate the mesiodistal angulations of teeth with greater buccal root torque and underestimate the mesiodistal angulations of teeth with greater lingual torque. The roots with buccal orientations may look more distal than reality and the roots with lingual orientations may look more mesial than reality.[44,58,16] Therefore if there is any concern about the availability of adequate space, periapical radiographs should be taken.

Today many devices are available for successful placement of TADs. Radiographs taken with orthodontic wires held with acrylic or silicone materials, surgical guides for TADs, and even 3D SLA models have been generated for the placement of TADs. These auxiliaries have some value, but recently more and more clinicians are using their clinical judgment and trust in the conventional radiographs for the placement of TADs.

Different systems favor different clinical protocols. The Ortho Implant system recommends locations with a minimum of 0.5 to 1.0 mm of bone around the circumference of the TAD. One method is to use a panoramic or periapical radiograph with direct clinical visualization to identify the site. In addition to the radiographic image, better clinical visualization and the use of the curved end of a periodontal probe or an explorer can be used to firmly indent the outline of the roots into the soft tissues before placement.

Anesthesia

Topical anesthesia applications seem to be adequate for placement of TADs on the facial surface. Clinicians have to be careful when using compounded pharmaceutical gels. Certain percentages of lidocaine, tetracaine, and/or phenylephrine are used in these gels. Prilocaine and benzocaine can also be added by different companies or by pharmacies. The use of these compounds is rapidly increasing TAD use by the orthodontist, not only for TAD placement protocols but also for isolated soft tissue laser applications. Whatever the compounds that are used, they should be checked against the group of compounds that have received a warning from the U.S. Food and Drug Administration. These compounds and guidelines for using intraoral topical anesthetics can be viewed on the FDA web sites.

A common compound that is used in orthodontics is the LTP gel. LTP stands for lidocaine (20%), tetracaine (4%), and phenylephrine (2%).

A commonly accepted method is to use 2 mL of topical anesthetic and leave it on for 2 to 3 minutes. However, locations lined with thick attached mucosa such as the palate may require longer application periods. Topical gels do have drawbacks.[37] They come in small jars, and, although maximum doses are still unknown, jars make it difficult to determine the dosing. The recommended usage is to cover the placement area with 2 mL of gel. However, clinicians should remember that the difference between effective and toxic dose is small. Compounds with tetracaine are more prone to cause allergic reactions, and compounds with high doses of phenylephrine are more prone to have hypertensive and vasoconstrictive effects. Tissue irritation due to prolonged administrations are by far the most common side effect.

Local solutions can be administered if topical compounds fail to provide adequate anesthesia and the patient is uncomfortable after the administration of the topical anesthesia. In some locations, the use of a topical anesthetic gel will either not provide adequate numbing or be impractical. These areas include various posterior locations, such as the infrazygomatic crest, retromolar areas in the maxilla, and the ascending ramus or the oblique ridge in the mandible. The use of local infiltration anesthesia is preferred in these locations. When local infiltration is used, block anesthesia is not used and administration is limited to the area of the TAD placement. One does not wish to anesthetize the tooth because the patient's response to potential TAD contact with the tooth can be detected by the patient as a slight discomfort.

Access Through Soft Tissue and Hard Tissue

Some self-tapping systems require a pilot hole before placement. Others recommend using a soft tissue punch. This provides a clean soft tissue margin that will surround TADs. It may also play a role in the healing process of the soft tissue around the screw. It is more advantageous to use a tissue punch on the unattached mucosa because this mobile soft tissue has tendency to wind around a predrilling bur and even around a TAD itself during placement. Flap surgeries are no longer used because they increase the healing time and thus delay the orthodontic force application.

The effectiveness of predrilling versus self-drilling (no drilling, drill free) applications has been debated. A self-drilling TAD is the type that has a sharp tip and a tapered body, which can be inserted to catch and lock to the bone surface and allow the screw to move the bone away from its path. Self-drilling TADs are a descendant of predrilling TADs, which needed a pilot hole before insertion. A bur with a 0.2-mm smaller diameter than the diameter of the TAD is recommended, and they are still used with several systems. In addition, depending upon the bone thickness, predrilling may still be necessary in drill-free systems.[6] Wang and Liou[68] reported similar responses to orthodontic forces in clinical situations for both approaches.

Effects of predrilling were discussed by Wilmes et al.[70] They tested two systems and measured the insertion torque for five TAD types (tomas®-pin [Dentaurum, Ispringen, Germany] 1.6 mm × 8 mm and 1.6 mm × 10 mm, and Dual Top [Jeil Medical Corporation, Seoul, Korea] 1.6 mm × 8 mm, 1.6 mm × 10 mm and 2 mm × 10 mm). The Dual Top System was a self-drilling system. They tested 1000 insertions, which were done on 36 pelvic bone segments on an animal model. The results indicated that insertion and removal torques increased with smaller predrilling diameters for all TAD types. In analyzing the effects of the predrilling depths, they were able to demonstrate a strong correlation to primary stability. They reported that self-drilling TADs (Dual Top) showed significantly greater primary stability. It seems that the deeper the predrilling, the lower the insertion torque and probably lesser primary stability will result.

Before Wilmes et al.,[70] a closer look by Kim et al.[33] reported on the histomorphometric and mechanical responses of the self-drilling TADs. They noted that screws in the drill-free group showed less mobility and more bone-to-metal contact. Although it was minimal, osseointegration was found in both groups they tested. Both of these studies concur with a more rigid feel of self-drilling TADs clinically compared with the types that require predrilling.

Limitations and Complications

Kravitz and Kusnoto[38] classified the complications with TADs and gave clinical examples. They listed four general areas: insertion, TAD material itself, patient's hygiene, and application of the TADs. They first dealt with complications during insertion and included trauma to the periodontal ligament. A few articles have looked at root injuries. The first animal study was published by Asscherickx et al.[2] who reported accidental damage to the roots during placement of three of 20 TADs. They showed that the defects with the periodontal ligament and the cementum completely repaired in 12 weeks after removal of the screws. In a prospective study, Fabbroni et al.[14] found that with 232 screws placed in 55 patients, 26 (11.2%) had major contacts (more than 50% of the screw hole diameter impinging on the root) with adjacent teeth, and 37 (15.9%) had minor contacts (less than 50% of the diameter of the screw hole). Only two screws were associated with complications in two patients. These authors concluded that screw-to-tooth contact did occur with transalveolar screws, but the incidence of clinically significant damage appeared to be low.

Kadioglu et al.[28] reported the results of their clinical study done on humans. They intentionally contacted TADs with two maxillary first premolars

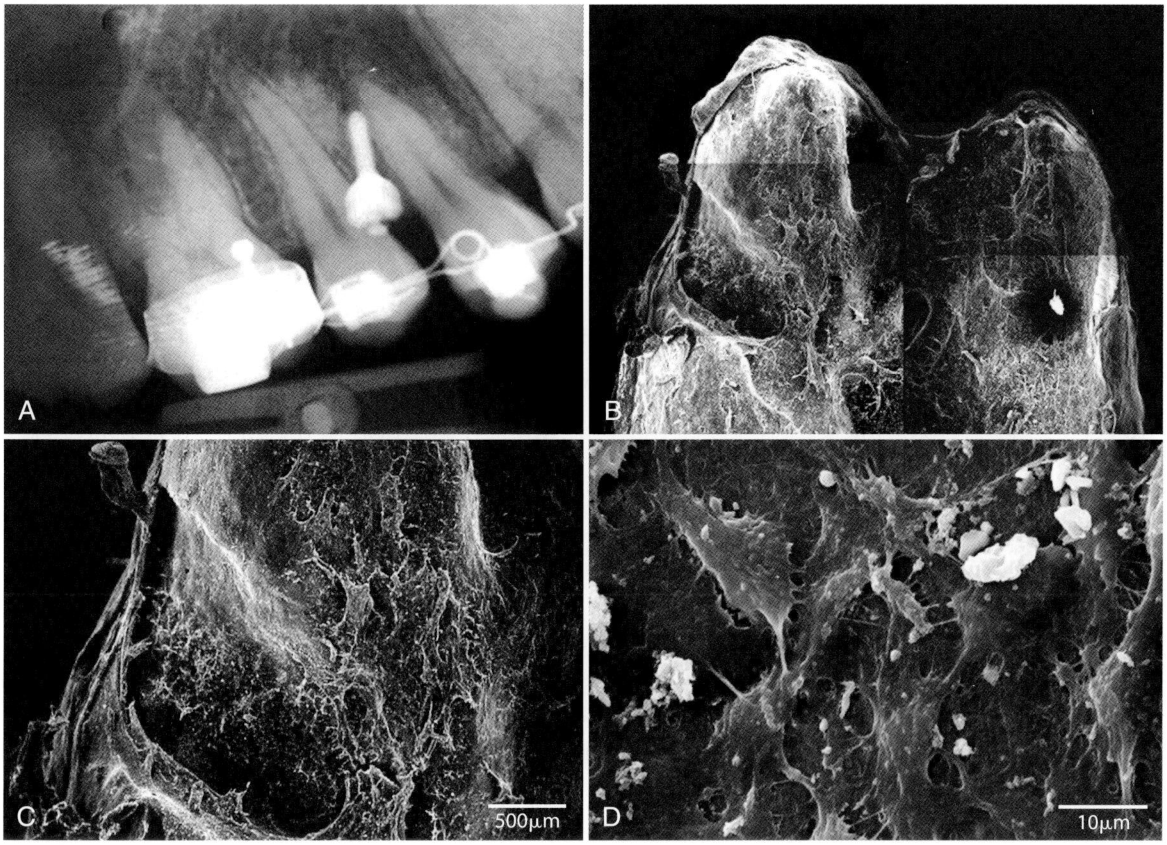

FIGURE 9-3. A, Periapical radiograph of the contact area of the miniscrew and the root surface after 8 weeks. B, Scanning electron microscope (SEM) evaluation after screw removal and 8 weeks of repair. See the fiber reorganization that is taking place at the bottom of the resorption lacunae. C, SEM evaluation after screw removal and 8 weeks of repair at a higher magnification. See the fiber reorganization that is taking place at the bottom of the resorption lacunae. D, SEM evaluation. New fibers are seen in the resorption lacunae at a higher magnification.

in orthodontic patients who were planned to have these teeth extracted as a part of their orthodontic treatment. There were five male and five female patients with a mean age of 15.8 years. They used tipping springs with a standardized force. Half the experimental teeth had contact with the screws for 4 weeks (mild resorption) and the other half for 8 weeks (severe resorption). In five patients, the screws were removed, and in the other five the springs were removed to allow the root to move back. The roots were allowed to recover for 4 or 8 weeks before extraction. The experimental groups showed signs of resorption with structural surface irregularities. No apparent denuded dentin surfaces after either healing periods were noted. They concluded that the root surfaces that touched the TADs showed swift repair and almost completely healed within a few weeks after removal of the screw or the orthodontic force (Figure 9-3).

Failing to fully engage the sharp tip of TADs may result in slippage over the bone surface and under the mucosal tissue along the periosteum.[38] The insertion angulation of the TADs may predispose this complication. The high-risk regions for this type of problem are sloped bony planes in alveolar mucosa, such as the zygomatic buttress, the retromolar areas, the buccal cortical shelf, and the maxillary buccal exostosis, if present.

Palatal applications may result in nerve involvement or sinus perforations. Although it is rare, one of the most likely locations for nerve involvement is the maxillary palatal slope due to the presence of the greater palatine nerve. The nasal sinus and the maxillary sinuses can be perforated during TAD placement. However, these heal with minimal consequences. As mentioned earlier, the palatal applications may also lead to excessive stress on the TAD, which might lead to breakage.

During orthodontic mechanics, failure of the TAD may occur. However, this is usually addressed by removal of the TAD and replacement to a different location. Liou et al.[42] clinically evaluated the stability of TADs. They used 17-mm long, 2-mm thick TADs and placed them in the maxillary zygomatic buttress. They noted significant forward tipping and extrusion of the TADs. They recommended a safety clearance of 2 mm from any anatomical structure or root.

Hygiene is extremely important for healthy peri-implant soft tissue. Patients having orthodontic treatment should present good hygiene and the ability to keep good hygiene. Melsen[45] reported that TADs should not be placed in heavy smokers and adults with systemic diseases.

Diagnosis and treatment planning is critical in preventing complications. Careful site preparation before placement of TADs is needed. This involves divergence of the roots neighboring the insertion site during orthodontic treatment. Also, one should delay the placement until ready to incorporate the TADs into the mechanics.

Future Considerations

Compliance is an issue in orthodontic therapy. TADs are not substitutes for patient compliance but are adjuncts to biomechanics. The effects on biomechanics are profound for most orthodontists due to the lack of reciprocal effects that orthodontists must deal with in treatment. Therefore the application of biomechanics needs to be reevaluated and highlighted. Patients who miss appointments and those with poor oral hygiene may have limited success with the use of TADs.

Extraoral appliances have their place in early treatment, especially for patients younger than 12 years old and where the use of TADs is not indicated. Teeth erupt at night so nocturnal application of headgear or facemask should not be dropped from the armamentarium of orthodontists.

TADs will not assist in correction of orthodontic problems in the transverse plane. Therefore the intervention of treatment for the transverse plane and the improvement of the axial inclination of the buccal segments with or without narrow arch forms necessitate other treatment modalities that are needed before cessation of dentofacial growth. The facemask and maxillary protraction need osseointegrated mini plates rather than TADs.

TADs with self-ligation systems in corrective or conventional orthodontics can assist in prevention of sagittal loss in anchorage in the mandibular arch. Those cases with partial banding and/or bonding might have some application with TADs, but this needs to be studied further. Its use in adjunctive orthodontics in correction of axial malposed teeth can be done on a case-by-case basis because adult treatment plans are highly individualized. For these cases, there would be less need for cross arch anchorage because of the TAD.

Studies comparing cases treated without TADs not only at the finish of the active phase but in terms of retention are needed. TADs might have only minimal beneficial effect related to relapse in tooth rotations, anterior deep bite, and anterior clinical crowding, all of which present challenges to orthodontists during the retention or postretention phase.

References

1. ADA Council on Scientific Affairs: Titanium applications in dentistry, *J Am Dent Assoc* 134(3):347–349, 2003.
2. Asscherickx K, Vannet BV, Wehrbein H, et al: Root repair after injury from mini-screw, *Clin Oral Impl Res* 16(5):575–578, 2004.
3. Block MS, Hoffman DR: A new device for absolute anchorage for orthodontics, *Am J Orthod Dentofac Orthop* 107(3):251–258, 1995.
4. Cha BK, Lee YH, Lee NK, et al: Soft Tissue Thickness for Placement of an Orthodontic Miniscrew Using an Ultrasonic Device, *Angle Orthod* 78(3):403–408, 2008.
5. Cheng SJ, Tseng IY, Lee JJ, et al: A prospective study of the risk factors associated with failure of mini-implants used for orthodontic anchorage, *Int J of Oral & Maxillofac Implants* 19:100–106, 2004.
6. Cope JB, Owens SE: Historical development and evolution of temporary anchorage devices. In Cope JB, editor: *OrthoTADs the clinical guide and atlas*, Dallas, TX, 2007, Under Dog Media, LP.
7. Cornelis MA, De Clerck HJ: Maxillary molar distalization with miniplates assessed on digital models: a prospective clinical trial, *Am J Orthod Dentofac Orthop* 132(3):373–377, 2007.
8. Cornelis MA, De Clerck HJ: Biomechanics of skeletal anchorage Part 1: Class II extraction treatment, *J Clin Orthod* 40(4):261–269, 2006.
9. Cornelis MA, Scheffler NR, Clerck HJ, et al: Systematic review of the experimental use of temporary skeletal anchorage devices in orthodontics, *Am J Orthod Dentofac Orthop* 131(4):52–58, 2007.
10. Creekmore TD, Eklund MK: The possibility of skeletal anchorage, *J Clin Orthod* 17(4):266–269, 1983.
11. De Clerck HJ: Class III Orthopedics Available at, http://www.hugodeclerck.net.
12. De Clerck HJ, Cornelis MA: Biomechanics of skeletal anchorage Part 2: Class II nonextraction treatment, *J Clin Orthod* 40(5):290–298, 2006.

13. De Clerck HJ, Timmerman HM, Cornelis MA: Biomechanics of skeletal anchorage Part 3: Intrusion, *J Clin Orthod* 42(5):270–278, 2008.
14. Fabbroni G, Aabed S, Mizen K, et al: Transalveolar screws and the incidence of dental damage: a prospective study, *Int J Oral Maxillofac Surg* 33(5):442–446, 2004.
15. Gainsforth BL, Higley LB: A study of orthodontic anchorage possibilities in basal bone, *Am J Orthod Oral Surg* 31(8):406–417, 1945.
16. Garcia-Figueroa MA, Raboud DW, Lam EW, et al: *Effect of buccolingual root angulation on the mesiodistal angulation shown on panoramic radiographs* 134(1):93–99, 2008.
17. Garfinkle JS, Cunningham LL Jr, Beeman CS, et al: Evaluation of orthodontic mini-implant anchorage in premolar extraction therapy in adolescents, *Am J Orthod Dentofac Orthop* 133(5):642–653, 2008.
18. Gracco A, Lombardo L, Cozzani M, et al: Quantitative cone-beam computed tomography evaluation of palatal bone thickness for orthodontic miniscrew placement, *Am J Orthod Dentofac Orthop* 134(3):361–369, 2008.
19. Gray JB, Steen ME, King GJ, et al: Studies on the efficacy of implants as orthodontic anchorage, *Am J Orthod* 83(4):311–317, 1983.
20. Herman RJ: Mini-implant anchorage for maxillary canine retraction: a prospective clinical study, Oklahoma City, 2004, Thesis for Master of Science, University of Oklahoma.
21. Herman RJ, Cope JB: Miniscrew implants: IMTEC mini ortho implants, *Semin Orthod* 11:32–39, 2005.
22. Herman RJ, Currier GF, Miyake A: Mini-implant anchorage for maxillary canine retraction: A pilot study, *Am J Orthod Dentofac Orthop* 130(2):228–235, 2006.
23. Huja SS: Mechanisms of bone adaptation to miniscrew implants. In Cope JB, editor: *OrthoTADs the clinical guide and atlas*, Dallas, TX, 2007, Under Dog Media, LP.
24. Huja SS, Roberts WE: Mechanism of osseointegration: characterization of supporting bone with indentation testing and backscattered imaging, *Semin Orthod* 10(2):162–173, 2004.
25. Huja SS, Litsky AS, Beck FM, et al: Pull-out strength of monocortical screws placed in the maxillae and mandibles of dogs, *Am J Orthod Dentofac Orthop* 127(3):307–313, 2005.
26. Jaffin RA, Berman CL: The excessive loss of Brånemark fixtures in type IV bone: a 5-year analysis, *J Perio* 62(1):2–4, 1991.
27. Kadioglu O: Assessment of Treatment of Class II Malocclusions Using Fixed Functional Appliances with Temporary Anchorage Devices in the Mandibular Arch. Thesis for Master of Science, Oklahoma City, 2008, University of Oklahoma.
28. Kadioglu O, Büyükyilmaz T, Zachrisson BU, et al: Contact damage to root surfaces of premolars touching miniscrews during orthodontic treatment, *American Journal of Orthodontics & Dentofacial Orthopedics* 134(3):353–360, 2008.
29. Kang S, Lee SJ, Ahn SJ, et al: Bone thickness of the palate for orthodontic mini-implant anchorage in adults, *Am J Orthod Dentofac Orthop* 131(4):74–81, 2007.
30. Kanomi R: Mini-implant for orthodontic anchorage, *J Clin Orthod* 31(11):763–767, 1997.
31. Keim RG: The Biomechanics of TADs, *J Clin Orthod* 42(5):261–262, 2008.
32. Kim HJ, Yun HS, Park HD, et al: Soft-tissue and cortical-bone thickness at orthodontic implant sites, *Am J Orthod Dentofac Orthop* 130(2):177–182, 2006.
33. Kim JW, Ahn SJ, Chang Y: Histomorphometric and mechanical analyses of the drill-free screw as orthodontic anchorage, *Am J Orthod Dentofac Orthop* 128(2):190–194, 2005.
34. Kim SH, Cho JH, Chung KR, et al: Removal torque values of surface-treated mini-implants after loading, *Am J Orthod Dentofac Orthop* 134(1):36–43, 2008.
35. Kircelli BH, Pektas ZO: Midfacial protraction with skeletally anchored face mask therapy: A novel approach and preliminary results, *Am J Orthod Dentofac Orthop* 133(3):440–449, 2008.
36. Kloehn SJ: Guiding alveolar growth and eruption of teeth to reduce treatment time and produce a more balanced denture and face, *Angle Orthod* 17(1):10–33, 1947.
37. Kravitz ND: The use of compound topical anesthetics: A review, *J Am Dent Assoc.* 138(10):1333–1339, 2007.
38. Kravitz ND, Kusnoto B: Risks and complications of orthodontic miniscrews, *Am J Orthod Dentofac Orthop* 131(4):43–51, 2007.
39. Kuroda S, Yamada K, Deguchi T, et al: Root proximity is a major factor for screw failure in orthodontic anchorage, *Am J Orthod Dentofac Orthop* 131(4):68–73, 2007.
40. Linkow LI: Implant-orthodontics, *J Clin Orthod* 4(12):685–690, 1970.
41. Linkow LI: The endosseous blade implant and its use in orthodontics, *Int J Orthod* 18:149–154, 1969.
42. Liou EJW, Pai BCJ, Lin JCY: Do miniscrews remain stationary under orthodontic forces? *Am J Orthod Dentofac Orthop* 126(1):42–47, 2004.
43. Liou EJW, Chen PH, Wang YC, et al: A computed tomographic image study on the thickness of the infrazygomatic crest of the maxilla and its clinical implications for miniscrew insertion, *Am J Orthod Dentofac Orthop* 131(3):352–356, 2007.
44. Lucchesi MV, Wood RE, Nortje CJ: Suitability of the panoramic radiograph for assessment of mesiodistal angulation of teeth in the buccal segments of the mandible, *Am J Orthod Dentofacial Orthop* 94(4):303–310, 1988.
45. Melsen B: Mini-implants: Where are we? *J Clin Orthod* 39(9):539–547, 2005.
46. Melsen B, Verna C: Miniscrew implants: the Aarhus anchorage system, *Semin Orthod* 11:24–31, 2005.
47. Melsen B, Petersen JK, Costa A: Zygoma ligatures: an alternative form of maxillary anchorage, *J Clin Orthod* 32(3):154–158, 1998.
48. Owens SE, Buschang PH, Cope JB, et al: Experimental evaluation of tooth movement in the beagle dog with the mini-screw implant for orthodontic anchorage, *Am J Orthod Dentofac Orthop* 132(5):639–646, 2007.
49. Paik CH, Woo YJ, Boyd RL: Treatment of an adult patient with vertical maxillary excess using miniscrew fixation, *J Clin Orthod* 37(8):423–428, 2003.
50. Park HS: The skeletal cortical anchorage using titanium microscrew implants, *Kor J Orthod* 29(6):699–706, 1999.
51. Park HS, Kim JB: The use of titanium microscrew implant as orthodontic anchorage, *Keimyung Medical J* 18(4):509–515, 1999.

52. Park HS, Bae SM, Kyung HM, et al: Simultaneous incisor retraction and distal molar movement with microimplant anchorage, *World J Orthod* 5:164–171, 2004.
53. Park HS, Bae SM, Kyung HM, et al: Micro-implant anchorage for treatment of skeletal Class I bialveolar protrusion, *J Clin Orthod* 35(7):417–422, 2001.
54. Park HS, Kwon OW, Sung JH: Nonextraction treatment of an open bite with microscrew implant anchorage, *Am J Orthod Dentofac Orthop* 130(3):391–402, 2006.
55. Park HS, Kwon TG, Kwon OW: Treatment of open bite with microscrew implant anchorage, *Am J Orthod Dentofac Orthop* 126:627–636, 2004.
56. Park HS, Lee JL, Jeoung SH, et al: Density of the alveolar and basal bones of the maxilla and the mandible, *Am J Orthod Dentofac Orthop* 133(1):30–37, 2008.
57. Park HS, Lee SK, Kwon OW: Group distal movement of teeth using microscrew implant anchorage, *Angle Orthod* 75(4):602–609, 2005.
58. Peck JL, Sameshima GT, Miller A, et al: Mesiodistal Root Angulation Using Panoramic and Cone Beam CT, *The Angle Orthodontist* 77(2):206–213, 2007.
59. Poggio PM, Incorvati C, Velo S, et al: Safe zones: a guide for miniscrew positioning in the maxillary and mandibular arch, *Angle Orthod* 76(2):191–197, 2006.
60. Power JP: Mini-implant system as orthodontic anchorage for mandibular retraction: a prospective study, Oklahoma City, 2005, Thesis for Master of Science, University of Oklahoma.
61. Roberts WE, Arbuckle GR, Analoui M: Rate of mesial translation of mandibular molars using implant anchored mechanics, *Angle Orthod* 66(5):331–338, 1996.
62. Roberts WE, Engen DW, Schneider PM, et al: Implant anchored orthodontics for partially edentulous malocclusions in children and adults, *Am J Orthod Dentofac Orthop* 126:302–304, 2004.
63. Roberts WE, Smith RK, Zilbernam Y, et al: Osseous adaption to continuous loading of rigid endosseous implants, *Am J Orthod* 86:95–111, 1984.
64. Shaar CM, Kreuz FP Jr: Manual of Fractures, Philadelphia, 1943, P. Blakiston's Son & Co, pp 3–53.
65. Smalley WM, Shapiro PA, Hohl T, et al: Osseointegrated titanium implants for maxillofacial protraction in monkeys, *Am J Orthod Dentofac Orthop* 94(4):285–295, 1988.
66. Thiruvenkatachari B, Pavithranand A, Rajasigamani K, et al: Comparison and measurement of the amount of anchorage loss of the molars with and without the use of implant anchorage during canine retraction, *Am J Orthod Dentofac Orthop* 129(4):551–554, 2006.
67. Thurow CR: *Edgewise Orthodontics*, ed 2, St. Luis, 1966, The C.V. Mosby Company.
68. Umemori M, Sugawara J, Mitani H, et al: Skeletal anchorage system for open-bite correction, *Am J Orthod Dentofac Orthop* 115(2):166–174, 1999.
69. Wang YC, Liou EJW: Comparison of the loading behavior of self-drilling and predrilled miniscrews throughout orthodontic loading, *Am J Orthod Dentofac Orthop* 133(1):38–43, 2008.
70. Wehrbein H, Feifel N, Diedrich P: Palatal implant anchorage reinforcement of posterior teeth: A prospective study, *Am J Orthod Dentofac Orthop* 116:678–686, 1999.
71. Wilmes B, Rademacher C, Olthoff G, et al: Parameters affecting primary stability of orthodontic mini-implants, *J Orofac Orthop* 67(3):162–174, 2006.
72. Yao CCJ, Lee JJ, Chen HY, et al: Maxillary molar intrusion with fixed appliances and mini-implant anchorage studied in three dimensions, *The Angle Orthod* 75(5):626–632, 2000.

Chapter 10

The Laboratory Technician's Key Role in MDI Prosthodontics

ANDREW JAKSEN JOHN KIRDAHY MURRAY SCHEINER LEONARD MAROTTA

Outline

Introduction by Dr. Victor Sendax

Just as vital to the success of the Mini Dental Implant (MDI) System—and comparable with the seminal role of the MDI Insertion Protocol—is the MDI Reconstructive Protocol, both of which are given equal attention in the original Sendax Patent granted by the United States Patent Office. The foremost firing line experience to be encountered in applying MDIs to clinical implant prosthodontics is the dental laboratory connection. This text has reserved an individual place of respect for the laboratory technicians who partner with doctors in establishing the specialized standards that apply to MDI restorations or reconstructions, whether for single tooth replacements, removable overdentures, or hybridized fixed bridges. The learning curve in restoring minis is subtle to much the same degree as mastering the essentially simple and typically straightforward intraoral MDI insertion steps, as long as attention is also paid to the often less obvious fine points. The imaginative and skilled certified dental technician (CDT) is often in the catbird seat (and occasionally the hot seat!) when it comes to refining those unique, hard-to-define MDI elements and taking them to full fruition. Our colleagues presenting herein are prime exemplars of this critical attribute.

The Laboratory Technician's Key Role in MDI Implant Prosthodontics:

Andrew Jaksen

The author and dentist-lecturer Dr. Benjamin Oppenheimer has been devoted to the process of consolidating advances in MDI laboratory coordination and work simplification via updated step-reduction techniques for fixed (and removable) applications and has pioneered in advancing MDI education with specialized seminars specifically oriented to the dental laboratory community. Rapidly evolving ceramic abutments for MDI fixed crown and bridge cases, along with CAD/CAM generated models, have also come to offer unique contemporary imaging and stent guidance approaches to esthetic restorative simplicity and affordability. Dr. Oppenheimer has been especially productive in presenting MDI educational seminars throughout the United States, emphasizing the close coordination needed between the laboratory staff and the implantologist to refine the essential MDI technology, with special emphasis on fixed crown/bridge applications.

The series of lab images (Figures 10-1 to 10-4) illustrates a typical multiunit Ponabut structure with ridge laps, embrasures, and flange elements designed to produce a secure and esthetically satisfying result. When inserted with self-cure resin cement, this fixed, splinted full-arch system can be made hygienically cleansable with a water irrigator lavage, preferably teamed up with a dedicated curved-bristle implant brush (e.g., ACCESS Implant Brush), for a well-emphasized labiolingual approach after meals and, of course without exception, before retiring at bedtime.

MDI fixed bridge-splint laboratory technology embodies MDI Ponabuts, which for multiple-unit fixed embodiments require a passive fit of the prosthesis overlaying the abutments and an easy draw without binding interferences, irrespective of any off-angle or nonparallel considerations. This requires the laboratory to block out sufficient relief room around the abutment heads on the working model (made chairside from a polyvinyl siloxane or polyether impression), with MDI analogs inserted, and poured in model stone or epoxy so that either individual castings can be fabricated, tried in and connected intraorally, or a one-piece cast

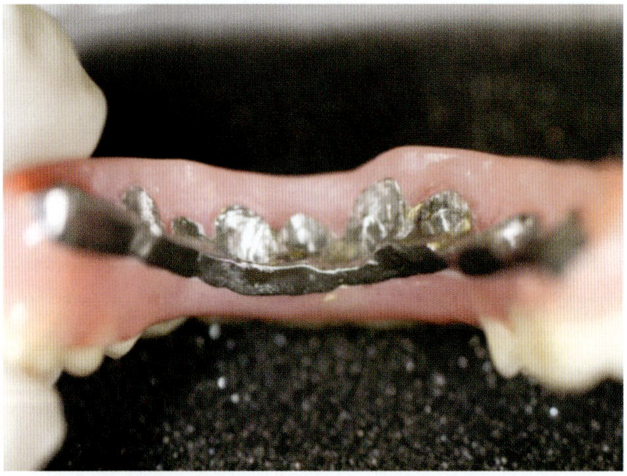

FIGURE 10-1. Ponabut prosthesis, lingual view.

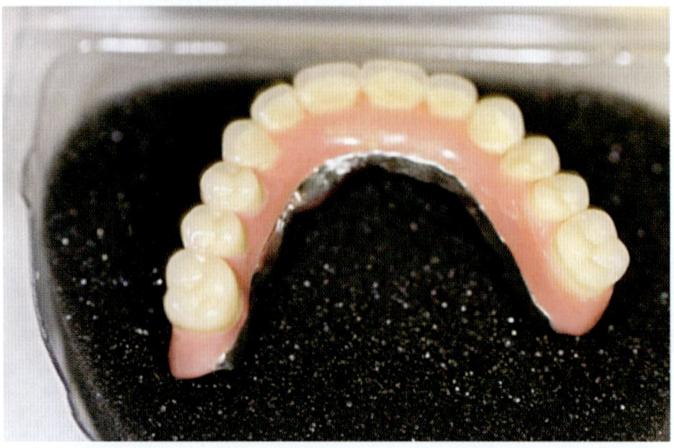

FIGURE 10-2. Full arch Ponabut palateless prosthesis, lingual view.

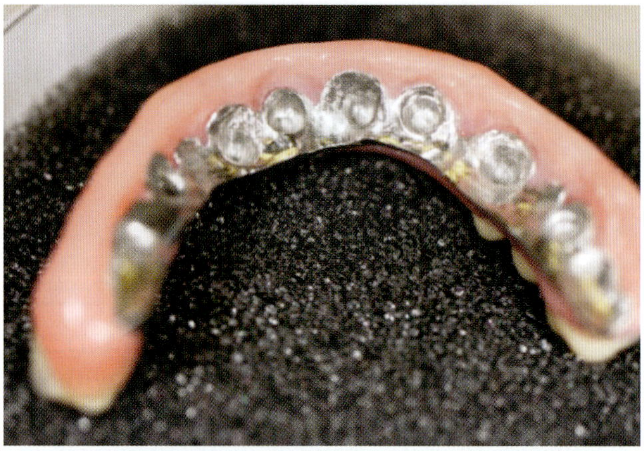

FIGURE 10-3. Ponabuts in the esthetic zone.

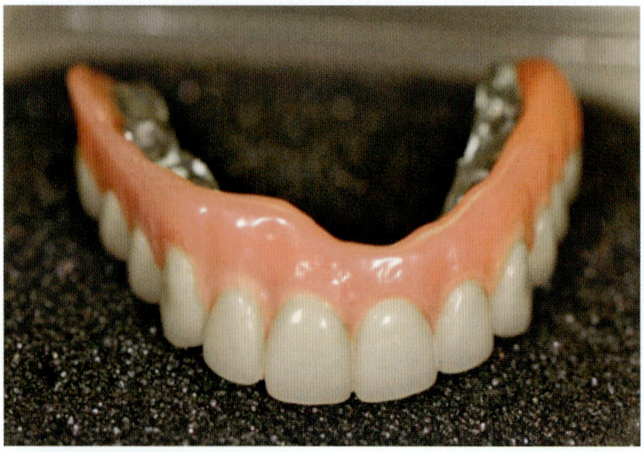

FIGURE 10-4. Final full arch Ponabut prosthesis, anterior view.

substructure can be manufactured and passively fitted intraorally. Bite registrations and records with any opposing jaw impressions are also produced to further the lab processing. Porcelain or composite resin is then layered and processed over the substructure. Various other techniques with or without an infrastructure are currently undergoing extensive development for both MDIs, conventional implant systems, and hybrid combinations and await additional studies and clinical case reporting to confirm their outcomes.

The updated Celara denture wax-up and duplicate modeling technology offers improved accuracy and directness in building the MDI-related removable prostheses and insertion guidance control for stent devices. Technician Andrew Jakson and dentist/associate Dr. Benjamin Oppenheimer, aided by Keith Henry of 3M-ESPE and a cross-section of MDI dentists and laboratories, have been instrumental in illuminating this user-friendly lab processing aid for conventional denture prostheses and removable MDI overdentures.

The Laboratory Technician's Key Role in MDI Prosthodontics:

John Kirdahy, Murray Scheiner

John Kirdahy, CDT, with pioneering forays into simplified MDI laboratory technologies and representative suggestions and tips, helped launch affordable MDI prosthodontic solutions.

John Kirdahy's Innovation Laboratory has consistently offered evolving lab techniques that have helped standardize the coordination of MDI chairside procedures with the implant-oriented dental laboratory and advanced the progressive design and processing of both fixed and removable MDI cases, two of which are represented in Figures 10-5 to 10-14.

Murray Scheiner, CDT, who has been Dr. Sendax's in-office personal lab technician for more than 40 years dating from the earliest MDI clinical trial cases, was initially exposed to the MDI restorative protocol at its inception in 1976, and since then has processed many fixed and removable MDI cases. Together with a consistent offering of the daily practical tips and suggestions that can be key to successful long-term case outcomes, Murray's benevolent contributions have been a highly-valued practice asset in developing and applying MDI laboratory technology advances and innovations.

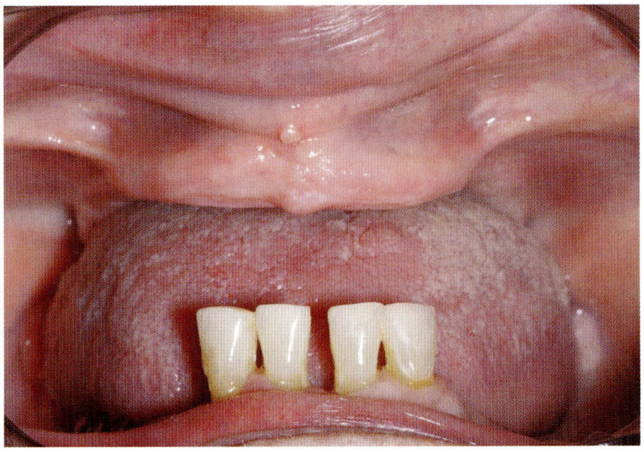

FIGURE 10-5. Maxillary and mandibular preoperative removable MDI Case No.1.

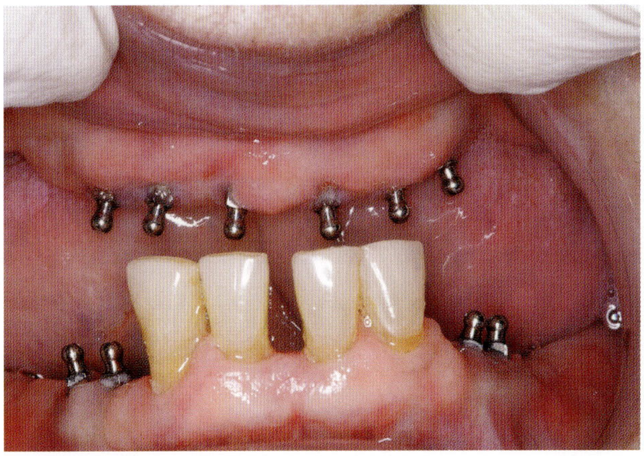

FIGURE 10-6. Maxillary and mandibular MDIs.

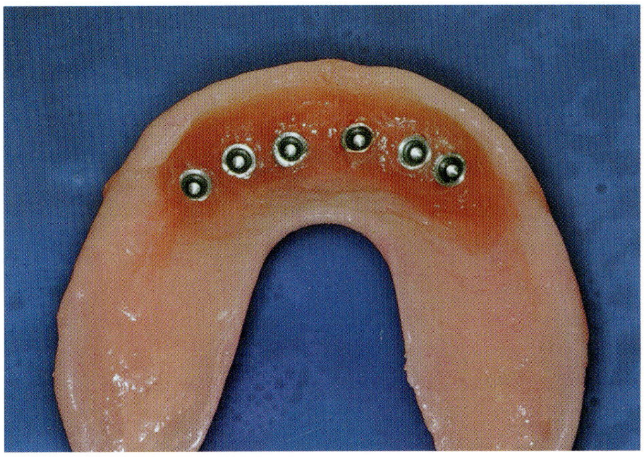

FIGURE 10-7. Maxillary 6 MDI O rings.

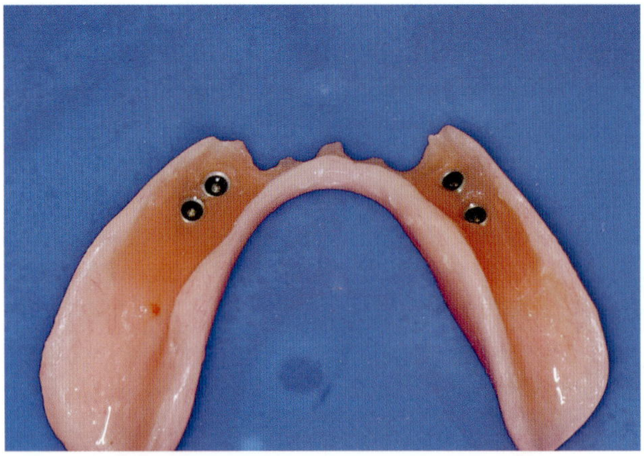

FIGURE 10-8. Mandibular 4 O rings.

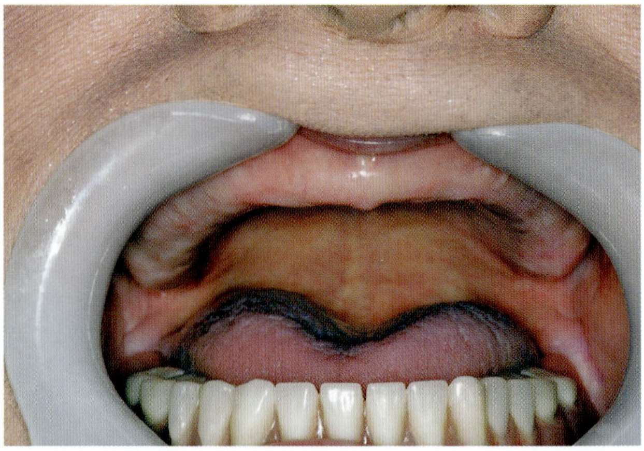

FIGURE 10-9. Maxillary Preoperative; MDI Case No. 2.

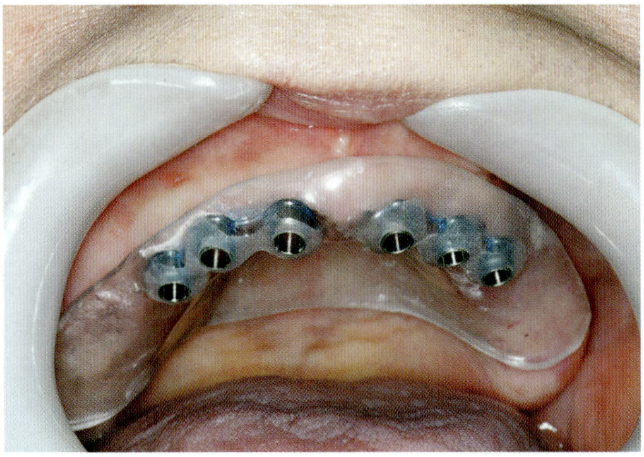

FIGURE 10-10. Maxillary MDI guide stent.

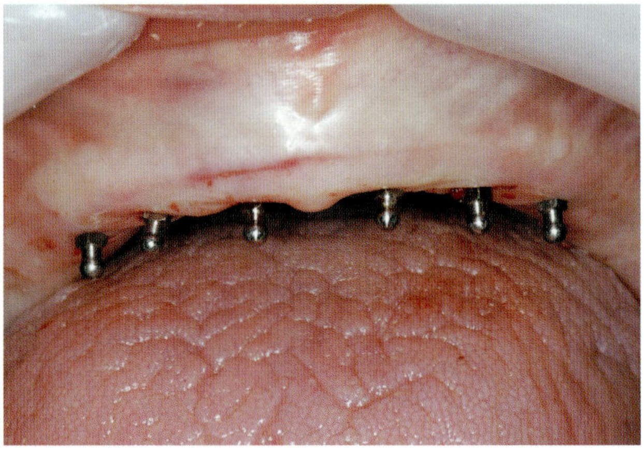

FIGURE 10-11. Maxillary 6 MDIs Postoperative.

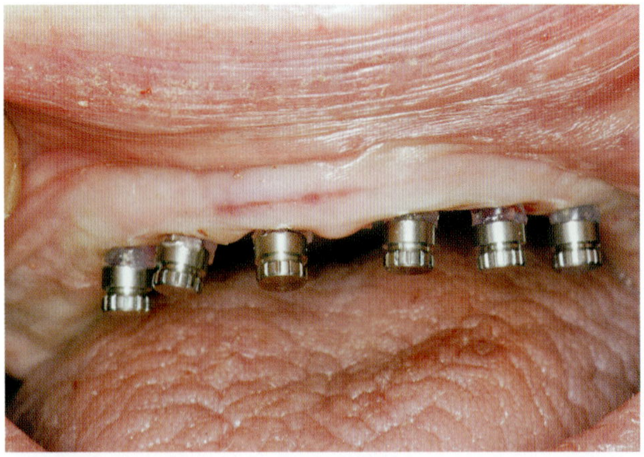

FIGURE 10-12. Maxillary 6 MDI O ring attachments.

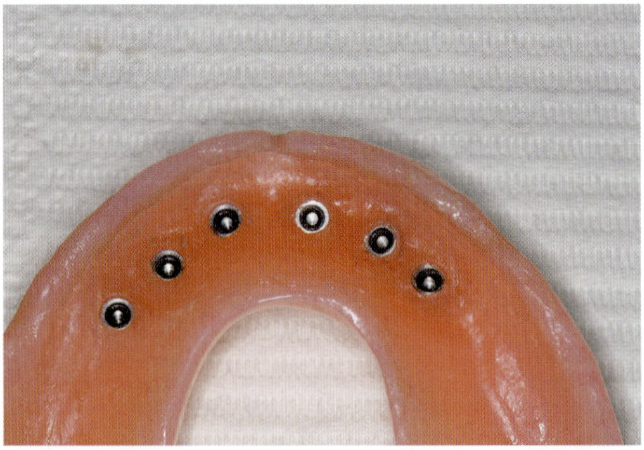

FIGURE 10-13. Maxillary MDI O ring attachments in removable prosthesis.

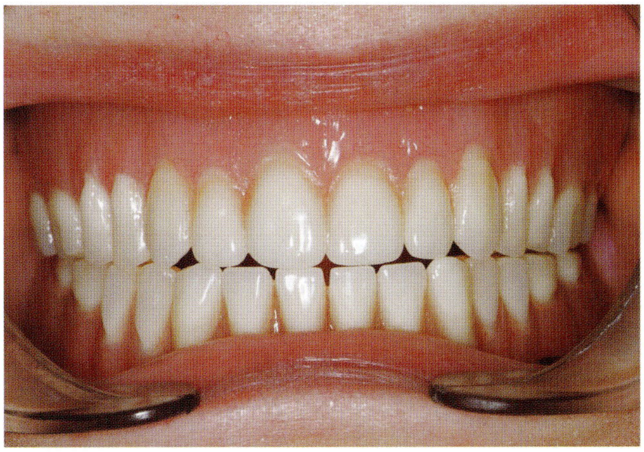

FIGURE 10-14. Maxillary and mandibular MDI postoperative; Case No. 2.

The Laboratory Technician's Key Role in MDI Implant Prosthodontics:

Leonard Marotta

The following images (Figures 10-15 to 10-47) illustrate the laboratory steps in fabricating an MDI fixed bridge and a comparable sequence for two single tooth fixed full-coverage restorations, all embodying the unique MDI "Ponabut" design that combines a pontic and abutment in a single entity.

MDI fixed bridge-splint laboratory technology embodies MDI Ponabuts, which for multiple-unit fixed embodiments require an atraumatic, unstressed fit of the prosthesis overlaying the abutments and an easy draw without binding interferences, irrespective of any off-angle or nonparallel considerations related to varied emergence profiles of the MDIs as they penetrate the crestal bone and soft tissues (through the periosteum and attached gingiva) into the oral cavity. This protocol requires the laboratory to block out sufficient relief room around the abutment heads on the working model (made chairside from a polyvinyl siloxane or polyether impression), with MDI analogs inserted, and poured in model stone or epoxy so that either individual castings can be fabricated, tried in and connected intraorally, or a one-piece cast substructure can be manufactured and then passively fitted intraorally. Bite registrations and records, with any opposing jaw impressions are also produced to complete the lab processing. Porcelain or composite resin is then layered and processed over the substructure. Various other techniques with or without an infrastructure are currently undergoing extensive development for both MDIs, conventional implant systems, and hybrid combinations and await additional studies and clinical case reporting to confirm their outcomes.

Single tooth replacement MDIs lend themselves particularly well to individual crown restorations with the Ponabut design as the underlying structural element. The Marotta Laboratory has produced herein a series of MDI case views that effectively illustrate the essentials when working with MDIs for individual crown and bridge restorations and define the sequencing steps, which basically follow conventional lab procedures but with several design modifications to simplify MDI fixed prosthodontics for both lab and doctor (Figures 10-48 to 10-59).

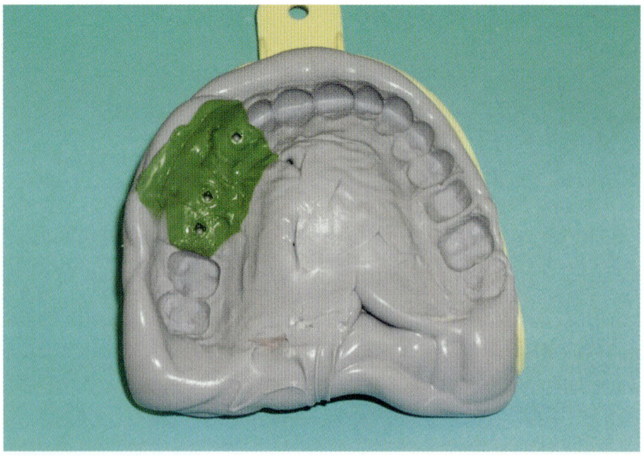

FIGURE 10-15. Polyvinyl siloxane O-ball implant impression.

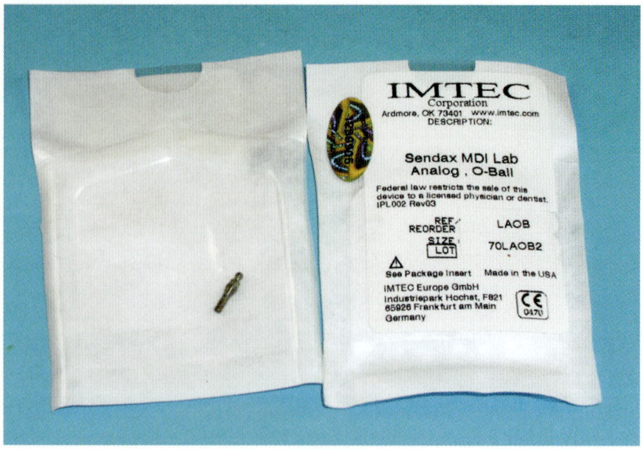

FIGURE 10-16. O-ball analog in packaging.

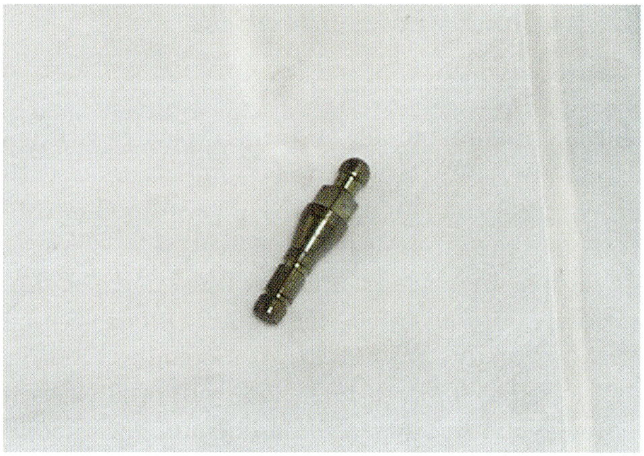

FIGURE 10-17. O-ball analog.

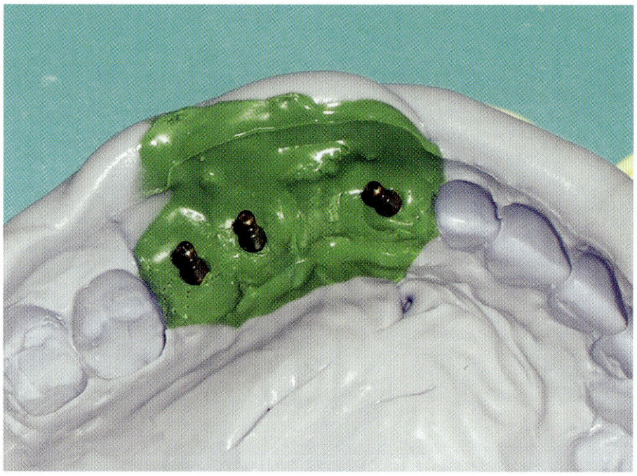

FIGURE 10-18. Three analogs inserted into polyvinyl sulfate impression.

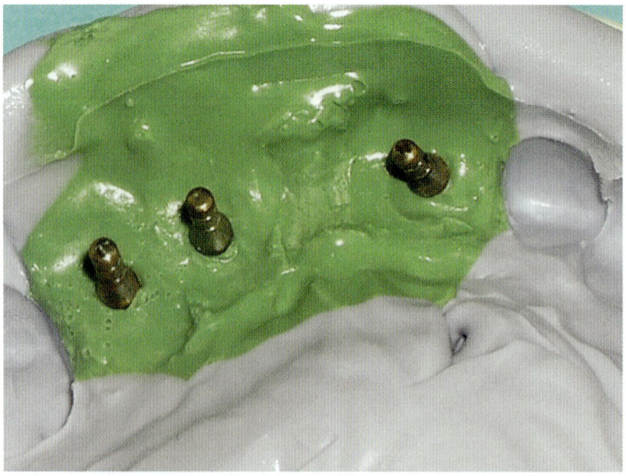

FIGURE 10-19. Three seated analogs.

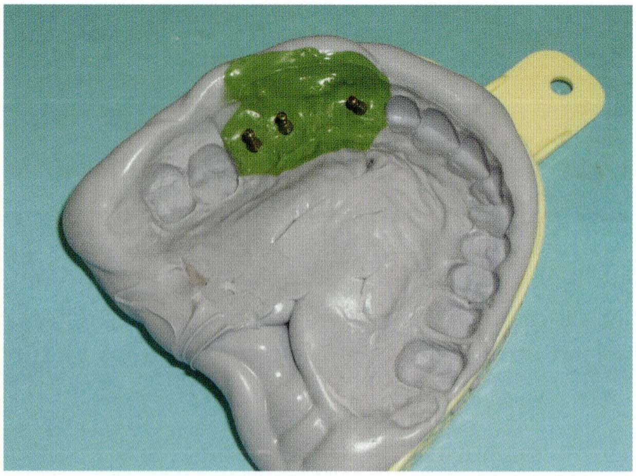

FIGURE 10-20. Full arch impression.

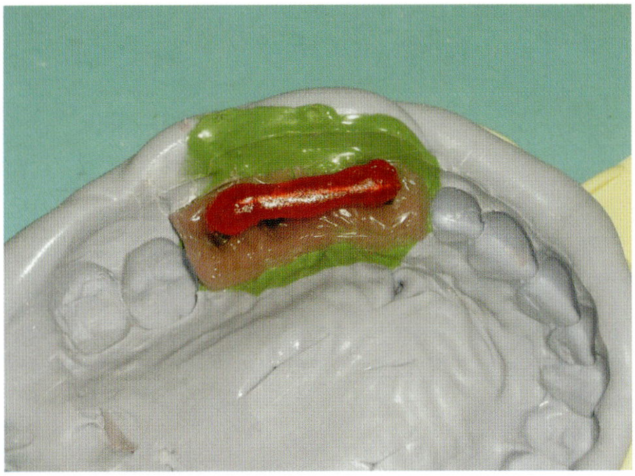

FIGURE 10-21. Duralay analogs antimovement reinforcement.

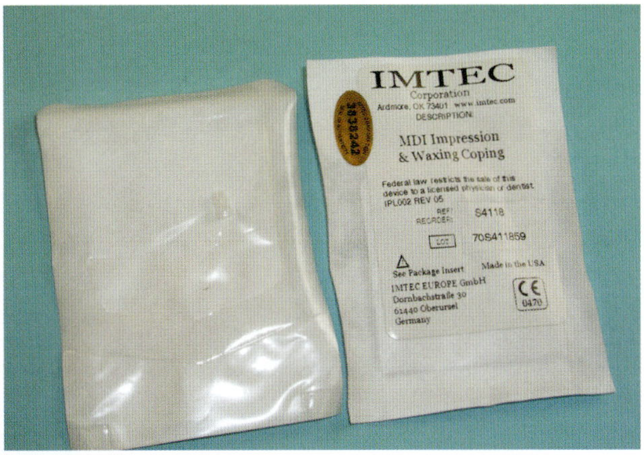

FIGURE 10-22. MDI impression and waxing coping in packaging.

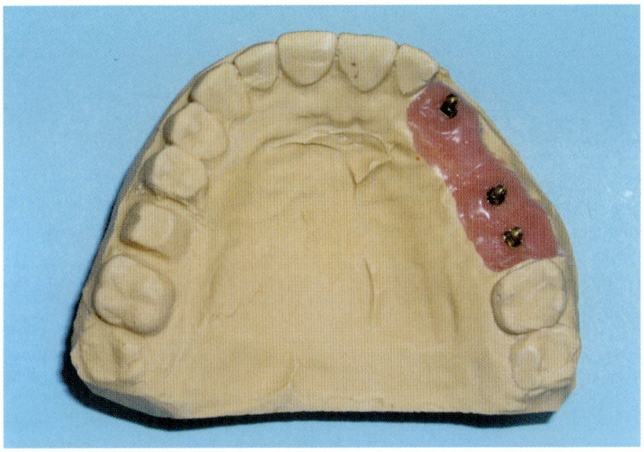

FIGURE 10-23. Model with soft tissue component.

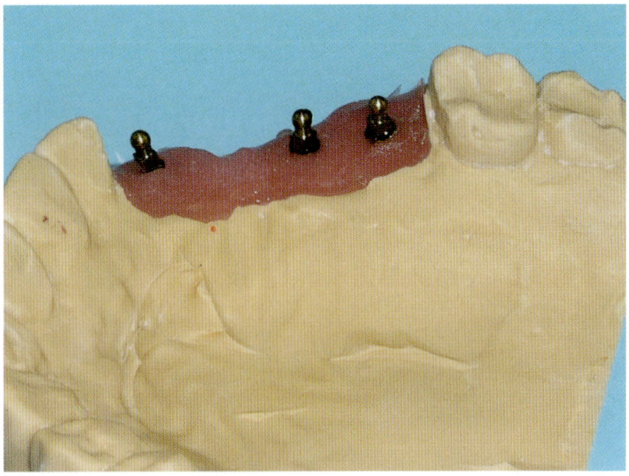

FIGURE 10-24. Before waxing.

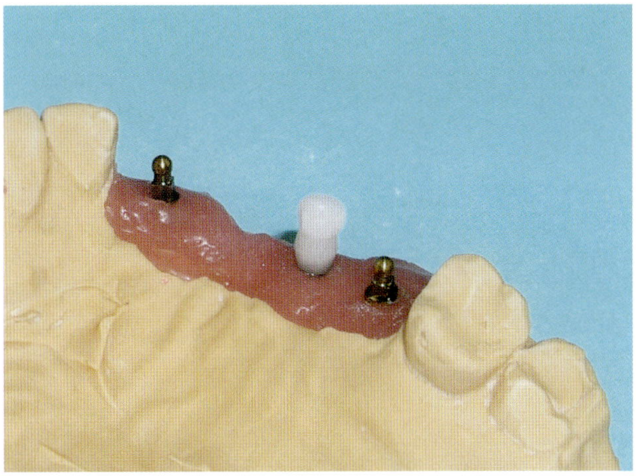

FIGURE 10-25. MDI impression and waxing coping.

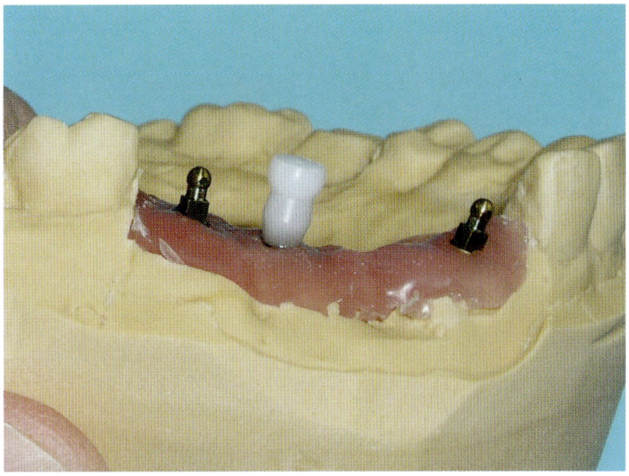

FIGURE 10-26. Waxing coping detail.

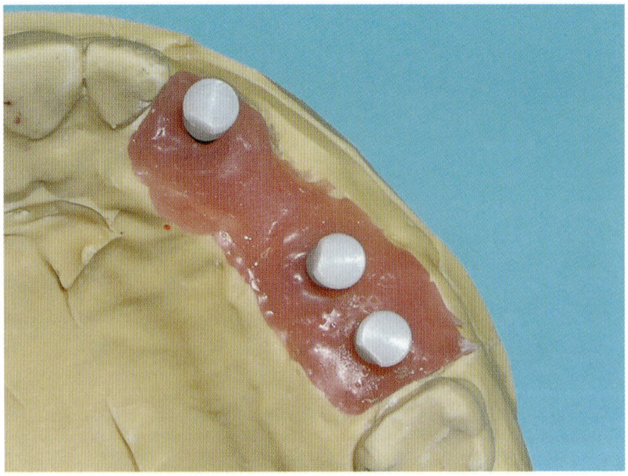

FIGURE 10-27. Waxing coping detail.

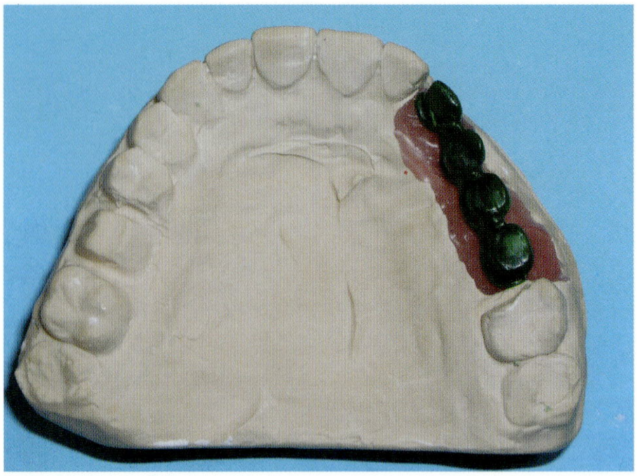

FIGURE 10-28. C & B Ponabut wax-ups, occlusal view.

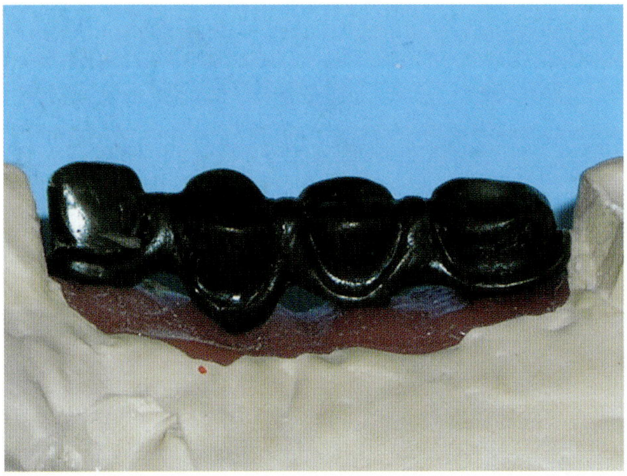

FIGURE 10-29. C & B Ponabut wax-ups, lingual view.

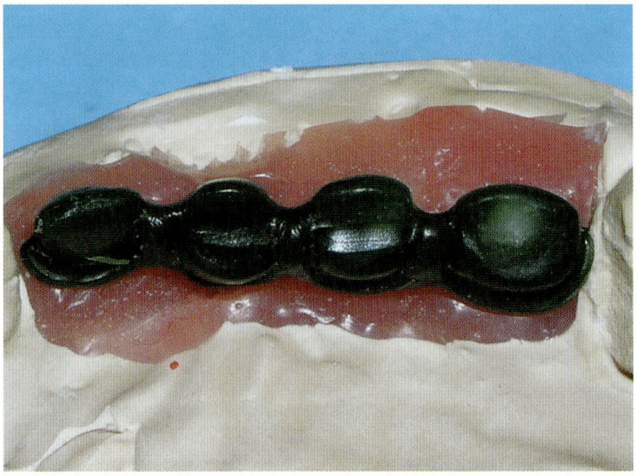

FIGURE 10-30. C & B Ponabut wax-ups, linguoocclusal view.

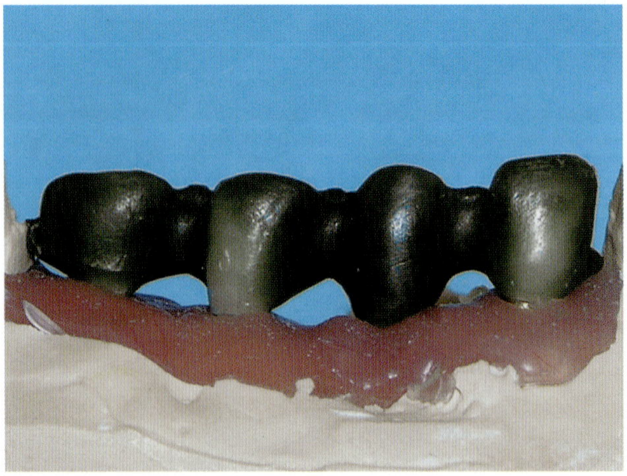

FIGURE 10-31. C & B Ponabut wax-ups, buccal view.

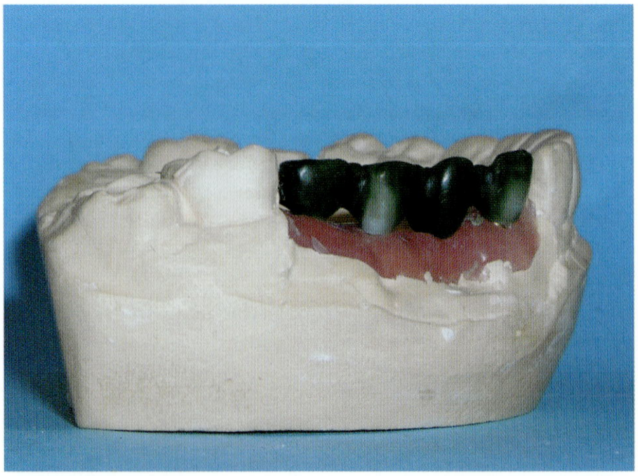

FIGURE 10-32. C & B Ponabut wax-ups, buccal view.

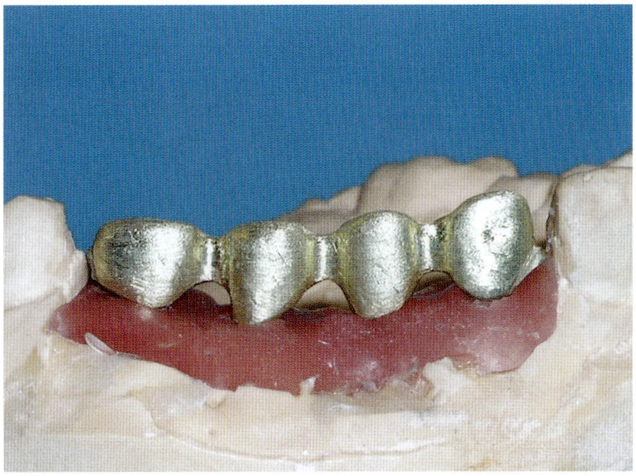

FIGURE 10-33. Ponabut cast framework.

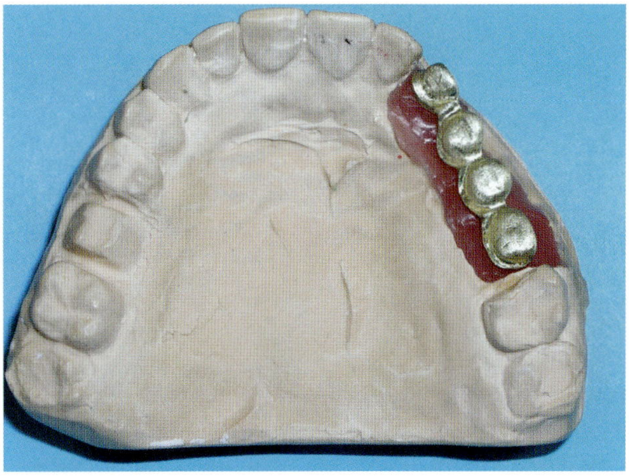

FIGURE 10-34. Ponabut cast framework, occlusal view.

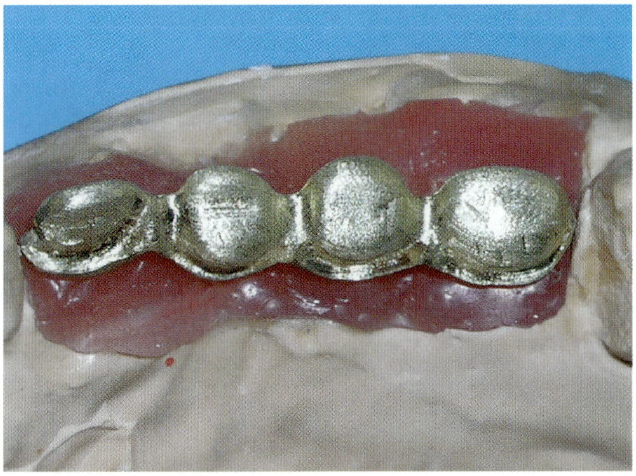

FIGURE 10-35. Ponabut casting framework, occlusolingual detail.

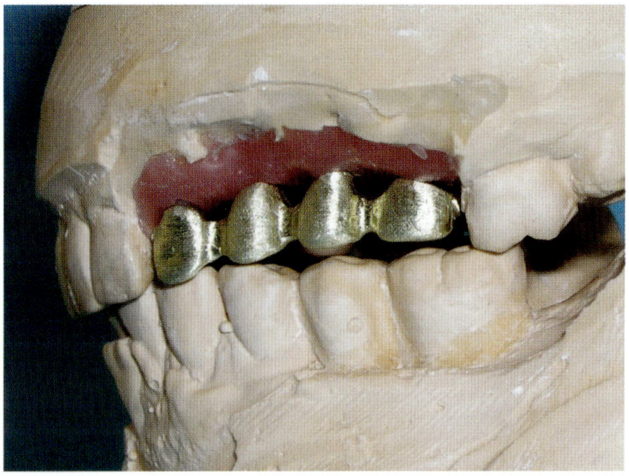

FIGURE 10-36. Ponabut cast framework, buccal detail.

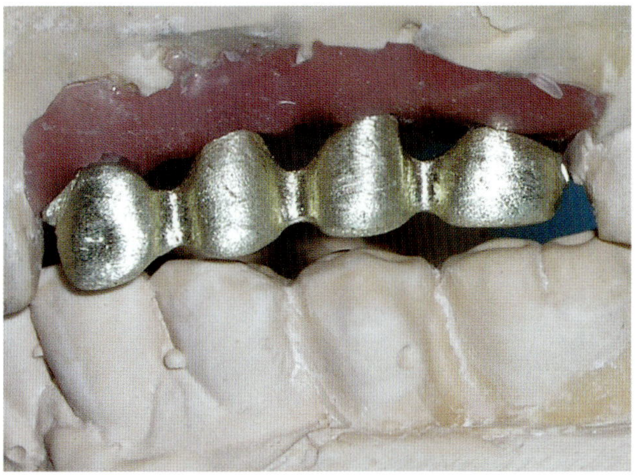

FIGURE 10-37. Ponabut cast framework, occlusal detail.

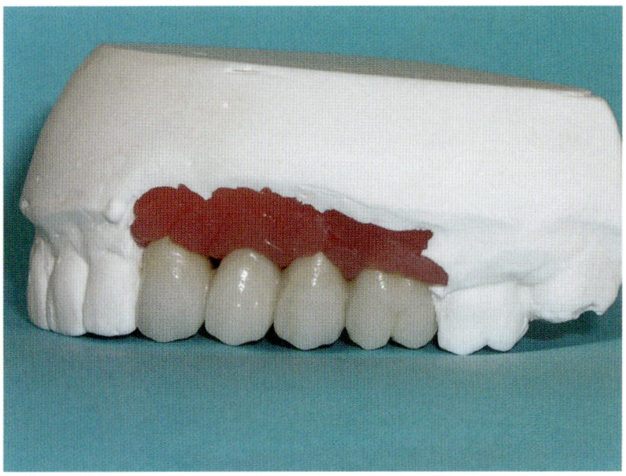

FIGURE 10-38. Porcelain Ponabuts, buccal view.

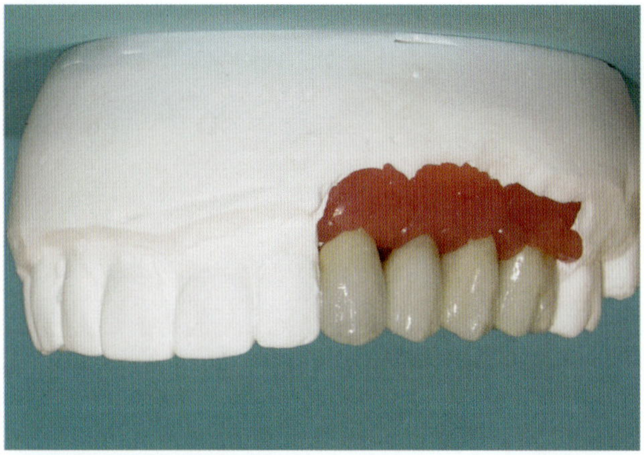

FIGURE 10-39. Porcelain Ponabuts, anterior view.

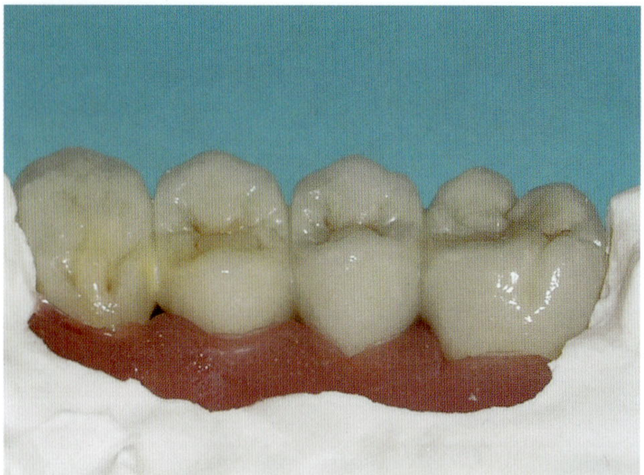

FIGURE 10-40. Porcelain Ponabuts, occlusolingual view.

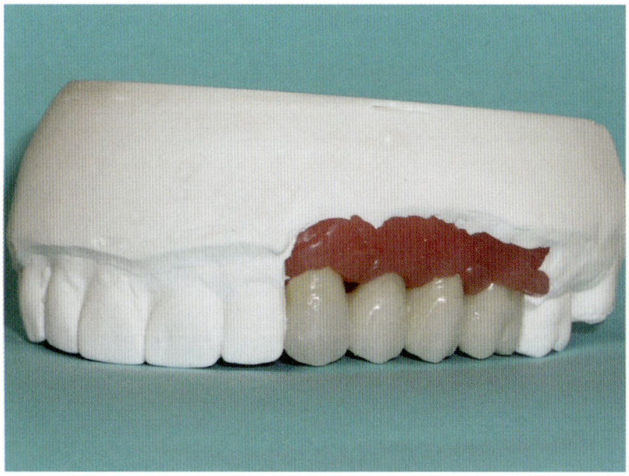

FIGURE 10-41. Porcelain Ponabuts, buccal view.

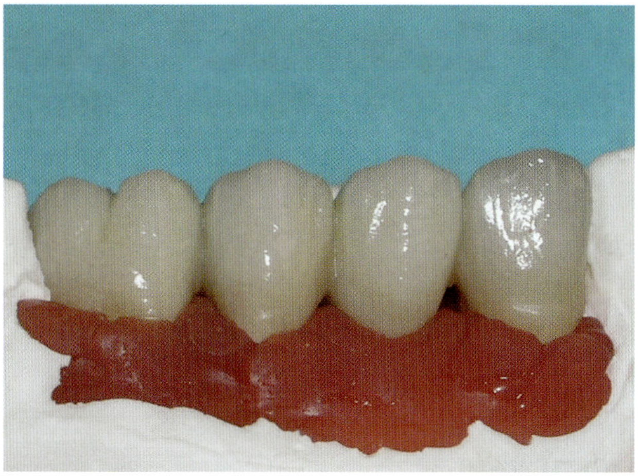

FIGURE 10-42. Porcelain Ponabuts, buccal view.

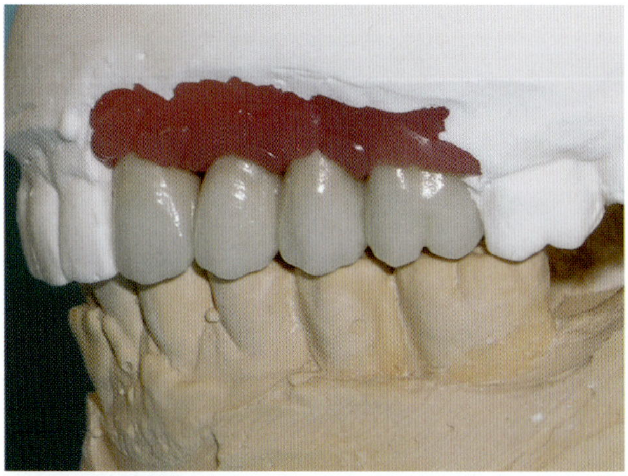

FIGURE 10-43. Porcelain Ponabuts, occlusion detail.

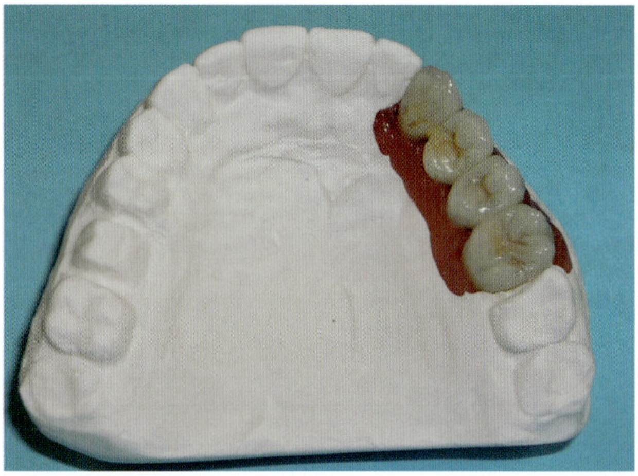

FIGURE 10-44. Porcelain Ponabuts, occlusal view.

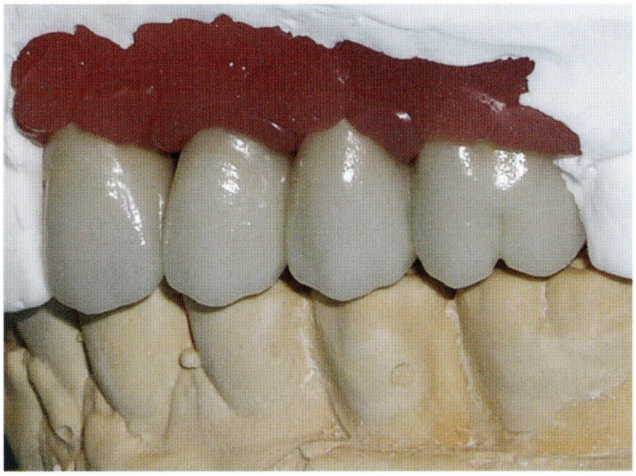

FIGURE 10-45. Ponabuts, buccal detail.

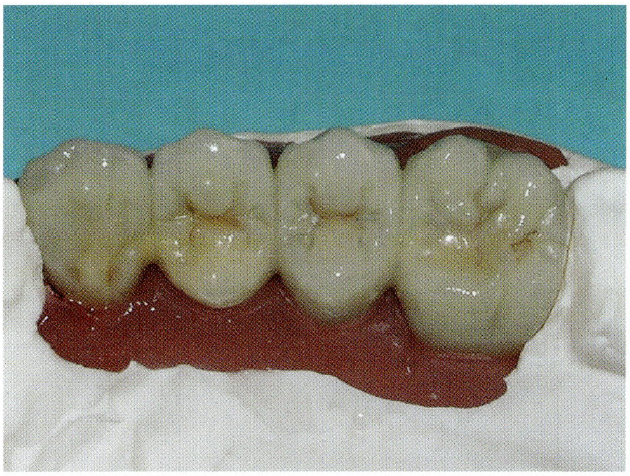

FIGURE 10-46. Porcelain Ponabuts, occlusal detail.

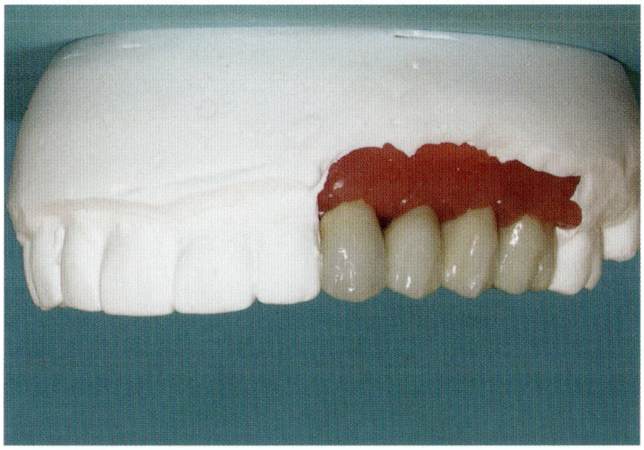

FIGURE 10-47. Glazed ceramometal MDI-supported fixed bridge.

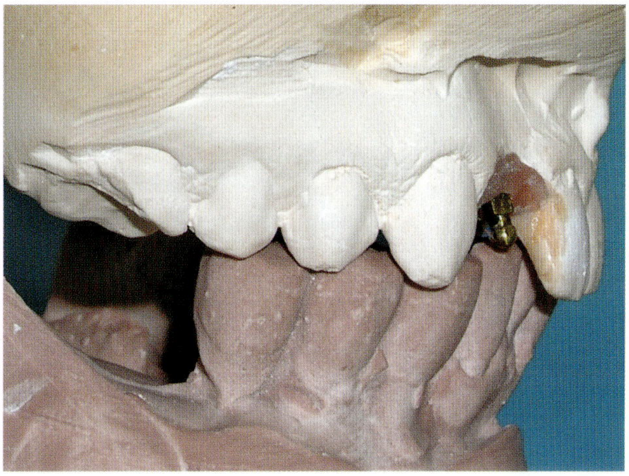

FIGURE 10-48. Single tooth replacement, right Ponabut view.

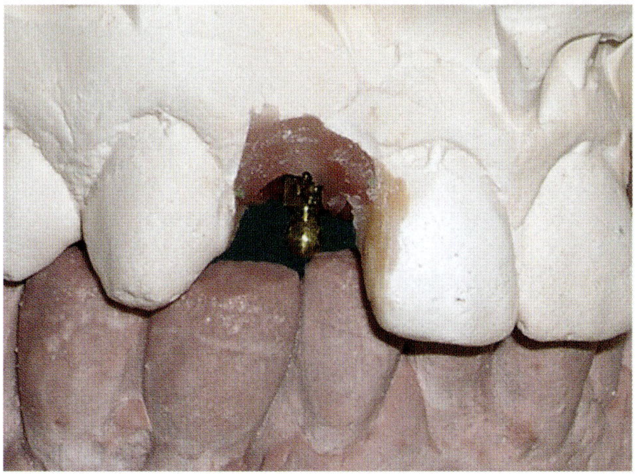

FIGURE 10-49. Single tooth replacement, right lateral incisor Ponabut.

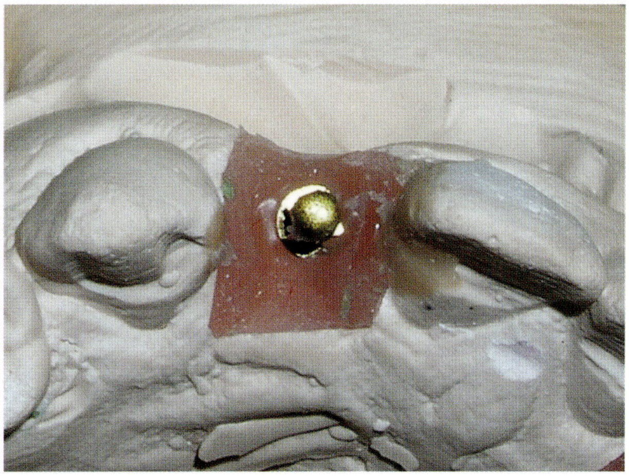

FIGURE 10-50. Single tooth replacement, right Ponabut.occlusal view.

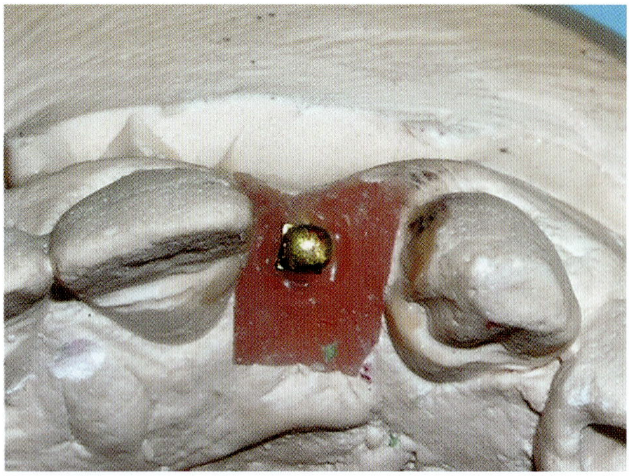

FIGURE 10-51. Single tooth replacement, left lateral incisor Ponabut.

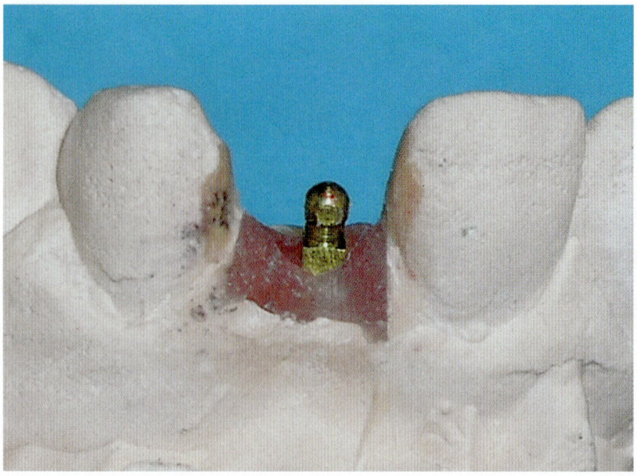

FIGURE 10-52. Single tooth replacement, left Ponabut view.

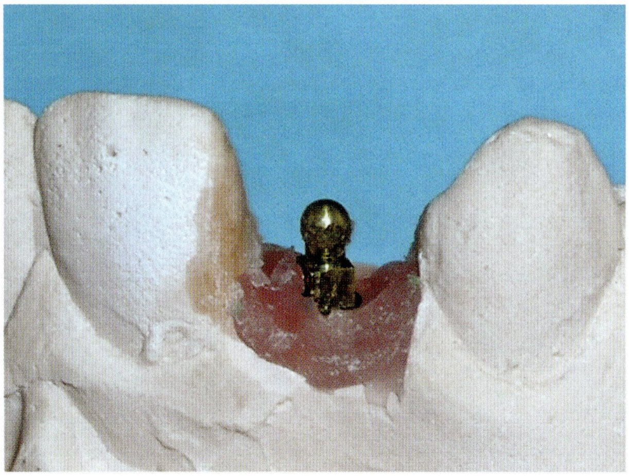

FIGURE 10-53. Single tooth replacement, close-up detail.

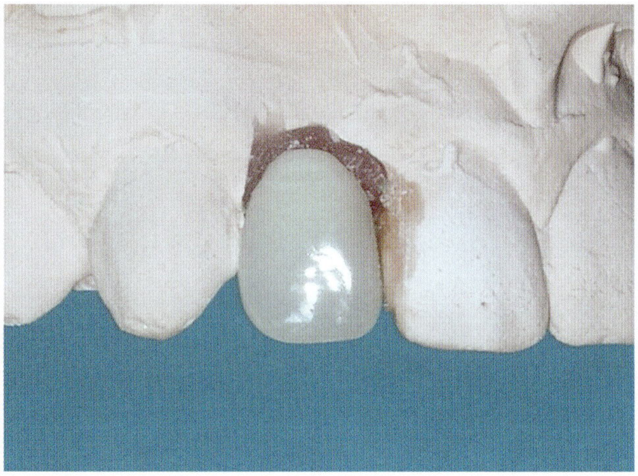

FIGURE 10-54. Right single tooth replacement, porcelain Ponabut.

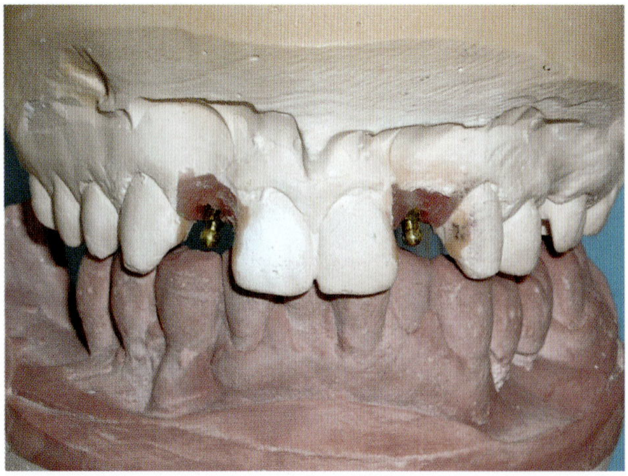

FIGURE 10-55. Right and left Ponabut single tooth replacements.

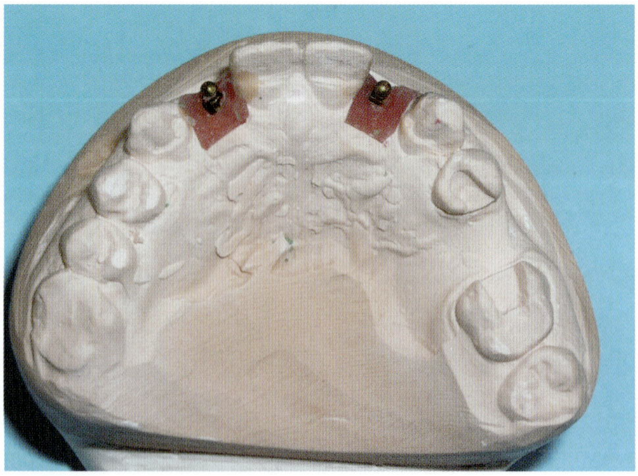

FIGURE 10-56. Right and left Ponabuts, occlusal view.

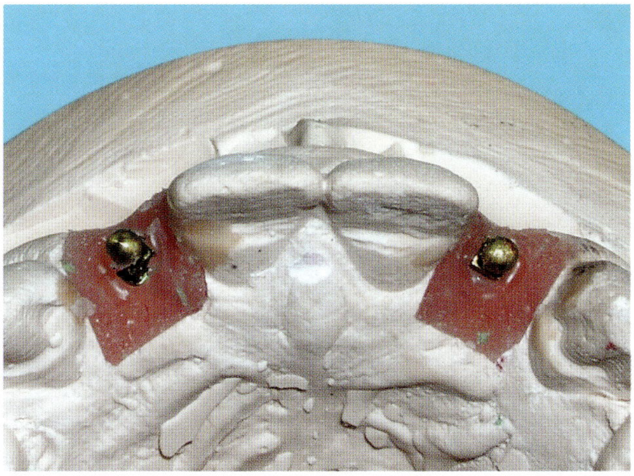

FIGURE 10-57. Right and left Ponabuts, occlusal details.

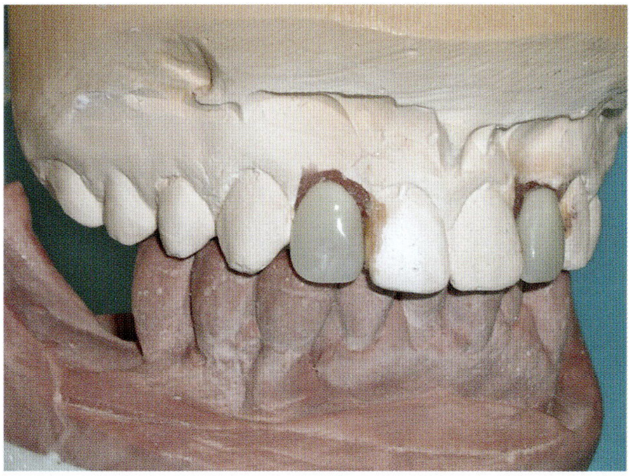

FIGURE 10-58. Single tooth replacement, right and left porcelain Ponabuts.

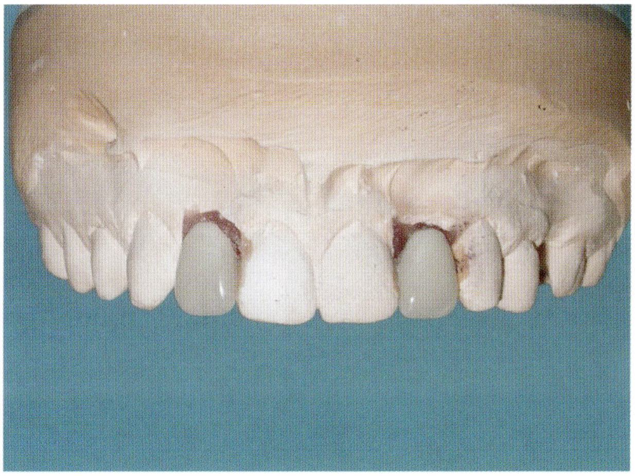

FIGURE 10-59. Single tooth replacement, right and left porcelain Ponabuts, anterior view.

Chapter 11

Concluding Postscript Analysis

STEPHEN M. TAUBENFELD VICTOR I. SENDAX

Outline

Positive Patient Psychology in Relation to Mini Dental Implant (MDI) Therapy

Stephen M. Taubenfeld

The psychosocial challenges faced by patients who experience uncompensated tooth loss are very real, and the consequences of missing teeth on self-esteem can be extremely debilitating. Simple activities of daily social life for an edentulous person, such as speaking, smiling, laughing, eating, and kissing, are rarely accomplished with total self-assurance. Replacing lost dentition is therefore not only essential to the maintenance of general medical health and bone preservation but can also have a profound beneficial impact on an individual's mental health stability.

The novel methodology of the mini dental implant (MDI) system is patient-friendly at its core. The nature of the procedure and follow-up care contributes to an overall positive experience for the patient. From a surgical standpoint, MDIs are so slender that they can be inserted directly through the overlying gum tissue and inserted into the underlying bone in a single minimal surgery. Many patients fear the relative invasiveness of conventional implants and associate them with a slow, painful recovery period. MDIs, however, are associated with significantly less postinsertion inflammation and soreness. Moreover, the relevant advantage of MDIs that evokes the most powerful psychological benefit is the fact that it is often possible to provide the complete implant service in a single office visit. Even in the rare event of a lost implant, the consequences, both physical and emotional, are measurably less severe than those of conventional tooth replacement systems, particularly when extensive grafting procedures are also necessary.

Some of the most profound clinical examples of positive mental health outcomes can be found in the adolescent patient population, a cohort not typically associated with edentulism. This elusively dynamic yet psychologically vulnerable stage of development is often characterized by multiple challenges to a young person's developing self-esteem. Symptoms of depression and anxiety in young adults are gaining increasing awareness in the mental health setting and are often attributed to the harsh, competitive environment in which teenagers play, learn, and mature. Consider the actual case of a teenage boy born with a defect that failed to manifest itself until the appearance of his other permanent teeth: anodontia of his lateral incisors. He was initially fitted with a space-maintainer (retainer) appliance, the type that some of his friends wore in conjunction with orthodontic therapy, which adversely affected his taste and prevented him from participating in sports that required a protective mouthpiece. The daily multiple cleaning rituals for an active teenager requires discipline and can be a tremendous obstacle. He began withdrawing from social situations in which he previously gained pleasure. The prospect of dating girls and experiencing kissing made him anxious. The next solution attempted was a "flipper" type of rudimentary partial denture fitted with prosthetic teeth. However, his active lifestyle resulted in several of them fracturing. When dental implants with transitional fixed resin teeth (allowing for interim jaw growth) were proposed to the young patient's parents, they immediately assumed that the cost would make them inaccessible, that the surgery would be lengthy, and that the recovery would be painful. With MDIs, the reality was quite the opposite, and he was fitted with two incisor MDIs in a single office visit. The implants gave him immediate biting function along with the morale-boosting sensation that they were his very own teeth, but most importantly they rehabilitated his confidence and restored his social freedom during a critical period of self-development.

The real-life emotional advantages of MDIs at times transcend the obvious clinical benefits to patients at every chronologic level, from teen to aged maturity, reinforcing positive self-image and practical functionality on a daily basis. There can be no question that this lifestyle enhancement has a parallel positive impact on ones' mental health status. Indeed, it is a medical milestone that we can share with our needful patients to help them achieve a healthier and more satisfying existence—less handicapped by debilitating tooth loss—and managed with minimal traumatic invasiveness.

The Role of MDIs in the Contemporary Imaging Evolution: A Current Assessment

Victor I. Sendax

With the recognition of bicortical stabilization techniques as the key to stable MDI longevity, it is useful to understand the role of imaging advances that have come to the fore and that significantly improve implant diagnostic and placement procedures.

Panoramic x-rays, tomographic modifications, and CT scans with volumetric collimated enhancements in tandem with computer-guided 3D surgery techniques have been skillfully designed to ease the pathway for mastering more complex and challenging maxillary and mandibular implant cases. Impressive scan views highlight the extensive scope of these digital imaging developments as they may apply to advanced MDI technology, to conventional implant applications, and to varied hybrid combinations of MDIs, conventional-width implants, and natural tooth abutments.

However, in this new era of increasingly sophisticated implant guidance devices and techniques, it is useful to remember that all of these visualization enhancements have a common purpose: namely, to render with more quantitative precision and accuracy the placement and ultimately the restoration of implant-supported prosthodontics, both fixed and removable.

It is equally important to recognize that the need remains to provide implant services to a large undercared-for patient population that could benefit enormously from a simplification of implant procedures leading to greater affordability and access. With this goal in mind, we see that the MDI can fulfill its role as a valuable niche procedure when patients need cost-effective dental implant therapy, particularly when medically compromised candidates are informed by their attending physicians that they are contraindicated for any invasive surgical procedures, including conventional dental implant insertions and extensive grafts. As minimally invasive and virtually nonsurgical entities, MDIs can usually gain physician acceptance when carefully planned and programmed by the implant-placing surgeon, allowing such patients to receive cost-effective, essential oral implant therapy with minimal significant health risk exposure, and with unequivocal medical clearance.

The sections of this textbook compiled by specialized hospital-based doctors such as Bohle, Lish, Peckitt, and Sussman attest to the consistent ability of MDIs to survive with minimal morbidity even under the most rigorous and threatening of local and systemic medical conditions. The conclusion that may reasonably be drawn from these graphic case examples is that if MDIs have long-term as well as routine shorter-term predictability, consistently demonstrated while under the cloud of such highly negative oral and systemic morbidities, it should confirm that MDIs can be considered on a par with conventional implants and, in select cases, may even surpass the usefulness of standard-width implants.

The enhanced ability to insert ultrasmall-diameter MDIs directly into narrow areas of bone without encroaching on vulnerable adjacent structures (e.g., sinus, nasal cavity, buccal or labial and lingual bony plates, neurovascular elements, & adjacent roots) has allowed the oral implantologist greater latitude in avoiding invasive hard and soft tissue grafting surgeries and associated flaps/sutures. Immediate functionality also implies less trauma to hard and soft tissues and vulnerable patient psyches, as well as reduced bone plate dieback and crestal bone loss. Although MDIs do not require routine use of CT technology (with its attendant costliness and radiation exposure risk) and have been typically placed with only basic periapical and/or panoramic radiographs, it is understandable that the more complex the case under consideration the more rational is the use of CT scanning as an ancillary aid to avoid vulnerable adjacent structures and to make maximum use of the available bone. This is especially the case when hybridized combined applications are being considered that may involve MDIs, conventional implants, and natural tooth abutments, and where the need is greatest to objectively evaluate the uneven morphology of the insertion sites in three dimensions and to critically assess the potential added value of partial and full flap surgery visualization and thereby enhance the precision of insertion.

The associated MDI benefits do not imply that MDIs are offered as a routine panacea or a cure-all substitute for conventional implants. Rather, the advocacy should be to fully consider hybridizing MDIs with conventional-width implants for more challenging treatment plans. In fact, the most sophisticated use of advanced digital imaging techniques is to help determine what implant system or hybrid combination is best adapted to the site-specific morphology of the area(s) under consideration and to correlate these findings with an affordable treatment plan, clearly embodying all the advances that have come to make oral implants an accessible mainstay of the modern dental profession and truly compassionate clinical practice.

Chapter 12

The Best of MDIs: Q and A

This anthology has been collected from an extended time span from the ongoing MDI Online Forum and selected blogs; it was assembled by Dr. Victor Sendax and associates with consultation with traditional academic resources as needed. It is in recognition of the fact that valuable and valid answers to often perplexing clinical conundrums may be gained via unsolicited e-mail commentary and queries from patients and colleagues who are on the clinical front line. The provided summary is deemed to embody some of the most constructive contributions from this vibrant resource, but it should not be construed as definitive answers to any of the posed questions.

Q. **What are the material components of mini dental implants (MDIs)?**

A. MDIs are made of high quality titanium alloy, consisting of Ti-6AL-4V. A 1997 test study at the University of Alabama at Birmingham clearly established that titanium alloy implants are significantly stronger than CP titanium products. More recently, a torque and dynamic loading study from the Medical College of Georgia at Augusta concluded that after 5,000,000 cycles of force, each ranging from 13 to 134 N at a sinusoidal rate of 8 Hz, no changes or fractures were detected in the submitted 1.8 mm × 15 mm and 1.8 mm × 13 mm MDIs.

Q. **What is the approximate distance from the inferior border of the mandible after the MDI is seated? Do I want the longest implant I can get in place without contacting the cortical bone on the inferior border? Or do I want to be half or three-quarters the distance? Secondly, is there any significance to the RPMs of the bur when penetrating the cortical plate and drilling into the cancellous space? I use intraosseous anesthesia regularly and am familiar with the feel of perforating the plate, but I am aware that most implant systems suggest a very slow rotation with a high-torque motor. Will a typical air-driven slow speed hand piece be okay, or do I need an electric motor with controlled speed?**

A. First of all, there is no exact specific length or distance recommended. Rather, the basic guideline should be to take advantage of as much available patient bone as possible. You are aware, however, especially in the anterior mandible, that the deep symphyseal bone can be very dense and hard to penetrate. In that event you would be better off not trying to overdo the length issue and settle for a shorter MDI rather than trying to aim for the inferior border. All you need is a crestal cortical penetration (using either a moderately high speed drill to break through or a slower speed drill if it can penetrate readily without excessive pressure or friction) only deep enough to provide a good starter opening to introduce the self-tapping implant. Then, it should be possible to readily auto-advance it with jaw support as you turn it with slow strokes into the medullary (and presumably more cancellous) bone.

Although the point is consistently not to over-instrument the patient's bone, it is also essential to remember that you must get a good initial penetration (at the right angulation, of course) for the starter opening to allow the MDI to take hold and work its way in effectively. Also, if the initial starter penetration needs to be accomplished at a slightly higher speed for better torque control, it is only in force for a few seconds, with simultaneous water spray and with a very narrow-width drill bit, so little initial bone damage is likely to occur.

If you then follow the classic placement protocol sequence with the finger driver, the more efficient winged thumb wrench, and finally the ratchet wrench if needed to attain the final biting depth, the length of the MDI becomes ultimately less important than its stability and solidity. After the implant is securely placed, it is a mistake to over-ratchet it in dense Type I bone. It is much better to settle for a somewhat shorter implant and with the abutment head consistent with the crestal bone and soft tissue level.

Q. How much postoperative pain should my patients with MDIs expect? I know this is a relative question but it will be commonly asked. For example, is it comparable with an extraction for this type of implant, or is it usually less painful? Whereas I may prescribe hydrocodone 5 mg for an extraction, would I also expect the same level of pain control needed here? What is your usual protocol for postoperative care?

A. If there was no previous inflammation or infection in the area under treatment, there should be little postoperative pain except for the needle injection sites. Low-level analgesics like aspirin, acetaminophen, ibuprofen, and comparable NSAIDs are the only usual postoperative medicines. Warm saline rinses are also beneficial to increase circulation and blood supply to the insertion site and speed the healing process.

Q. After inserting MDIs, do you only use O rings seated in the denture or do you ever use one of the newer soft liners directly over the implant?

A. You can use chairside, immediate soft-liners over the O-ball abutment heads as the kindest, gentlest retainers until your own comfort level with the technique convinces you that, in your own hands, the Sendax MDI technique works as described. Then you can substitute O rings for more secure retention after you are convinced that the MDIs are solid and secure. You can often acquire sufficient retention with only two or three implants as well as four; therefore my recommendation is to avoid limiting yourself to any exact number in advance and allow the individual case variables help you fashion a customized decision, which also allows for what I consider a more professionally desirable complete case fee to be presented rather than the typical shopping list of charges.

Q. If you load immediately, why don't you produce a fibrous encapsulation at the implant interface and thus possible clinical mobility?

A. A fibrous tissue response down the line is possible with an implant if it is subject to consistent traumatic lateral movement. Even ongoing micro-movement can be destructive to bone healing physiology. However, MDIs are placed directly through the crestal gum tissue into the underlying medullary bone with a very small starter opening, just enough to promote a self-tapping "take" and permit the auto-advancement thread design to then virtually draw the implant into the bone. This means that there is no conventional "healing period" because nothing requires a period of repair. The direct contact of implant surface to bone (osseoapposition) is accomplished immediately with minimal surgical intervention. No significant amount of bone is lost by drilling it away, as would be the case in a typical implant osteotomy procedure. The only bone loading force during a slow turning insertion phase is mostly compressive, which bone is uniquely able to tolerate within reasonable limits.

Most fundamentally, the threaded surfaces of MDIs do not have to first grow into contact with the bone; it's already there from day one by direct osseoapposiiton, and it is mature support bone. How well the implant then bears up under diverse loading conditions may have more to do with peripheral systemic issues like medical profile and heredity. More than two decades of clinical experience with MDIs has proven the integrity and legitimacy of this unique insertion protocol and made it possible to achieve immediate and sustainable loading without significant bone loss or mobility. This is possible even in medically compromised patients in long-term applications.

Q. How about single tooth replacement?

A. MDIs work very well as single tooth replacement implants where space is insufficient between tooth roots for a conventional implant. MDIs can be considered long-term implants if the patented insertion protocol is followed precisely.

Q. Have you used this implant for replacement of a single mandibular incisor? I am a periodontist treating a 23-year-old woman with a congenitally missing #26 that is presently restored via a repeatedly debonded Maryland bridge. The adjacent #25 and #27 are essentially virgin teeth. Interradicular space slightly less than 4 mm makes placement of a conventional narrow diameter fixture problematic. Her restorative dentist is open to any options. Have you managed similar cases?

A. This is actually an ideal application for the MDI and we have been successful in cases with congenitally missing teeth and narrow interradicular space, with or without a previous failed Maryland bridge. Assuming you have experience in placing MDIs, follow your previous steps, taking a little extra care to get the angulation on target by taking a few progress periapicals and making any midcourse corrections as needed. A temporary crown can be placed on top of either the rectangular head or O-ball head abutments until the definitive crown is made. Some dentists are now using the CAD/CAM CEREC and comparable techniques to fabricate crown restorations over MDIs as well as via the more traditional crown techniques.

Q. I would like to place MDIs in my patient's anterior mandible. She only has 8 mm of bone height. I was going to place the 10-mm MDIs and possibly have 1 mm through the inferior cortex. Comment please.

A. There is nothing intrinsically problematic about this strategy. The primary difficulty I see is trying to self-tap the MDI through the last few millimeters to reach the inferior cortex of the extradense symphyseal bone, leading to the likelihood of either stripping the bone or burnishing it. Also, if you do manage to penetrate or perforate through with great effort, you run the risk of the patient experiencing bone necrosis and abscess. It's better to stop when you hit too dense a layer of apical anterior bone and even to allow a few MDI threads to remain uncovered by bone and/or gingiva if necessary. Remember, don't over-instrument the bone! A significant number of failures can be attributed to over-instrumentation.

Q. I have a patient with a very heavy bite who has a history of fracturing several of his upper dentures. He's asked me about MDIs. Also, what do you suggest insofar as protocol when an MDI fails? Do you replace it with a longer one? Do you go adjacent?

A. For heavy bite and temporomandibular joint parafunction cases I recommend starting with a soft liner in the O-ring caps that have been incorporated into the denture. Remove the rubber O-rings from the caps, and use a nonrunny soft liner (either powder/liquid mix or automix) in each minicap and rebase the entire intaglio (soft-tissue bearing) surface. Insert the prosthesis in the patient's mouth over the O-ball abutment heads in centric and vertical occlusal and allow to set over the MDIs. This will give the patient a reasonably stable overdenture in which the heavy occlusion will be born mostly by the soft liner and will protect the MDI bone support from functional and/or parafunctional overloading. Eventually you can convert some or all of the O-ring caps to regular O-ring retainers as needed by the patient and if the MDIs are stable and comfortable.

As for implants that are loose or exfoliated, I recommend replacement without charge within a reasonable time frame after insertion, especially if I feel that poor bone resource is the likely cause for failure. Each clinician must be responsible for formulating a replacement charge policy based on his/her learning curve status. It applies to length, location, and number of such replacements or repositionings. It's basically your call because you know from your x-rays and working the region far better than someone else how to proceed with reasonable confidence.

Incidentally, doctors sometimes ask if they should refund the cost for a failed MDI if the patient is unhappy. Again, this is an individual call, but I would advise approaching refunds cautiously because there is a suggestion or hint of error on your part. It's better to focus on replacement without charge on the basis that you are still in the exploratory stage of determining where the best quality of bone for MDI support is located.

Q. I know fees vary greatly by region, but could you give me an idea of the fees currently being charged for placement of four MDIs and modification of an existing complete denture?

A. Fees do vary greatly and a lot of factors come into play. Clinicians at seminars talk about fees ranging from $250 to $750 per MDI depending on all the usual factors clinicians are accustomed to.

Q. I just placed my sixteenth MDI and everything went well once again. To me, the MDIs are almost scary. They're so easy! Plus, my patients LOVE them. I've been charging $500 per implant and another $200 to pick up the O ring into the denture (per implant). My practice is located in a Boston suburb. Am I charging fairly? I can place two MDIs and pick up the O-ring caps in about 90 minutes start to finish.

A. Of course it's fair if the patients think so, too. However, I would note that we typically recommend a minimum of four MDIs in the anterior mandible. One or two posterior MDIs can add significant additional retention and stability if there is available bone without the risk for encroachment on the neurovascular bundle or mental foramen.

Q. Should I have a patient having MDIs placed go without his or her dentures for any period of time after the surgery or treat it more like an immediate denture? If he or she wears it immediately after surgery, should I wait until the next day to remove it or should it come out that same evening?

A. There is no need to let the patient go without his or her prosthesis at any time unless the prosthesis itself is causing iatrogenic pressure ulcers or other comparable problems that you cannot resolve chairside by basic denture border and internal adjustments.

Q. What is your favorite sequence for placing MDIs? For example, do you work from one side to the other or do you place the two center implants first or the two outside implants first?

A. Each case is different, as you well know. Keep in mind that you need to stay well mesial to the vulnerable mental foramen and associated nerve "loops" and distal to (and superior to) any extremely dense symphyseal bone in the midline. We recommend you present the procedure to your patient as an exploratory process to test the bone quality and quantity rather than as a "tentative implant placement." This is a professional approach, is truthful, and, importantly, less stressful for you and your patient.

Q. On a full lower denture, I placed four MDIs: three 13 mm and one 10 mm. I placed them too close together to use one of the abutment posts, allowing only three metal housings. I felt I was placing the implants into the body of the mandible through the little attached gingival I had. When I finished and was placing the housings, they were all lingually inclined, impinging on the lingual tissues. The one that could not be used because it was too close to the other implants was also so lingually inclined that it couldn't have had a housing cap on it anyway. After 1 week the 10-mm MDI was lost. (It was positioned farthest to the left and supported one of the retention caps). Clinically I feel I had left too much cold cure acrylic around the implants and/or she bit on her denture too hard during set, which caused pretty severe tissue irritation and probably loosened the implant. Currently there are three solid implants, two with metal housings (both positioned on the right side) and one with no housing. The retention of the denture is good but the right side is solid and the left "lifts a little" during eating, making it uncomfortable to the patient. I would like to place one or two more implants on the left side to balance the retention. I would like someone to look at the case and show me the optimum position and other suggestions. The patient is fine with placing the other implants. I have a lateral cephalometric x-ray, a panoramic x-ray, and

a lower study model. Please advise me how I could discuss this with someone.

A. The best bet when you want to progressively load MDIs is to use at the outset only a soft liner rebase over the implants and the entire tissue-bearing surface of the denture. This would have eliminated any starting complications in your first case by giving you time to evaluate the viability of the MDIs before committing yourself and the patient to the more efficient O-rings in their encapsulations. In fact, I use this sequencing myself in most of my own cases. Be careful to use the silicone elastomeric shims on the square 4-mm base portion of the abutment to avoid the excess acrylic locking on during O-ring cap pick-ups (*that obviously would be the wrong way to give a patient a fixed bridge!*). Also, I recommend that you enroll in a Mini Residency or MDI Seminar, if you haven't already done so, at which time you might bring along your diagnostic materials for evaluation.

Q. **How do I determine the amount or length of available bone to determine if I have enough or what length implant I would want to use? I do not have a panoramic x-ray machine, but have access to one through my local orthodontist. Would you please explain how I could take x-rays and make this evaluation for maxilla and mandibular arches? Also, could you expand on what parameters you use to judge the quality of bone? I am looking forward to using the system a lot and am already advertising for patients.**

A. You have raised many pertinent questions that relate to both conventional implants and MDIs. All types of x-rays are useful guidelines for bone quality (density), quantity, and height. A panoramic unit is basic if you do implant therapy, whether it's your own by purchase or rental, for maximum visualization ability. CT scans, tomograms, lateral plates, etc., can also be useful, but keep in mind that all these methodologies are approximations and therefore none of them give you a truly foolproof answer. Consequently, the best advice is to gain experience in estimation by doing the MDI procedures and taking evaluation x-rays to check your progress. Make mid-course corrections as needed to maximize use of available medullary and cortical bone without encroaching on any vulnerable structures, such as neurovascular bundle, mental foramen, labial, buccal and lingual plates of bone, and floor of sinus or nasal cavities. The most useful learning tool is experience doing the procedure and carefully monitoring the results. You'll be surprised and gratified by how rapidly you'll master the learning curve for a procedure that's essentially simple but still embodies variable and occasionally challenging elements.

Q. **How long can I predict to patients that their MDIs will last?**

A. All implants, including MDIs, will last as long as they remain bone-integrated without mobility or infection. MDIs are the only implants on the market that can be deemed integrated immediately after insertion due to their unique, patented insertion protocol. Operating as a minimally invasive, totally self-tapping procedure, a MDI does not require a conventional osteotomy to ream out a considerable amount of bone that must be regenerated into contact with the implant surface before supportive integration can reasonably be expected. Histologic human studies have confirmed that MDIs demonstrate direct bone contact without any intervening soft tissue, and, most importantly, ongoing clinical experience has shown the ability of an integrated MDI to be able to bear functional intraoral loading without loss of integration. However, all implant systems can potentially lose bone anchorage from occlusal overloading, especially during habitual bruxism and other parafunctional, nonphysiologic activity, and local and systemic disease. Smoking has also been shown to be a prime negative factor in connection with osteoporosis and periimplantitis, leading to a greatly increased likelihood of implant failure.

If you use only a minimal starter cortex penetration and progress only 3 to 4 millimeters into underlying medullary bone, you'll find that the MDI device auto-advances into the remaining bone until it is rock solid. This totally self-tapping, virtually nonsurgical insertion protocol will provide immediate integration without an intervening healing period. That is the core rationale for any assumption of MDI longevity.

No one can simply claim longevity. A clinician must gradually develop the essential "comfort level" required. You'll quickly find the MDI works not only for short-term but long-term, on-going applications as well.

For implants in general as well as Sendax MDIs in particular, there should be no specific cutoff date for implant survival if the implants are in direct bone contact support. This is called osseointegration by the Brånemark definition, or as we prefer to call it, *osseoapposition*, because direct bone contact with MDI threads occurs immediately upon auto-advancement insertion rather than by the slow healing and bone regrowth/repair process characteristic of conventional implant systems.

Q. How do I restore the implant prosthetically? I can see that the implant has the O-ball head for a denture. What if I want to use the implant for a three-unit bridge or for a single crown? Also, are they recommended for bridges or single crowns?

A. You can still use the same O-ball head for fixed applications by blocking out the complete length of the abutment with an elastomeric shim before wax-up and casting to permit an easy "draw" of the pattern from the abutment analog. This also avoids undercut or parallelism problems. Of course, you can also use the rectangular "preppable" head MDI abutment as well as the O-ball type.

Q. I'm using the MDI Max for replacement of an upper lateral incisor. You frequently mention the use of a "shim" for casting to block out undercuts. Is the shim placed on the MDI intraorally before the impression is taken for a crown, or should I send the shim to the lab and instruct them to place it on the master plaster cast before wax-up? Will the final crown have a "positive" seat if the shape of the implant was altered by use of the shim and therefore rotates when tried in instead of fitting with a "definite" seat? You also mention that the MDI can be shaped to allow for occlusal clearance or parallelism. Any problem doing this directly in the mouth using high speed drill with water or is generation of heat from high speed drilling a concern? Comments, please.

A. The usual sequence of procedure for fixed single or multiple restorations is to take an intraoral impression in polyvinylsiloxane or comparable material, place an IMTEC analog in the MDI location, then pour up the model. (An elastomeric shim would only be used intraorally if you were doing a direct O-ring/cap pickup.) A shim can also be placed over an O-ball analog in a model to provide a spacer and undercut blockout for a wax-up. Make intraoral adjustments with moderate speed and water spray.

Q. Please comment on the MDI system's applicability for provisional use.

A. After placing O-ball MDIs, you can easily retrofit an existing maxillary or mandibular denture (or bridge) by hollowing out the acrylic for relief over the MDI(s) and following up with a soft chairside liner. When set, this will provide moderate anchorage without compromising the MDIs bone support. After you have attained your own comfort level with the system's ability to be put into immediate function, you can switch over to the more secure O-ring retention attachments, which are included with each O-ball MDI. You might also think about O rings for medium and longer-term use rather than only as a short-term transitional solution, but that will come about naturally in the course of your familiarity and experience with the entire MDI insertion and reconstructive protocol.

Q. If I'm certain I'm going to do a "fixed" case, should I use the square- (rectangular) headed MDIs as opposed to the ball type? Also, do you often have the laboratory place the O rings at the bench rather than doing it chairside, especially for a new denture?

A. You can use either rectangular head or an O-ball head for fixed applications because they both retain well. Be sure to use the elastomeric shims for any easy draw and undercut blockout when doing direct intraoral pickups. O-ring caps can be picked up directly intraorally, or indirectly, by means of a poly impression and analogs, then lab processed.

Q. I have a lab question. I visited a dental lab in New York recently. The lab technician had a few of my MDI cases. He mentioned that on

a new removable partial denture, after I place the MDIs before final impression, I can place the O-ring cap on the implants and withdraw it in the impression, place analogs inside the O-rings, and they'll process the case. Supposedly this would save chair-time but can it be as accurate? He thinks yes; what do you think?

A. It's apparent that your lab tech contact knows a lot about restoring MDIs. This technique works just fine, but when you ask if it's accurate, I would respond by asking you: Accurate as compared with what other technique? An alternative would be to take a full arch heavy-bodied polyvinylsiloxane (PVS) or polyether impression of the entire jaw. A good supplemental tip is to eject some PVS medium-bodied material directly over the O-ball abutment heads before taking the impression so you get a more fully-detailed seat for the analogs. Remember that you must also get a good bite registration at the same visit that you take your PVS impression (and a counter alginate or PVS impression).

Q. I would like to expand the use of the MDI system in immediate extraction cases. I have seen emphasized the importance of having mature cortical bone for success in the symphysis region. I'd like to know what your recommended protocol is in handling immediate cases. I have thus far told my patients that we need to wait about 6 months after an extraction before we place the MDI. I would appreciate a quick response because I have several immediate cases coming up and want to provide timely service to my patients.

A. I'm afraid there is no infallible "protocol" for handling immediate extraction cases. You are on your own with this issue because it is the residual bony architecture that is most important after extractions, not how long you need to wait before MDI insertions are contemplated. If the interseptal bone is there to receive a 1.1-mm starter drill opening (and with no infection and only minimal inflammatory soft tissue), it is possible to insert MDIs on the first day. You must also be the one to evaluate the patient's insertion site and decide if the area is stable enough to proceed with good access and visibility.

Q. Would you have any reservations about using the MDIs for the maxillary edentulous patient exhibiting severe hyperplastic ridges (soft, spongy, and movable tissue)? I have a patient who currently wears a full upper denture with several unsuccessful reline attempts. She claims the spongy tissue was removed surgically several years ago, leaving her with a flat upper ridge. I am considering four MDIs in the maxilla, similar to recommendations for full lower denture MDIs. The tissue is approximately 3 mm thick and very movable. Can I place the MDIs into this soft tissue (and of course into bone) without worrying that 3 mm of the implant screw might be in soft tissue, not bone, because of the 3 mm thickness of tissue? Is there a higher risk for failure or periimplantitis?

A. I generally advocate that, where possible, MDIs (as well as conventional implants) should emerge through keratinized, attached ridge gingiva, rather than through unattached mucosa. It is well accepted that tough, keratinized tissue is much more resistant to bacterial invasion and pericementitis, as well as periimplantitis, than loose mucosa; it is reasonable to apply this to MDIs as well. The advantage of the MDI insertion protocol is the fact that this ultrathin MDI has such a small footprint that it can readily be accommodated in even a small patch of keratinized ridge tissue. This makes it much more likely that the MDI can be accommodated in very sparsely keratinized atrophic ridges compared with the relatively bulky traditional implants that often end up in unattached mucosa. This does not mean that implants placed through nonkeratinized tissue are doomed to failure, but the prognosis is always better for emergence through attached gingiva. Because we also advocate placing our insertions directly through soft tissue and into the underlying medullary bone with a minimal "starter" opening without incisions, flaps, or sutures, in most cases we can assume a more stable soft tissue profile surrounding the MDIs without worrying about significant remodeling, die-back, or loss of our original keratinized crestal tissue.

Q. I have placed two mini O-ball implants as posterior abutments to a four-unit bridge. The

implants are in tooth #30 area, well integrated, with healthy natural teeth #28 and #29 as the anterior abutments. My lab has some questions about how to handle these implants: (1) How should we finish the gingival margin because there is no "true" margin on these implants, only the head of the implant itself? (2) Coming up from the gingival, what type of emergence profile shall we use? (3) What type of cement would you recommend, assuming the metal frame of the bridge is nonprecious metal?

A. The basic concept with MDIs for fixed bridge applications is to treat all ridge lap areas as normal pontics with normal ridge laps and embrasures, but with openings into the tissue side for the O-ball head to reside passively inside without any internal contacting surfaces. We call these hybrid pontic/abutment combinations *Ponabuts*. Consequently, there are no gingival margins in the usual sense (except for normally narrow lower anteriors where the MDI crown margins finish at the gingival terminus of the O ball or rectangular abutment) or where a conventional emergence profile may actually be considered.

As for cementation options, any cement that you routinely use and find works is the best choice. Problems only occur when a new and untested cement is used, and setting time, film thickness, etc., are question marks. I prefer zinc oxyphosphate cement, which works well for me but may be alien to another operator's experience and comfort level. Also, if fit needs to be improved after internal etching, a chairside reline of the internals with a bonded resin (self-cure or light-cure) works well if you remember to slightly strip the internals after bonding (using a bullet-shaped diamond with water spray) to provide an easy but precise fit before final cementation.

Q. I can't say enough good things about what the MDI system has done for my patients. The system works! I do need your input concerning a patient, however. I placed twelve MDIs in her mouth, six up and six down. I placed three MDIs distal to her lower existing teeth (cuspid to cuspid) on each ridge. No implants are in the mandibular canals or the mental foramen. However, the patient complains of cold sensitivity from the middle implant on the left side. I spoke with Dr. Charles English about this and he said that he had not seen this problem before. Have you? Please let me know if you can figure out what might be causing this phenomenon.

A. Thanks for your gracious comments about the MDI system. I must say though that I have never encountered the apparent cold sensitivity you describe. If natural teeth were present in the area of interest I could understand such a temperature reaction, but with only MDIs in the affected region it is difficult to draw any inference from what you describe. I suppose if the implant is in close proximity to some neurologic focal area it could conceivably transmit cold sensitivity, but admittedly that's awfully hypothetical.

Q. Should I use a standard informed consent office form with patients receiving MDIs?

A. We recommend a standard informed consent form that is custom-tailored specifically for the MDI procedure. However, you might also consult with your personal legal counsel before using any particular consent form.

Q. I know it's possible to use well-integrated MDIs for ongoing, long-term, fixed ceramometal bridge restorations as well as the typical shorter-term transitional prosthesis, but how do you provide a good fit and a smooth, polished finish to the ridge lap of the Ponabut in the area of the MDI emergence through crestal soft tissue?

A. A step-by-step protocol to accomplish this important procedure is as follows:

1. The finished, glazed ceramometal bridge, crown, or splint is tried to confirm proper occlusion, contacts, and basic fit. Use of elastometric shims should permit an easy "draw" bypassing or clearing any angulation or undercut variations.
2. The interiors of the Ponabuts (and the ridge laps, if there are any and they need small additions to compensate for soft tissue remodeling changes) are etched with a microetcher to provide a reliable bonding surface.
3. Any high-quality, lite-curable composite resin paste, shade-compatible with the porcelain, and with good flow characteristics, is introduced into the interiors of the Ponabuts to the level of the ridge laps.

4. Restoration is inserted over the abutments intraorally, and the patient is instructed to bite slowly but firmly into a guided centric occlusion, with extruded composite excess teased away from the cervical margins.
5. Restoration is removed from the patient's mouth, leaving uncured composite resin inside the surface-etched Ponabuts. Any excess is trimmed away, with any voids touched up with additional composite resin paste. Restoration may be reseated and adjusted until inspection reveals an acceptable result, with easy draw and smooth compensation for any abutment angulation variations.
6. Composite resin is light-cured until surfaced hardened. Internals may be fine tuned with slow speed bullet shaped diamonds (with copious water spray) to provide an easy fit intraorally.
7. When all occlusal, contact, and internal adjustments are finalized, the ridge laps of the Ponabuts are brushed with a micro-fill composite resin glaze and light-cured until completely surface hardened. A time saver that ensures a complete bonding cure at this final stage is to employ a standard curing light unit.
8. Restoration may now be temporarily cemented with ease of removal. If the fit is snug, and ease of removal is questionable with so-called "temporary" cements, then a reasonable alternative is a mix of antibiotic ointment (such as Neosporin) with a denture adhesive (such as Fix-O-Dent) for a good transitional seal. Final cementation may be accomplished with zinc oxyphosphate or materials of your choice. On a personal note, I prefer the classic zinc cement because of the ease of removal of the hard-set excess from all margins.

Q. Please discuss what I can expect insofar as mobility is concerned.

A. Good question. Mobility (looseness) of MDIs occurs typically in the first few weeks after insertion, and is almost always associated with over-instrumentation of bone at time of drilling procedure (osteotomy). After the learning curve for the MDI procedure for bone site preparation, subsequent mobility is rarely encountered if self-tapping, bone-to-implant integration is accomplished at the outset. Steady bone stability is then routinely encountered.

Moreover, mobile implants were encountered in clinical trials over a 4-year period primarily when the MDI was placed in an extremely osteoporotic bone site where only a limited quantity and quality of osseous resource was available.

Q. How important is the strict following of the recommended insertion and reconstructive protocol? Also, please comment on fracture rates.

A. The protocol is critical. Long-term experience has demonstrated a consistent record of safety and effectiveness of the original concept that these devices, when placed using a strict insertion and reconstructive protocol, have the ability to function both for transitional and long-term applications. As for fractures, they're minimized when the titanium alloy (Ti6A14Va) is utilized instead of CP titanium. Records of clinical trials have proven that the optimal resistance for final seating of a MDI is 35 NCm. Any value beyond 45 NCm could result in a fracture of the implant, but lateral forces placed on the implant during insertion can also cause fracture. Fracture can also be more readily controlled by careful occlusal management.

Q. Please discuss placement issues insofar as parallelism of the MDIs is concerned.

A. Parallelism questions primarily depend on how many implants are involved. A greater number of implants requires greater degree of parallelism because it gets more difficult to insert and remove the prosthesis if multiple angulation problems are present. The best rule is to try to insert the MDIs as nearly parallel as possible, and, if angulations are excessive, the best approach is to use a soft liner rather than O-ring retention in such areas, especially with multiple MDIs (more than two). Simply tease out the O ring with an explorer or comparable tool from its retaining cap and fill it with self-cure soft liner over the O-ball head intraorally. When set, a modest degree of retention will still be present but without excessive binding, even with less than ideal angulation. Another approach is to slightly strip the internal fit of an O ring with a tapered bullet-shaped diamond instrument at moderate speed and light water spray. This relief should reduce the tendency for the O ring to bind on the O-ball head when inserting or removing a full or partial prosthesis when off-parallel MDIs are present.

Q. **I have recently started treating cases using the MDI and am very excited about the prospects. I have chosen to use one in a case in which I will be placing a few root form implants where appropriate, but I want to use a MDI for a site (with minimal buccolingual width) and restore with a Ponabut. My question is: how exactly do I make the prosthesis? I have IMTEC's FAQ on your system and think I can picture the prosthesis; however, I'm not sure about any special considerations for preparation and impressions and instructions for laboratory work. Thanks for your input.**

A. I would not get too upset about the Ponabut design. Just design a normal pontic with normal ridge lap, normal proximal contours and contacts to maximize esthetics, phonetics, and occlusion. Then simply think of the tissue-contacting surface of the pontic having a small receptacle in it (i.e., a hole) to receive the MDI abutment head wherever it emerges through the ridge soft tissue (hopefully, through keratinized attached gingival) and enters the underbelly of the Ponabut. In other words the final product is both pontic and abutment and therefore called a Ponabut, combining both features in one entity, and totally unlike any other implant system. Composite resin or resin cement then fills in any marginal voids around the entry area of the MDI abutment head into the Ponabut during final cementation.

Q. **I recently placed four MDIs in a patient on her mandibular using no incision. She had a knife-edge ridge with a ridge of tissue on top. After placement, the tissue grew over the implant heads and the denture won't seat. I placed the implants until they were snug. Should I have removed the excess tissue, or perhaps not have seated the implants so deeply?**

A. As much as I like to retain any attached, keratinized ridge tissue around MDIs, you may have to do some gingivoplasty to expose the implant abutment heads. You might try putting a soft liner in the prosthesis first and see if the tissue might remodel sufficiently on its own without surgery to expose the heads. Most important of all is to be sure you have well integrated MDIs, so I wouldn't be concerned about seating the implants too deeply.

Q. **I'm an oral surgeon and have a patient who I think is a good candidate for MDIs. She's 71 years old and was recently diagnosed with Parkinson disease. Her mandibular denture is unstable due to severe alveolar resorption, and the patient is having more difficulty with it now that she's developed significant tongue thrusting motions. I think I could place four 13-mm MDIs, but wonder if her tongue movements would doom them. Any experience with that, or any thoughts? Also, how critical is angulation for these implants with O-ball attachments?**

A. The patient sounds like a plausible candidate for MDIs. As for the prognosis question, there should be no special concern about tongue thrusting and immediate stability, even in a patient with Parkinson's disease, if the MDIs have been placed according to the proper insertion protocol. Using only a minimal starter opening through the crestal soft tissue and underlying cortical bone and for approximately a third of the length of the threaded portion of the MDI into medullary bone should provide sufficient entry for the MDI to be totally self-tapping. Using the finger wrench, winged thumb wrench, and finally the ratchet wrench for a few turns should secure a rock solid MDI, braced immediately by compressed bone without any conventional healing period needed. The low-profile abutment head also minimizes lateral iatrogenic loading pressures. Moderate angulation variations provide few insertion or removal problems with the gentle but retentive MDI O rings.

Q. **I have now placed 37 MDIs. I have had a total of five become mobile, two in the past 2 weeks in the same patient. I realize every case is different, but what would be the main reasons for that to happen? I believe in one case where both came loose, it was a lower full**

denture; I don't think I had the patient's existing denture seated all the way down to the ridge when I attached the O rings. I also think the metal housings were in contact with the inside of his denture, so all of the occlusal forces were on the implants, with no tissue bearing areas. One of the other three that came loose was a 13-mm MDI that I was not able to screw all the way down. Some threads were exposed, which I try not to have happen even if I have to change the length or type of implant. So maybe it was too heavy.

Also, with lower overdentures, do you usually place more than two MDIs? Do you always try to use the existing denture so long as the base is thick enough to accommodate the O rings? I find myself using the micro-metal housings more than the regular housings that come with the implants. My best results have been with a new denture over four MDIs. Comments please.

A. Thanks for the update, even with some negative reports regarding loosening and exfoliations. The best advice I can give you about using a patient's existing denture is that these cases must be relined with a hard or soft liner for stability, preferably before picking up O-ring encapsulations. In fact, it may be best to simply remove the existing hard acrylic overlying the MDIs and provide sufficient relief (clearance). Then reline the entire denture including the MDIs with soft liner to avoid overstressing them from lateral traumatic contacts, especially if you have some reservations about the integration of the MDIs at this stage. Defer O-ring loading pickups until your confidence level is adequate.

As to length of the MDIs, we always recommend not overscrewing into dense Type 1 bone and to either use a shorter implant or try to deepen your starter drilling by pecking away a little more of the apical bone to get a better take. You can use only two MDIs if the bony integration is solid and secure, but clearly three or four gives you a better margin for error or exfoliation. In a short bite, limited interarch space situations the micro O rings are indeed a better bet, which is why we offer them as an option.

Q. I am an oral and maxillofacial surgeon practicing in Westchester County. I have yet to use the MDI system. A patient recently presented to my practice for placement of a dental implant into site #7 that is congenitally missing. Having gone through considerable orthodontic treatment, there is only approximately 4 mm of interradicular bone in this site. The orthodontist does not believe they can create any additional space. Obviously, this is insufficient for a conventional 3.25-mm MDI. I am hopeful that your MDI may work as a long-term restoration. My concern obviously is esthetics in this anterior area. I am requesting your advice on how a natural emergence profile can be obtained with this implant system.

A. The Sendax MDI system works extremely well in areas of limited spacing often encountered in congenitally missing sites because it is a 1.8-mm width implant, approved by the FDA for both transitional and long-term applications. As to emergence profile and related esthetic considerations, there should be no concern because the prosthetic tooth/crown replacement is essentially a pontic with a ridge lap access opening for the small 1.8-mm abutment head (either square or O ball). We call it a Ponabut because it incorporates features of both a pontic and an abutment and therefore permits ideal esthetic design. It's a little hard to visualize this concept at first until you are more familiar with the MDI system, but your restoring colleague should have no trouble with it after a modest learning curve.

Q. Can the square head of the MDI be used in the posterior area in the cuspid or molar position, or is it ideally used for a lateral?

A. It can be used anywhere and prepped as needed to conform to incisal or occlusal clearance and angulation considerations. Keep in mind that the O-ball abutment head can also work in the same situations anteriorly or posteriorly. Additionally, the O-ball head provides excellent retention even in low profile/low clearance situations and offers O-ring retention for removable applications.

Q. How can the MDI be used to save a failing bridge?

A. Salvage procedures are one of the great uses for the MDI, both rectangular head and O-ball abutment head types.

Q. Can the O ball be used for a removable partial? Fixed?

A. Absolutely. It's suited for both types of applications. Just be sure to always use the elastomeric shims as spacers and to prevent inadvertent lock-on during fabrications.

Q. Is the alveolar nerve the only reason the MDIs are placed in the anterior portion of the mandible or can they be placed in the posterior if a clinician is careful about nerve location?

A. Both anterior and posterior applications are appropriate with a level of care.

Q. Can the MDIs be placed in the posterior area of the maxilla? How careful should one be of the sinus cavity?

A. The only concern about the sinus is that if you penetrate into the sinus cavity, there is no supportive bone and therefore a waste of implant surface. It's best to place MDIs just anterior or posterior to the sinus walls (maybe "biting" into these walls or the sinus floor, all of which are good supportive cortical bone for MDIs).

Q. As far as office equipment is concerned, to place the MDI is a panoramic x-ray sufficient?

A. Both panoramic x-rays as well as periapical (and even occasionally bite-wing) x-rays have their place diagnostically and for important implant placement detail, both preoperative and postoperative.

Q. How many degrees can you be off on parallelism? Should you start over or compensate another way?

A. Moderate off-angle placements will work when you consider that abutment heads can be prepped or that O-ball heads have the rubber O rings that are forgiving unless extreme angulations are involved (soft linings can be used in such extreme unparalleled situations). Rubber O rings can be relieved internally with a tapered bullet-shaped diamond under water spray for an easier retention and release.

Q. When using two square heads at an angle, how do you keep bacteria from the V-shaped area?

A. Best with an *Access* implant toothbrush to gain the requisite interface access!

Q. What can I tell my patients to expect about recovery time after MDI placement?

A. There is no significant recovery time after insertion because it is a minimally invasive procedure. The most typical reaction is a little gum soreness for a few days from the minimal local anesthetic injection sites. MDIs typically go into immediate function and, depending on the type of tooth replacements on top of the MDIs, patients should function immediately after placement with few side effects.

Q. I have now placed 29 MDIs and know how easy the procedure is. My only problem has been with the patient that has less than 1-mm width at the top of the mandibular ridge. It's obvious that 1.8-mm implants will not penetrate a 1-mm ridge. (A) Do you open these patients up and remove bone to a suitable width level? (B) If so, can you still put the denture in place knowing that there will be considerable swelling? (C) Or, do you do the leveling first as a separate procedure and let it heal before placing the implants?

A. The issue of what to do about very thin crestal bone is to essentially ignore it as long as it widens inferiorly as do most ridge anatomies, even very atrophic ones. Just initiate the process by lightly tapping a very thin starter drill in this delicate bone until the ridge widens sufficiently to encompass the 1.8-mm width with a millimeter or two to spare labially (buccally) and lingually. I like to use a very thin tapered diamond drill for this purpose in a friction grip. A conventional high speed air turbine, ratcheted back using the foot controller with care, will in most cases allow a controlled access to thin crestal anatomy and make it unnecessary to reduce the ridge as a separate surgical procedure, which might result in excessive crestal bone loss and remodeling. Also, if one spot proves inadequate, it is only necessary to move down the line to the next adjacent location until you find a more usable site.

Also, as to postoperative morbidity, edema can be minimized by drilling only through attached, keratinized crestal gingival. The only discomfort usually reported by patients is in the area of the needle sticks for local infiltrations. From a prosthodontic standpoint, there is no reason why the implants can't be put into immediate function with O-ring attachments. You can hedge this if you are concerned about postoperative complications by simply using a soft liner temporarily in the O-ball receptacles and softly reline the entire prosthesis simultaneously for maximum initial comfort and negligible chair time.

Q. **I had the pleasure of taking your 1-day clinical seminar in February. I learned a lot and am now much more comfortable in placing MDIs.**

I have a clinical question and I invite your comments. I am treating a 90-year-old woman who has muscular dystrophy. Her anterior teeth have extensive cervical decay. Treatment options generally result in extraction with a removable partial denture or four root canal therapies followed by crown lengthening and porcelain/metal crowns. Because of the moderate bone loss, the second option is not only very expensive to patient but also has only a fair prognosis.

I remember seeing in a dental journal some time ago an innovative idea of placing MDIs through the mandibular incisors and several millimeters into the alveolar bone. A crown is then placed on each coronal portion of each implant. Your thoughts, please.

A. What you are referring to are endodontic stabilizers, meaning that you must do root canal therapy before you can do this kind of procedure; even then it is technique-sensitive and may result in a guarded prognosis. Your best bet is to try to save teeth in a 90-year-old patient and supplement any lost teeth with MDIs as necessary, which is much less traumatic for the patient.

Q. **I'm an oral surgeon; in our implant study group we have an orthodontist with young children who are congenitally missing most of their adult teeth. The oldest is 14 years old and he has been limping along with various orthodontic appliances to replace these teeth, but this is no longer working. He will need extensive bone grafting and implant reconstruction when it is age appropriate but is in need of something to get him by while in high school. We discussed flippers until he is finished growing, but he and his orthodontist father would like something more fixed. I had mentioned possibly using transitional implants, but I am not aware of any that are indicated for this type of situation. Could you give me your input on this and let us know your thoughts? Also, how can orthodontic tooth movement be enhanced by using MDIs?**

A. The Sendax MDI system is the first minimally invasive implant system approved by the FDA for transitional and long-term applications. It should be an ideal solution to the problem you describe and could conceivably function long-term and for the interim pedodontic application you envision. Replacing congenitally missing dentition is in fact one of the most beneficial potential uses of the MDI concept. By all means investigate this approach. In answer to your last question, orthodontic tooth movement may definitely be enhanced by using MDIs, which work as anchorage units. The patient's orthodontic appliances may be attached directly or indirectly to a MDI to apply forces that facilitate and aid in tooth movement.

Editor's Note: See the Orthodontic Section of this textbook for an in-depth profile.

Q. **Please comment on the following case and appropriate MDI applications. My patient is a 16 year-old boy with congenitally missing #7. #10 is a peg-shaped lateral incisor. The patient is nearing completion of 2 years of orthodontic treatment by an orthodontist who has moved #6 into correct position and opened up space for replacement of #7. The patient is a member of his high school football team and won't wear a retainer or flipper. The oral surgeon during implant cases with me suggests it would be advisable to wait to place an implant for #7 until the patient is at least 18 years of age because the alveolar bone and gum position in the area of #7 will not mature until the patient is 18 or older.**

Would a MDI be advisable here? I realize that another standard option would be a Maryland type retainer bridge, but I'm unhappy with long-term retention of the Maryland bridge procedure. Another option would be a tooth added to the orthodontic retainer, but the patient's parents feel he's not the type that would cooperate in wearing a retainer.

Could I present the MDI as an interim type replacement for 3 to 5 years that would be cosmetically acceptable and which might need to be replaced with a conventional implant several years from now? If the MDI needs to be replaced with a conventional implant in the future, can it be retrieved without extreme disfigurement of the architecture in that area?

A. MDIs can be ideal transitional or long-term replacements for congenitally missing teeth at any age and can typically be retrieved without difficulty if that becomes desirable at some stage. Keep in mind though that the MDIs might, quite reasonably, suffice for long-term support. As a minimally invasive implant, the IMTEC Sendax MDI in no way compromises the site it inhabits, and, if it ever needs to be removed, it in no way diminishes the use of the same site for any root form implant.

Q. **I'm a general practitioner in South Florida, and I have been using MDIs for more than 2 years in overdentures with great success. I was wondering if MDIs could be used as an abutment under a cantilever to save a bridge or maybe to replace a lateral incisor? I would also like to know if you have used them before or if you have any recommendations for usage besides denture retention for a transitional stage for permanent implants?**

A. The "salvage" use you describe is perfect for Sendax MDIs. Other ideal applications are single tooth replacements and under failed Maryland bridges, etc. Also, take a look at Dr. Gordon J. Christensen's excellent videos for more concepts and applications.

Q. **I attended your mini-residency in NYC recently. I have placed eight MDIs so far with no concerns or problems. A question: When you are working with a processed acrylic crown and bridge temporary and you want to attach some MDIs to it, do you put a shim over the implant and add jet acrylic to the abutment area and cement the temporary over the implant? I have several with Coe-Soft denture reline material temporarily but I want to convert it to something more retentive. Also, if you're working with a fixed porcelain to metal bridge and wish to add a MDI, what do you use in the hollowed out pontic area to attach it to the implant? Composite? Jet? Do you use the shim to avoid undercuts?**

I'm very impressed with the system, having also placed conventional implants for 12 years.

A. You are on the right track with the critical use of the elastomeric shims in all the applications you referred to. In addition, to get good bonding of jet acrylic or composite to acrylic, metal, or porcelain, you should invest in a micro-etcher. The aluminum oxide etch powder will provide an enhanced bonding potential for your cases. You'll have to try out several techniques until you arrive at the preferred method.

Q. **I've purchased insertion tools and implants and am now surveying candidate patients. One problem that I frequently encounter in association with the severely resorbed mandibular symphysis when placing "conventional" implants relates to the difficulty in establishing a zone of immobile gingiva through which the intended implant(s) will emerge. With respect to the Sendax O-ball MDI for use in lower overdenture cases, we sometimes find that the minimal width zone masticatory mucosa that might exist crestal to an edentulous ridge is displaced lingually to the desired exit point of the implant. Thus, absent a soft-tissue graft effort, the implant placed "nonsurgically" will be placed through mucosa. Have you found this to impact either prognosis or comfort?**

A. Attached keratinized gingival is always desirable for both short- and long-term applications. That said, there are exceptions to the rule, but there is always the risk for after-insertion mucogingival complications, including tender, vulnerable periimplant soft tissues (especially where muscle attachment "pull" is evident labially or lingually). The best approach, if topography is too hard to read, is to bite the bullet and do a limited incision to visualize the location of the most usable underlying bone for pilot entry and be less concerned about immobile gingiva because it probably is virtually nonexistent in the case you describe. Fortunately, the minimal 1.8-mm footprint of the MDI is much less vulnerable to periimplantitis problems than larger, bulkier conventional implants.

Q. (1) How many months would you wait to place a MDI into an extraction site after the extraction? (2) Would the waiting period be altered at all if you placed a freeze-dried bone graft into the socket immediately after the extraction? (3) What was your diamond drill of choice (size and shape) that you used in your high speed handpiece to create the pilot hole for the MDI?

A. MDIs do not require a specific socket healing time before placement if you can find a solid septum of bone in or around the socket periphery that will accept a 1.8-mm width MDI or if the socket depth is so minimal that apical to the socket there is a substantial height of uninvolved virgin bone to receive the pilot drill opening. Waiting for initial socket healing is also a reasonable approach. Of course, placement of bone graft matrix material (with or without a barrier) in the actual socket hole is an acceptable ancillary procedure to level out the defect after MDI insertion, but this should not really affect immediate MDI placement at the time of extraction. Any coarse-grained, long, thin, tapered diamond drill should work well to make the initial pilot starter opening.

Q. Have any independent agencies or groups researched the 1.8-mm diameter MDI and reported their findings?

A. Yes. Clinical Research Associates of Provo, Utah, a nationally recognized research organization headed by Gordon J. Christensen, DDS, MSD, PhD., in Vol. 25, Issue 1, January, 2001 of *CRA Dental Products Buying Guide*, entitled "Trends Evident From Outstanding Products Studied in 2000" states that "Mini implants [less than 2-mm diameter] are increasing in use for patients with minimal bone. They can provide both excellent transitional and long-term service." Dr. Christensen also demonstrates the Sendax MDI in one of his excellent teaching videos entitled "The 'Mini' Implant for General Practitioners" (Item C900A) and the new DVD "Mini Implants for Your Practice" (Item D2317) that are available through 800-223-6569 or www.pccdental.com and at his many seminars, lectures, and workshops internationally.

Q. Are there any indications for immediate placement of the MDI after extractions in the mandible? If not, how long do you suggest waiting postextraction before placement?

A. The basic guideline for MDI placement after extractions is to avoid placing them directly in any area of inflammation or infection. If you can find an adjacent region without inflammatory issues, you can feel comfortable about placement of the MDIs at any time. The longer you wait for such inflammation to subside, the better the prognosis.

Q. I've been using MDIs the last few months with few failures as yet. I recently had a case of a patient with knife-edge ridges, and I was unable to get a good start with a 1.1-mm drill because it kept bouncing off the ridges and being deflected either lingually or facially. I thought about doing a crestal incision and flattening the ridges to get a start with the drill, but I hate to sacrifice bone. Any suggestions?

A. The best approach to narrow ridges is to use a high-speed conventional turbine for better control with a friction grip, thin tapered diamond drill. If you use medium speed via the foot controller with water spray, you can tap the crest until you feel solid cortical bone just below what I would have to assume is minimally thick crestal soft tissue. If the chosen site is poor, move on to another adjacent spot with attached gingiva and continue the straight up and down tapping through the cortex into medullary bone a few millimeters in depth with constant water spray. If you continue to feel medullary bone contact, proceed for a few more millimeters of up and down gentle drilling and stop. If your angulation is reasonable, try your implant into this "starter" opening and see if you have a good self-tapping "take." If it's okay, then continue to auto-advance the implant with the finger driver and thumb wrench followed by the ratchet wrench, as required by bone density, to full depth.

Q. I had the first MDI I inserted come out today. I must have over-instrumented the bone. It sounded solid and lasted approximately 1 month. Is this the learning curve you mention? Anyway, I was disappointed. A question: How long after an extraction should we wait for the bone to heal to insert a MDI in the general area?

A. Sorry to hear about your first exfoliated MDI but, as you pointed out, that is indeed part of the learning curve. The question is also best answered by acknowledging that although over-instrumentation may have certainly played a part, other considerations also might have been negative factors. Poor quality and/or quantity of bone? You make no mention of location, height, or length. Healed site or recent extraction site? Immediate or progressive loading? Soft liner, O-ring retainers, cemented (provisionally or finally)? What kind of occlusal management, number and type of other abutment supports, and muscle dynamics/habits/fixed versus removable, etc? As you can see, it's not such an easy analysis. Don't despair; just keep all the variables in mind.

As to healing time before MDI placement after extraction, there is no best answer because this is another tough judgment call, with a long list of variables—for example, residual bone circumferentially around the postextraction socket periphery and height of residual bone apically before you reach vulnerable sites. Theoretically, if no infection and minimal soft tissue inflammation occurs, you can try to insert a MDI immediately. However, the longer you wait postoperatively, the easier it is to analyze these factors and have the best prognosis.

Q. I read Dr. Ron Bulard's article on use of the Sendax MDI in the July 2001 edition of *Dentistry Today* and it raises a question. I am heavily involved with the CEREC system that, as you know, has the ability to make single crowns chairside. Is there any reason why I can't use the MDI system to replace teeth in one visit, such as preparing a premolar CEREC crown over a MDI? Because my practice is mainly fixed restorative, this is primarily the area that interests me. The literature I've received from IMTEC describes the full denture application. If so, it seems that it will be able to push the envelope of restorative dentistry much further. Also, from the insertion protocol, it seems that no special surgical skills are necessary, which would make this system accessible to a wide range of general dentists.

A. Your basic concepts are right on target as to the intrinsic fixed crown and bridge prosthodontic potential for the MDI system. We made a strategic decision at the outset to introduce the concept to the profession as a removable solution to the unstable and unusable lower (and in many cases the upper as well) denture problem that plagues so much of the world population. After the learning curve and essentially simple technique is mastered, it is a logical progression to incorporate fixed prosthodontics as well, which is what I am personally doing in my practice. Also, the CEREC concept should certainly be applicable to the MDI system, along with some of the newer all-ceramic CAD/CAM techniques.

Q. I have reviewed the Sendax MDI system and am impressed. I have an 85-year-old woman with substantial bone loss. I'm enclosing her panoramic x-ray. Please comment as to her eligibility for the MDI system. Also, she's asked, "Is this treatment permanent?" What should I tell her?

A. This should be a workable case to treatment plan for the Sendax MDI system. I've reviewed your panoramic x-ray, and it reflects that the anterior mandible (symphysis region) seems to have adequate bone for the MDIs. Because this is a minimally invasive system, it should be safe and effective for her. As for the patient's question about permanency, as you know, nothing in the world is "permanent" so I counsel clinicians to never use that word in describing dental care in general or implant care specifically. As to basic durability, the FDA has granted clearance to market the Sendax MDI for transitional and long-term applications, which essentially means as long a term as a patient's case requires. That should cover any short-, medium, or long-term uses you may have in mind for the MDIs. For that particular elderly patient, I would say you have a reasonable prognosis.

Q. I attended your MDI course in Dallas in August. I have a patient with a congenitally missing #21. I am considering placing a MDI to restore it. Have you any thoughts on the implications of this treatment? The patient is a 23-year-old woman and can't afford conventional implants. The teeth on either side are virgin. Thanks in advance for your help.

A. Restoring congenitally missing teeth are ideal MDI applications for all the reasons you suggest with respect to this young adult patient. Of course, without seeing periapical and panoramic x-rays of the area in question, it's difficult to be very specific or definitive.

Q. I attended the late Dr. Charles E. English's MDI seminar in Chicago and have a primary concern: How much torque will the MDI withstand? I am aware that there is a learning curve here, but some subjective guidelines would be helpful. There were several instances of broken implants in the seminar class while using a wood medium. Is a broken implant a common mistake, or were we just being "ham handed"? What do I do in event of a sheared MDI? Finally, I do not use a water cooled low speed hand piece in my clinic. Is this essential, or is a conventional low speed unit with a light touch acceptable? Forgive the elementary questions, but I am eager to stabilize those dentures I made many years ago. This is an exciting concept that I find very attractive. I have practiced for 45 years and have resisted, until now, learning anything about implants; however, this idea is irresistible. Congratulations on developing such an invaluable contribution. I learned of it from Dr. Christensen a while back.

A. MDIs inserted in dense wood technique blocks should be placed with care because wood does not have a comparable level of viscoelasticity as living bone and may indeed make the MDIs more vulnerable to fracture than in typical cancellous bone environments. Most fractures in living bone typically occur when the tip end of the implant gets apically embedded in very dense Type I bone and is over-instrumented by use of excessive force in an attempt to seat an over-long implant fully up to its abutment neck. A more realistic approach is to simply back out the implant and use the next shorter length MDI that should then be readily insertable without exerting extreme torquing forces. Final ratcheting should only be used for a few slow turns to provide a solid MDI and with distinct recovery pauses between partial ratchet turns.

As to drilling equipment, low or high speed can work equally well, with assistant-directed or internal water spray both effective, considering that only a very brief minimal "starter" opening is required to gain a self-sustaining purchase for the auto-advancing MDI.

As to any broken titanium elements left in the jawbone after fractures, it is rarely necessary to trephine out such tiny, benign elements; they are best left behind and may actually help retain bone in the insertion site.

Q. I attended a mini-residency at your Manhattan office in October and have my first MDI case this month. Please clarify a few things for me about sequencing:

My patient has teeth #20 and #21 and nothing more posterior. She presented with a failed cantilever bridge—#20 splinted to #21 with a very small pontic hanging off #20. The vertical space is extremely limited in the area of the cantilever. So far I have redone the post and core on #20 and performed a root canal on #21. I am planning to do the following at the next appointment and in the following sequence: Post and core #20; final prep #20 and #21; insert two MDIs in the space of #19; and cement a temporary (#20, #21, #19). Questions: (1) Do I have to do the soft reline for the Pontabut with a cold cure soft acrylic or can I cement the temporary with temporary bond? (2) Do I need to wait longer than 2 weeks to take the final impression? Is it advisable to take a final impression at this insertion appointment?

What is the code used for the MDIs? Is it the same code regardless what is put over it? In other words, is there a different code for a Sendax MDI used in a denture attachment than for under a bridge? Further, what are the codes used for the crown and pontic placed over the MDI? Also, do you use a different charge for a crown over one of the MDIs than for a crown over a natural root?

Thanks in advance for the information. I'm very excited about these MDIs and hope they will work.

A. My suggestion is to use temporary bond for the tooth preps #20 and #21, but reserve a soft liner for the O-ball MDI abutments that you want to be sure of, as to stability and integration, before inserting prosthesis with a temporary cement.

This is just a precaution when initially using MDIs as bridge abutments so as not to inadvertently pull out an incompletely integrated implant when removing the temporary. As to waiting time before taking impressions, I don't see any reason to delay unless you are unsure of stability and full bony integration. If they sound solid when tapped, I would proceed with impressions. The basic MDI concept is that the MDIs should be ready to function from day one.

On the matter of codes, there is no special code for MDIs. Use the regular code for endosseous implants, but remember that implants are rarely covered by dental insurance. Codes for full coverage and pontics involving MDIs would be the same as for any routine crowns and pontics. But, again, if insurance companies are made aware of the presence of implants under crowns or pontics as supports, they may try to exclude coverage. Check your patient's insurance benefits booklet for details. Obviously, you must decide whether or not the extra benefits you expect from implant-supported bridge prosthodontics warrant additional fees.

Q. **I have placed three Sendax MDIs, all 15 mm on lower left as a support for a five-unit bridge between #17 and #21 as a transitional prosthesis; 2 months after insertion, a radiograph shows at least 2-mm bone loss around the three MDIs. They are not mobile, but I am concerned that I may not be able to use these as supporting posts under the new bridge. The patient did not have any pain or infection after the surgery.**

I have placed conventional implants in the past and followed good surgical protocol. The patient in this case cannot have a permanent replacement until after the first of the year, so we have a couple of months before the final bridge. I will evaluate the bone level at that time. How much bone loss will it take to load the stress under the bridge? What could be done to prevent such bone loss? I realize that these MDIs are not intended to be used as bridge abutments. However, in this case it was not used as a terminal abutment, but rather for support of the bridge. Also, the patient is a heavy smoker. Comments, please.

A. When you said the patient is a smoker it reminded me that smoking is a strong potential negative for both bone and soft tissues around implants and natural teeth. You might very well be encountering this significant factor in the bone loss you describe around your MDIs. Try to get the patient to break this malignant habit by also emphasizing the cancer risk.

As to bone loss levels, we do not typically see significant bone loss around MDI sites unless there have been recent extractions, soft and hard tissue inflammation, or infection. Also, check the occlusion carefully to avoid traumatic deflective contacts during excursive movements and centrically. A remarkably "steady state" of bone is more routinely observed. Also, we do indeed consider these integrated MDIs usable as ongoing bridge abutments after convincingly integrated with bone. After your own comfort level with the procedure is a reality, you should be in a position to ethically recommend this procedure for longer-term fixed bridge applications.

Q. **I'm a Canadian doctor. Is the MDI approved here?**

A. Yes. Health Canada in Ottawa has accepted the MDI for both transitional and long-term use.

Editor's Note: Since this textbook material has gone to publication, the IMTEC Corporation, which was the Ardmore, Oklahoma implant company originally licensed by Dr. Victor Sendax to manufacture, market, and distribute the Sendax MDI System, has been acquired by the 3M Corporation in St. Paul, Minnesota, which markets MDIs exclusively as part of the 3M ESPE dental products brand. All components of the IMTEC/Sendax MDI System will presumably continue to be available directly from 3M, along with the Access oral home care brushes.

Summation and Future Horizons

The MDI Latter-Day Equation

VICTOR I. SENDAX

An inescapable conclusion from the preceding sections detailing the extensive scope of this MDI modality is its significant potential for expanding the impact of oral implantology on an international scale. This is especially true for a worldwide populace that is often unable to receive the many health benefits of implant dentistry owing to its typical high cost, which puts such critical care beyond patients' means. As we have observed, such regrettable inaccessibility has been only obliquely addressed by the dental profession to date, and dental implant therapy has been generally, and rather heedlessly, accepted as a benefit largely limited to relatively well-off members of the international community. In fact, the most desperately needful patients are just as often citizens of impoverished third world and emerging societies where vast numbers of people are edentulous or suffering from untreated major oral disease entities. For that matter, not everyone in America is so fortunate as to be able to afford implant benefits either, where dental insurance carriers may refuse to even partially cover such expense by arbitrarily assuming that it is too costly an elective "luxury." Insurance premiums are basically designed to provide bottom-line profits for the industry rather than to expand benefits. Paradoxically, the extension of coverage for MDI therapy could actually in the long-term reduce the substantial costs of insuring untreated oral disability and systemic health comorbidities for an increasingly aging and often fully or partially edentulous global population.

Various research and ratings groups have consistently charted the rapid growth of global markets for dental implants, focusing on the United States, Canada, Latin America, and Europe, but also more recently Russia, India, China, Japan, both the Near and Middle East, Southeast Asia, and Hawaii. What is of special significance to the scientific community is the startling degree to which the MDI (ultra-small-diameter implant), starting from zero, has caught the imagination of clinicians in both less developed countries and wealthier societies. This is in no small part due to the clear affordability of the MDIs for average patients in these more modestly endowed communities, especially in light of the worldwide economic recession that appears to have been at least as deep and unforgiving as some previous downturns.

In addition to cost-effectiveness, one can include the minimally invasive insertion process and the immediate (real-time) functionality of MDIs in the list of benefits, and it becomes obvious why these streamlined MDIs have become a powerful force for the rapidly growing international acceptance of this patient-friendly oral implant modality.

It is the hope and presumption that the advent and acceptance of MDI technology, with its exceptional affordability, will pave the way to a much wider accessibility for just those very needy patients who have heretofore been written off on the presumed basis of nonaffordability. Broader access to implant therapy is now envisaged as being far more achievable by the generous application of MDI principles globally.

We have noted with appreciation the prescient comments and the perspectives of distinguished periodontist Dr. Michael G. Newman, which were given in an editorial in the *International Journal of Oral and Maxillofacial Implants.* He offered a challenge to the dental health community to shoulder greater responsibility and apply the benevolent benefits of contemporary oral implantology to an aging population's edentulism problems, but at an affordable level for all classes, rather than focus primarily on the upper strata of financially well-endowed members of society.

We have come to believe that applied MDI therapy can be a major factor in helping to level the playing field for essential oral implant therapy, with special emphasis on developing nations and our own unaddressed domestic needs. As costs and fees continue to increase for increasingly expensive implant-related procedures, it is a unique attribute of the simplified MDI technology that cost-containment is one of its most essential attributes and virtually alone addresses the critical issue of access as a matter of public conscience.

To turn this philosophic, quasiexistential concept into a realistic clinical strategy, the need to develop a comprehensive MDI delivery system that could fulfill the desired therapeutic level at a meaningful cost/benefit ratio for the broadest range of off-shore (and domestic) economies was perceived. With an eye to bringing well-trained general practitioners into this field and taking specific advantage of the remarkable convergence of the latest digital and imaging technologies, the concept of dedicated MDI centers, embodying turnkey multinational operations, has evolved into a workable reality with the introduction of a cooperative franchise-structured business model. This often has the potential for productive development when seed financing may emerge from newly empowered governmental health agencies, operating on the basis of enlightened self-interest, in an effort to accommodate a rising middle class hungering for government to help provide some of the comparable benefits previously reserved for only wealthier communities.

First enunciated in a 1996 pilot format, a detailed Sendax Business Plan for Mini Dental Implant Centers designed specifically to deliver dedicated minimally invasive implant services in the United States has been formulated and is in the process of being introduced into the worldwide therapeutic arena, with unique modifications to address the pressing and uniquely specialized oral implant needs of previously underserved global societies. This gradually evolving business model based on shared patient and professional acceptance offers the hope that the benefits of implant dentistry can be expanded internationally via the constructive and sensitive applications of MDI therapy on a scale with a substantial enough volume to make it realistically achievable. If volume can be expanded and effectively delivered, the costs will inevitably decline and access assured. This suggests that an enlightened partnership between competing implant device manufacturers, dental laboratories, dental schools, insurance companies, governmental agencies, and the international patient population is essential if the obvious benefits of dental implant therapy are to be made available on an equitable basis worldwide.

The advent of an innovative new delivery system in the form of dedicated MDI centers should provide a welcome key for unlocking greater public accessibility to implant therapy that has proven elusive in the past. The new delivery system offers the same challenge now being faced by both the United States and its global allies and partners when contemplating how best to deliver and fund more equitable universal health care for the needful patient population and for the committed health professionals charged with providing such essential human services.

Alternatively termed Sendax MDI or minimally invasive implant (MII) centers, put forward to encompass a wider range of useful implant sizes utilizing the Sendax Insertion and Reconstructive Protocol, are optimally positioned to provide the basis for a "new age" delivery system, emphasizing affordable dental implants both domestically and off-shore. They could conceivably serve as ideal bellweather pilot locations for launching global MDI or MII projects, which have the potential to grow to include all affordable contemporary implant services, customized to the needs of the communities they are designed to serve.

GLOSSARY

Access implant brush:
A uniquely curved-bristle collis-type toothbrush design originally brought to the attention of the IMTEC Corporation and named Access by Dr. Victor Sendax as it was modified to serve as a dedicated oral hygiene access aid for mini implants. Subsequently found to be comparably effective, and recommended, for routine conventional implant maintenance as well as natural dentition prophylaxis. Access brushes have been most recently available from the 3M Corporation as part of the ESPE-3M line of dental products, St. Paul, Minnesota.

Auto-advancement:
The process of slowly feeding a MDI like a wood screw (as first described by Dr. Burton Balkin) into a minimal starter opening directly through soft-tissue and crestal bone, and then, with the subsequently added assistance of a modified reverse-buttress thread design, allowing the ultra-narrow width MDI to feel while being turned with light pressure as if it is being drawn into the underlying medullary bone without the need to exert great insertion force. (Self-tapping of conventional-width implants typically requires an extensive osteotomy and considerably more torque effort, owing to the greater width and consequent bony resistance to the insertion process, with the possible exception of ultra-cancellous Type IV bone.)

Elastomeric shim:
The elastic silicone-based spacer designed to block out the 2-mm square MDI base during the hard acrylic pick-up of O-ring encapsulations for removable applications to prevent unwanted acrylic flash bonding to the MDI. The spacer can also be used by the laboratory technician or dentist covering the full 4-mm rectangular abutment head when fabricating temporary or definitive restorations so that an easy "draw" may be realized when removing or inserting one or more restorative units, especially when there are angulation or parallelism issues to be bypassed and overcome.

Fixture:
Term first advanced by Brånemark and associates to characterize the specific device inserted in the jawbone after a surgical osteotomy and anchored by a hypothesized "osseointegration" process. As manufactured and promoted by the Nobelpharma company (Tokyo, Japan), the complete device originally was limited to a 3.75-mm width screw fabricated of pure titanium, with an external hex platform mated to a screw-affixed hexed abutment. The "fixture" term is less in vogue currently, having generally given way to the less ambiguous use of the term *implant*.

Immediate function:
MDIs can go into immediate function mode as soon as inserted, with the following caveat clearly in mind: *Bicortical stabilization* must be secured if long-term predictability is to be reliably achieved. For small-diameter MDIs that term refers to the penetration of the crestal cortical bone layer (most often directly through attached crestal gingiva without a flap) and after auto-advancing through varying densities of medullary bone coming to rest apically, by biting into a dense bone layer to achieve rock-solid primary stabilization, which is in contrast with conventional diameter implants that typically aim to gain a degree of bicortical stabilization buccolingually or labiolingually, without necessarily anchoring into a dense apical cortex. That dense cortical bone layer may be found at the floor of the maxillary sinuses, the floor of the nasal cavity, the midline suture region, the walls of the tuberosities, and in the mandible the external oblique ridge buccally, the mylohyoid ridge lingually, or the very dense anterior symphyseal bone, often accessed well before reaching the mandible's inferior border.

Implant prosthodontics:
The basic glossary of prosthodontic terminology (developed by the now defunct Federation of Prosthodontic Organizations) originally made no reference to oral implant restorative prosthodontics as a distinct component. At a FPO workshop for Directors of Postgraduate

Prosthodontic Programs, Dr. Sendax (then director of the Columbia University Postdoctoral Implant Research and Training Program) introduced a new term—*implant prosthodontics*—to describe the evolving field of implant-supported fixed and removable restorations, which was subsequently accepted for inclusion in the updated FPO *Glossary of Prosthodontic Terms*.

MDI implant prosthodontics:
This term encompasses the evolution of the now well-documented implant prosthodontics term to include the Sendax MDI System's prosthodontic modifications and specialized chairside and laboratory technologies.

MDI outcomes:
Implant outcomes are best judged by relative assessments of short-, medium, or long-term successful longevity and in relation to quality of survival. Because nothing in our existence is scientifically *permanent,* it is preferable not to apply that inviolable standard to any oral implant and that includes MDIs. A considerable body of well-documented evidentiary studies and anecdotal case reports demonstrates that MDIs have comparably beneficial outcomes to conventional implants when applied with judicious care and skill, based on appropriate training and experience.

Micro-gap:
The connection between an abutment post and the implant body that is characteristic of two-piece dental implant systems. Although engineered to be maximally close-fitting to avoid micro-leakage (and associated microorganism infiltration), such a connection may be implicated as a potential source of infection and periimplantitis (soft and hard tissue breakdown), especially if the connection becomes loose or separates under function. A comparative advantage of the one-piece solid MDI is its avoidance of any micro-gap vulnerability, and thereby it is not subject to screw-loosening, Morse-taper connection failure, or thread-overhauling problems that may be encountered with two-component implants. On the other hand, one-piece implants may be vulnerable to the problem of abutment angulation and parallelism issues, especially in connection with multiple implant applications.

Mini dental implant (MDI):
Ultra-small-diameter, endosseous root-form, machined titanium alloy, and reverse-buttress-threaded implant, inserted preferably via a minimally invasive (nonosteotomy) starter drill preparation, most often directly through keratinized crestal soft tissue followed by a dense subperiosteal cortical bone layer, and then auto-advanced (self-tapped) with specialized drivers until it passes through mature medullary bone and finally "bites" into dense apical bone to achieve primary bicortical-type stability that permits immediate clinical function. Functionally compressive *osseoapposition,* rather than a conventional delayed osseointegration process, characterizes the unique Sendax MDI Insertion Protocol that earned the distinction of having the U.S. Patent Office acknowledging it as the only nonsurgical insertion method ever granted for dental implant intraoral placement.Clinical trials have shown a 1.8-mm to 2.1-mm width dimension to be the most efficient for atraumatic MDI auto-advancement through average density medullary bone without the need for a conventional surgical osteotomy.

Osseoapposition:
See *mini dental implant (MDI)* definition above for a discourse on how this process is unique to mini implants placed according to the Sendax proprietary insertion protocol, effective from first day of insertion, compared with gradual osseointegration (ad modem Brånemark), and makes possible the immediate clinical functionality of the MDI.

Ponabut:
The combined *pontic* and *abutment* that represents the prime MDI reconstructive element for fixed mini implant applications, sharing features of conventional pontics and crown abutments. The intaglio surface of the Ponabut has an opening large enough to permit the abutment head of the MDI to penetrate into the undersurface of the Ponabut as the abutment emerges through the crestal soft tissue ridge, This connection is typically secured with either a temporary cement, soft-liner, adhesive, or a final resin cement. The Ponabut can be connected to natural tooth abutments, pontics, conventional implant abutments, and other Ponabut elements in fixed or removable applications.

MDI Ponabuts have specialized esthetic considerations because the Ponabut can be considered an optimal cosmetic unit. Whereas considerations of "emergence profile" and "biologic width" may play critical roles in the cosmetic challenges of conventional implant prosthodontics, the MDI's simplified Ponabut design frees the general practitioner or prosthodontist from many of the esthetic and angulation dilemmas raised by typical implant installations in both maxilla and mandible.

Combining the flexible attributes of both pontic and abutment configurations eliminates many of the potentially troubling design conflicts often associated with both simple and complex conventional implant cases.

Small-diameter implants:
In contrast to the original 1.8-mm width MDIs, so-called small-diameter implants are implants that are essentially too wide to be routinely auto-advanced through anything but Type IV poorly trabeculated, ultra-cancellous bone. Any implant with a wider than an approximately 2.1-mm diameter cannot realistically be considered a mini implant, while those from 2.5 mm to 3.25 mm wide are fundamentally small-diameter implants that require substantial bone drilling, clearly resulting in a deep osteotomy excavation. In addition, if this small-diameter implant is also a one-piece design combining implant body and abutment, it emerges into the oral cavity upon insertion and becomes immediately vulnerable to micro-movement from tongue, lips, and cheeks and occlusal and parafunctional forces. The erratic waiting period for classic osseointegration to produce a viable bony support requires any osteotomy-inserted implant be given an extra measure of cautionary postinsertion management to avoid premature destructive overload forces. The valid MDI, in contrast, having the benefit of immediately supportive osseoapposition buttressing its auto-advanced threaded shaft, may be less vulnerable to such early-onset micro-motion liability, and this may help to account for the ability of MDIs to function predictably even as immediate, stand-alone, single tooth replacements—literally from day one—if placed according to a dedicated Sendax Insertion Protocol.

Mini Views

Personal Essays on Diverse MDI Topics

Connecting Natural Tooth Abutments to Mini Dental Implant Abutments

Investigation of bending stiffness variables could serve as the key to understanding the apparent ability of mini dental implants (MDIs) to be mated with natural tooth abutments without the morbid complications occasionally reported when conventional-width implants are comparably splinted to teeth intraorally. Research studies are under development designed to confirm that the ultra-narrow 1.8-mm Sendax MDIs have a degree of latitude in their bending stiffness analogous to the stress-breaking effect derived from a tooth's periodontal ligament and thereby may serve as a protective mechanism, helping to safeguard the restorative system from the unequal loading and mobility, anecdotally observed when natural tooth abutments are connected to unyielding, virtually ankylosed conventional-width implants.

(For additional commentary on this related subject matter see Dr. Frank Spear's article, "Connecting Teeth to Implants," J Am Dent Assoc, Vol. 140, May 2009.)

Critical Evaluation of Competing "Small-Diameter" Implant Systems

Any analysis that purports to offer a fair rating of the growing numbers of manufacturers offering a competitive product to the MDI must first address the fundamental distinction that exists between the multitude of marketed widths that claim to replicate what the studies, reports, and anecdotal evidence on MDIs have shown to be reality.

The FDA standard for small-diameter implants had for many years been established at 3.25 mm wide. After 10 years of informal clinical trials involving three cooperating centers, Dr. Sendax appeared before FDA advisory committees on two successive occasions to advocate for the ultra-small diameter 1.8-mm width as the most favorable width capable of self-tapping and auto-advancing its way into most bone types, after a minimal starter drill penetration through crestal keratinized mucosa and crestal cortical bone and a limited distance into the underlying medullary bone. The main FDA concern, aside from whether the reduced surface area of a MDI (as compared to a conventional width implant) might be insufficient to gain a strong enough osseous interface, was the concern that the MDI might be susceptible to fracture under heavy loading conditions.

Ongoing clinical experience demonstrating the validity of a solid one-piece 1.8-mm MDI to be comparable in fracture-resistance to a hollow two-piece 3.75-mm conventional implant and effectively resistant to exfoliation during function helped answer concerns about the ability of the MDIs to hold their own in the often hostile oral environment. Fractures were acknowledged as occasionally occurring, but the frequency of such failure was comparable with conventional implants and moderate enough to be considered statistically insignificant. The considered explanation that in the case of these failures either too few abutments were expected to carry too large a payload or too rapid and heavy-handed an insertion technique had been employed reduced the FDA's intrinsic cautionary approach before approving the MDI and its 1.8-mm underlying width as an acceptable diameter for typical clinical applications. Although initially approving MDIs for transitional use only, after the analysis of follow-up data submissions from Dr. Sendax and associates, the FDA granted approval for ongoing fixed and removable applications and, with additional favorable studies, ultimately acknowledged that the MDI could be used for long-term cases; this was a major breakthrough for the ultra-small diameter device and for its unique, minimally invasive, and immediately functional insertion protocol that made it all possible—which was never, in at least one estimation, fully comprehended by competing manufacturers that failed to grasp the critical core basis for long-term MDI predictability. As a direct consequence of such conceptual lapses, these competing product lines never fully qualified as enduring long-term entities and to this day survive in the market-place essentially as transitory devices despite the FDA's proforma device designation of 510-K: "substantial equivalence."

An additional caution is that, as increasingly larger-width "small-diameter" implant modifications (approximately 2.5 mm to 3.00 mm) have come into the market as immediate-load implants, they characteristically cannot be readily self-tapped in the same way as the streamlined 1.8-mm (or up to possibly 2.4-mm) MDI in any bone type much denser than Type IV because resistance increases greatly without an invasive extended-length surgical osteotomy.

Limited primary stability may still be gained, but—an equally important cautionary note—a one-piece implant-abutment protruding from a typical osteotomy site is more vulnerable than a two-piece (two-stage) device to immediate lateral overload and micro-movement from tongue activity and other potentially destructive parafunctional forces, even if masticatory function is kept to a minimum. Concomitantly, immediate osseoapposition is no longer plausible when a standard, almost full-length, invasive osteotomy is drilled, and a variable waiting period for classic osseointegration to occur must be observed before nondestructive loading can be predictably deployed. Although temporary splinting will mitigate iatrogenic overload, any measurable micro-movement at this vulnerable stage makes for a more guarded prognosis. None of this denigrates the use of wider small-diameter implants, but these are not the same devices as the approximately 1.8-mm MDIs with the proprietary insertion protocol, and thus these may have different functional outcomes. The trick is to understand these variables and to know how to work with them experientially in a complex clinical setting, which often implies a newly modified learning curve before one can take salutary results for granted. Attempts to ignore this guideline may already have accounted for some reported integration failures.

While on the subject of wider modifications to the original 1.8-mm "standard" width MDIs, another innovative approach that may bear some fresh attention is the renewed role to be explored for hydroxyapatite surfaces and hydroxyapatite's potential role for MDI application.

Hydroxyapatite Coating of Implants: Pros and Cons

In studies, hydroxyapatite (HA) coating has shown an ability to enhance the speed and density of bony integration; on the negative side, the presence of any conventional two-component implant's micro-gap at the interface of abutment and implant body could be incriminated as a possible causative agent in the idiosyncratic breakdown of HA surfaces, particularly in the presence of gram-negative anaerobes that could conceivably emanate from a micro-gap source of infection. In the history of HA-coated oral implants, this sporadically encountered potential of HA coating to be associated with periimplantitis seemed to offset some of its clearly positive osseoconductive advantages. However, when considering HA-coating for a one-piece, no-micro-gap, small-diameter implant, there could be less wariness about using HA, which deserves further investigation. Indeed, the HA coating might very well spell the difference between success and failure outcomes when immediately loaded after the osteotomy-type surgery needed for an atraumatic insertion of increasingly popular wider-diameter one-piece fixtures (with their usefully greater surface area). The added cost of HA-coating might be a limiting factor for understandably bottom-line-oriented manufacturers; however, if HA really provides significant predictability benefits without potential morbidity, it clearly warrants further scientific scrutiny as an enhancement for the more initially vulnerable midsize one-piece small-diameter implant, particularly if the trend towards wider-width small-diameter implants perseveres.

In the meantime, it is worth reemphasizing that the immediate osseoapposition of a properly inserted, bi-cortical stabilized, 1.8-mm standard Sendax MDI gives it a high survival potential in the face of immediate function, even without the reputedly enhanced osteoconductivity benefit of HA-coating. In other words, it always pays to conceptually go back to the basics before venturing too rapidly into relatively uncharted waters.

(For additional background details on HA-coated dental and orthopedic implants, see *Dental Clinics of North America,* Vol. 36, No.1, Jan 1992, compiled and edited by Dr. Victor Sendax.)

Improving Access to Implant Dentistry

Access to dental implants for a needful public has always been on the mind and conscience of the dental profession. But how to implement this worthy abstraction has turned out to be an elusive accomplishment.

For early-on forthright enlightenment on this accessibility subject we need only turn back to the editorial by Dr. Michael Newman published March 1994 in *International Journal of Oral and Maxillofacial Implants,* in which he decries the frequent inability for patients of limited means to avail themselves of the proven advantages and benefits of oral implantology, which carries an implied warning that failure of organized dentistry to broaden access to this benevolent therapy will encourage outside forces (e.g., government, private industry, insurance companies, and regulatory agencies) to either step in and intrusively fill the vacuum left by professional inaction or just sidestep the issue.

In a more recent recognition of this access problem, Dr. Bernard Touati, the Editor-in-Chief of *Practical Procedures and Aesthetic Dentistry,* wrote in an editorial opinion column entitled "Benevolent Dentistry" that "Patients have begun to cut back on elective, and even required, care because of financial constraints. While it has been generally accepted that improved access to comprehensive and preventive dental care is essential both throughout the U.S. and globally, particularly in developing nations, dental professionals are now being challenged to consider patients' needs in their own communities as well."

Providing MDIs alone or hybridizing MDIs in combination with conventional implants and/or natural tooth abutments represents one practical technique for making implant dentistry more accessible. Each MDI put into the overall rehabilitation equation substantially reduces the total cost of therapy and makes it more likely that a patient can afford to accept an oral implantology treatment plan instead of settling for chronically loose full or partial dentures that may represent less than desirable outcomes, functionally and psychologically, for many needy beneficiaries. In addition, MDIs may often permit frugal salvaging of existing failing prostheses that might otherwise be irrevocably lost and require costly remakes (as so aptly noted in this textbook's foreword by Dr. Gordon Christensen and in many of his instructional DVDs, seminars, and lectures). At the very least they may provide an affordable transitional solution that might otherwise be realistically out of reach. In any event, access is a subject that will not readily go away or be brushed under the rug.

Of course the key to the acceptability of this MDI approach rests on the credibility of the underlying durability and functionality of the MDI system. One of the occasional arguments advanced against MDI use is the claim that MDIs are essentially temporary implants and should not be considered on the same plane as conventional-sized osseointegrated implants. However, the documented experiences of many of our contributors (for a good example see Coler-Goldwater Hospital's outcomes for the most extreme medically compromised cases under the jurisdiction of periodontist Dr. Harold Sussman) have consistently demonstrated MDI longevity, confirming the long-term data submitted to the FDA, which gave its primary approval to market ultra-small-diameter MDIs as minimally invasive long-term devices if scrupulously placed according to the Sendax proprietary insertion protocol.

Standard of Care Issues as Applied to MDIs

Although the *standard of care* term has been bandied about extensively and applied both broadly and narrowly to the dental implant special field of interest by various practitioners and groups, it has remained an elusively controversial descriptive label because there are literally dozens of approaches to oral implantology and an ever-growing variety of implant devices; thus it is a supreme challenge to try to define a "gold standard" that will have any assurance of acceptance by the dental profession at large—which has never, it should be recalled, given the official American Dental Association (ADA) stamp of approval to implant dentistry as a clearly defined specialty but instead has permitted it to be subsumed within other existing components of the profession.

The best the profession has been able to do, at least to date, is to acknowledge that virtually all the recognized dental specialties have at least some claim on the field, but as the ADA has concluded to date, none have any exclusive rights. More recently the profession has come to respect general practitioners' often key role in overseeing the entire implant therapeutic process for prospective patients rather than passing on responsibility for coordinating the often complex issues underlying implant decision-making, sequencing, and ongoing follow-up maintenance, especially when troubleshooting problems intrude into the long-term picture.

What constitutes a source of authority in this complex arena has likewise proven to be a challenging search. Each of the subspecialties may vie for claims of superior wisdom, but in the final analysis the only standards that stand up to scrutiny are the experiential front line backgrounds of the claimants and the amount of continuing postdoctoral education absorbed by them over a substantial timeline because undergraduate implant training is still a slowly evolving component.

It is not uncommon to find practitioners with little or no training in MDI technique nor, for that matter, any actual insertion and restoration experience, offering seemingly definitive commentary on whether MDIs can be considered "standard of care" for varied removable and fixed applications. Whether the motivations for such statements are purely altruistic or are subtexts to justify monetary compensation biases, the ultimate result is confusion for patients who already have enough issues to confront and consider in deciding what therapeutic approach best suits their needs.

It is with these considerations of paramount concern that the author/editor and publisher of this first textbook on MDIs hope to offer a rational guide to their use without making unreasonable claims of superiority and without desire to supplant and/or replace any existing modality that has stood the test of time. Along this line, it is instructive to remember that when the original Brånemark studies from Sweden many years ago pointed to osseointegration as a working definition of successful implant therapy, it was offered only to the oral surgery community and was literally banned by commercial fiat for training to periodontists, prosthodontists, and generalists, thereby arbitrarily suggesting that acceptable standards of implant placement could only be fulfilled by the specialty of oral and maxillofacial surgery. Today, that restrictive limitation no longer exists, and all members of the dental profession are free to receive training and develop skills in oral implantology. The original Brånemark-type implant likewise no longer represents an unchallenged standard because design and insertion techniques have long since been modified, evolving to meet current real needs and applied research.

MDIs are therefore to be considered neither panaceas nor foolproof devices but rather components of an ever-growing family of oral implant options and choices that can be fairly rated as to standard of care only if evaluated by colleagues with specific MDI training and background experience to render valid informed opinions. It is just as incumbent upon the profession to inform patients of the availability of MDIs and conventional implants as it is to suggest the availability of long-standing therapeutic alternatives to implant-supported prosthodontics. Standards of care in the oral implant arena evolve just as they do for other components of the profession and are intimately connected to the degree of training and experience of its practitioners. This applies in equal measure when evaluating the role of MDIs in the overall therapeutic equation.

Conclusion

Most significantly, the specialist and generalist contributors to this volume have demonstrated a proven record of viable MDI placements in some of the most severely debilitated patients, often in hospital and clinic centers catering to the management of just such a cross-section of advanced and even terminal cases. The positive outcomes of MDI therapy for these otherwise hapless individuals unequivocally render plausible the claim for impartial acceptance of the modality's ongoing validity. If MDIs have been consistently shown to work predictably for such a medically challenged patient population, MDIs should certainly be valid for the healthy, uncomplicated implant candidate and should be rated not only as comparable, but in certain instances of anatomic and clinical variability, might be considered a superior choice over conventional implant options, both with or without hard and soft tissue grafting enhancement.

INDEX

Page numbers followed by *f* indicate figures; *t,* tables; *b,* boxes.

C

D

I

N

O

T

U

V

W

X

Y

Z